Research Methods in Nursing and Health

Research Methods in Nursing and Health

Sonya Iverson Shelley, Ph.D.

*Professor, Center for Research, University of Maryland
School of Nursing, Baltimore*

Little, Brown and Company, Boston/Toronto

Library of Congress Catalog Card No. 83-82830

ISBN 0-316-78474-5

Printed in the United States of America

DON

To *Philip*

for loving: understanding, cajoling, supporting, brainstorming, critiquing, rewriting, strategizing, caring—and mentoring. What more could I ask?

Contents

About the Author and Contributors

Sonya Iverson Shelley, Ph.D.

Professor, Center for Research, University of Maryland School of Nursing, has taught research methods to undergraduate and graduate nursing students for over 10 years. In 1975, she started the Center for Research and was its director for 7 years. She has consulted to numerous government agencies and health researchers in the areas of research methods and program evaluation and conducted research in sexuality, patient compliance, stress/coping, and instrument development.

Peggy Parks, Ph.D.

Assistant Professor, Center for Research, University of Maryland School of Nursing, has taught research methods to undergraduate and graduate nursing students for 6 years and edits *RSVP,* a biannual newsletter from the Center for Research. She has conducted research on early childhood, parenting, and children's rights and consults in this area with local agencies.

Eleanor Reiff-Ross, Ph.D.

Formerly Assistant Professor, Center for Research, University of Maryland School of Nursing and now a clinical psychologist in private practice, taught research methods to undergraduate and graduate students for 8 years. She has conducted research in fetal alcohol syndrome, antecedents of female alcoholism, and suicide among young adults.

Mary L. Wolfe, Ph.D.

Assistant Professor, Center for Research, University of Maryland School of Nursing, has taught research methods to undergraduate and graduate nursing students for 7 years. A mathematical statistician, Dr. Wolfe has conducted research in numerous aspects of research methods, math anxiety, and attitudes of health professionals. She is also an expert in program evaluation.

Preface

Because nursing research has evolved from a stage emphasizing consumerism to the current emphasis on practice, it is hoped that this textbook will represent the first of a new generation of research methods texts focusing on practice, or the *methods* of nursing research. The issues relevant to the practice of nursing research—finding a suitable topic, placing the topic into a theoretical framework, exploring the role of theory in nursing research, conceptualizing a problem, and conducting a literature review—do not command individual chapters in this "new generation" research text. Instead, these topics are integrated throughout the book, whenever they are relevant to the research *methodology* being presented. It is presumed, of course, that these subjects are major topics of discussion in nonresearch courses as well. As state-of-the-art knowledge is presented in other nursing "content" courses, the gaps where research is needed should become readily apparent.

This text also reflects a substantial change in content as far as inferential statistics is concerned. Power analysis to detect type II error rate when a null hypothesis is not rejected is presented at the introductory level, as are methods for estimating the magnitude of any statistically significant effects. The role of sample size is implicit in this material. It is hoped that this more comprehensive approach *in the very beginning* of a researcher's education will minimize the abuse and hocus-pocus associated with so much of statistical "significance." It also provides concrete tools for evaluating the practical significance of research reported in the journal literature.

No longer are two or three books necessary as required reading for a single research methods course. This text covers all aspects of the research process in sufficient detail so that it alone is necessary: from the brief overview in Chapters 1 and 2; to design and threats to internal and construct validity; to descriptive statistics and epidemiologic methods; to sampling, procedures for human subjects, and threats to external validity; to measurement and instrument credentialing and development; to inferential statistics, threats to statistical conclusion validity, and power analysis; and, finally, to pulling it all together to interpret and communicate results.

A number of premises and beliefs guided development of this textbook in addition to the aforementioned ones:

1. This book is intended for use at *both* the introductory and intermediate levels of research education. It is suitable for both undergraduate and graduate students and is based on the author's more than 10 years of experience teaching research methods to nurses at *both* of these levels. Self-starting or honors undergraduates often need more than the typical syllabus provides, and there are topics of this nature included (e.g., instrument credentialing, multivariate statistics). Also, the research they may be conducting as part of their course requirements often entails knowing more in a certain area (e.g., testing for a significant difference between two correlations) than the typical syllabus provides, and most of these likely topics are included. Graduate students, on the other hand, often need to review basic concepts (e.g., research design, summary statistics) if more than 2 or 3 years have passed since their introductory course as an undergraduate.

2. Just as learning to swim requires getting into the water, learning to do research requires actually doing research. While nonswimmers, well coached at poolside lectures, can give literate commentary on swim meet activities, so *might* nonresearchers well versed from an introductory research text give literate commentary on a report of research. In all likelihood, however, both would be too critical and lacking the depth of understanding that comes only from hands-on experience. Therefore, this book is a how-to-do-it book. It provides practical advice for researchers and is intended to be used in combination with participation in a research study. Such a study may take the form of a single project in which an entire class participates, or it may involve many individual studies within a single class. The choice might depend on whether introductory or intermediate study is involved. With both, the instructor usually acts as Project Director and guides students through the process, minimizing mistakes that might have been avoided had the entire book been digested before the project began. The experience of *gathering data* for a study and then *analyzing these data* to discover the results is exciting. Then, rather than merely being viewed as required reading, this book suddenly becomes a gold mine of useful information, a wonderful tool for doing what you never thought you could. So, too, is the instructor no longer just another teacher but, rather, a catalyst and tour guide for a fascinating adventure.

3. This book focuses upon quantitative methods. Quantitative methods must be learned prior to the more difficult qualitative methods, if qualitative research is to have the rigor and objectivity it deserves. In this way, the need for both control and objective/systematic measurement/observation is learned and is therefore impinged upon research that could otherwise have become too subjective to yield adequate data. Therefore, the need to master quantitative methods in order to do good qualitative research is discussed in several chapters, so that the reader is aware of other approaches to research. Similar reasoning has caused experimental designs to be placed ahead of descriptive designs in this book. The additional control required for experimental designs can then be brought to descriptive designs, thereby enhancing their rigor and ultimate utility.

4. An attempt was made to write this book in an informal style—appropriate, perhaps, to this period of history that considers designer jeans as a proper and sometimes necessary part of virtually everyone's wardrobe. After all, the generation of new knowledge is a creative endeavor loaded with unforeseen challenges along the way. A more relaxed attitude *without sloppiness* is good insurance against ulcers for a researcher who is creatively meeting those unforeseen challenges.

5. Care has been taken to include essential statistical techniques. We know that, traditionally, students have been "turned off" to research because of the statistics involved. Therefore, for a time, statistics was minimized or omitted in favor of courses that critiqued research articles and emphasized design and measurement without their concomitant statistical analysis. It was thought that statisticians could be hired to do the data analysis at the appropriate time. Conceptualization and design were all that was believed important. As one statistician called in to salvage data gathered by those who subscribed to this approach, I saw with painful clarity that it would not work. For example, each year a few researchers thought they were following a pretest-posttest design only to find out after their data were gathered that group means were simply not enough. Pretest and posttest scores for *each* subject needed to be linked. Other researchers failed to incorporate additional independent variables into their design and instead left them to confound the study, increase error, and otherwise obscure results. Where a few multivariate hypotheses could be tested, pages of bivariate hypotheses were generated. In others, many variables were measured among too few subjects. Most of the time, data were not salvageable. Therefore, this book presents an integrated approach to research that presumes statistics to be an essential element among many. Research designs are meaningless without the statistical techniques to analyze them. Without some notion of the various options for analysis available (and their requirements), we cannot even design a study for a statistician to analyze. In this book, mathematical derivations have been minimized and conceptual formulas emphasized, since actual computations are usually done via computers. Thus, it is hoped that this integrated approach will provide sufficient information to enable "turning on" students to the need for *good* research and give them the necessary tools to do it in a nonthreatening way.

6. Lists, labels, and diagrams abound in this book as various aspects of research have been synthesized into a logical organization for presentation. However, they are not sacred or carved in stone. You are encouraged to organize in other ways if they are more meaningful to your research situation.

7. Suggestions for critiquing research that are understandable early in the course are presented in Appendix I. The research outline that is included is also understandable early, although it takes on added meaning as additional knowledge is achieved. As an appendix, rather than a chapter that can be read and "finished," it is hoped that it will be referred to often throughout the course of study. Similarly, resources for use in reviewing the literature are presented in Appendix II.

This book would never have been completed without the help and encouragement of Philip E. Shelley, Ph.D., and Betty Shubkagel, R.N., Ph.D. Their contributions, amounting to many hours of work freely given, are gratefully appreciated. Appreciation is also expressed to Shirley Damrosch, Ph.D., Mary Wolfe, Ph.D., and Mildred Kreider, R.N., Ph.D., for critiquing Chapters 3, 4, and 9, respectively. Also, special appreciation is due Karen Soeken, Ph.D., who reviewed the entire manuscript for statistical accuracy (as well as an unknown reviewer who was most encouraging). Their helpful comments were incorporated whenever possible. In addition, the help of Sandra Wach, Sharon Lichtenberg, and Cathy Haynes at various stages in manuscript preparation is acknowledged. They typed multiple drafts with care, patience, and good humor. Finally, I am grateful to the Literary Executor of the late Sir Ronald A. Fisher, F.R.S., to Dr. Frank Yates, F.R.S., and to Longman Group, Ltd., London, for permission to reprint four tables from their book *Statistical Tables for Biological, Agricultural and Medical Research* (6th ed., 1974).

S. I. S.

I: *Introduction*

Unit I introduces the research process and basic vocabulary needed by a researcher. It also provides some advice about group projects that should be considered before you embark on a research adventure. Chapters 1 and 2 provide a superficial background, in order to prepare students for planning and implementing a research study (with an instructor or a mentor) as they progress through this book. Chapter 1 describes the origins of research ideas, the three kinds of information available (i.e., theory, research results, and clinical experience), the so-what and doable tests, and the research process. A continuing review of literature is emphasized rather than a review that is just one step in the process. To provide an overview of the research process and a base from which to begin more in-depth study, many concepts (e.g., reliability and validity of operational definitions) are mentioned and defined only briefly, since large portions of subsequent chapters treat these concepts in much greater detail. Finally, peer review and accepted practices regarding authorship credit are discussed.

By using six examples of actual nursing research studies, Chapter 2 presents kinds of research, types of variables, hypotheses, research questions, and objectives. The chapter concludes with levels of measurement, dummy variables, and Likert scaling.

Basic vocabulary words are found at the end of most chapters. The first time the word is used in the discussion it is usually in boldface print, to emphasize the need to fully understand its meaning and to locate it if later reference to it is needed. If you understand the basic vocabulary in a discipline, you are well over halfway toward mastering the basic content in this discipline. Therefore, it is suggested that, as a self-evaluation, you do the following:

1. For each vocabulary word, define it, use it in a sentence, and give two examples of its use.
2. Meet with one to four of your classmates to exchange responses to item 1. You might correct and grade someone else's responses, return papers, and discuss each answer with the group. If you still have questions, discuss them with your instructor, or ask them at your next research class meeting.

This approach to learning the vocabulary of research is best utilized throughout the book and course of study. When words are repeated from chapter to chapter, often added meaning is given to them in a subsequent chapter.

In addition to your work with vocabulary words for this unit, you will want to practice scoring Likert scales, develop hypotheses of your own, and practice categorizing measures according to their level of measurement. These skills are basic to mastery of later chapters.

1: *The Research Process*

The best way to learn how to conduct research and how to critique the research of others is to do it yourself. How many people have learned to swim or ride a bicycle by reading a book or even observing lecture-demonstrations? How did you learn to administer medications or catheterize a patient? *Guided* experience *in doing* is essential. Therefore, begin learning the research process by selecting several researchable questions. The first part of this chapter tells you how to do this. If you must write a term paper for another course you are taking or do extensive reading for a work-related project, you could select a researchable question on the same topic, in order to do one large review and bibliography rather than two separate, smaller reviews of literature. Then as you progress through this book, apply the principles you are learning to your topic area. When you finish, you also will have finished a research study—or at least developed a detailed plan (called a research proposal) which you can implement.

As a novice researcher, you will need a **mentor**—an experienced researcher with whom you can discuss your ideas and from whom you can get advice. For students enrolled in a research course, your instructor is your mentor, or project director. A research instructor who acts as a project director anticipates pitfalls and takes steps, based on past research experience, to avoid them. Being creative in helping to design, analyze, interpret, and communicate the research is all part of a project director's function. Expertise in research methods and the content area also is needed. When the content area is not in your instructor's specialty, a consultant in this area is usually secured.

If you are not enrolled in a research course, you will still need to find a mentor to follow this plan of action. After you have read this chapter, look for researchers in your locality. Talk with a researcher in your area of interest about the possibility of acting as your mentor, and negotiate a "contract" whereby you *both* benefit from the association. Beware of arrangements in which you are given all the work (for the chance to learn) and none of the glory. Materialistic as it sounds, glory, in terms of communicating your research results, is one of the rewards of doing research. Aim high. Try to be a coauthor, not a footnote. Then you can always compromise to a footnote rather than anonymity.

Finding a Researchable Question

Research ideas are everywhere. We are constantly bombarded with problems or ideas or things that need exploration. For many, we need more information than is available, no matter how much time we spend in the library or talking to experts. This need to discover new information is the essence of research. Research is, in fact, the generation of new knowledge.

As we look for ideas to research, we should look for patterns of events. Does the same problem situation occur frequently? Is it related to another aspect in the larger situation? Is there a pattern to the occurrence of the problem?

We ask questions everyday. Some relate to our personal or family lives. Are marriages better if the couple has cohabitated beforehand? How many persons will drop out if dues are raised $5? What activities should be offered on campus that would give commuter students a greater feeling of identity with the college? Which suntan lotion promotes better tanning?

Questions that relate to your professional life as a nurse are the concern of this textbook. These might involve the education of nurses, patient care, administration of nursing service, client behavior, the changing role of nurses, or any other areas of interest to nurses.

Is there a difference in the level of achievement between students who select nursing as their initial career and those who select it later? What are the effects of social and psychological factors on the job performance of married and unmarried nurses? Why do diploma nurses return to school to obtain their B.S.? What is the role of the school nurse in teaching death education in secondary schools? Why do nurses choose to specialize in community health nursing? Are nurses who work in community health nursing different in any respect from those who choose to work in hospitals? What effect does increased violence in a community have on the community health nurse in providing care? How do the attitudes of emergency room personnel toward certain types of patients (e.g., psychiatric, alcoholic, women, blacks) affect the care they give these patients?

What nursing actions are conducive to a patient having a good night's sleep? Does evening care affect the patients' ability to sleep? How can self-care be promoted in nursing homes? Does greater self-care increase patient comfort and wellness? Does primary nursing require more time per patient than team nursing? What are the benefits to patient care and nursing service of primary nursing? How effective are nurse intern programs in relation to their cost, what nurses learn from them, and retention of nurses? Do nurses become careless about methods of medication administration several years after graduation? Does socioeconomic status affect a client's view of her or his right to health care? What effect does personal contact with the nurse have on patient compliance with the prescribed therapeutic regimen? Does the time of day when clinics are open affect whether people keep their appointments? Does the personality of the provider affect compliance with the therapeutic regimen? What nurse actions will motivate people to assume responsibility for their health care? Does including a patient in determining his or her health care goals increase the probability of meeting these goals? Do diabetics who are hospitalized when they are initially taught insulin therapy view their disease differently and respond to it differently from those who are taught insulin therapy at home? How do patients' expectations of treatment compare with what they actually receive?

These areas are a sample of researchable ideas listed by both undergraduate and graduate nursing students after the first session of their class in research methods and statistics. The ideas come from their experiences in nursing. Some included hunches about the answers. As a professional nurse, it is perfectly respectable to give testimony, based on your education and clinical experience, about the answer. Often it is all you have to go on. Eventually, though, you also must find out what others have to say about it. This entails a trip to the library.

Usually, when a researchable idea occurs to you, it involves a number of concepts and complex relationships. It covers a broad territory. In your search for theory or reports of research that shed light on your question, you discover many possible avenues of pursuit. In using the various bibliographic indexes, such as the *International Nursing Index* or *Index Medicus,* you find many relevant key words. At this point, you might narrow your topic to fewer concepts. Even so, before long you have a huge stack of books and journals to read and synthesize. You begin by reading appropriate sections of three or four textbooks. These give you an overview of the area. Next you look at theories that attempt to explain the phenomenon of interest, reports of clinical experience, and articles describing research studies.

To many, the library literature search and subsequent synthesis of all the available information are considered research. In other courses, this process is even called a research paper. This is not what is meant by research in this book. **Research** is viewed here as the *generation of new knowledge,* not the synthesis of existing knowledge. However, the synthesis of existing knowledge is the first step in the research process. Once you are an expert on the topic you have chosen (and, believe it or not, your synthesis of existing knowledge qualifies you as having some expertise), you will know what you do *not* know. You will know those questions for which there are either no answers or dubious answers. These are the researchable questions from which you can choose. Your original question may or may not be among them. In any event, your perception of it will have changed.

As you synthesize the literature relating to your idea, look for unexpected findings from research studies. Note the populations or related characteristics that have *not* been studied. What suggestions for further research are made by the authors, and what would they do differently next time? How were the characteristics measured or described? Are there research results that support a *correlation* between characteristics which could be researched further to test a *cause-and-effect* relationship between them? Furthermore, is there a theory that explains the problem you are exploring? Do theories about it conflict? Has research been conducted to test various parts of the theory or to see which of several competing theories appears more valid?

Finally, look for research approaches, carried out over years, that have not produced significant results. One or two replications of unproductive research results can be justified to confirm the previous finding that the area is unproductive. Repetitions beyond this cannot be justified and usually suggest that the researcher did not adequately review the literature.

It is appropriate here to explore the type of "knowledge" you must synthesize. Generally, it comes from three sources: theory, the results of research, and clinical experience. All these sources can be either valid or dubious. You must be the judge. **Theory** is a broader view of many separate, researchable question-and-answer pairs. Sometimes the basis for theory includes years of clinical experience, the same experience you may have. A theory, then, is a creative integration of known facts and observations that, in addition to explaining the phenomenon, predicts events to come. Theories can be disputed. They are not carved in stone. They are, for the time being, one of the best explanations available for the observed phenomenon that includes your research idea. However, research results more closely approach being carved in stone if the research methodology is sound and the results have been replicated or found by other researchers as well. This is rarely the case, however. Moreover, research studies cover a much smaller territory than theories, often testing one small part of a theory.

We do not explore in this textbook various theories related to nursing. These are amply covered in other nursing courses. Nor are we going to explore theory building except to say again that it is a creative integration of research results, clinical experience, and hunches. Research as described in this text plays an important part in **theory building** as well as **theory testing.** A research idea that eventually evolves into a researchable question with a theoretical basis in predicting the answer is golden. Not only does it shed light on your clinical problem, but also it tests a theory. A research study whose results support one of two conflicting theories is equally interesting. In addition, the theoretical basis, or framework, of a research study helps you interpret your results. If this sounds like a plug for a theoretical basis for your research, it is. In so doing, you are building on the work of others—the most efficient way to build an integrated body of knowledge. Do not, however, give up a perfectly relevant research question because you cannot relate it to an existing theory. You can always discover "theoretical considerations" as a result of your literature search. You may even be taking the first step in generating theory. Finally, some questions are very pragmatic and simply do not need a theory to suggest answers. Many additional factors must be considered when you select from the many researchable questions generated by your search and synthesis of literature.

At some point, you must declare your *initial* literature review finished. This is harder to do than you think, because there are always related areas to pursue. Time constraints and the generation of many specific research questions will signal that it is time to pause, reflect, and select from the questions that need answers. In selecting three or four possibilities, the so-what and doable tests are applied. You may be aware of a United States Senator's Golden Fleece Awards bestowed on federally funded researchers. He took issue with the **so-what test.** Is the research worth doing? Will the information generated make a difference? How will it benefit nursing? What will be the implications for nursing practice? Which questions are in greater need of answers?

The **doable test** is very pragmatic. Can you do this research in the time available? Do you have the financial resources required? Is there available a study population of subjects from which you can sample, and do you have a good way of gathering information to describe variations in the concepts and characteristics you wish to study? How will you get from your question to the answer? Finally, are you really interested in it? A great deal of a researcher's time and psychic energy is involved in the research area. It must meet your personal so-what test. Otherwise, you will become bored before you have finished—if you finish.

Sometimes this process of refining a series of possible research questions must be repeated. The questions emerging from your literature search may not meet your so-what or doable tests. But, you say, I have done all the library work. Is it all for nothing? Perhaps. Clearly the knowledge you have gained can never be called nothing. To pursue an area that no longer interests you or has severe limitations truly would be working for nothing, because the initial literature search is only the top of the iceberg. More is to come. Make sure you have worthwhile research questions.

Eventually, you are faced with selecting from several compelling questions. How do you make the final choice, and then how do you find the answer? That is the purpose of this book—to provide you with the various techniques for finding the answers. In the process, you will begin to look at questions in a different way–to see them in a *quantitative* framework. As your repertoire of creative ways to *quantify* and seek answers expands, you will easily select from your researchable questions the one that best meets your personal doable test.

Quantitative Research—What Is It?

Quantitative research is concerned with the measurement of phenomena, characteristics, concepts, or things. It seeks to describe *how much* of a characteristic is present. For example, how many persons in your class have brown eyes? If 18 percent have brown eyes, then 18 percent is the quantification of eye color. When a number or numbers are attached to blood pressure, dosages, temperatures, and weights in daily clinical practice, the numbers are their quantifications. Most phenomena, characteristics, concepts, or things have in common a capacity to *vary*, or, in other words, to have more than one number that describes them. Thus, they are called **variables,** a much more efficient way of describing phenomena, characteristics, concepts, factors, traits, things, entities, items, objects, constructs, and so forth.

The method by which you quantify or measure a variable is called its **operational definition.** For example, body temperature must be quantified by the calibration lines on a thermometer placed under the tongue of a patient. Your **instrument,** or operational definition, is the thermometer. Diabetic patients' knowledge about diet may be operationally defined by a pencil-and-paper test consisting of 20 questions, or **items.** The test is your instrument. Some variables that are easily observed, such as eye color or sex, need no special instrument to operationally define them. Another way of viewing an operational definition is as the "operations" needed to measure and thus quantify a variable.

Quantitative research involves attaching to variables, by means of operational definitions (or instruments), numbers that indicate *quantity.* Thus it is called quantitative. Not only can you describe variables by quantifying them, but also, after two or more variables are quantified, the researcher can manipulate (by adding, subtracting, multiplying, and/or dividing) the numbers according to certain clear-cut procedures to describe a relationship, if it exists, between the variables. This manipulation is known as *statistical analysis,* and it has an undeserved reputation as difficult, anxiety-provoking, and worse. It is actually a helpful way to simplify and summarize research.

The quantification of a variable implies that more than one measurement is needed if we are to describe accurately the variable as it occurs in the world. Thus, if you wish to describe the amount of anxiety in preoperative patients, you would not do well to quantify the anxiety of only one patient. That patient might happen to be very different from others. Your chances of being correct are greatly enhanced if you measure the anxiety of many preoperative patients. (The issues of how many patients and how to select them are considered in later chapters.) As a result, though, you end up with many datum points, each point being the quantification of one patient's anxiety. You could report all of the numbers. However, this would be not only clumsy but also very uninformative. Therefore, through statistical analysis all the data are summarized in a single number that represents the average of scores and another that describes how much the scores of the entire sample vary from the average. This class of procedures describes what is observed and so is known as **descriptive statistics.** The other class of procedures, known as **inferential statistics,** allows you to compare, for example, the averages from two separate groups to discover whether they are significantly different. It allows you to infer characteristics of a population from the characteristics you observe in a sample from that population. Each inferential procedure has certain assumptions, or conditions, that must be met before you can use it. Then, if they are met, you simply follow a series of steps, essentially a mathematical formula, and eventually find a number(s) that, when compared with values in a table, indicates whether you have real, or significant, differences. How do you know which statistical procedure to use? That is relatively simple also. Usually only one or two procedures are appropriate for each combination of (1) the kind of number used to quantify a variable and (2) the type of relationship between variables being examined. You select the procedure whose rules, or assumptions, you can meet. Subsequent chapters in this book cover this topic in detail.

Research Process

Statistical analysis, or number manipulation, plays a relatively small part in the research process in terms of time expended, although the exact opposite seems to be true when you begin. Because it is newer to you and more complex than other parts of the research process, often statistical analysis requires more of a *beginning* researcher's time and effort. For example, it takes up a large portion of this book. Once you have mastered the basic principles of statistical analysis, however, a much smaller portion of your research time will be devoted to it.

The research process consists of a series of steps, or tasks, as described in Exhibit 1.1, that are followed to conceive, implement, and communicate the results of a research study. The use of the word "steps" is misleading, because it implies that you finish one and then move on to another. That is not the case in the research process (although it is usually true with statistical analysis). Sometimes you are working on more than one step at a time. At other points, you might go back to redo or rethink an earlier step. Finally, the literature search is ongoing, even though it appears confined to steps 2 and 4a, because you always must keep abreast of the latest information in your area. Moreover, you will return to reread certain research studies to get ideas for sampling, operational definitions, research designs and procedures, and even ways of displaying and analyzing your data (e.g., graphs and figures).

As you become more familiar with the techniques of quantitative research, you will see new flaws in some of the published studies. Wherever possible, you will try to avoid them in your design, although some compromise between perfect design and real-world conditions is always necessary in research. These compromises, in turn, result in flaws in even the best of study designs. For example, human subjects must give informed consent to participate in your study. Thus your study is flawed to the extent that volunteers may be different from the target population to which you wish to generalize or apply your results. Your ingenuity and creativity, given substantial help from your literature review and these pages, will determine the number and magnitude of flaws with which you live.

The first three steps in the research process are discussed at the beginning of the chapter. Essentially, they involve the location of several researchable questions that meet the *so-what test*. Appendix II describes the major indices available for use with your literature review. Step 4, gathering information for your doable test, is divided into two parts, because it involves two simultaneous activities that are helping you make a final selection from your researchable questions. Continue to review the literature, primarily to locate a theoretical framework or theory to help you predict the answer to a researchable question and to search for similar research studies worthy of emulation. Exhibit 22.1 illustrates a review form that can be used to record notes about each article you review. You also may wish to talk with experts and researchers who have published in the area. At this step you are particularly concerned about finding operational definitions and **subjects (Ss),** the participants in the study. Beginning researchers do best to find existing instruments (operational definitions) that are **reliable** and **valid** for their research rather than developing their own.*

---

*Reliability refers to the consistency, equivalency or stability of a measure. Reliability is required for validity. *Validity* refers to the fact that the instrument measures what it is designed to measure. If a thermometer always measures 98.6°F on a healthy person whose body temperature remains constant, it is reliable. If it measures 97, 101, and 98°F on a healthy person whose body temperature remains constant, it is not reliable. If it were used to quantify skin secretions, however, it would not be considered valid. It would not be measuring what it purports to measure. There are several types of reliability and validity. These are discussed in detail in Chapters 11 and 13.

Exhibit 1-1. The research process.

Aspects generally not involving number manipulation

Aspects involving some number manipulation (among other things)

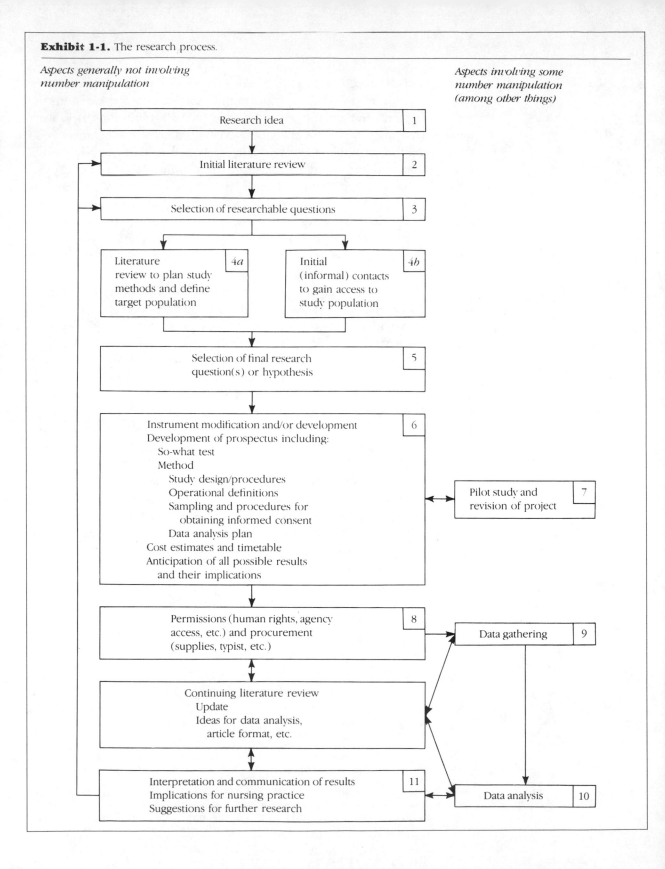

The process of instrument development is complex and a research endeavor in its own right. Gaining access to subjects is a key factor. If you wish to study patients with coronary bypass surgery (your **target population**—the one to which you wish to generalize your results), you must get local hospital and physician cooperation to conduct your study with patients having the surgery in hospital *X* (your **study population,** from which you will select your **sample** of patients). Sometimes their cooperation and consent involves time-consuming approvals of a written research prospectus or proposal by hospital review committees. Student research projects that are part of course requirements and thus considered part of the educational process are occasionally either excused from some steps in the hospital review process or hurried through them. Your task, on this fourth step of the research process, is to informally find out what is required to gain access to subjects if the institution is receptive to such a request. Rely on your nursing instructors and friends working within the agency for helpful advice.

Step 5 involves selection of your research question and generation of a research hypothesis (see Chap. 2), if appropriate. Usually your choice is obvious at this point as a result of your work in step 4. Now you can limit further your ongoing review of the literature and begin to focus on the "nuts and bolts" of implementing your research project.

Step 6 is where your library work and conversations with persons who have published or are doing work in the area pay off. It is also where your ingenuity and creativity become apparent. Hopefully, at this point, you are not developing a totally new **measurement instrument.** This is too complex a task if you are just learning the research process. You may, however, need to develop a questionnaire or interview schedule to gather demographic data (i.e., sex, age, income, educational level, marital status, and so forth) and other survey data (see Chap. 14). Also you might need to adapt an existing instrument for use with your target population. In this case, depending on the extent of your modifications, you may need to do item analysis and establish new reliability and validity coefficients (see Chaps. 11 and 13). Then the final methodology for your research (i.e., study design and procedures, operational definitions, sampling technique, and data analysis plan) will be summarized succinctly in a two- or three-page **prospectus.** Some examples are shown in Exhibits 1.2 and 1.3. The prospectus focuses on the so-what test and essentially sells your research to others. It also summarizes the research as concisely as possible. In the prospectuses in Exhibits 1.2 and 1.3, the first paragraph describes the importance of the topic area. The second paragraph quickly presents the state of the art (from research and theory) in terms of knowledge about the topic, citing only those few references that have the most direct bearing on the topic, and it ends by describing what small piece of the larger topic area the researcher is taking as a project. Note how in just a few lines the reader is led quite logically from the larger topic area to the researcher's smaller piece. Next, the purpose and hy-

Exhibit 1-2. Prospectus to compare personality characteristics of critical-care and other nurses. R. Boggs, J. Boxall, P. Dietz, M. Harvey, A. Killen, P. Pallett

The nursing shortage crisis—especially in critical-care areas—has generated considerable interest in not only how to attract but also how to keep qualified staff. A low turnover rate promotes the proficiency of the individual, the stability of the work environment, and the productivity of the group. It also reduces the cost of new staff orientation, the stress of shortages, and the distress of waste. Achieving this desirable condition is partly a matter of matching work and worker. This requires knowing what distinguishes the best-suited individuals in each employment area. The identification of salient characteristics would be useful not only to staff recruiters but also to graduate nurses uncertain about employment choices and to nursing school curricula developers.

The analysis of personality traits of nurses has been focused primarily on attempts to distinguish nursing students from nonnurses in order to solve the puzzle of the high attrition rates of nursing schools (Adams and Klein 1970; Bailey and Claus 1969; Bry and Marisco 1980; Burns et al. 1978; Levitt et al. 1962; Lewis 1979; Long and Gordon-Crosby 1981; Stein 1969). The findings tended to be inconclusive or to contradict other studies except that nurses throughout the 1950s and 1960s tended to show higher needs than their nonnurse controls for order, deference, endurance, abasement, and nurturance. They also showed low needs for achievement, dominance, and autonomy. The later studies of nursing students showed a lower ranking of needs for order, deference, and abasement (in keeping with the changes in feminine identity prompted by Women's Liberation), but achievement and autonomy still ranked low. The few studies of nurses already in practice (Cohen and Edwards 1965; George and Stephens 1968; Lentz and Michaels 1965; Navran and Stauffacher 1957, 1958; White 1975) compared public health nurses, medical-surgical nurses, and nurse practitioners with psychiatric nurses. Psychiatric nurses seem to be the preferred comparison group, because they were the first specialty group studied (Navran 1957). Again, these groups ranked achievement low on their need scale, but they differed in the rankings of order, endurance, dominance, and deference. *There are no studies of critical-care nurses.* The critical-care nurse has been described as assertive, autonomous, and achievement-oriented, but the description was qualified as "only common sense" and "without absolute evidence" (Smith 1980). It has also been proposed that the critical-care nurse is a risk taker. It might be expected that there would be considerable differences between critical-care nurses and nurses of other areas.

Therefore, this study is proposed to determine the personality traits of critical-care nurses and compare them with nurses in obstetrics/gynecology, psychiatry, and general medical-surgical areas. The following hypothesis will be tested: Critical-care nurses differ from other nurses in their needs for achievement, dominance, autonomy, and change.

A convenience sample of 200 nurses (50 from each specialty area) from six hospitals in a large metropolitan area will be used. A modified Edwards Personal Preference Schedule (EPPS) will be used as the measurement instrument for personality. The EPPS has been widely used to describe the personalities of nursing students and nurses because of its lack of maladjustive connotations and its design for fake response prevention. The EPPS was chosen for this study because of the relevance of its measures and ease of comparison with related studies. Other data obtained include age, sex, education, and approximate years of experience in their area and in nursing. The data will be analyzed by using analysis of variance. About 4 weeks will be required to complete data collection and analysis.

Exhibit 1-3. Prospectus for research investigating a relationship between parental visitation and premature infant growth. P. Coccaro, D. Powanda, S. Reed, M. Symanski, R. Thompson

---

The parent-infant bonding process has proved to be of value to both parent and baby (Klaus and Kennel 1976). As a result, family-centered maternity care evolved. Premature infants pose a special problem since they must spend time in the hospital away from their parents. Despite liberal visitation policies, for various reasons some parents do not visit their hospitalized infants. This knowledge has led researchers to study the later development of hospitalized infants and behaviors of their parents. Lack of visitation to hospitalized infants by their mothers has been linked to child abuse, failure to thrive, and other "mothering disorders" (Fanaroff et al. 1969). In other studies, tactile stimulation of premature infants in the hospital was related to increased growth and development of the child and to better maternal behavior when the handling was done by the mother (Skoff et al. 1969; Powell 1974).

Research on premature infants and parental contact thus far has addressed mainly the psychosocial effects of infant visitation by their parents and the physical effects of tactile stimulation. We believe there is a need to research the possible physical effects on the infant of parental contact or lack thereof. This would describe the importance of parents visiting their premature infants in the hospital. It would also provide a sound, scientific reason why great efforts should be made to find parents or foster parents for children placed for adoption as quickly as possible.

The purpose of the study is to test a relationship between parental visitation and the growth of premature hospitalized infants. The following hypothesis will be tested: Premature infants of 32 to 34 weeks gestation whose parents visit frequently grow faster than those whose parents visit infrequently.

A record search will be conducted at five hospitals in a large metropolitan area. By using the neonatal admissions logbooks as screening tools, 20 infants per hospital will be randomly selected according to a subject protocol. The protocol is designed to eliminate as subjects those infants with complex and devastating medical complications, a possible confounding variable. Then data will be collected from each chart. The data will include date of birth, birth weight, gestational age, daily weight, head circumference per week, number of parental visits per week, feeding methods, length of hospital stay, and any medical complications.

The data will be analyzed by using correlational techniques. It is predicted that there will be a positive correlation between the frequency of parental visits and increased rate of growth of the infants in the study. It is anticipated that it will require approximately one day per hospital to gather the required data. The study will be completed in 2 months.

---

pothesis, if any, of the research are presented. The fourth paragraph describes the research methods to be used. This section and the selection of particular references in the second paragraph establish the researcher as having expertise and being capable of conducting quality research. Finally, the last paragraph describes data analysis plans, time frame, and other details that must be included.

The prospectus is often sufficient when you are seeking funding support from foundations and for agencies within which your proposed study population is located. A much more detailed research proposal is required when government funding or a thesis or dissertation is involved. In this case, a prospectus (or abstract) is still needed at the beginning of the paper.

Step 6 of the research process includes two tasks that often are overlooked by researchers. The first involves cost estimates and a timetable. List the important steps for your project, who will perform them, and dates by which each is supposed to be completed. Then the costs for each step can be estimated. Do not forget travel and photocopying. The second task in step 6 involves anticipation of all possible results from your study and finding possible reasons for them. Expect the unexpected. Play the devil's advocate. What if your data result in differences in the opposite direction? What if a large percentage of potential participants refuse to participate? What if your subjects all respond in the same way; for example, what if you find only compliant subjects? If none of your hypotheses are supported, how can you "milk" the data? That is, will your data yield new information in spite of the fact that you failed to support your hypothesis? Are other explanations or variables responsible for your results (see Chap. 4)? How can agency personnel sabotage your study? By anticipating pitfalls, often you can accommodate them in your methodology. Assumptions and limitations of your study that emerge must be considered when you interpret your results. This, in turn, may affect your so-what test.

The **pilot study,** step 7, is very important. It should simulate as nearly as possible your anticipated research setting, even down to the day of the week and perhaps hour of the day. Note how your subjects respond to your questions. If they have trouble with some, change the questions. This is your last chance to make changes. How much time does your experiment take? Is it reasonable, or do your subjects complain? Perhaps you will have to shorten your procedure or divide it into segments. Try analyzing the data you have gathered. Do you have all the information you need? Did something in the setting distract or put off subjects? Do subjects tend to leave some questions unanswered or drop out before the study is completed? Often it is useful to ask the individuals who participate about their reactions to and general impression of the project. Also ask them for suggestions to improve the procedure. On the basis of information gained from your trial run, make changes in your methods. If extensive alterations are made, you may want to do a second pilot study. Thus, at this point you may move back and forth between steps 6 and 7.

Step 8, securing formal permission from agencies to use their facilities and approval of any committee(s) that must review your procedures for safeguarding the human rights of participants in your research also may become part of steps 6 and 7 if you must obtain these permissions to conduct your pilot study. Often informal permission and approval are granted if fewer than nine subjects are involved. However, it is your responsibility to find out the regulations in your targeted setting.

Once permissions have been received and you have procured your instruments and supplies, you are ready for the big event—data gathering. Be sure no unplanned changes in your procedure occur that might alter your data. In studies that extend over a period of time, this may not be easy. Sometimes, in spite of great care, changes do occur. For example, an agency staff member might be called away on emergency leave, thereby reducing the number of patients available or introducing a new (substitute) health care provider. Or the patient load may be spread over the remaining staff, thus increasing waiting time or pressure on the staff. If changes do occur, carefully record them in a **log book** and refer to them during data analysis and interpretation of results. Do not forget to record events that fail to occur, especially those that you anticipate might cause problems.

Many researchers believe that once they have gathered their data, they are almost finished. In actual practice, you are only half to two-thirds done in terms of your time involvement. However, you can now breathe a big sigh of relief. You now control your destiny. Outside events, such as many refusals by potential subjects, can no longer deter you. You are ready to analyze your data, step 10 (see Units III and VI) and interpret your findings (see Chap. 21). Next you communicate your results (see Chap. 22). Hopefully, the generation of suggestions for further research will have sparked your interest, and you will return to step 2 or 3 to begin the research process again. The generation of a body of knowledge is not accomplished by a single research project. It is the result of a series of studies by you, the expert, and those who later come to study and do research with the expert.

Note the extra box in Exhibit 1.1 that is below step 8 and above step 11. It reminds us that the literature review is continuous as we keep track of the latest developments in our topic area and look for research models worth emulating.

One further point should be noted about the research process. As diagramed in Exhibit 1.1, steps 1 through 6 involve logical thinking with words, not numbers. Number manipulations, mathematics, is utilized only in steps 9 and 10 to quantify the variables and describe their relationships. We do this because mathematics is the basic language of all phenomena. Can you imagine multiplying or dividing one word by another? In any event, the final step, step 11, again involves logical thinking with words. If you think this is a plug to reduce any anxieties about statistics you have learned, it is. Relax, unlearn your anxiety, and learn to make statistical analysis work for you. Statistical analysis is a pussycat, not a tiger, when you not only know why you are using it but also have written its job description. To do this, of course, first you must know what statistical analysis can do. This book will show you.

Working as a Research Team and Peer Review

Research teams, instead of researchers working in isolation, are prevalent. Several creative intellects addressing a research question often produce better research. More persons to do the work, especially the literature search and data gathering, allow a larger project. Sometimes work proceeds faster. It is also more fun to do research when you have someone with whom to brainstorm and share daily ups and downs. In large, complex funded research projects, there is simply too much work for one person to do. Expertise from too many different professional disciplines is required.

With rare exceptions, thesis and dissertation students in academic settings are required to conduct a research project alone, and its successful completion is considered a demonstration of their qualifications for graduate degrees. In most cases, thesis and dissertation committee members extend their role beyond the traditional one of an examining committee to one of an advisory committee that gives considerable help to the student. The chairperson, in fact, often acts as a project codirector, providing a great deal of time, expertise, and creativity. Sometimes the chairperson has ongoing research in which a student becomes involved, conducting one part of a larger study. These arrangements are forms of team research.

When research studies are conducted by students as part of a research course during a semester or quarter (a practice the author strongly advocates), usually the team approach is most efficient in terms of completing the project on time, keeping the student workload as low as possible, and providing maximum instructor input into the research. This is another type of research team.

Working as a team in any of these ways is a stimulating, challenging way to do research. It can be education made enjoyable. However, occasionally a team member does not do his or her fair share of the work. When this or other interpersonal problems develop, what could have been a joyful experience turns into just another job to finish as soon as possible or, worse, a nightmare. For that reason, some form of team review is recommended.

For a group of students working as a team in a research course, the review process, called *peer review,* can be fairly simple. At midterm and again at the end of the term when the team's written report is submitted, each member also submits a separate and confidential peer review statement to the instructor. In the peer review statement, each member, including the person submitting the statement, is listed and given a letter grade (A, B, C, D, or F) and a share of 100 points, which are distributed among the members of the team. The grade and points are based on that person's contribution to team efforts. Next a paragraph is written about each member, detailing that person's contributions to the team project and the reason(s) for the grade and share of points. At midterm, the instructor summarizes the individual statements for each team in such a way as to keep individual statements confidential and yet still give feedback regarding the strengths and weaknesses of the team effort. This written summary is given to each team to use as appropriate. In no way do these midterm peer reviews affect student grades in the course. They have always, in our experience, helped a team with problems to heal itself. Often those perceived as not doing their fair share or not doing quality work are unaware of this evaluation by their peers, and when they are made aware, they either put forth more effort or negotiate with the team to assume different responsibilities better suited to their capabilities. If a team is unable to solve a problem at that point, they involve their instructor who seeks a solution. Occasionally a team breaks into two separate teams.

The final peer review in a research course setting is often utilized differently. The instructor generally uses this to mediate the grade that individual students earn on the research project. For example, if a project receives a B and peer review indicates that one student did more work than the others, the student who did more work would earn an A while the others earn the project grade B, unless they did very little. Conversely, if a project graded B had one team member who did very little, that person would receive a C or lower while the others would receive the project grade of B.

Team or peer review in other settings will require modification of this procedure, perhaps in terms of merit salary increases or authorship credits. The point is that some process for constructive review halfway into a project (or sooner) may prevent it from being abandoned, sabotaged, or considered inferior. Asking for a review after a problem has developed is not nearly as effective as planning one as part of the "contract" when the team is being formed. Another issue that should be settled early in the life of the team is authorship of any publications resulting from the research.

Authorship Credits

In practice, the author of a publication is the person who conceptualized the idea, created the design, supervised data collection and analysis, and wrote the article—not necessarily the person(s) who actually *implemented* the research (e.g., data gathering, computer programming and statistical analysis, and library search for related literature). Those who contribute significantly to the *implementation* of the research are generally acknowledged in footnotes. When several people share authorship, the order in which they are listed (e.g., first, or senior, author; second, or junior, author; third author; and so forth) usually is determined by the magnitude of their total contributions. Some teams devise other approaches, such as alphabetical order, when all contribute equally.

Two research studies have surveyed psychologists [2] and nurses [3] about authorship credits. The majority of respondents in each study agreed that the design of the project was the most important contribution, followed by writing the article for publication, *assuming responsibility* for analyzing the data, and setting up the procedures and *assuming responsibility* for data collection. These four contributions usually qualify individuals for authorship. Moreover, a number of significant contributions to research were defined that generally deserve footnote acknowledgment:

1. Contributing the research idea which is used without any other major involvement in the project
2. Testing and interpreting projective tests and other very specialized assessment procedures
3. Designing and building equipment for the project
4. Conducting interviews to obtain data
5. Serving as an administratively responsible investigator (e.g., budget) without involvement in the research process itself
6. Searching the literature for related studies
7. Running subjects through research procedures called for in the design, under close supervision
8. Doing statistical analysis, under close supervision

In addition, the following contributions do not require acknowledgment (although it is certainly not prohibited):

1. Testing subjects with pencil-and-paper tests involving simple instructions
2. Extracting data from files under supervision without being involved in the planning or design of the project
3. Typing
4. Performing other clerical tasks (e.g., appointment making)

The two studies about authorship credits [2, 3] involve a series of vignettes describing various research situations for which respondents select the best authorship credit alternative. They are good resources if you find yourself in an unusual situation. In terms of student research, some guidelines can be developed from the results of these two studies. Thesis or special-problem students who design their studies with little input from their faculty advisors and also write their own articles with minimal suggestions usually do not need to acknowledge the faculty in any way. When faculty contribute significantly to the idea, design, or implementation, that contribution is acknowledged by footnote. If the contribution is great enough or involves writing all or part of the article, coauthorship is expected. Faculty generally expect second authorship with the student receiving first authorship unless the faculty member carried most of the responsibility for writing the article in addition to making major contributions to the idea, design, and data analysis. In this case, the faculty member would expect to be senior author. There is a fine line between collaboration (hence coauthorship) and consultation (hence a footnote).

Classroom research is yet another kind of research in which students become involved. When projects like the IDIR model [1] are employed,* faculty analyze

---

*Instructor-directed research (IDIR) model projects are generally a composite of data collected by up to eight separate classes (i.e., sections) of students by the time data are subjected to more sophisticated analysis (than in separate classes or sections) on which the faculty publication is based.

and publish, as sole authors, data collected by students who are doing a class research project designed and supervised by their instructor. In effect, students receive instruction via an apprenticeship approach by participating in their instructor's research. This is one of the best ways to begin learning the research process. Instructors are project directors, so to speak. When occasional students make contributions beyond the call of duty, faculty generally acknowledge it through footnotes and occasionally coauthorship, depending on the contribution. While the two research studies about authorship credits [2, 3] support faculty use of data gathered (or generated) by students, they also expect students to be told beforehand that the data may be used for this purpose. Classroom research is also expected to have a relationship to the course objectives.

There are many gray areas in determining authorship and order of authorship. In some work settings, department supervisors automatically are given authorship by those they supervise, even though they contribute absolutely nothing to the research. In others, this is considered unethical. When you are in doubt, ask. Just as friction between members of a team is deadly, so is ambiguity regarding authorship credit.

The best approach is to determine authorship credit when the study begins and attach a caveat regarding flexibility should the nature of contributions change. Authorship credits in a mentor situation are less clear since so much depends on unique aspects of the situation. It is, therefore, even more important to determine the policy for authorship of any papers or presentations of data in the beginning of your relationship.

Vocabulary

Authorship credits	Prospectus
Descriptive statistics	Quantitative research
Doable test	Research
Inferential statistics	Research process
Instrument	Sample
Instrument reliability	So-what test
Instrument validity	Study population
Item	Subjects
Logbook	Target population
Measurement	Theory
Mentor	Theory building
Operational definition	Theory testing
Peer review	Variables
Pilot study	

References

1. Shelley, S. I. Beat the Publish or Perish Syndrome. In B. Thomas (ed.), *Methods of Teaching Nursing Research* (conference proceedings). Iowa City: University of Iowa College of Nursing, 1982.
2. Spiegel, D., and Keith-Spiegel, P. Assignment of publication credits: Ethics and practices of psychologists. *Am. Psychol.* 25:738, 1970.
3. Werley, H. H., et al. Research publication credit assignment: Nurses' views. *Res. Nurs. Health* 4:261, 1981.

2: *Research Concepts*

In Chapter 1, quantitative research is described as fact finding in which variables are defined by using numbers. This, in turn, allows us to use a single number to describe many different measures of the same variable. For example, we can summarize and make sense out of many different scores by obtaining the average, or mean, score.

Research Statements

Sometimes the relationship between different variables is described by manipulating those numbers. The type of relationship between or among the variables, if any, that is being described is dictated by the type of quantitative research statement being investigated—causal, correlational, comparative, or descriptive. Often more than one type of statement is examined in a single research study.

Causal Statements

When making causal statements, as the word "causal" implies, researchers wish to demonstrate that *X* causes a change in *Y*, for example, that preoperative teaching causes a reduction in patient anxiety, or that weekly quizzes in a nursing research course result in higher grades on the final examination, or that inhalation of cigarette smoke causes a rise in the blood pressure of nonsmokers. Generation of a causal statement is the purpose of **experimental research** in which variable *X*, the causal agent, or **independent variable,** is manipulated by the researcher (experimenter), and then the effect of this manipulation on variable *Y*, the **dependent variable,** is observed. Suppose half of a group of available patients are randomly assigned to receive preoperative teaching and the others are not. If those who received preoperative teaching, the **experimental group,** were observed to have less anxiety than those in the **control group** who were not taught, you would conclude that the teaching had an **effect** on anxiety—assuming that you had carefully planned your experimental design to avoid **rival hypotheses,** or equally good explanations besides preoperative teaching, for the difference between the experimental and control groups.

Correlational Statements

When investigating correlational statements, researchers are unable to manipulate an independent variable. Instead, they can observe only two (or more) variables as they occur, or vary in quantity, in a group of subjects. If changes in one variable occur when changes in another variable occur, you can conclude that the two variables are correlated, or related, if no rival hypotheses exist. In correlational research, a single group of subjects would be given, for example, a test of their knowledge about surgical procedures and assessed for anxiety, or each subject is assessed for anxiety and has a blood pressure reading recorded. Researchers cannot control the amount of knowledge, number of quizzes, amount of anxiety, or blood pressure. Thus they cannot conclude that *X* causes *Y*. They can, however, conclude that *X* and *Y* are correlated. If *X* and *Y* both increase or both decrease, it is a **positive correlation.** If one variable increases and the other decreases, it is a **negative,** or **inverse, correlation.** Thus the anticipated, or hypothesized, correlation between knowledge and anxiety would be negative, or inverse, while the anticipated correlation between level of anxiety and blood pressure would be positive.

Correlational research can go one step further toward causal research by predicting a score on one variable given scores on one or more other variables. This is called **regression analysis.** In fact, several complex procedures are available which, based on correlations among a series of variables, attempt to predict changes in scores on one variable based on changes in other variables. The variables being used to predict a **criterion variable** are called, logically enough, **predictor variables.** Moreover, less logically, sometimes criterion variables are called dependent variables, and predictor variables are called independent variables even though no causal statement can be tested and the independent variable cannot be manipulated.

The important fact to remember about correlational research is that no independent variables can ever be manipulated by the researcher in order to make a causal statement. The best that correlational research can do is predict. In causal or experimental research, the study sample is assigned randomly to at least two groups, one of which either does not receive the independent variable because the researcher withholds it or receives it in a different form. In correlational research, the study sample is not divided into smaller groups, nor is the researcher able to control the quantity of a variable that the subjects might have (except by selecting for the study sample only those with certain characteristics). You simply describe the relationships among preexisting amounts of the variables as found in the study sample. Correlational statements, therefore, are considered a form of descriptive research.

Comparative Statements

Comparative statements, like correlational statements, do not involve the researcher's manipulation of an independent variable. Are you beginning to wonder why the independent variable is called *independent?* Certainly not because it is independent of the researcher who manipulates it. It is, however, independent of the subjects. In theory, the independent variable does not occur naturally in the study sample. The researcher introduces it to the study (and removes or withholds it) according to a plan called the research design. It is manipulated. Suppose that hospital A has a strong preoperative teaching program while hospital B teaches when there is time available, which is seldom. Is this a ready-made experiment? Use hospital A for introduction of the independent variable and hospital B for the controls. Suppose teacher A gives weekly quizzes and teacher B does not. Is this a ready-made causal research design? No, on all counts. These investigations can yield only comparative statements because the researchers have not *manipulated* the independent variable. The variable already occurred naturally in half the sample. To test a causal statement, all study subjects should have an equal chance of receiving the independent variable, although only some actually experience it. This is the essence of **random assignment** to groups. When you find significant differences between *preexisting* groups, such as students of teachers A and B, you can only suggest the quizzes as a *possible* explanation. Other explanations also would be possible causes. Only with a good experimental research design would you know for certain.

Of course, many variables can never be manipulated. Persons cannot be randomly assigned to sex or age, for example. In these cases, comparative or correlational statements are all that can be tested. Nor can a random half of a group be given cancer or pneumonia, although animals have been used for this purpose in some studies. As with correlational statements, comparative statements are part of descriptive research, because differences between groups as they occur naturally in the total sample are being described, not manipulated.

Descriptive Statements

Descriptive statements simply describe variables. The average midterm examination grade describes a class's knowledge of the material covered by the examination. The letter-grade **cutting points,*** further, describe the percentage of those receiving passing and failing grades. The cutting points, moreover, are determined by the researcher, hopefully on some rationale basis. Descriptive statements, of course, are also part of descriptive research and often are called **survey research.**

To summarize, four types of statements or questions can be addressed by quantitative research methods: causal, correlational, comparative, and descriptive. Each statement is represented by number manipulations.

Descriptive statements typically may include a number that represents an average score on a variable for a group of subjects, a number that represents how much individual scores vary from the group average, and the percentage of subjects fitting into various categories of a variable. Categories either may occur naturally in the population, such as sex or disease, or may be determined by cutting points established by the researcher or current practice, such as passing or failing scores on a R.N. licensure examination or moderate versus average versus severe disability.

Correlational statements describe, on a scale of 0 to 1, the amount of overlap between two variables. In most cases, the square of the reported correlation indicates the percentage of overlap.† Negative correlations, represented by a minus sign in front of the correlation (for example, $-.84$), indicate that as one variable increases, the other decreases. Positive correlations (for example, .84 but not $+.84$) indicate that the variables increase or decrease in the same direction. Correlations involving more than two variables are still described on a scale of 0 to 1 where 0 means no correlation and 1 means a perfect correlation.

---

*The *cutting point* is sometimes called a *cutoff* or *cut point*. Use whichever term best suits you or your instructor/mentor.
† If a correlation of .80 is reported, the percentage of overlap is .64, or 64 percent [$(.80)^2 = .80 \times .80 = .64 = 64\%$].

If the correlation is large enough, as determined by a statistical test, it is declared **statistically significant,** which means there is a strong probability (usually 95 percent) that it exists in real life. If the percentage of overlap seems **practically significant** to the researcher, then the research findings should lead to either additional research, preferably to test causal statements between the variables, and/or changes in clinical practice.*

Comparative statements compare at least two groups within the study sample. Often they are naturally occurring subgroups. The comparison may be based on numbers representing group averages on the dependent variable, the variation of subjects from the average of their group, correlations within each group, percentages of subjects in various categories within each group, and so forth. If the difference is large enough, as determined by a statistical test, it is declared statistically significant. Again, you must decide whether the difference is practically significant. In many cases, the difference between groups can be converted to a correlation that describes the magnitude of the relationship between membership in a specific subgroup and the dependent variable. This number, in turn, helps you assess the practical significance by estimating the overlap between the two variables. It is known as a **magnitude estimate.**

Causal statements are represented by the same number manipulations as comparative statements. The distinction between them is the use of a randomly assigned control group (from whom the researcher may withhold the independent variable) and the interpretation of results. Causal statements, when supported, can conclude that X causes Y. Comparative statements can conclude only that there are differences between groups and then speculate on the reasons why.

Another distinction should be apparent now. The two types of quantitative research, descriptive and experimental, differ in only one area—causal statements. Experimental research tests causal statements, and descriptive research cannot.

Other Ways to Cut the Cake

There are other ways of labeling research, such as laboratory, longitudinal, retrospective, and evaluation research. While the various labels at first may seem confusing, if not unending, they are organized easily according to the five W's— who, what, when, where, and why. *Who* refers to the target population to which your results should apply and your rationale for selecting the study population as representative of the target population. *What* refers to the kinds of statements you are making about variables or the relationships between variables. We

---

*In behavioral research, correlations of .30 (or 9 percent overlap) often are statistically significant. Because of the problems in measuring behavioral variables, such as anxiety, researchers have been content with these low correlations and have sought to combine them with other variables to increase the overlap.

described these and have further distinguished between them by classifying them as experimental or descriptive research.

Retrospective and Prospective Research

When refers to the time frame over which data will be gathered. **Retrospective research** involves going back over time to examine various relationships. The use of records to gather data is retrospective in nature because the events have occurred already, the variables have been measured. A study of myocardial infarction (MI) patients that seeks to describe various events during the year before the MI is retrospective. A study that involves asking breast cancer patients how many self-examinations they made the previous year is retrospective. Retrospective studies have the advantage of covering long periods without losing subjects and having research results available quickly. The disadvantage lies in errors or omissions in record keeping and subject recall. **Prospective research** (also called **longitudinal research**) studies, however, follow subjects over a period of time. The advantage of this type of study is its greater objectivity because the outcome is unknown, whereas retrospective studies often begin with an outcome and work backward to test correlations. Prospective studies can test causal statements because an independent variable can be introduced into the setting. They have the disadvantage of potential loss of subjects over time, potential changes in the independent variable or introduction of rival hypotheses, and much greater cost. Although no clear-cut time interval is defined, research that follows subjects over a 6-month or greater period generally is accepted as longitudinal. A study is prospective if subjects are followed over any time period. But **cross-sectional research** studies involve gathering data from subjects at only one time. These have an advantage in that subjects are not lost, extraneous events have less chance of disrupting data collection or results, relatively less cost is involved, and research results are available sooner. Correlational and comparative statements generally are tested by utilizing a cross-sectional approach.

Laboratory and Field Research

The *where* of research refers to the laboratory or field settings in which the research is conducted. **Field research** takes place in a natural setting where the study population would be located, such as an outpatient clinic if hypertensive patients are being studied. Thus far, nursing research has been conducted primarily in the field. Some, however, do utilize **laboratory research.** For example, many sleep studies are conducted in laboratories equipped with sophisticated monitoring devices rather than in the subjects' bedrooms. Alcohol consumption and sexual behavior studies often are conducted in a laboratory. **Simulation studies,** such as attitude responses to case studies which are described to subjects to simulate real-life situations, usually are considered a form of laboratory research.

Evaluation Research and Clinical Practice

The *why* of research not only includes the so-what test, but also separates clinical practice, evaluation, and research:

... nursing process is essentially a decision-oriented procedure, which aims to collect data for a nursing diagnosis and for subsequent interventions that will affect a client's well-being. Given this definition, nursing process is easily distinguished from research, which aims to enhance the knowledge base from which decisions are made, and from evaluation, which illuminates effectiveness against a set of generalized criteria (Downs [3]).

The distinction between clinical practice and research was debated extensively by the National Commission for the Protection of Human Subjects of Biomedical and Behavioral Research, because research, not clinical practice, requires institutional review board approval. *Practice* was finally defined as interventions (1) that have a reasonable expectation of success and (2) that are designed solely to enhance the well-being of the *individual* patients or clients. In *research,* moreover, we test hypotheses from which conclusions are drawn, thereby contributing to knowledge as expressed in theories, principles, and statements of relationships. Innovative or novel practices designed solely for an individual patient are not considered research, even though they might not be validated practices (tested sufficiently to have a reasonable expectation of success). Such practices, however, if sufficiently radical, should come under the auspices of clinical practice committees and supervisors.

The distinction between research and evaluation is sometimes less clear, because evaluation research generally utilizes quantitative research methods. It involves generalizing to only the study population, however. Causal statements are rarely tested, because the program being evaluated is ongoing and rarely under the control of the evaluator. Usually, an independent variable cannot be manipulated. Instead, the program's output or product is measured and compared with a preexisting set of measurable objectives formulated prior to program development which, in turn, incorporated practices already validated by research. The rapid development of social programs over the past 25 years, largely for disadvantaged groups or those being trained to work with them, occasioned incorporation into program delivery a number of practices not validated by research. Therefore, research to test many of these practices is either incorporated into program evaluation or occurring concurrently. Opportunities to conduct research as part of a program evaluation should not be overlooked. **Formative evaluation** refers to ongoing evaluation to ascertain how well the program is doing and to suggest areas in which change in delivery is needed. **Summative evaluation** refers to evaluation at the end of the program period.

The following are descriptions of actual research studies conducted by nurses. As you read them, answer the questions of who, what, when, where, and why.

1. Pulse rates, considered indices of stress reactions, of 25 myocardial infarction patients who were exposed to resuscitation procedures on other patients were compared with 12 patients not similarly exposed. Data were gathered over a 4-month period (Sczekalla [8]).

2. The diarrhea sometimes associated with nasogastric tube feeding often was attributed to the cool temperature of the formula. To test this assumption, the effects of three temperatures of liquid diet and water feedings on gastric mobility and emptying were studied by surgically implanting a Walton-Brodic strain gauge and feeding tube in rhesus monkeys. With the monkeys awake and restrained, researchers infused constant volumes of water and liquid diet formula at the three temperatures of warm, 36°C; room, 23°C; and cold, 5°C (Williams and Wallke [9]).

3. The effect of position, upright or recumbent, on the intensity and frequency of uterine contractions in the primigravidae during first- and second-stage labor was studied by placing an electric monitor on the maternal abdominal wall. It indicated the intensity of contractions, relaxation time, and contraction durations as well as rhythm and rate (Giambra [5]).

4. To survey the basic knowledge of syphilis and gonorrhea held by school nurses, a 52-item questionnaire was mailed to 170 nurses. Of these, 129 (or 76 percent) were returned. Questions that were answered incorrectly by 30 percent or more nurses were examined (McGrath and Laliberte [7]).

5. A random sample of clinic outpatient records, consisting of 202 clients evaluated over a 2-year period, were examined to determine the rate of compliance with keeping the first psychotherapy appointment following evaluation in the clinic and to identify factors (e.g., time between evaluation and first appointment, sex, age, diagnosis, referral source, and evaluating therapist) related to compliance (Cone and Stephens [2]).

6. The effect of simulation gaming on the authoritarianism and social restrictiveness toward mental illness of 60 nursing students was explored. Each of two games consisted of seven rounds where one of seven subjects took her turn to play the role of a mental patient or ex-patient. The "patients" were asked to convince the rest of the group that they were ready for discharge or some new responsibility. Ten days following the games, a researcher cohort administered the posttest (Godejohn et al. [6]).

The *who* of all examples except the second is obvious—myocardial infarction patients, primigravidae, school nurses, psychiatric clinic outpatients referred for treatment, and nursing students. In each, the study population is clearly representative of the target population. In the second example, however, rhesus monkeys were utilized as the study population while the target population was humans undergoing nasogastric tube feeding.

The *what* of research refers to the kind of statements being tested. Causal statements are being examined in examples 2, 3, and 6. This is readily apparent by observing the use of the word "effect." It implies the manipulation of an independent variable and use of controls. Example 5 involves correlational statements when identifying factors related to compliance. The rate of compliance is descriptive. A comparative statement is tested in example 1, and a descriptive statement is made in example 4. Four independent variables and one possible group of predictor variables are mentioned. Can you find them and their corresponding dependent, or criterion, variables?

The *when* of five of the examples is prospective, because data are gathered over time. However, none last long enough to be considered longitudinal. Moreover, examples 1 and 4 are actually cross-sectional since subjects are measured at only one time and no time period, such as measures during first- and second-stage labor, is involved. Example 5 is retrospective.

The *where* of examples 1, 3, 4, 5, and 6 is the field. Laboratory research is used in example 2 where monkeys are implanted with strain gauges and feeding tubes. Example 5, the record search, is a special case of field research in which actual subjects are never observed.

The *why* of these six research examples should be obvious. All seek to generate new knowledge by examining research statements, and all appear to meet the so-what test. Examples 2 and 3 examined areas for which no evidence to support current clinical practices existed. Determination of a single clinic's rate of compliance over a 2-year period (example 5) most likely would be considered evaluation. To generate knowledge upon which clinical decisions are made, rates for more than one clinic would be needed. However, the identification of factors related to compliance is research; as such, the compliance rate for the clinic is useful in describing the research setting.

Hypotheses and Research Questions

Research Hypothesis

The who, what, when, where, and why of your research relates to your hypothesis, objective, or research question. It focuses on a specific aspect or relationship from your larger topic area or researchable question. (Note that a researchable question is different from the research question, which is described in this section.) Your focus can be worded as a statement, known as a hypothesis, as an objective, or in the form of a research question. In experimental research you always use a research hypothesis, which is then supported or rejected. It is the traditional way of establishing causality. In descriptive research, however, you can use a hypothesis, an objective, or a question. It often depends on whether theory or prior research suggests the nature of the relationship or difference. Frequently questions and objectives are appropriate when the results of research are used to build theory. Hypotheses are used to test existing theory.

The **research hypothesis** is a short statement, a sentence or two in length, that describes the who and what of your research. It is the piece of knowledge that you wish to add to the larger body of knowledge. (Whether this piece is actually added depends on the results and the credibility of your research methodology, such as the use of valid and accurate measures to quantify your variables, selection of a design that controls rival hypotheses, sampling of an appropriate study population, the when and where of your research, and so forth.) For example, the research hypotheses for the six examples cited earlier might be as follows:

1. Myocardial infarction patients who are exposed to resuscitation procedures on other patients, as compared with those who are not, exhibit stress reactions.
2. Diarrhea among those with nasogastric tube feeding is caused by the cool temperature of the formula.
3. Body position, upright or recumbent, during first- and second-stage labor of primigravidae affects uterine contractions.

   or

   Upright position, as compared with recumbent position, during first- and second-stage labor shortens the duration of labor and reduces the perception of pain intensity by primigravidae.
4. Basic knowledge of syphilis and gonorrhea held by school nurses is adequate.
5. Outpatient compliance with keeping the first psychotherapy appointment following clinic evaluation is associated with length of time between the evaluation and appointment, sex, age, diagnosis, referral source, and evaluating therapist.
6. Simulation gaming reduces authoritarianism and social restrictiveness toward mental illness among nursing students.

These research hypotheses have five characteristics in common:

1. They are written in the present tense.
2. They include no statistical jargon, such as "statistically significant," "random assignment," "control group," "subjects," and so forth.
3. They allude to the target population to which the piece of knowledge would apply, rather than the study population.
4. They are simple and concise, generally including only one relationship or difference to be tested (although a string of dependent variables might be used for which a series of very similar statistical tests are required). Furthermore, the description of the relationship specifies the direction of change or differences, if known.
5. They are amenable to testing by using quantitative methods.

Some researchers use the future tense instead of the present tense. While this is a minor point not worthy of extended debate, the present tense is more logical and appropriate, because if it is supported by your results, your piece of knowledge is worded as a relationship that exists *now* and not one which will occur in the future. The relationship is in the tense of the theory from which it is taken. The present tense also translates directly to the statistical hypothesis and alternate, which are basic to the theory underlying inferential statistics. The absence of statistical jargon in research hypotheses is reasonable when you recall the discussion and diagram of the research process in Chapter 1. The translation of your research to numbers and number manipulations occurs after generation of your hypotheses. Thus, statistical jargon is out of place. Moreover, the piece of knowledge you contribute to the body of knowledge should be understandable to all, not just to those acquainted with the language of quantitative research.

Inclusion of the target population with the relationship being tested makes the statement more precise. Inclusion of only one relationship allows acceptance or rejection of a very specific piece of new knowledge. If many relationships were included, you would stand a good chance of supporting only part of your statement, thus revision into single statements would be required anyway. As you have noticed, most of the research hypothesis examples specify how the variables will change or differ. Even the descriptive statement about the level of knowledge about syphilis and gonorrhea specifies "adequate" as a prediction of results. Of course, the researcher must define "adequate" in her or his methodology as 90 or 100 percent correct or whatever, and the consumer of the research must, in turn, agree with the rationale for defining "adequate." Example 3 has two hypotheses, depending on whether the researcher can specify the nature of the difference beforehand. There is a slight statistical advantage if the direction is specified in advance; that is, the chances of obtaining significant results are slightly greater. However, if results are in the opposite direction, however large the change or difference, the research hypotheses will not be supported. Prior research results or theory should guide your decision to specify **directionality.** If previous work is conflicting, you may do better to use a **nondirectional** hypothesis. In what other ways might the six examples be worded to specify either another direction or none at all?

The last characteristic of hypotheses is that they are quantifiable. This may seem superfluous at first. It is not. Many obvious causal relationships, as we have stated previously, cannot be tested. In addition, questions of morality can be addressed only through the opinions of others. The attitudes of nurses toward euthanasia can be measured, but the ultimate goodness or badness of it cannot be measured. We can observe the healing effects of the laying on of hands, but we cannot (as yet, anyway) quantify the psychic exchange of energy that is reported to occur. How do you quantify the will to live?

A final word about research hypotheses is needed. Most often a research hypothesis specifies that a relationship does exist, although directionality might not be specified. On rare occasions a research hypothesis specifies that no relationship exists. This is permissible, when it is adequately justified by theory and prior research, and requires a slight change in the procedure used for the statistical test.* It should not be confused with the null hypothesis.

---

*If a conventional hypothesis utilizes $\alpha = .05$, the table of critical values is entered at $\alpha = .20$ or $.25$ (instead of $\alpha = .05$). See Chapter 15, which explains the use of statistical tables.

Null Hypothesis

For every research hypothesis there is a **null hypothesis.** The opposite of the research hypothesis, the null hypothesis states that there is no relationship, change, or difference. Technically, the null hypothesis is tested with inferential statistics. If it is rejected, the alternate, or research, hypothesis is supported. Conversely, if it is not rejected, then the research hypothesis is not supported. The null hypothesis can never be said to have been *supported,* only *accepted* or *rejected.*

Research Questions or Objectives

Research questions or objectives include all parts of the hypothesis except the anticipated results. They are useful in place of a research hypothesis when there is no clear indication of the results to be expected. The **research question,** as the name implies, is worded in the form of a question whereas the **research objective** is a statement preceded by "The purpose of this research is . . ." or "The objective of this research is to examine . . . ." The six examples are now worded as questions and objectives:

1. Do myocardial infarction patients who are exposed to resuscitation procedures on other patients, as compared with those who are not exposed, exhibit stress reactions?

   or

   The purpose of this study is to compare stress reactions of myocardial infarction patients who are exposed to resuscitation procedures on other patients with those who are not exposed.

2. Does the temperature of the formula used in nasogastric feeding cause diarrhea?

   or

   The purpose of this study is to investigate the effects, such as diarrhea, of the temperature of the formula utilized in nasogastric feeding.

3. What effect does body position, upright or recumbent, during first- and second-stage labor of primigravidae have on uterine contractions?

   or

   The objective of this study is to examine the effects on uterine contractions of body position, upright or recumbent, during first- and second-stage labor of primigravidae.

4. What is the basic knowledge of syphilis and gonorrhea held by school nurses?

   or

   The purpose of this survey is to assess the level of basic knowledge about syphilis and gonorrhea held by school nurses.

5. What factors are associated with outpatient compliance with keeping the first psychotherapy appointment following clinic evaluation?

or

The objective of this research is to describe factors associated with outpatient compliance with keeping the first psychotherapy appointment following clinic evaluation.

6. Does simulation gaming reduce nursing students' authoritarianism and social restrictiveness toward mental patients?

or

The objective of this research is to explore the effects of simulation gaming on nursing students' authoritarianism and social restrictiveness.

The questions and objectives can be worded in other ways. The important point to remember is that they still specify a research statement and target population. They simply do not predict results.

The decision to use a research hypothesis, question, or objective is determined by the circumstances of your research. Among our six examples, a research question or objective might be more appropriate for the survey of school nurses and search for factors associated with psychiatric patients' compliance. Example 2, which examined a long-standing assumption of nursing practice, might have been worded best as an objective.

As further practice in delimiting a research topic, study the following hypotheses. Do they fulfill the criteria? What types of research statements are being made? Who is the target population? Is directionality specified? If necessary, reword these statements for greater clarity. Convert each to a research question and objective. Finally, select the most appropriate format—research hypothesis, research question, or research objective. How do the when, where, and why of the research influence your decision?

1. There will be a statistically significant difference between the control group of subjects receiving regular medication by a nurse and the experimental group who administer their own medication even though subjects are randomly assigned to groups.
2. A correlation will be found between having had a course dealing with terminally ill patients and doing a better job with them.
3. Institutionalized adults in state mental hospitals located within 1 mile of a body of water are restless and get into more trouble during a full moon because the full moon changes their auras to a slightly brownish hue.

Operational Definitions

Earlier we referred to the quantification of variables. This process of measuring a variable and thereby attaching a number to it is called *operationally defining* a variable. The number that results is termed the **operational definition.** It is the translation of your research into numbers. Two things related to an operational definition must be considered. The first involves estimating the accuracy/error of the number, and the second involves the nature of the number itself.

Reliability and Validity

Reliability of an operational definition refers to its consistency or stability over time. If you weigh 125 lb on one scale and 135 lb on another one, you conclude that either one or both are not accurate. At least one is not a *reliable* operational definition of your weight. If you weigh yourself every hour on the same scale and register 125, 135, 120, 130, and 115 lb over a 5-hour period, you also conclude that the scale is not *reliable*. However, if your weight varies by only 1 lb or so over 5 hours and you are normally active during that time period, you probably conclude that scale is reliable.

Validity refers to whether the instrument or scale is quantifying what it claims to. You have no problem believing that the weight scale does, in fact, measure your body weight. However, what if the weight scale were used to operationally define your body temperature? You would say it was not *valid*— the resulting number is not my body temperature. The weight scale lacks validity as an operational definition of body temperature.

Researchers must present evidence that their operational definitions are reliable and valid. Reliability usually is described in terms of a correlation coefficient which, as you recall, varies on a scale from 0 to 1. Only in the case of a reported reliability coefficient is the overlap indicated by the value of the correlation itself. You do *not* need to square a reliability correlation as you do for its other uses. Validity is sometimes described in terms of a correlation (which must be squared) with other valid measures of the same variable. Often, unfortunately, the evidence is limited to testimony by experts. In addition, reliability is necessary before validity can be established. At the risk of oversimplification, reliabilities as low as .60 are generally permitted for research purposes. Reliability of .90 or better is needed for clinical diagnosis. Rater agreement is usually acceptable at .85. Finally, be aware that a validity correlation can never be any larger than the square root of the reliability correlation. The process of operationally defining variables is discussed at length in Unit V, in which the wide variety of instruments available for use and ways to establish reliability and validity are discussed.

Levels of Measurement

Once you are satisfied that a variable will be (or has been) operationally defined reliably and validly, you must assess what kind of number it is in order to select the appropriate statistical test. There are three classes of numbers. Each has associated with it a collection of statistical procedures.

Interval or Ratio Data

Interval or ratio level numbers are the highest level of measurement. They indicate *how much* of a variable, or the quantity, a subject has. Usually it is a score. Body temperature, blood pressure, and a score on a midterm examination all qualify for treatment in this category. Interval data get their name from the fact that they represent points along a continuum which has equal distances, or intervals, between the points. The continuum is metric. The distance between midterm scores of 85 and 90 is the same, theoretically at least, as the distance between scores of 91 and 96. They each have intervals of 5 points. The difference between 3 and 4 inches is the same as the difference between 10 and 11 inches. Time, age, blood pressure, and the number of analgesics consumed during the nightshift are other examples of this type of data. These data are considered superior because more statistical procedures are available for use with interval and ratio data. With these procedures you generally have greater capability of controlling rival hypotheses as well as requiring fewer subjects than comparable procedures designed for use with lower levels of measurement.

Ratio level is distinguished from interval level by having a zero point that really means zero. A final examination score of zero would not be considered a ratio measure, for example, because a zero could not be considered an absence of *all* knowledge. So final examination scores would be considered interval data. A temperature of zero is not the absence of temperature. Temperatures, therefore, are considered interval rather than ratio data. In research, the distinction between interval and ratio measurement is rarely needed, because both use the same statistical tests. Therefore, it is more efficient to group them in one category.

Ordinal Data

Ordinal data consist of categories of a variable that are rank-ordered according to a predetermined standard. For example, clothing size, military rank, contest winner (e.g., first, second, third) are ordinal data. A ranking of patient behaviors according to how often they occur during a given period is another example. Although there are no equal intervals between points represented by the categories being ranked, rank data do have a relative order between categories. Interval or ratio data can be converted to ordinal data according to the magnitude of each score. However, ordinal data cannot be converted to the higher interval or ratio levels.

Nominal Data

Nominal data consist of different categories of a variable into which each subject's response is placed. Then the number of (subject) responses is summed to give percentages, or the number of subjects in each category, also known as a **frequency count.** The categories have no relative standing or order among them like ordinal data. This is the lowest level of measurement. Sex, eye color, and type of disease are nominal level variables. Ratio, interval, and ordinal level data can be converted to nominal level if a researcher desires. However, nominal level data cannot be raised to higher levels.

Examples of Data Levels

Exhibit 2.1 illustrates the levels of measurement. Ratio is separated from interval to show how they differ. The pulse rates of 10 subjects have been taken. Since a zero pulse does indeed mean an absence of pulse, it is appropriately considered as ratio level. It has both equal intervals and a zero point. If we remove the zero point as an indicator of the absence of the variable but retain the equal intervals, we have data at the interval level of measurement. In this example, we did this by making the lowest pulse equal to zero* and then converting the others according to the number of intervals they were above 38, the lowest pulse: 43 is 5 intervals above 38, and 88 is 50 intervals above 38, and so on. These scores still place subjects on a continuum, or ruler, of equal intervals relative to one another. However, we have lost the zero point. An interval level pulse score of 117 has no intrinsic meaning, since it does not mean the number of beats per minute. It has meaning only in relationship to the other scores.

We can reduce our pulse measures further to ordinal level by rank-ordering them from highest to lowest, where the highest rank receives a 1. Now we have lost the equal intervals, or continuum, on which scores were placed. Therefore, we no longer can observe that subjects D and E were farther apart than subjects E and F. All we can observe now is that D had a faster pulse than E and E had a faster pulse than F. Subjects still have positions relative to one another, but their nature or magnitude can be observed no longer.

We can reduce these data one step further to nominal level by placing subjects in categories according to their scores. If we can agree that a pulse below 50 or above 150 is not normal, we can divide the subjects into two categories: normal pulse and not-normal pulse. Since not-normal pulse includes both very low and very high rates, these data have lost their ordinal nature and can be considered nominal.

In this example, we were able to convert higher-level data to lower-level data. This is always possible. However, you can never convert lower-level data to higher-levels, except in the case of dichotomous data, which we discuss later. Therefore, higher is better. Try for at least interval level data and settle for less only if you must. Interval and ratio data have much more sophisticated statistical procedures associated with them which allow testing more complex kinds of hypotheses. This is very desirable in research with humans, who are complex indeed.

One more example must be presented in a discussion devoted to levels of measurement, because of a widespread and outdated belief. Exhibit 2.2 presents 10 items from a scale developed by Ashton [1] for her nursing research study about adolescent attitudes toward sexuality and contraception. Subjects respond to the items on a *scale* of 1 to 4, where 1 means "strongly agree," 2 means

---

*Any number, not just zero, can be used. When zero is used at the interval level like this, it no longer means the absence of the variable. Try using 1 or 5 to convert the numbers. They will still have the same intervals.

Exhibit 2-1. Pulse according to levels of measurement.

Subject	Ratio	Interval	Ordinal	Nominal
A	170	132	1	X
B	155	117	2	X
C	135	97	3	N
D	120	82	4	N
E	100	62	5	N
F	88	50	6	N
G	64	26	7	N
H	50	12	8	N
I	43	5	9	X
J	38	0	10	X

Note: Although it is hard to get experts to agree on cutting points, pulses below 50 and above 150 are considered not normal and so are marked X in the nominal level column.

ordinal

Exhibit 2-2. Likert scale measuring sexual attitudes.

Directions: For each of the following statements, write a 1 if you strongly agree, a 2 if you agree, a 3 if you disagree, and a 4 if you strongly disagree.

1	2	3	4
Strongly Agree	Agree	Disagree	Strongly Disagree

Interval. 5 words except two extremes

_____1. There is nothing wrong with engaging in sexual relationships out of wedlock.

_____2. Using contraception takes away the fun of sex.

_____3. A woman should feel free to begin a sexual encounter with a man.

_____4. In general, women do not enjoy sex as much as men.

_____5. When I have sex, pregnancy is just the chance I take.

_____6. Sometimes I really worry and wonder about my ability to get pregnant when I take chances and still do not get pregnant.

_____7. Sexual feelings and urges in unmarried persons are generally abnormal and unhealthy.

_____8. Consistent birth control can increase sexual enjoyment.

_____9. Abortion is acceptable only when birth control methods fail.

_____10. Unwanted pregnancy only seems to happen to other people who are careless at birth control.

Abridged from Ashton [1] with permission.

"agree," 3 means "disagree," and 4 means "strongly disagree." This type of scale is known as a **Likert scale,** and according to current accepted practice, it yields interval level data, not ordinal, as too many textbooks suggest. The response scale of 1 to 4 for each item is *assumed* to represent an equal interval continuum, and thus the sum of responses is considered interval data. Moreover, by presenting the **response alternatives** in the form of a ruler (continuum), as shown in Exhibit 2.2, the researcher emphasizes the interval level nature of the data.

About half the statements on Likert scales are worded as positive toward the topic, and about half are negative. This prevents response bias in which some subject may tend to agree (or disagree) with all items. When items are so worded, meaningful total scores cannot be obtained by simply adding all responses. Instead, only the half that is negatively worded is summed. Then responses for those items that are positive are subtracted from a constant (number) which is 1 more than the highest possible number response. Then these values are added to the sum for negative items. In Exhibit 2.2, items 1, 2, 8, 9, and 10 were considered positive items (according to Ashton's theoretical framework). Since 4 was the highest possible number response, the constant from which positive item responses are to be subtracted is 4 + 1, or 5. The process of subtracting the response of the positively worded items from a constant is known as **flipping.** The fact that items can be flipped adds credence to the interval nature of the data obtained. With an equal-interval continuum, flipping can occur.

Suppose you have a subject's responses to the scale in Exhibit 2.2 as follows:

Item 1: 2
Item 2: 3
Item 3: 2
Item 4: 4
Item 5: 2
Item 6: 4
Item 7: 4
Item 8: 2
Item 9: 1
Item 10: 1

To obtain a total score, responses to the negatively worded items (2, 4, 5, 6, and 7) can be summed: 3 + 4 + 2 + 4 + 4 = 17. Next responses to the positive items must be subtracted from 5:

Item 1: 5 − 2 = 3
Item 3: 5 − 2 = 3
Item 8: 5 − 2 = 3

Item 9: 5 − 1 = 4
Item 10: 5 − 1 = 4

Now they can be added to the sum of negatively worded items: 17 + 3 + 3 + 3 + 4 + 4 = 34. This subject's total score is 34 on a Likert scale ranging from 10 (10 items with responses of 1) to 40 (10 items with responses of 4) where a score of 25 would be the middle of the **possible range of scores.** In Exhibit 2.2, higher scores suggest more positive attitudes and lower scores suggest more negative attitudes.

With Likert scales, the definition of positive and negative, the decision about whether 1 means "strongly agree" or "strongly disagree," and the decision about whether a high score will be positive or negative (or important or not important) depend on the researcher. (Be sure you know these things before you use someone else's scale.) From these decisions comes identification of the items that must be flipped. In addition, some Likert scales have a scale of responses from 1 to 5, where 3 means "undecided." Still others have ranges from 1 to 7 or 1 to 3. Some researchers do not use an "undecided" alternative, because they want to force respondents to "take a stand." With children, alternatives are sometimes "YES," "yes," "?," "no," and "NO." There are numerous possibilities. The decision is up to the researcher.

Finally, Likert scores can be converted to ordinal level data by rank-ordering subjects according to their total scores. They even might be categorized into "favorable," "unfavorable," and "undecided" according to their scores. The researcher's purpose must be the deciding factor regarding how scores will be handled. At least with interval level scores you have options. More is said about your many options for data analysis in the rest of this book.

Dichotomous Data

A special case exists for data that fall into only two categories. Although these data ordinarily might be considered nominal level (e.g., pass-fail, sex), they also can be treated as interval level in many statistical tests, because the variable either has an underlying continuous characteristic, such as pass-fail, or is changed conceptually to represent, for example, the presence or absence of femaleness. Moreover, this practice is further justified by researchers who cite experts such as Gaito [4] who argues that the concept of levels of measurement itself may be overemphasized.

Statisticians have gone so far as to create **dummy variables** by converting a nominal level variable to a set of dichotomous variables in which *each* new variable represents one of the response alternatives and is coded as 1 if the subject selected it and 0 if the subject did not. The entire set of dummy variables is then analyzed as a single group with multivariate statistical procedures (e.g., multiple regression). For example, suppose patient diagnosis, a nominal level variable, had five response alternatives in a research study (i.e., myocardial infarction, diabetes, hypertension, colostomy surgery, and spinal cord injury).

By using the dummy-variable method, each diagnosis would be considered a separate variable with a response of yes or no. Then the entire set of five dummy variables would be combined in multivariate analysis (see Chap. 20) or used as separate variables in a less complex analysis—if and only if doing so made sense in a given research situation.

The best approach in planning research is to select, if possible, variables that can be measured at the interval or ratio level. Then all options are available to you. The use of dummy variables is an advanced procedure which requires very careful use.

Statistics and Levels of Measurement

There are different comparative statistical procedures, used with both causal and comparative statements, for *each* level of measurement. Also there are correlational statistical procedures, used for correlational statements, for each level of measurement. Likewise, there are descriptive statistical procedures, used for descriptive statements, for each of the levels of measurement. With knowledge about the kind of statement and the level of measurement, the selection of the appropriate statistical procedure is straightforward. Once it is selected, you simply follow directions for the mathematical procedures until you have computed a number, called the **test statistic.** This test statistic is compared to a **critical value** in a statistical table to ascertain if you have found statistical significance. Units III and VI explain the commonly used statistical procedures.

V*ocabulary*

Causal statement	Formative evaluation
Comparative statement	Frequency count
Control group	Independent variable
Correlational statement	Interval level data
Criterion variable	Laboratory research
Critical value	Levels of measurement
Cross-sectional research	Likert scale
Cutting points	Longitudinal research
Dependent variable	Magnitude estimate
Descriptive statement	Negative (or inverse) correlation
Dichotomous data	Nominal level data
Directionality	Nondirectional hypothesis
Dummy variables	Null hypothesis
Effect	Operational definition
Evaluation research	Ordinal level data
Experimental group	Positive correlation
Experimental research	Possible range of scores
Field research	Practically significant
Flipping	Predictor variable

Prospective research

Random assignment

Ratio level data

Regression analysis

Reliability of measurement

Research hypothesis

Research objective

Research question

Research statement

Retrospective research

Rival hypothesis

Simulation studies

Statistically significant

Summative evaluation

Survey research

Test statistic

Validity of measurement

References

1. Ashton, R. S. Teenage girls' knowledge and attitudes of reproduction, sexual activity, and utilization of contraception. University of Maryland Master's thesis, 1981.
2. Cone, B., and Stephens, N. E. Compliance with beginning therapy in a psychiatric outpatient clinic. Unpublished manuscript. University of Maryland School of Nursing, 1978.
3. Downs, F. S. Clinical and Theoretical Research. In F. S. Downs and J. W. Fleming (eds.), *Issues in Nursing Research.* New York: Appleton-Century-Crofts, 1979.
4. Gaito, J. Measurement scales and statistics: Resurgence of an old misconception. *Psychol. Bull.* 87:564, 1980.
5. Giambra, N. A study of the effects of maternal positioning on characteristics of contractions and the length of labor. University of Maryland Master's thesis, 1980.
6. Godejohn, C. J., et al. Effect of simulation gaming and attitudes toward mental illness. *Nurs. Res.* 24:367, 1975.
7. McGrath, P., and Laliberte, E. B. Level of basic venereal disease knowledge among junior and senior high school nurses in Massachusetts: A survey. *Nurs. Res.* 23:31, 1974.
8. Sczekalla, R. M. Stress reactions of CCU patients to resuscitation procedures on other patients. *Nurs. Res.* 22:65, 1973.
9. Williams, K. R., and Wallke, B. C. Effect of the temperature of tube feeding on gastric motility in monkeys. *Nurs. Res.* 24:4, 1975.

II: *Research Design*

The three chapters in this unit present the most common research designs, including some with more than one independent variable. Chapter 3 begins with a clinical problem involving compliance to the therapeutic regimen among kidney dialysis patients. Preexperimental, true-experimental, and quasi-experimental designs are considered for use with this problem. Multiple measures of the dependent variable are utilized in the examples, although the rationale for multimodal measurement is not actually discussed until Unit V. The importance of control via random assignment, manipulation of the independent (i.e., experimental) variable, and use of control (or comparison) groups is stressed. Although only two groups are utilized in the examples, the use of three or more groups for many studies is more appropriate. Chapter 3 concludes with a brief overview of single-case (i.e., n of 1) designs.

Chapter 4 continues the design diagrams introduced in Chapter 3 as time series and factorial designs are presented to control possible rival hypotheses. Threats to both the internal validity and the construct validity of research designs are explored as well as ways of minimizing them. Chapter 5 presents a number of descriptive designs utilizing the same format for diagraming them as was developed in Chapter 3.

Basic vocabulary words are listed at the end of each chapter, and they might well be treated as suggested in the introduction to Unit I. In addition, after you have read this unit consider the following hypotheses:

1. Sensory stimulation and orientation techniques by the nursing staff decrease disorientation and incidence of black patch syndrome among patients who have both eyes tightly patched following retinal surgery.
2. Patients continuously receiving nasogastric tube feedings differ in the incidence of diarrhea and aspiration from those receiving the feedings intermittently.
3. Intensive care units with no visiting restrictions have less anxious patients than those with inflexible visiting restrictions.

How might these hypotheses be tested? Which designs are appropriate? Select one hypothesis, modify it when necessary, and demonstrate how each design presented in this unit could be used to test a hypothesis in the general problem area. Point out the threats to the internal and construct validities of each of your design examples. If you should support (or not support) your hypothesis, what conclusions could you draw—considering the threats and rival hypotheses you have found?

Maria Langley, R.N., works in a 20-bed kidney dialysis unit at a large urban teaching hospital. She is concerned about the high percentage of patients who do not come in for treatment as regularly as they are scheduled. Patients often express pessimism about the effectiveness of their dialysis treatment by saying they still do not feel as well as they would like to, even after treatment. They consider themselves as not being of much benefit to their families. Others cite fear of the dialysis treatment itself. Still others hold erroneous beliefs about their condition and its treatment. Patients living alone or without an apparent support person are referred to the medical social work department. However, nothing is being done for those who are living with their families.

Maria decides to try doing something for those with families. She develops a 1-hour slide presentation which includes factual information about kidney disease and its treatment, as well as testimonials from family members attesting to the need for and many benefits provided by dialysis patients to their families. She plans a 2-hour evening session in which she will present her slides and answer any questions. The hospital director agrees to pay transportation expenses for those who need it. She hopes her program will result in a change in patient attitudes and behavior.

Maria holds her meeting, and all seems to go well. Patients applaud at the end of the slide presentation, and after an uneasy first 5 minutes, they eagerly ask questions and even volunteer answers to the questions of others. As they leave, they thank her for the interesting evening. Many say they learned something new. Maria feels good. She has done something to help her patients. It was a success. Or was it? Has she really established a causal relationship between her presentation and a change in the attitudes or behavior of the patients? No. Although the willingness to ask questions and answer them on the part of some patients may be satisfying to observe, it does not necessarily relate to a change in attitudes or behavior. Neither does having an interesting evening. Did the patients really learn something new, or were they being polite? Perhaps what they learned will not relate to attitudes or behavior. What percentage stated they learned something new? Maria really cannot remember.

Maria has not assessed the effects of her experimental variable. When the hospital director asks if his money was well spent, what can she say? Her experimental design looks like this:

$$E \rightarrow ?$$

The box stands for her group of subjects. The symbols within it represent what happened to her research subjects. Symbolically, E represents the experimental variable or program in question, the arrow stands for "followed by," and the question mark is self-evident. This design, unfortunately, is often used.

One of the most critical components in experimental research is the selection, before a project begins, of an appropriate design. Without this design, it is impossible to determine whether the **experimental variable** (also called either the **treatment** or **independent, variable**) is responsible for any measured **effect** on the **dependent variable.** Only with a good design can a **causal statement** be inferred from statistically significant results. The following descriptions present both inappropriate and appropriate designs commonly found in experimental research. By understanding each of these you will be able to better plan your own research as well as judge the quality of research studies you encounter.

Preexperimental Design

Single-Group Posttest Design

The single-group posttest design follows administration of the experimental variable with an appropriate measuring device, *M*. It is shown in Exhibit 3.1 in its most simple form. Maria's slide presentation is aimed at clearing up misconceptions about kidney disease and its treatment, changing attitudes, and ultimately altering behavior. So she decides to ask patients to complete a short test of knowledge *K* and an attitude scale *A* at the end of the session. She also decides to follow patient records for 6 months to see whether they become more regular in their treatment *B*. She will use a ratio of appointments kept to appointments made. Her design is shown in Exhibit 3.2. Each of her three measures is listed: *A* symbolizes her attitudinal measure; *K*, her knowledge measure; and *B,* her behavior measure. In parentheses following each measure is the level of measurement. Nominal level is indicated by a 1; ordinal, by 2; and interval or ratio, by a 3. In this example all measures are ratio or interval. Since the same statistical procedures apply to both interval and ratio measurement, labeling can be simplified by using a 3 for both levels. The "6 mo." above the arrow between *E* and *B* represents the 6-month period required between the experimental program and computation of the behavior ratio. (When the arrow does not have a time period with it, the measure is taken immediately after administration of the experimental variable.)

Maria has now measured the variables of interest. But what can she say? Have attitudes changed? Did knowledge increase? Have patients become more regular with their treatments? She cannot say. All she can do is describe the attitudes, knowledge, and behavior after she administered her experimental variable. She does not have evidence to support change. Again, her design is faulty.

Single-Group Pretest-Posttest Design

The addition of a pretest before her program would strengthen her design. Had she pretested, she would know whether attitudes and knowledge changed. Had she measured appointment-keeping behavior for 6 months prior to her pro-

---

Exhibit 3-1. Simple single-group posttest design.

$$E \longrightarrow M$$

Exhibit 3-2. Single-group posttest design.

$$E \left\{ \quad \xrightarrow{} \begin{cases} A(3) \\ K(3) \end{cases} \right.$$
$$\xrightarrow{(6\ mo.)} B(3)$$

gram, she would know whether behavior had changed. Her design is shown in Exhibit 3.3. The arrows outside the box indicate which measures are being compared. Here pretest and posttest measures are compared. A_1 is the attitude pretest, and A_2 is the attitude posttest. Similarly, K_1 and B_1 are pretests while K_2 and B_2 are posttests. The word "comparisons" directly above the box indicates that comparative statistical procedures appropriate to the levels of measurement are to be used. All experimental designs use comparative statistics.

In this design, each subject's pretest score is compared with the same subject's posttest score. Then the sum of all differences (for each subject) is used for statistical analysis. You must link the pretest and posttest scores for each subject if you wish to use this design. Usually tests are coded to give confidentiality to subjects. If you were to average all pretests and all posttests without linking them for each subject, statistical analysis would be far less precise. To repeat, pretest and posttest scores should be linked for *each* subject if you use this design.

Unfortunately, if a change had occurred in our example, Maria would not know for certain whether her program caused it or other factors, rival hypotheses, brought about the change. She may have evidence of a change, but she has no evidence of what caused it. Therefore, the design is **preexperimental.** For example, fatigue or boredom could have produced the change. Perhaps some patients who did not change became bored and left the program before the posttest was given. Or some patients may have been hospitalized during the 6-month follow-up period, thereby improving their appointment-keeping behavior since it was no longer under their control. The many possible rival hypotheses are discussed further in Chapter 4.

Exhibit 3-3. Single-group pretest-posttest design.

Comparisons

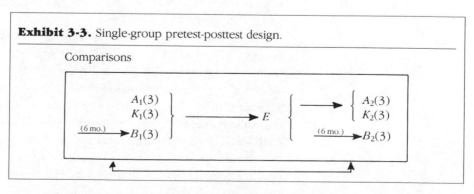

T*rue Experimental Designs*

How do you control for rival hypotheses? You use a control or comparison group and random assignment. A **control group** is another group that is identical in all respects to the experimental group with one exception. The control group is not exposed to the experimental variable. A **comparison group** receives a different version of the experimental variable. If subjects are **randomly assigned** to groups, the rival hypotheses are assumed to fall randomly to all the groups. Control group subjects could become fatigued or bored also. Some subjects might have left before the posttest was given. Control group subjects might be hospitalized during the 6-month follow-up period. Any observed differences, then, between the groups can be attributed to the experimental variable. Of course, records must be kept to ensure that these possible rival hypotheses did occur about equally in both groups.

A **true experiment** in which most rival hypotheses are controlled so that a causal relationship can be inferred has three characteristics. First, a control or comparison group is used. Second, subjects are randomly assigned to each of the groups. This may involve one experimental and one control group, or it may involve several experimental groups, each receiving a slightly different version of the independent variable. Quite often control groups receive something, even if it is routine nursing care, standard medical treatment, or a placebo. It is rarely "nothing." For example, an experiment designed to assess the most effective treatment for breast cancer could not have a control group of patients who received no treatment at all. This would be unethical. Instead, patients might be randomly assigned to radical mastectomy, modified mastectomy, or lumpectomy. There would be three levels of the experimental variable. The point is that each group or level of the independent variable is compared with the others. If differences are found and rival hypotheses are not present, cause is inferred. Differences found in the three treatments for breast cancer lead to the conclusion that the nature of treatment *affects* recovery.

The third characteristic of a true experimental design is that the independent or experimental variable is manipulated by the researcher. The researcher systematically controls and varies the subject's exposure to the independent variable. For example, Maria would *control* who received her special program and who did not by virtue of whom she randomly assigned to the experimental group. The control group, in this case, would receive routine patient education. If she wished to assess the effects of gender as well, she would be able to use gender only as a **blocking variable** since she could not randomly assign human beings to be either male or female. She could not *manipulate* gender. To block, she would first divide subjects into groups according to the blocking variable of sex, then randomly assign subjects of one sex to levels of the experimental variable, and next randomly assign those of the other sex. In this way each level (or group) of the **manipulated** experimental variable would have an equal proportion of males and females. If gender differences were found, Maria could conclude only that there is a difference between the sexes. She could not conclude that gender *caused* the observed difference because that independent variable was not manipulated. Chapter 4 discusses blocking variables in greater detail.

The use of randomly assigned experimental and control groups is illustrated in the following three true experimental designs. For simplicity, one experimental group and one control group are used. In reality, however, more groups could be employed in each design.

Pretest-Posttest Control Group Design

The **pretest-posttest control group design** is diagramed in Exhibit 3.4. Although the diagram of the pretest-posttest control group design may look complicated at first, conducting the design actually involves little effort beyond the single-group pretest-posttest design and provides much stronger evidence to support or reject a research hypothesis. The only addition is an extra box to symbolize a second group of subjects, the control group (C). The broken line separating the two groups indicates random assignment of all subjects to one of the two groups.

Random assignment means that each subject could have been assigned to either the experimental or the control group. Final assignment to a group depends on chance alone. This could be accomplished in a number of ways. To illustrate, suppose 60 patients accepted the invitation to the program. Before the time of the meeting, Maria could go down the list of names, tossing a coin as she came to each one. If the coin came up heads, the patient would be put in the experimental group; if the coin came up tails, the patient would be put in the control group. Given an unbiased coin, any patient has an equal opportunity (a 50-50 chance) of assignment to either group. Maria would not use this simple technique, however, since she wants the same number of subjects in each group and she realizes that in 60 tosses she might not get 30 heads and 30 tails.

Instead, she chooses to use a technique that is equally simple but a little more difficult to describe. She uses a table of random numbers similar to Table A in

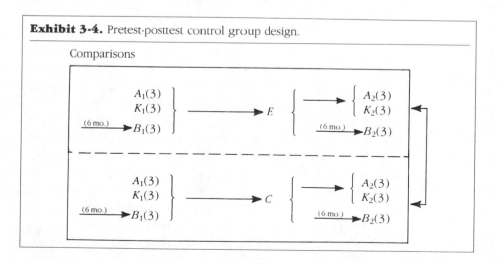

Exhibit 3-4. Pretest-posttest control group design.

Appendix III. She assigns each patient a two-digit number from 01 to 60. She then decides to use the last two digits in the number groupings in the table to identify subjects and to read down the columns. With the table of random numbers in front of her, she closes her eyes and places her finger anywhere on the table. Next she reads the number under her finger. The patient with this number is put in the experimental group. Maria, going down the column, now reads the next number, and the patient with that number is assigned to the control group. The next is assigned to the experimental group, and so forth. Maria could have read across the rows or down the columns or wherever she wished as long as she decided on the order in which she would read beforehand and adhered to her plan. If she came to a number larger than 60 or one she had encountered before, she would skip it and go on to the next. If you would like to try this process, turn to Table A in Appendix III and randomly assign 60 patients to experimental and control groups. Remember to decide how you will read numbers from the table before you begin.

Do not confuse **random assignment** with **random sampling.** They are two separate processes. *Random assignment* refers to what you do with your subjects once you have them. *Random sampling* refers to the method you use to select your subjects from the population of all possible subjects. Random sampling is discussed in Chapter 10.

In Maria's design there is a dilemma about what to do with the control group. She could use a less promising program or nothing at all. Maria chose the first option. The control group could not be expected to make a special trip to the hospital for nothing. She therefore used a **placebo.** Control group subjects were given a tour of the hospital and a demonstration of how the dialysis equipment worked. Then they received refreshments and were greeted by hospital administrators. While this placebo itself may have produced some changes, any changes above and beyond this would be due to Maria's more focused program.

If she had wanted to use the second option, nothing at all, Maria would have had to change her procedure for collecting data. Perhaps all pretesting and posttesting could have been done as both experimental and control patients came to the unit for their regular appointments. This might introduce other rival hypotheses, however. For example, patients unwilling to make an extra trip to the hospital for the program might be included in the control group. Then the control group would differ from the experimental group in more ways than just the experimental variable. If she could argue the absence of any rival hypotheses, preferably with some evidence, the second option might well be used to test her causal hypotheses.

The behavioral observation measure presents another possible problem. Since it will be based on the 6 months after treatment, Maria must make sure that experimental subjects are not inadvertently treated in a special way that enhances their performance. Researchers often allow for this by having the experimental variable administered by someone who does not work in the clinical setting and/or by concealing the identity of experimental and control subjects from the staff. When subjects do not know whether they are in the experimental or control group, as when a placebo is used, this is known as a **blind** experiment. When experimenters or staff do not know who is in which group and subjects do not know either, the experiment is described as a **double-blind.**

In Maria's study, both the experimental and control groups were pretested and posttested with the same measures. Instead of exposing all 60 patients to an unproved experimental program, Maria saved time and money through a sound application of research principles. By comparing the posttest scores, she would be able to determine the effects of her experimental variable. If her program produced significant differences, the control-group subjects could be exposed to the program at a later date. By comparing pretest scores, Maria knew for certain that her random assignment resulted in groups that were about equal on the dependent variable. The pretest also allowed her to observe changes in both groups. If the experimental group changed considerably more than the control group, this difference could be attributed to the experimental variable unless some other rival hypothesis were present.

Posttest-Only Control Group Design

Maria probably did not need to pretest the patients in her study. Since she was able to randomly assign them to the experimental and control groups, she could have assumed with 95 percent confidence that both groups were equal in their knowledge, attitudes, and behavior before the project began. Random assignment allows you to *assume* pretreatment equality between experimental and control groups. Not only will both groups have the same information about kidney disease, but also their average I.Q. and attitudes about it probably will be quite similar, too. Of course, the probability is usually that the groups will not be equal in 5 percent of the cases, even though we have randomly assigned subjects to them. Researchers generally accept this small probability of error.

The **posttest-only control group design,** shown in Exhibit 3.5, is simpler

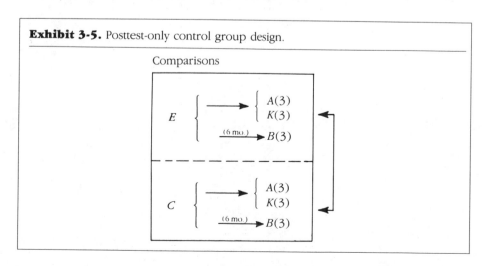

Exhibit 3-5. Posttest-only control group design.

Exhibit 3-6. Indications for using a pretest.

You are unsure about the randomness of assignment.

Your measure is not conspicuous or reactive.

You are interested mainly in whether your program works, rather than attempting to generalize your results to the larger population.

You are interested in change rather than just differences due to the independent variable.

There are fewer than 60 subjects.

Alternate forms of the test are available.

---

to carry out than the pretest-posttest control group design and is considered superior because you do not have to be concerned that the pretest also may have caused an effect. You do not have to be concerned about limiting the generalizability of your results to a pretested population. Pretested control group subjects may be different from the population from which they came simply because they had the pretest. While the behavior measure could not change them, it is possible that just taking the attitude and knowledge pretests could change them so that their posttest scores would no longer reflect the unpretested population. For example, not knowing some answers might have caused them to seek the answers. Then their posttest scores would show more knowledge than if no pretest had been given.

With the posttest-only control group design, however, in spite of random assignment, the probability is that the control group will differ initially from the experimental group in some experiments. Had the control group had less knowledge and poorer attitudes and behavior, a weak experimental variable would have appeared to produce change. However, had the control group known more or had better attitudes and behavior, even the best experimental program might have failed to yield significant differences. For these reasons some researchers use a pretest. Exhibit 3.6 contains considerations which may help you in deciding between these two experimental designs. These problems are solved by the next, more complex design. It, however, presents another difficulty.

Solomon Four-Group Design

The problems involved in using a pretest are addressed in the **Solomon four-group design.** In this design, shown in Exhibit 3.7, subjects are randomly assigned to one of four groups. Two groups receive the same experimental variable, but only one has a pretest. Similarly, two other groups serve as controls, with only one receiving a pretest. Although the design has more prestige and controls the effects due to pretesting, statistical analysis of results is slightly more complicated, since no single statistical procedure can simultaneously use all six sets of measures.

Selecting one of these three experimental designs involves tradeoffs. The

Exhibit 3-7. Solomon four-group design.

Comparisons

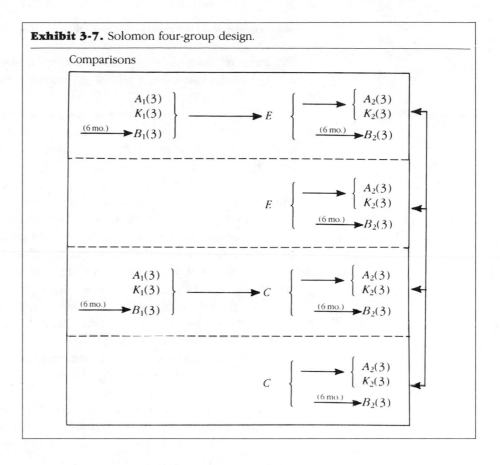

circumstances surrounding your specific research study undoubtedly will help in making your decision. The use of control groups, random assignment, and experimenter manipulation of the independent variable is central to testing causal hypotheses via experimental designs. If you understand these as they relate to controlling or avoiding rival hypotheses, your creativity in designing the best study for your circumstances will be enhanced.

Quasi-Experimental Designs

Quite often, nurses in the real world find themselves party to inflexible conditions. They may not have the opportunity to randomly assign subjects to experimental and control groups, or they may be told that all available subjects must receive the experimental treatment. If you find yourself in such a situation, there are several quasi-experimental designs you might consider. Although they do not offer as much control over rival hypotheses as the three experimental designs just discussed, they are considerably better than the two preexperimental designs. As long as you anticipate the possible rival hypotheses, document their presence or absence, and then consider those present while you interpret your results, they are very respectable designs. Many of the most important behavioral research studies, especially those in field settings, have used quasi-experimental designs. They still have been able to draw causal conclusions when documentation was available to disqualify rival hypotheses.

Split-Group Pretest-Posttest Design

The **split-group pretest-posttest design** is shown in Exhibit 3.8. It can be used when there is no option of dividing the sample into experimental and control groups. Restraints such as "everyone must be exposed to the program" or "the program can be conducted only once" may require using this design. For example, suppose Maria could not present a placebo program for the control group. Furthermore, scheduling difficulties and staff shortages precluded her pretesting and posttesting in the clinical setting. Perhaps the time for some subjects between testing and the experimental programs was too great. Therefore, she could use this design. As patients came into the room, every other person could be pretested (assuming their order of arrival was random). Then she could conduct her program. Those who were not given the pretest would be given the posttest. Differences found between the pretest and posttest scores could show that her experimental variable had an effect.

This design does have some weaknesses. For example, extraneous events occurring while her program was being conducted, such as news of the death of a recalcitrant dialysis patient, might change attitudes. (However, if this news came to only one of the groups during the implementation of one of the three experimental designs, it, too, could be a rival hypothesis.) Fatigue might contribute to changes in attitudes or knowledge. Disinterested patients might leave early, thereby biasing the results toward positive effects. Although this design is not quite as strong as the experimental designs, it is better than the preexperimental designs. It is highly recommended for exploratory or pilot research.

Exhibit 3-8. Split-group pretest-posttest design.

Comparisons

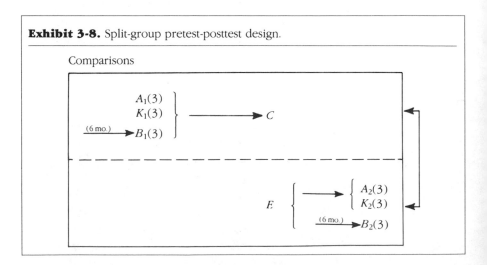

The **nonequivalent control group design,** shown in Exhibit 3.9, differs from the pretest-posttest control group design in that subjects are not randomly assigned to the experimental and control groups. The solid line between the groups indicates that the researcher is dealing with **intact groups.** In other words, rather than patients being randomly assigned to experimental and control groups, one group of patients might have been selected for the experimental program, and the results compared with those of other patients available in the clinical setting. The appropriateness of this design is directly related to how strong a case can be made that the experimental and control groups were equivalent before the program began. For example, those willing to make the extra trip to the program may differ from other members of the clinic population. The time of day during which the attitude and knowledge tests were administered might affect the results on those two measures. A daytime group might include more homemakers and/or severely disabled while an evening group would include more wage earners.

The strongest nonequivalent control group design would consist of intact groups impartially formed from the same or similar populations with the researcher having the option to flip a coin to determine which group received the experimental program. Similarity on the criterion or dependent measure as demonstrated by the pretest as well as similarity on crucial demographic characteristics would strongly document an argument of equivalence.

The greater the deviation from the spirit of this model, the less confidence you can place in the results, especially in making causal statements. Quite often, when the case for equivalence is weak, the best approach is to consider the research study as descriptive-comparative. Statistically significant results would be interpreted as indicating a difference between groups, but a causal statement would not be made. When this design does not involve a pretest, it becomes a

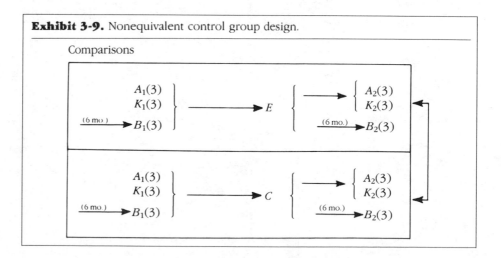

Exhibit 3-9. Nonequivalent control group design.

Comparisons

$A_1(3)$
$K_1(3)$
(6 mo.) $\rightarrow B_1(3)$ $\longrightarrow E$ $\rightarrow$ $A_2(3)$
$K_2(3)$
(6 mo.) $\rightarrow B_2(3)$

$A_1(3)$
$K_1(3)$
(6 mo.) $\rightarrow B_1(3)$ $\longrightarrow C$ $\rightarrow$ $A_2(3)$
$K_2(3)$
(6 mo.) $\rightarrow B_2(3)$

much weaker preexperimental design, called the **static group comparison design.** This design is not featured in the presentation of designs for this chapter, because it is especially weak as a test of causal hypotheses in nursing and health behavior.

Split Intact Groups Pretest-Posttest Design

The split intact groups pretest-posttest design, shown in Exhibit 3.10, is a combination of the preceding two quasi-experimental designs. It is used relatively rarely. However, when a researcher is using a very reactive pretest, one which might cause change, this design is appropriate. Two intact groups are used. The researcher flips a coin to decide which is the experimental and which is the control. Then, by using random assignment, half of each group is pretested and the rest are posttested. To establish equivalency of the two intact groups, the pretest results are compared. If they are equivalent, the posttest scores are compared to determine experimental effects. Can you think of any rival hypotheses in this design?

Additional quasi-experimental designs are discussed by Campbell and Stanley [1] and Cook and Campbell [2]. However, unless the circumstances or constraints of your research situation are very unique, the designs already discussed and the time-series designs in Chapter 4 should offer enough flexibility. To

Exhibit 3-10. Split intact groups pretest-posttest design.

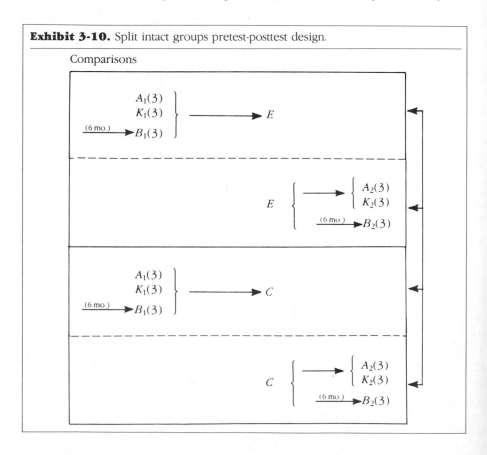

repeat, reality often prevents use of the three experimental designs. This should not stop your research. Some of the best and most prestigious field research studies utilizing human subjects in many topic areas have used quasi-experimental designs.

Individual Administration of the Independent Variable

Suppose Maria could not administer her experimental variable to all her patients at the same time. Instead, she had to administer it on a one-to-one basis as they came for dialysis. The severity of their conditions might have prevented their making an additional trip to the hospital. Perhaps not enough patients would be available at a single time. Or she may not have wanted her control group to have a placebo. Since control group subjects would have been tested individually in the clinical setting on a dialysis day, she may have believed a rival hypothesis, the setting, might account for differences between the groups if the experimental group were tested on a day when they came to the hospital for the special program instead of for dialysis.

This often happens in health research. As a result, the experimental and quasi-experimental designs do not seem to fit the reality of the research situation, since they *appear* to be designed for administering the independent variable to a group of subjects at the same time. While some modifications of these designs to allow individual administration of independent variables to experimental group subjects have turned up in the literature, unfortunately teaching of the principles of experimental design has remained focused on group administration, perhaps because the principles are easier to communicate. In actual practice, individual administration rather than group administration may be an even stronger design (see Campbell and Stanley [1]) since the effects of group process are removed as rival hypotheses. The modifications to allow for individual administration of the independent variable are relatively simple.

Describing the Independent Variable

The first thing that must be done is to describe in detail the independent variable. (This is just as important when it is administered to groups, because other researchers must be able to replicate the experiment.) It is important also to present evidence that the independent variable does not change over time. It must remain the same for all subjects.

Maria's 1-hour slide presentation seems to fit this requirement. If she fears that the commentary accompanying the slides might vary beyond safe limits, she could tape-record it and, in effect, develop a self-administered slide-tape program for patients. But what about the second hour in which patients ask questions? Will the results not be affected by the nature of a patient's questions? Yes, they could be. However, if all patients were given 30 or 60 minutes (the time should be the same for all patients) to ask questions of Maria, she must assume that this question time dealt with the unique problems of each patient. This part of the independent variable would be described as 30 or 60 minutes, on a one-to-one basis, of discussion based on concerns and questions of the patient. By using a large sample of patients, she will assume that they average to her definition.

With independent variables which include such components as Maria's 30 minutes of individual questions where some uncertainty about sameness exists, you would do well to keep detailed tape recordings or notes (e.g., the questions asked by the patient) about each administration. Thus you can either document the sameness of the procedure or, when extreme variations occur, remove them from the study or cite them to explain ambiguous results.

Administering the independent variable individually to 30 patients is a lot more work than just presenting it to a large, single group. Therefore, Maria might decide to have another nurse on the unit help her. This introduces another possible rival hypothesis. The two nurses might differ in how they present the independent variable. In an extreme case, one could cause a positive change and the other could cause a negative change. The overall results, however, would show that there was no change! Therefore, evidence must be offered to establish the sameness of the delivery of the independent variable by each nurse.

Of course, the interplay between patients in a group is lost unless Maria uses many small groups of two or three. She can do this or anything else she wants, as long as all patients assigned to the experimental condition receive the same experimental program.

To summarize, the independent variable must be described in enough detail that other researchers could duplicate (i.e., replicate) it. When the independent variable is administered many times, evidence of the sameness of administration must be presented. If several experimenters administer the independent variable, the sameness of their delivery must be documented. The discussion of reliability in Chapters 11 and 14 will help you explore this further.

Random Assignment

Maria's population of patients is relatively stable. She knows that about 60 patients come in regularly. New patients are added slowly. Her behavior measure requires that patients have been in treatment for at least 6 months. Thus she lists all patients eligible for her study. This is called **prelisting.** Since she hopes to include 50 patients in her study, she decides to include all available patients, the entire study population, rather than selecting a smaller number from her prelisting. She reasons that some patients may not wish to participate and others may be lost during the 6-month follow-up.

At the time she obtains consent to participate, she pretests all her subjects. Then she randomly assigns them to an experimental or a control group. All experimental subjects are exposed to the independent variable 2 weeks after pretesting. They are posttested at its conclusion. All control subjects are posttested 2 weeks after pretesting. Within 1 month she has tested 50 patients twice and administered 25 independent variables. This busy schedule probably required additional experimenters, each testing both experimental and control subjects. Her experiment is finished; now she is free to organize her data, analyze the attitude and knowledge tests, and wait 6 months to complete her behavior measure.

But what if she did not have anyone to help her? She might have followed the same procedure except for one step. After prelisting, she would randomly divide the population into three or four groups of 14 patients each and then randomly decide an ordering of the four groups. Next, with the first group of 14 patients, she would secure permission, pretest, and randomly assign to experimental and control groups as before. After administering the independent variable to 7 subjects and posttesting all 14 subjects, she would proceed to the second group of 14 patients. In this way, her workload would be eased.

The important consideration is to have *both* experimental and control subjects included in the study at the same time. Another important factor is that the period between pretesting and posttesting remain the same for all subjects. Similarly, the period between pretesting and administration of the independent variable should be the same, as should the time between the independent variable and posttest. If impossible, a **time frame,** a span of time, should be used. For example, the experimental variable might be administered 2 to 3 weeks after pretesting. Whenever a time frame is used, it must be described and your rationale for doing so presented when the results are reported. A large variation in time, of course, might seriously weaken your study, especially if there were a different time frame for experimental and control group subjects.

If Maria were using only her behavioral measure, appointment keeping, she would need less patient contact, of course. She would secure cooperation, obtain any demographic data she needed, and randomly assign the patients to experimental or control groups. Then the remainder of her patient contacts would be limited to administering the experimental variable to half the patients.

If she is using only her behavioral measure, why should she secure consent to participate from the control group? She does not absolutely have to. However, several factors may favor her doing so. First, the hospital ethics committee for research involving human subjects may believe that it is necessary to comply with recent federal legislation. Let them be the judge. That is why they exist. In cases such as our example, probably they would not consider it necessary. However, each situation is unique. The second reason for securing patient consent (since only their records of appointments are used) involves the researcher's need to gather demographic and other information not included on the medical chart. Third, the control group could become different from the experimental group if a significant number of patients refused to participate in the experimental group. Those who would have refused would not be excluded from the control group if permission were not sought.

Another restriction might be present. Maria could not administer the independent variable to experimental subjects in the unit while control subjects were also present and thus aware of or even observing administration of the experimental variable. In this case, she would have to change the random assignment of subjects to the random assignment of days. Each day would be randomly assigned to either experimental or control. On any given day, then, she would include all patients who came in as either experimental or control subjects. This is not as strong as complete random assignment, but it is still better than nonrandom methods.

One last problem in random assignment might lie in the reality of a research setting other than Maria's. Perhaps you cannot prelist all subjects before your study begins, because you do not know who will become patients during the time frame of your study. For example, your independent variable may be primary nursing in an emergency room (ER) setting. You can set up a time frame for your study based on census figures describing ER use. During the month of your study, you may have to assume that patients arrive in random order and simply assign every other patient who enters to the experimental group. If this assumption is not tenable, you can randomly assign 20 numbers, representing, in order, the first 20 patients, to an experimental or a control group. As patient 1 arrives, she or he is given whatever assignment the number 1 was given. Patient 2 receives the assignment given to the number 2, and so forth.

Combinations of the preceding random assignment methods may be used. Modify them to fit your situation. Whatever your method, keep in mind its purpose—to be objective and allow an equal probability to all subjects for inclusion in the experimental group.

S*ignificant Differences*

There are usually some differences between experimental and control groups. Statistical analysis allows you to determine how likely it is that a given difference occurs by chance or random error versus being due to the experimental variable. You use a statistical test appropriate to your level of measurement and research design. Sometimes the size of your sample is a factor, since some statistical tests are not very effective with a small number of subjects. Exhibit 3.11 lists inferential statistical tests for each design and level of measurement. These are meant as guides rather than rules. The circumstances of your study may make them inappropriate. Once you have found a statistical test that seems to apply to your situation, you should look it up, study its assumptions and limitations on use, and only then make your final decision to use it.

After you run your statistical test, you may be faced with another decision. Is the statistically significant difference large enough to be of **practical significance?** Sometimes, particularly with large sample sizes, a small difference may turn out to be "significantly different" statistically. For example, say that the difference between the experimental and control groups is 4 points on a 40-point scale. That is a 10 percent difference. Even though this difference may prove to be statistically significant, you must ask whether it is really worth the time, effort, and expense of implementing your experimental program in the clinical setting. Does a 10 percent change mean significant improvement for a patient? Only you can decide. There are no tables or mathematical procedures to help you determine practical significance.

Single-Subject Experimental Designs

Often in nursing research, a nursing intervention may be appropriate for only one patient. Obviously, scientifically testing the effects of such an intervention with a single patient is impossible if you are using the experimental and control group approach of the classical experimental designs just described. Although rarely used thus far in nursing research, **single-subject experimental designs,** as used in behavior modification and some educational research, may be useful in such situations. This approach involves only one or very few subjects who are measured or observed many times, both before and after the intervention is employed. The measures before the intervention are called the **baseline.** Although in group research 30 subjects may be measured once (i.e., the post-test), in single-case research one subject may be measured 30 times. To a limited extent, the number of times a single subject is measured is similar to the number of subjects included in a group research design.

Basic ABA Design

The basic design in single-case experimentation is known as the **ABA design,** where A indicates the **time periods** in which the intervention is absent (baseline and **withdrawal**) and B indicates the time period during which an intervention is employed. Each time period (A and B) includes many observations or repeated measurements, usually 10 or more. This is a form of time-series research in which one subject is used and acts as his or her own control (Chap. 4 presents time-series designs for groups of subjects). The key ingredient, of course, is being able to delay the intervention long enough to get baseline measures and then later being able to withdraw the intervention to demonstrate a return to baseline conditions. Withdrawal must occur early enough to render the return to baseline possible. This return to baseline compares to control group observations in group research and is the basis for making causal inferences after replication with two to five other, similar patients.

Suppose Susan, a liaison nurse, wished to test the effects of giving physical care (versus conversations only) with a cancer patient undergoing chemotherapy. Staff nurses complained that the patient was demanding and uncooperative. Multiple dependent variables include (1) the acting-out behaviors of excessive use of the call light, shouting, and refusal to eat, as recorded on a behavioral observation checklist; (2) patient anxiety, as measured by a short self-report measure; and (3) a sweat index physical assessment taken every 4 hours from 8 a.m. through 12 midnight for 2 days. These established the baseline. During the third and fourth days, Susan offered and then gave physical care during her morning and afternoon visits. On the fifth and sixth days, she called a staff nurse to give any physical care requested by the patient, as she did during baseline. The results are displayed in Exhibit 3.12.

Exhibit 3-11. Experimental designs and suggested analysis procedures.

Design	Ratio/interval data	Ordinal data	Nominal data
Single-group posttest design	Generally, no analysis is possible (except for "eyeballing" sample in comparison to other group norms). If comparison to the population is valid, a t or z test is used.	Generally, no analysis is possible. If comparison to the population is valid, the Kolmogorov-Smirnov One-Sample Test or the One-Sample Runs Test is used.	Generally, no analysis is possible. If comparison to the population is valid, the Chi-Square One-Sample Test or Binominal Test is used.
Single-group pretest-posttest design	t test for Dependent Groups.	Wilcoxon Matched-Pairs Signed-Ranks test or the Sign Test.	McNemar Test for the Significance of Change.
Pretest-posttest control-group design	Repeated-measures analysis of variance (ANOVA) or analysis of covariance (ANCOVA) with the pretest as a covariate.	Analysis is unclear because there is no procedure which will use all measures. In the analysis, pretest scores could be used to ensure sameness, and results could be based on posttest scores by using procedures for the posttest-only control group design.	Analysis is unclear because there is no procedure which will use all measures. In the analysis, pretest scores could be used to ensure sameness and results based on posttest scores with procedures for the posttest-only control group design.
Posttest-only control-group design	Analysis of variance (ANOVA) or t test for Independent Groups.	Kolmogorov-Smirnov Two-Sample Test, Mann-Whitney U Test, Median Test, Wald-Wolfowitz Runs Test, or the Moses Test of Extreme Reactions.	Chi-square for Two Independent Samples.
Solomon four-group design	Analysis is unclear. No procedure makes use of all six measures. Often the pretests are used to ensure "sameness" of groups. Then results are based on the t test or analysis of variance (ANOVA) with posttest scores. Factorial ANOVA with pretesting and experimental variable as factors on posttest scores is also used.	Same as pretest-posttest control-group design.	Same as pretest-posttest control-group design.
Split-group pretest-posttest design	Same as posttest-only control-group design.	Same as posttest-only control-group design.	Same as posttest-only control-group design.

Design	Ratio/interval data	Ordinal data	Nominal data
Nonequivalent control-group design	Same as pretest-posttest control-group design if linear regression between groups can be assumed to be homogeneous before administration of the independent variable; otherwise, same as posttest-only control-group design.	Same as pretest-posttest control-group design.	Same as pretest-posttest control-group design.
Split intact group pretest-posttest design	Same as Solomon four-group design.	Sameness of pretests and then comparison of posttests permit analysis described for posttest-only control-group design.	Sameness of pretests and then comparison of posttests permit analysis described for posttest-only control-group design.

From Exhibit 3.12, it appears that giving physical care made a difference. Note how one of the measures, in this case the self-report anxiety scale, was last in demonstrating change. This often happens in research and is discussed further in Chapter 11 when measurement methods are presented. The failure to completely return to baseline conditions during withdrawal may be due to the **carryover effects** (i.e., duplicating) of the intervention. **Replication** of this

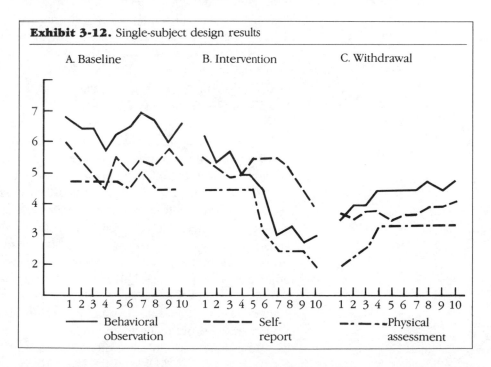

Exhibit 3-12. Single-subject design results

design with other patients would lend further support to this interpretation. Finding these same results while using one of the other single-subject experimental designs also would lend support.

Single-case designs, in addition to not requiring many subjects, have several advantages. They allow exploration of individual differences that might be masked through use of group averages. For example, under stress one subject's 17-hydroxycorticosteroids may decrease while another's may increase. The designs also allow greater flexibility to extend baseline time periods or modify interventions as the researcher monitors the *ongoing* results of the experiment. Researchers usually examine several measures of the **target behaviors** which the intervention is designed to modify as well as **carryover effects** on related variables. Although research utilizing groups could and should use multiple measures also, sometimes multiple measures are more manageable when fewer subjects are involved.

In establishing a baseline, enough time must be allocated to establish a **stable line.** If the line is moving gradually upward or downward in the desired direction, there will be no way of knowing whether the intervention or spontaneous remission is the causal agent. Ideally, the time periods for baseline, intervention, and withdrawal are equal. Sometimes, to get a stable baseline, this rule is ignored, especially if a similar extension of the intervention time period would magnify the effects so that return to baseline during withdrawal would be impossible. The withdrawal time period in some research is called **reversal** when the opposite of the intervention is employed. Since physical care was still available, albeit from another person, the term would not apply to Susan's study.

Finally, the very flexibility of these designs to alter the baseline or intervention time periods makes them more vulnerable to attack by more classically oriented (i.e., group) researchers. Therefore, it is not only important to replicate results with other single-subject trials but also advisable to consider, once the time periods and interventions are standardized, using a group design to further demonstrate cause and effect.

Other Designs

Other single-case designs, all variations of the *ABA* design, have been used. The **ABAB design** allows return to the intervention to again demonstrate its effects and also end with the intervention still in use. Other designs test the effects of more than one intervention, such as **ABABCBA designs.** In these, care must be taken to introduce only one new independent variable or intervention at a time and then to withdraw it to establish return to baseline, or prior, conditions. A danger in designs such as the *ABABCBA* is **multiple-treatment interference.** For example, the effects of *C* might be due to the fact that *B* preceded it rather than due to *C* itself. In this case, replications in which the order of introducing *B* and *C* is changed would counter this rival hypothesis.

An interesting single-subject quasi-experimental design (*BAB*) was used in a psychotherapy experiment about empathy by Truax and Carkhuff [4], because they were unable to ethically withhold treatment long enough to establish a baseline. They explored the effect of warmth and empathic understanding on three patients' intrapersonal exploration, measured on a 10-point scale where zero indicated no personally relevant material occurring (such as a discussion of appointment hours). During the 20-minute *A* phase (i.e., baseline) after 20 minutes of relatively high conditions, the therapist withheld the best empathic and unconditional positive warmth responses. That is, he held back and did not reflect to the patient his better guesses of what the patient was experiencing or feeling. To address ethical concerns regarding negative impact on the patients of withholding these responses, at the beginning and end of the baseline *A* phase, the therapist answered a knock at the door to converse briefly with another therapist in order to establish a cover story of extreme concern about another patient. Each of these 1-hour first psychotherapy sessions was tape-recorded, and separate raters analyzed the sessions, using the Depth of Intrapersonal Exploration Scale, Accurate Empathy Scale, Unconditional Positive Regard Scale, and Therapist Self-Congruence Scale. The independent variable was assessed as well as the dependent variable to validate withdrawal of empathic and unconditional positive warmth responses. Results were in the expected direction for two patients. The third patient was so distraught that the therapist chose not to withhold his responses. Although this study had some methodological problems, such as no baseline, it does suggest that single-case experimental designs assessing variables such as empathy are possible.

Ethical considerations in nursing research may prevent withdrawal or reversal of the intervention or treatment. In this case, there is one design that might be considered: the **multiple baseline across subjects design.** In this design four (or more) patients are included over five (or more) time periods. The first time period is a baseline of about 10 observations for all subjects, and the next four time periods each introduce one of the four patients to the intervention. Subjects are randomly assigned to time periods 2 to 5 for exposure to the intervention and remain as baseline, acting as controls, until it is their turn. Once given the intervention, a patient continues it until the end of the experiment. The disadvantage of this design, of course, is that the intervention must be withheld through four time periods for the patient randomly assigned to the last phase. This multiple-baseline approach also can be used across settings (e.g., work versus clinic versus home) or behaviors (e.g., various self-care activities) for a single patient where the settings or behaviors are randomly assigned to each time period.

Statistical Analysis

There are two schools of thought regarding statistical analysis of single-subject experimental design data. To date, most research using this approach has been conducted in clinical settings with specific target behaviors, such as overuse of call lights, not eating, shouting, or withdrawal, which needed modification. Clinicians, therefore, argue that change in target behavior is the only criterion of success. And this gross change in behavior, of course, would be more than highly significant *statistically*. On the other hand, many researchers believe interventions that produce less dramatic yet statistically significant effects still might be useful, especially if they could be combined with several other less dramatic interventions so as to produce even greater change. Subtle changes in related behaviors, such as personality change after large weight loss, might be of interest also. Thus some believe statistical tests to determine change are beneficial.

Statistical analysis is fairly straightforward if **autocorrelations,** strong relationships between the repeated measures, do not occur. Then the repeated measures can be treated like "subjects," and averages for baseline, intervention, and withdrawal can be compared by utilizing the same statistical techniques as in comparing three groups. Problems arise when autocorrelations occur, and most of the time they do. Statistical analysis then is complex, necessitating a computerized time-series approach beyond the scope of this text. For the time being, the clinicians' approach, which does not utilize statistical analysis, is suggested for beginning researchers. A fuller discussion of single-subject experimental designs is available in Herson and Barlow [3].

In summary, single-subject experimental design offers an alternative if you have few subjects. Because many repeated measures are taken over time, the researcher often is dependent on the staff to help make observations. Sabotage from clinic personnel is not uncommon, and often it has greater impact in single-case than group research. Be certain you secure complete cooperation before you begin.

▼ocabulary

ABAB design	Manipulated variable
ABABCBA design	Multiple baseline across subjects design
ABA design	Multiple-treatment interference
Autocorrelation	Nonequivalent control group design
BAB design	Placebo
Baseline	Posttest
Blind	Posttest-only control group design
Blocking variable	Practical significance
Carryover effects	Preexperimental designs
Causal statement	Prelisting
Comparison group	Pretest
Control group	Pretest-posttest control group design
Dependent variable	Quasi-experimental designs
Double blind	Random assignment
Experimental group	Random sampling
Experimental variable (treatment)	Reliability of independent variable
Experimenter reliability	Replication
Independent variable	Reversal
Intact groups	Rival hypotheses

Single-group pretest-posttest design
Single-subject experimental design
Solomon four-group design
Split group pretest-posttest design
Stable line
Static group comparison design

Statistical significance
Target behaviors
Time frame
Time period
True experimental designs
Withdrawal

References

1. Campbell, D. T., and Stanley, J. C. *Experimental and Quasi-Experimental Designs for Research.* Chicago: Rand McNally, 1963.
2. Cook, T. D., and Campbell, D. T. *Quasi-Experimentation: Design and Analysis Issues for Field Settings.* Chicago: Rand McNally, 1979.
3. Herson, M., and Barlow, D. H. *Single Case Experimental Designs.* New York: Pergamon, 1976.
4. Truax, C. B., and Carkhuff, R. R. Experimental manipulation of therapeutic conditions. *J. Consult. Psychol.* 29:119, 1965.

In chapter 3, rival hypotheses often were suggested as possible explanations, instead of the experimental variable, for changes observed in dependent variables. A substantial number of patients leaving the evening program before Maria administered her posttest might have changed the experimental group results. Having 25 females, who are often considered more compliant, assigned to the experimental group while only 5 were included in the control group might account for differences instead of Maria's intervention. The possibilities are numerous. This should not discourage you, however. Instead, you must anticipate the rival hypotheses in your study and then document the presence or absence of these threats.

An experiment is not invalidated by the mere *possibility* of rival hypotheses. Only *plausible rival hypotheses* are invalidating. Random assignment and the use of a control group in the experimental designs are potent antidotes to many threats. Even then, care must be taken to document and control possible rival hypotheses. With the quasi-experimental designs, rival hypotheses are much more common. Rather than giving up and refusing to use your data because of lack of control, you should generate plausible rival hypotheses by informed critique of your design in your setting; then do supplementary research to test these hypotheses. How many persons left before the evening program was completed? Were their pretest scores different from those of the people who remained? How many males and females were assigned to each group? If unequal, can you redo your random assignment by **blocking** on the sex variable? That is, can all females and then males be randomly assigned in equal numbers to each group?

Anticipating a rival hypothesis often can lead to your controlling it or, at the very least, measuring its presence or absence. Sometimes, then, statistical analysis can be used to hold constant the effects of that variable. Less can be done when you discover a rival hypothesis after the study is completed. Finally, after all threats that can be controlled are circumvented, others might remain that simply must be lived with. Your interpretation of results should account for them. There has never been a study designed that was perfect in all respects. Some have been much stronger than others, however.

Threats to Internal Validity

Researchers (e.g., Campbell and Stanley [2]; Cook and Campbell [1]) have defined a number of rival hypothesis categories which provide for a more orderly critique of an experimental design. One group is referred to as **threats to internal validity** because they interfere with the internal aspects of the experiment—the causal link between the independent and dependent variables. Another group is called **threats to construct validity,** because they refer to how well the words and constructs of your hypothesis are converted or operationalized into quantitative research parts. These are both presented in this chapter. A third set of threats, threats to external validity, refers to aspects outside the experiment, the generalization of your research results to the target population, other settings, and other times. These are explained in Chapter 10, which deals with how you sample the population. The fourth set, threats to statistical conclusion validity, which deals with errors related to statistical analysis of data, are presented in Chapter 15, which introduces inferential statistics. Thus, an experiment needs construct validity to ensure it was operationalized correctly, internal validity to ensure that the causal link is between the independent and dependent variable, statistical conclusion validity to ensure that the data were analyzed correctly, and external validity to ensure that you can appropriately generalize your findings from your sample to the larger population of people, places, and times. The first group of these, threats to internal validity, follows. These concern rival hypotheses which may also account for observed differences between the control group and experimental group(s). Thus, this group is primarily applicable to experimental research while the other three groups of threats are applicable to all kinds of research.

History

History refers to events other than the independent variable that occur during the conduct of an experiment. Do not confuse this term with the more common use of the word "history." It is used here to mean events *during* the experiment, not events before it or "back in history." If a group of subjects are given learning materials on venereal disease by a school nurse and a posttest demonstrates increased knowledge, it is possible the materials produced the learning. However, history is a threat if a television show on venereal disease was aired during the time the subjects had the materials.

The single-group pretest-posttest design is most vulnerable to history. The only thing a researcher can do is try to shorten as much as possible the time period during which the independent variable is administered. Generally, these history events are beyond the researcher's control. When you become aware of them, you must judge whether the event has a high probability of influencing results and report this and the rationale for your judgment.

A special kind of history threat, known as **intrasession history,** refers to group dynamics within a single group that might cause an effect rather than the experimental variable. For example, if the outcome measure is empathy and the experimental variable includes experimental training in this skill, a group (even a **placebo** group) in which there is a "click," or sudden and lasting cohesiveness, might show an effect on the dependent variable because of this click. When intrasession history is a serious threat, group administration of the independent variable is avoided in favor of one-to-one administration.

Maturation

Maturation refers to biologic and psychological processes that naturally occur within subjects to produce changes, such as hunger and fatigue. You might expect better performance from a group assessed in the late morning than one assessed in the late afternoon. Therefore, if their performances were compared and a difference occurred, maturation (in this case, fatigue) would be a plausible rival explanation and thus a threat to internal validity. The effects of spontaneous remission or other natural changes in health status are also possible maturation threats.

Longitudinal studies with a single group that is pretested and posttested are particularly vulnerable to maturation. The use of a randomly assigned control group, of course, is the best antidote for this threat as well as most others, because the control group also would be affected. Thus, any differences that remain most likely would be due to the independent variable.

Selection

Selection refers to **bias** in the method by which comparison groups are obtained. For example, suppose the first 30 patient volunteers were used for an experimental presurgical readiness program, and the rest of the surgical patients, including those who refused to participate, were used as a control group. Selection would be a rival hypothesis in explaining group differences, because the two groups were not the same to begin with. This threat is usually present in quasi-experimental designs that use intact groups and rarely present with *randomly assigned* control or comparison groups.

Earlier methodologic approaches often used **matching** as a way of equalizing groups. In addition to the many problems involved in matching on all relevant variables, this procedure did not take advantage of the fact that group comparisons rather than individual subject pair comparisons were being made. Group variation is an essential aspect of the traditional statistical analysis of differences, and utilizing random assignment to groups acknowledges that group performance rather than individual performance is the focus. Extensive controversy remains on the subject of matching individual pairs of subjects to obtain a control group that is equal to the experimental group.

Mortality

Mortality, as the word implies, means loss of subjects during an experiment. If there is bias in those who are lost, this is a possible rival explanation for observed group differences. For example, if those who leave a weight reduction program are those who are unwilling to limit caloric intake, the program might well appear more successful than it is. Patients who do not keep appointments have long been considered noncompliant and their chronic disease assumed to be unstable. If this assumption is true and a significant number of patients break the appointments at which their posttests were scheduled, mortality might account for the observed beneficial effects of an intervention.

Hawthorne Effect

The famous **Hawthorne effect** refers to a change in subjects because they know they are "guinea pigs" in a research study. The experimental setting, informed consent, change in routine care, more individual attention, incentives such as money or free physical examinations, and myriad other factors might make subjects feel special and so affect their performance. It is a threat to internal validity when the experimental group has this special treatment and the control group does not. This interjects a systematic difference between the groups in addition to the experimental variable. Researchers often try to use a **placebo** or alternative treatment with the control group to avoid this systematic difference. Removing the Hawthorne effect generally is considered about impossible. Therefore, it remains a threat to external validity when you generalize your results (see Chap. 10).

Closely related to the Hawthorne effect, subsets of it, are demand characteristics and experimenter bias. **Demand characteristics** refers to a subject giving the response he or she thinks the researcher wants rather than a true one. Separating the dependent variable(s) from delivery of the independent variable, as well as using unobtrusive measures, is one means to counteract this. A **blind experiment** in which subjects do not know to which group they are assigned is also helpful. **Experimenter bias** refers to behavior by the researcher that may influence subjects to respond in the hypothesized direction. A nurse unknowingly may spend more time with a patient in an experimental group or give more encouragement. A **double-blind experiment** is sometimes utilized in which neither the experimenter nor the subjects know who are control and who are experimental subjects. In addition, naive experimenters, who do not know the true purpose of the study, have been used in situations where it is permissible ethically. To repeat, these threats compromise internal validity when they are responsible for *differences* between the experimental and control groups. They can compromise other kinds of validity when they produce other effects, such as external validity when all subjects including controls know they have participated in this "famous" study.

Testing

Testing is the effect of taking a pretest on the scores of the posttest. Typically, there is a gain of a few points when a test is retaken, due only to having taken the test previously. In personality tests, the change is usually in the direction of better adjustment. Thus, if a pretest is used in a study, modest changes on a second testing might be due to the pretest and not due to the independent variable.

This brings up the problem of the **reactivity of measures.** The process of measuring may bring about behavior change. In a study of therapy for weight control, the initial weigh-in itself might be a stimulus for change. Placing an observer in a patient's room to observe a nurse's preexperimental interactive style itself might change the nurse's style. Tape-recording an interaction could change the way subjects behave. Thus, the use of nonreactive measures whenever possible is strongly recommended. If the reactivity of a measure is considered a possible threat, a disguised administration of it or a design that also measures this effect should be considered. Reactivity of measures is discussed in greater length in Chapter 11.

Instrumentation

Instrumentation refers to changes in a measuring device during its use that result in different scores for equivalent traits. For example, observers getting better at observing as they practice during a study, or getting tired or bored as they work over time, could account for differential effects. Change in the method of scoring a test (especially essay questions) is also an instrumentation threat. Changes in the calibration of physical assessment measures, of course, also are possible. In addition, consider the problem of different raters interpreting the color gradations used for the acetone urine test with diabetic patients. Frequent comparisons of raters evaluating the same test or observation period and/or repeated comparisons over time of single rater's evaluation of the same test or videotaped observation assess the impact of this threat. This is known as the **reliability** of a measure and is discussed in greater detail in Chapters 11 and 13.

Regression

Regression is a statistical effect by which a group selected on the basis of extreme test scores (either high or low) will tend to have less extreme scores if it is tested again, either on the same variable or another, related variable. Persons selected for an educational program in health care (e.g., basic hygiene, nutrition) on the basis of very low scores on a test measuring their knowledge about basic health care would tend, for example, to improve somewhat on a later measure regardless of whether the program was effective. Nursing research often utilizes "extreme" groups of patients as the target population for interventions. Fortunately, most regression threats can be controlled by using a control group and with statistical analysis using appropriate computation of gain scores or analysis of covariance.

Interactions with Selection

It is possible that an additional, unique threat to internal validity may be presented as a result of combining two of the preceding threats. **Selection-maturation** is an example. This refers to differential maturation in comparison groups due to bias in their selection. For example, a study involving an experimental program of rooming-in for neonates using two different hospital maternity units might be invalidated if one unit composed mostly young primiparas and the other included older multiparas. Older, more experienced mothers might be expected to learn faster and adjust more quickly to this new approach. A **selection-history interaction** could occur if comparison groups came from very different settings, some (or one) of which had an effect on the dependent variable. Attitudes toward collective bargaining could be influenced if a comparison group of nurses came from a hospital setting where nurses had just gone on strike. A **selection-instrumentation interaction** can occur when a measure is not calibrated to measure the highest or lowest scores in a group. These are known, respectively, as **ceiling** and **floor effects** of measures. This phenomenon could certainly cause groups to appear more alike if extreme scores went undetected.

*Diffusion of Experimental
Conditions*

Diffusion of experimental conditions occurs when experimental group subjects tell control group subjects all about their experiences in the study. Blind experiments and use of placebos help to counteract this threat.

*Compensating Equalization of
Controls*

Compensating equalization of controls occurs when either the controls or someone else tries to make up for their missing this new, exciting program. Double-blind designs are the most effective antidote.

*Rivalry and Demoralization of
Controls*

Rivalry (also known as the *John Henry effect*) and **demoralization of controls** occur when control subjects believe they are missing something. When this affects their performance on the dependent variable, internal validity is jeopardized.

*Limitations of Random
Assignment*

Random assignment to experimental and control groups can be *assumed* to successfully counteract most of the preceding threats. They remain as major considerations, however, when preexperimental or quasi-experimental designs are used. To repeat, when randomization is impossible and these designs must be used, the researcher is responsible for gathering evidence to demonstrate that these threats were not present prior to concluding support for a causal hypothesis. All this should be laid out during the planning and pilot test stages. There is no substitute for careful planning.

Even with random assignment, some threats may remain. In fact, in most experiments the probability is 1 in 20 that random assignment will result in unequal groups. In addition, random assignment cannot control diffusion of experimental conditions, compensating equalization of controls, or rivalry and demoralization of controls. The design must do this. Nor can randomization prevent differential mortality from the experimental group. When a pretest is used, the impact of differential mortality can be estimated sometimes by comparing the pretest scores of those who remained with those of the people who dropped out.

Threats to Construct Validity

Construct validity has to do with *how* you operationalize and/or quantify the variables being studied. It concerns the appropriateness and adequacy of (1) how the independent variable is operationalized and (2) the procedures used to implement the research design as well as (3) how well the dependent variable(s) is measured. In other words, construct validity is concerned with the fit, or link, between the theory or causal construct being tested and the manner in which it is done. For example, suppose you are interested in the effects of touch. Perhaps the experimental group is to be touched by their physician on the upper arm with a gentle, circular movement for 30 seconds at the end of a short visit to each patient's hospital room. Or touch may be operationalized as the primary care nurse holding a patient's hand during a specified instruction period. Or touch may mean a massage. The possibilities are endless, and the correct choice is sometimes difficult. Touch must be operationalized as it is defined or assumed to exist in the theory that guides the research and dictates the research hypotheses. If it is not, there is a problem with construct validity. Of course, all three examples of the operationalization of touch may be permissible under the theory. If two have the predicted effect and one does not, research will have provided information with which theory can be made more precise, because it will have indicated that one of the operationalizations does not belong in the theory.

Unlike the threats to internal validity pertaining to experimental research in which causal hypotheses are tested and which are, in large part, beyond the control of the researcher, construct validity is more under the control of the researcher and is a significant concern in *all* kinds of research. In addition, construct validity can involve detection and assessment of confounding variables, side effects, and variables that do *not* correlate with those under scrutiny. Whether a health care provider smiles or frowns while touching a patient may have an effect. Thus this could be a confounding variable. Or touch may lead to eye contact which leads to tears which leads to encouragement which leads to greater compliance and so on. Thus, construct validity concerns an accurate representation of the theory and continued vigilance to help improve the theory.

Chapters 11 and 13 discuss construct validity as it relates to the measurement of variables. Construct validity, of course, also relates to the *design* of a research study. Cook and Campbell [2] described 10 threats to the construct validity of a research design that provide a convenient checklist for researchers designing a study. They are not sacred. There are other less prevalent threats which may not be listed, and some of those listed may be threats to other aspects of the research process as well. Their labels are not sacred either. Other researchers may refer to a threat by another name.

Inadequate Explication of Constructs

Inadequate explication of constructs involves poor elaborations or definitions of variables and constructs within a theory. The clearer and more specific the **constitutive definition** of a variable, the one that uses words, the easier it will be to determine a good **operational definition** for a variable.

Mono-Operation Bias

Mono-operation bias involves only a single operation or measure of a variable instead of several. Since almost all operationalizations contain irrelevancies and fail to contain all aspects, or characteristics, of the variable being studied, use of only one measure (or operation) lowers construct validity. No single measure is perfect. There is little excuse for using only one measure of the dependent variable since additional measures generally do not add much effort or expense to the research. This is not always true with adding either more independent variables or more levels of the experimental variable, however. When possible, more variations of the experimental variable (hence several experimental groups instead of one) should be added to enhance construct validity.

Mono-Method Bias

Mono-method bias involves multiple measures or operations that still use only one method, such as self-administered pencil-and-paper tests, as multiple measures of the dependent variable. Failure to randomly alternate correct answers as both true and false might introduce this threat also. Thus, manipulations or measures should be selected to include multiple delivery modes whenever possible.

Hypothesis Guessing

threat to int. validity

Hypothesis guessing is just what the name implies. Informed consent requires that research subjects know the purpose of the research. If this leads easily to accurate or even inaccurate hypothesis guessing and actions based on this guessing, the construct validity is threatened.

Evaluation Apprehension

Int. Val.

Evaluation apprehension can result in subjects attempting to present themselves as competent, psychologically healthy, and anything else that may result in a favorable evaluation by the researcher. In longitudinal research in which experimenters become part of the woodwork, so to speak, perhaps this is not a problem.

Experimenter Expectancies

Int. val.

Experimenter expectancies sometimes have been shown to influence the data obtained. This threat can be reduced by using double-blind procedures.

Overlooking Interactions

Overlooking interactions means that with certain variations of the experimental variable you may conclude that X does not cause Y. If, in reality, X does cause Y under other levels or variations of the experimental variable not included in the research, a misleading conclusion is drawn. The construct validity was flawed when the research was designed without the important levels or variations of the experimental variable.

Multiple-Treatment Interference

Int. Validity

Multiple-treatment interference occurs when subjects participate in a series of research studies. These may have cumulative effects independent of those of each separate study and thus may bias results and restrict their generalization to populations other than the sample. This is more of a problem in laboratory research and experiments with college students.

Interaction of Testing and Treatment

Interaction of testing and treatment involves the effects due to a pretest or even multiple posttests. To the extent that these testing effects are confounded (i.e., mixed) with the observed effects of the experimental variable, the results are misleading and construct validity is compromised.

Restricted Generalizability Across Constructs

Restricted generalizability across constructs occurs when too few relevant outcomes or dependent variables are assessed. The practical significance of the

I.S. Orig. model

research is limited because the impact of the experimental manipulation on a number of important variables was never assessed.

Time-Series Example

Suppose that in 1981 your State Nurses Association (SNA) became alarmed about the high rate of death originating from breast cancer within the state. A decision was made to offer free breast examinations and instruction in self-examination at shopping centers and other locations throughout the state. Volunteer nurses provided the services. In the second year of this activity, the rate was down 25 percent. Exhibit 4.1 summarizes the results.

The SNA jubilantly concluded that the extensive program had made a difference and therefore wanted to continue their efforts. They decided to ask for

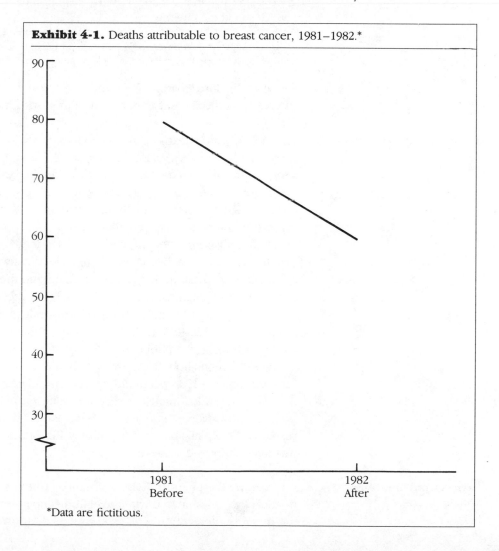

Exhibit 4-1. Deaths attributable to breast cancer, 1981–1982.*

*Data are fictitious.

funding from state health department officials, who unfortunately were not as impressed by the effects of the SNA program. Their critique included the following threats to *internal* validity:

History: During the same time period, a national organization conducted a nationwide media campaign about the warning signs of cancer. It emphasized the high probability of remission with early detection. Certainly part of the drop could be due to this factor.

Maturation: Death rates have been decreasing because of new advances in treatment and safer life-styles of the public.

Testing: In 1981, for the first time, the state publicized the high death rate from breast cancer. Although the testing threat generally involves the test itself as an agent of change, the fact that this was the first data collection so publicized does suggest it as a rival hypothesis.

Instrumentation: The base for the per capita rate changed from 1981 to 1982 owing to new census figures. The state population has grown, and thus the new base may account for the drop in 1982. Of course, this might be ameliorated by better reporting as a result of the publicity.

Regression: If 1981 were an extreme year, the rates would reduce in 1982.

Selection-Regression Interaction: Your program could be a result of the high rate in 1981. Thus, a high year was selected, which produces spurious results for 1982.

The state health department, nevertheless, funded the program for 3 years, admonishing the investigators to return then with more conclusive data.

Single-Sample Time-Series Design

The most obvious next step was to go back 5 years to look at prior rates and to carry forward for the 3 additional years of funding. This is known as **single-sample time-series design** and is illustrated in Exhibit 4.2. It greatly improves the single-sample pretest-posttest design. The trend over time was now evident. Indeed, 1981 was an unusually high-rate year. Regression and the selection-regression interaction are possible threats. However, the continued downward trend, though not as steep, for the 3 subsequent SNA program years suggests that these threats have been ameliorated. The downward trend, of course, could be due to either maturation (a natural decline in the population death rate) or the media campaign. Also it could be due to the nursing intervention. It is unlikely that the 1981 publication of death rates would continue to exert an influence beyond 1982. In fact, continued publicity of the reduction in rates might even make the public more complacent, thereby causing a rise in rates.

The instrumentation threat owing to new census data was studied next. Rates for 1982 through 1985 were computed by using the old base. They are shown as a broken line in Exhibit 4.3. A very small effect due to instrumentation appears possible. However, it is not considered large enough to seriously affect the results or be a plausible rival hypothesis. Furthermore, the 1981 ratio probably was inflated for the same reason.

Comparison Time-Series Design

To examine the unknown effects of history (the media campaign) and maturation, data were compared with those from a neighboring state that did not have the nursing intervention. This is known as the **comparison time-series de-**

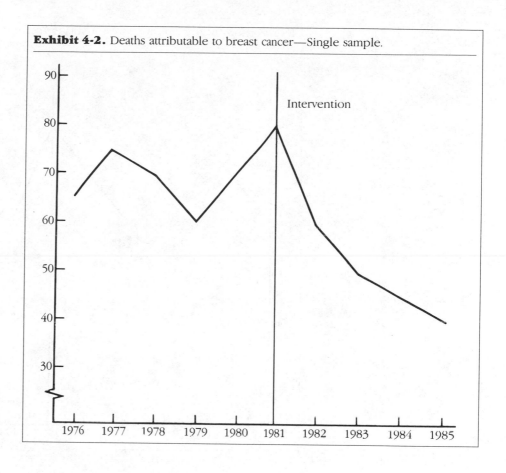

Exhibit 4-2. Deaths attributable to breast cancer—Single sample.

Intervention

sign (also known as the *control series design,* or the *multiple time-series design*). Results of this tabulation are shown in Exhibit 4.4. Just as the single-sample time-series design is an extension and improvement of the single-group pretest-posttest design, the comparison time-series design extends and often improves the quasi-experimental design called the *nonequivalent control group design.* By extending the observation period before the intervention, both designs provide baselines against which the observations during and after the intervention can be compared.

A **baseline** provides additional control, the essence of experimental research. Thus even greater control is provided by the comparison time-series design, because the baselines for the experimental and comparison groups can help establish their equivalency. Then comparison of both groups after the intervention can infer effects due to it.

As is apparent in Exhibit 4.4, the nursing intervention had an effect over and above that of the media campaign and alleged decline in death rates. This conclusion, of course, is dependent on the equivalency of the two groups. In what other ways does Exhibit 4.4 provide data to refute rival hypotheses?

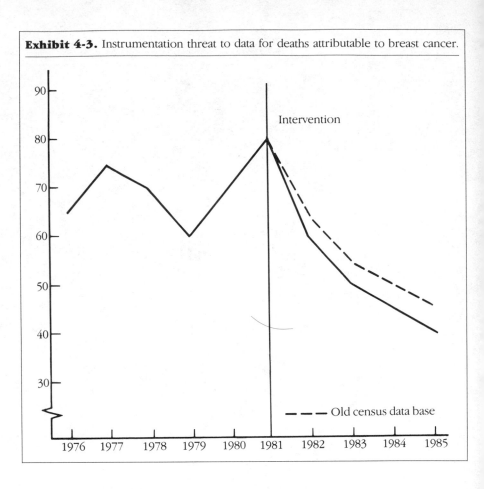

Exhibit 4-3. Instrumentation threat to data for deaths attributable to breast cancer.

Cluster Research Studies

During the 3-year funding period for the breast examination program, researchers, in all likelihood, would be investigating other aspects of the problem area and generating a cluster of studies. Probably they would want to investigate whether the lower death rate was related to breast self-examinations or other rival hypotheses. This might take the form of a survey of newly diagnosed patients. A longitudinal study of some participants in the SNA program might be undertaken, hopefully with a comparison group. The likelihood of a bona fide control group might be ethically impossible, unless funds and other resources could not cover services for the entire state.

Early detection might result in not only lowered death rates but also an increase in cases reported. A comparison time-series design might be used to compare cases reported and actual deaths for each year, instead of the data from the two states. If a larger difference were observed during the intervention period, the SNA program would be further validated. Perhaps other variables were affected by the intervention. The attention to breast cancer may have influenced health behavior in other areas, such as obtaining regular Pap tests.

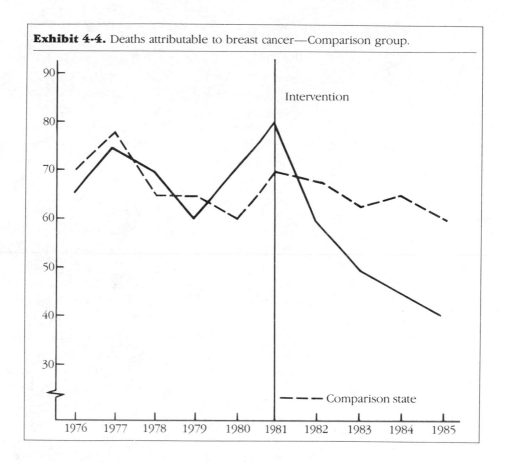

Exhibit 4-4. Deaths attributable to breast cancer—Comparison group.

Perhaps subgroups within the population (e.g., by age, parity, ethnicity) were affected differentially.

Did the independent variable change over the 4-year period? Adequate descriptions of the intervention as well as changes that occurred must be made. Perhaps these changes can be linked to changes in the dependent variable(s). The possibilities are endless. Keeping a detailed log of events, especially regarding the stability of the independent variable, is essential.

Controlling Confounding Variables

Potential confounding variables not covered by previous lists of threats are another category of rival hypotheses which usually threaten either construct or internal validity. They are sometimes called extraneous variables, mediating variables, moderator variables, suppressor variables, or anything else an author may select or invent. Unfortunately, authors of different books and articles label, define, and classify the variables differently. For simplicity, this test considers this group as **confounding** (your study is messed up); **intervening,** or **block-**

ing (you recouped by incorporating a potentially confounding variable into your design); or **controlled** (its effect has been eliminated or held constant). So the designation of a variable as confounding, intervening, or controlled depends on how you handle it in your research. This group includes all those variables that cannot be classified among the other threats and yet must be considered as rival hypotheses or explanations for observed effects on the dependent variables. Often they are unique to a particular study. Finding them requires creative thinking and detective work. Now we describe ways of controlling probable rival hypotheses.

Factorial Designs

Suppose you wished to study the effect on (1) complications during pregnancy and delivery, (2) attachment behaviors, and (3) social isolation of small group meetings which provided (a) social support and (b) education in parenting to a group of unwed teenage primiparas. If you planned only one experimental group (receiving both social support and education) and one control group, your independent variable would be confounded already, because you could not tell whether your results were due to the social support, the education, or a combination of the two. Therefore, four randomly assigned groups would be more appropriate, one receiving social support through weekly group meetings, one receiving education in parenting via programmed materials utilized at home, a third utilizing the programmed materials and receiving social support, and a fourth group to act as a control group. The two aspects of the original independent variable no longer would be confounded. Instead, they would be separated into two independent variables in order to test the effects of each as well as their combined effect. It would be similar to conducting three studies at the same time. The research not only would have greater precision and control but also would yield more information.

This approach is known as a **factorial design,** because it has more than one independent variable. It is diagramed in Exhibit 4.5. As you recall from Chapter 3, the broken lines represent random assignment, in this case to one of four possible groups. Each group is represented by one cell in the table. Indicated within each cell are measures of the dependent variables. $C(3)$ stands for complications summed during pregnancy and childbirth. The (3) indicates that this variable is operationalized as an interval level measure with a score that sums the product of weighted (according to severity) complications times duration of occurrence(s). The " $\xrightarrow{\text{(6 mo.)}} B(3)$ " represents an interval level observation of parenting behaviors associated with attachment measured 6 months *after* delivery, and $S(3)$ represents an interval level self-report scale measuring social isolation administered shortly after delivery.

With the original two-group (experimental and control) design, only one comparison was possible. By adding an additional independent variable, or factor, three comparisons are possible:

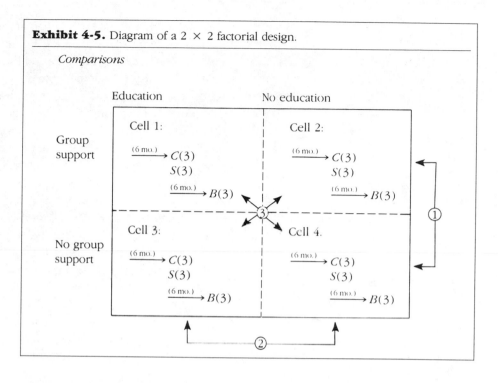

Exhibit 4-5. Diagram of a 2 × 2 factorial design.

1. The effects of weekly group meetings for social support are assessed by comparing the average of combined cells 1 and 2 with the average of combined cells 3 and 4.
2. The effects of parenting education are assessed by comparing the average of combined cells 1 and 3 with the average of combined cells 2 and 4.
3. The effects of both group support and education versus group support only versus education only versus nothing at all are assessed by comparing the averages of each of the four cells. All four cells are compared at once.

The first two comparisons are known as **main effects.** These could be made by conducting two separate experiments, each with one of the independent variables. The third is known as an **interaction,** because it compares different combinations of the two independent variables. This comparison can be made only when a factorial design (two or more independent variables) is used. In our example, the interaction effect will tell us, for example, whether the effect of group support is dependent on parenting education. Likewise, it will tell you whether the effect of parent education differs according to whether support was present. Interactions are a welcome bonus to the careful researcher, especially since the complexities of human behavior and thus behavioral research involve many interactions.

In spite of the use of factorial designs, other confounding variables are still possible. Suppose 80 percent of the control group subjects happened to be living alone, without family ties, while less than 40 percent of the experimental subjects did so. Living alone, rather than the independent variables, might account for observed differences and so confound the study. Even if the percentages of those living alone were about the same in all groups, an assumption (not certainty) of random assignment, one might hypothesize that the weekly group meetings to provide social support would have greater impact on those who lived alone. Therefore, observing the effect of living alone on the hypothesized causal relationship between social support and the dependent variables would cause it to be used an an intervening, or third, independent variable. Doing this, in all likelihood, would add even greater depth and sophistication to the study. The diagram of the study is shown in Exhibit 4.6. The design now has eight cells. The solid line separating those who live alone from those who do not represents two intact groups, because random assignment to living alone is not possible. Instead, subjects are **blocked** on this variable by dividing them into the two living arrangement groups before random assignment to one of the four experimental (manipulated) conditions. This form of factorial design, in which

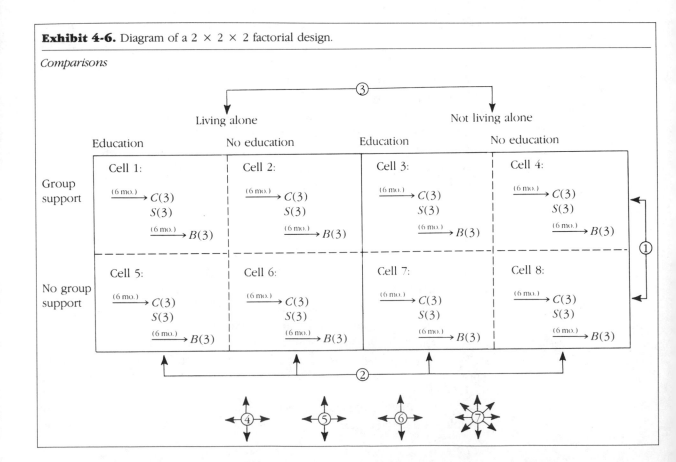

Exhibit 4-6. Diagram of a 2 × 2 × 2 factorial design.

the researcher cannot randomly assign subjects to different categories of a variable, is known as **randomized blocks design.**

Seven comparisons are now possible—three main effects and four interactions. The interactions are included in the diagram only as symbols, because inserting arrows to the variables involved would only confuse the diagram. These comparisons are possible:

1. The effects of group support are assessed by comparing the average of combined cells 1, 2, 3, and 4 with the average of combined cells 5, 6, 7, and 8.

2. The effects of parenting education are assessed by comparing the average of combined cells 1, 3, 5, and 7 with the average of combined cells 2, 4, 6, and 8.

3. The effects of living alone are assessed by comparing the average of combined cells 1, 2, 5, and 6 with the average of combined cells 3, 4, 7, and 8.

4. The interactive effects of group support and education are assessed by comparing the average of combined cells 1 and 3 with the average of combined cells 2 and 4 with the average of combined cells 5 and 7 with the average of combined cells 6 and 8. This is a **first-order interaction** because two factors, both independent variables, are involved. Four means, or averages, are compared with one another. To explain in another way, the interactive effects of group support and education are assessed by (a) comparing the average of cells 1 and 3 with the average of cells 2 and 4 and (b) comparing the average of cells 5 and 7 with the average of cells 6 and 8. If, for instance, comparison (a) shows a significant positive effect of education while comparison (b) shows no effect or a negative effect, you conclude that the effect of education differs according to whether group support was present. In a similar manner, comparing the average of cells 1 and 3 with the average of cells 5 and 7 and then comparing the average of cells 2 and 4 with the average of cells 6 and 8 will show whether the effect of group support depends on whether education was provided.

5. The interactive effects of group support and living alone (the new hypothesis) are assessed by comparing the average of combined cells 1 and 2 with combined cells 3 and 4 with combined cells 5 and 6 with combined cells 7 and 8. If the comparison of combined cells 1 and 2 with combined cells 3 and 4 indicated that those who lived alone and had group support had fewer complications and fewer feelings of social isolation, the research hypothesis would be supported. This is also a first-order interaction between two factors, an experimental variable and a blocking variable, are involved.

6. The interactive effects of education and living alone are assessed by comparing the average of combined cells 1 and 5 with combined cells 2 and 6 with combined cells 3 and 7 with combined cells 4 and 8. This is also a first-order interaction.

7. The last interactive effect is a **second-order interaction** because three factors—two experimental variables and one blocking variable—are involved. All eight cells are compared with one another. It is often difficult to interpret interactions this complex, and so researchers sometimes ignore them when interpreting results. However, in this example, if those who lived alone and received neither of the experimental variables did as well as those living alone and receiving only group support, a decision might be made to not spend the money and time involved in delivering the group sessions.

Eventually, of course, you must stop adding variables to the study design, in order to avoid making it too complex. Not only can it become impossible to interpret higher-order interactions, but also more subjects will be required as more cells are added to the design. As a rule of thumb, most factorial designs of this type require as a bare minimum 10 subjects in each cell.

Sampling

If other probable confounding variables emerge that random assignment might not control, such as younger subjects within each group being positively affected while older subjects are negatively affected (thereby canceling the effects of each other and showing no change for the group as a whole), the potential culprit might be eliminated by careful sampling. A variable, confounding or otherwise, is a variable only as long as it can vary. If only one value or category of a variable is included in the sample, such as younger but not older subjects, or only those living alone, then the potential confounding variable has been controlled through sampling. It cannot vary, because it has only one value. This is a useful technique when you do not have enough subjects to use a factorial design. However, it limits the generalizability of your results in that they can apply only to, say, younger subjects or those who live alone.

Statistical Control

Sometimes it is not possible to control a probable confounding variable by sampling, random assignment, or inclusion in a randomized blocks design. The data may not be available before the research begins, or you may have no interest in a variable as a block. Suppose you fear that other social stressers, such as a pressure to marry, loss of job, eviction, and so forth, might confound the study of teenage primaparas described earlier. However, you will not have information about these until after the study begins. Data still can be gathered to document the nature of these social stressers, and then by calculating a social stress score according to one of the several methods currently in use (e.g., Sarason, Johnson, and Siegel [3]), the variable can be controlled statistically. Chapter 20 explains some of the multivariate statistical techniques, such as analysis of covariance, which can help in this situation.

To summarize, four strategies can be used to control potential confounding variables. First, random assignment most often distributes these variables equally to all groups. When comparison groups are used because random assignment is not possible, matching on relevant variables is suggested by many researchers. This is acceptable if none of the other strategies will work. Second, when the variable can be eliminated from a study, sampling in such a way that only one category of the variable is included will successfully eliminate it. Third, if the measurement of a variable is not possible before a study begins, often measures of it can be used later in statistical analysis to remove or hold constant its effects. Fourth, when the variable is of interest to the researcher, it can be incorporated into the design as an additional factor, or independent variable. Chapters 5 and 20 discuss intervening variables as they are found and used in correlational research.

Additional Control Considerations

The concept of control means the elimination of competing explanations for the differences between experimental and control groups which you are attempting to quantify. The following control guidelines should be followed whenever feasible:

1. Train others to conduct the experimental program rather than yourself. Select them randomly from the population of available experimenters, and once they are selected, randomly assign them to treatment and control groups. Do not bias the experiment by telling them which approach you believe is best. *Or* allow each experimenter to conduct both experimental and control conditions. The first procedure minimizes the influence of experimenter bias, and random assignment reduces the effects attributable to differences in ability among experimenters. The second procedure controls only the differences among experimenters.

2. Utilize a traditional, or placebo, program with the control group instead of simply withholding the experimental variable. Just as sugar pills sometimes produce a positive change in health, one might occasionally expect a weak intervention to produce changes. Learning that your intervention is "better" than an alternate might be more valuable than learning that your intervention is simply better than nothing at all. Furthermore, if your study takes place over time, your placebo treatment may help keep your control group subjects available for the posttest. Loss of many control group subjects over time could result in your randomly assigned experimental and control groups no longer being equivalent.

3. Sometimes you cannot get the information you need to eliminate categories of a variable from your sample before you gather data. In that case, enlarge your sample, gather the necessary information, and later disregard the responses of those not fitting your subject protocol. Whenever possible, of course, this action should be avoided, because subjects later discarded are, in effect, wasting their time by responding. Ethical issues, therefore, must be considered.

4. When a potential confounding variable has been eliminated through sampling, replicate your study utilizing a different category of that variable.

5. Pilot testing your design often reveals potential confounding variables and threats to internal validity as well as problems in sampling, measurement, and procedure.

6. When you use one of the quasi-experimental designs and assume a possible threat to internal or external validity is not present, gather data to support your position. Similarly, gather data to assess the magnitude and influence of a threat you believe may be present.

7. Replicate. The value of replicating your research cannot be overstated. **Replication** under the same conditions with similiar subjects supports your research findings. Replication with other settings, times, or target population makes the research more generalizable if your results are supported and provides valuable information to modify the theoretical underpinnings of the research if the findings are different. Construct validity is enhanced when in a replication a different operationalization of an experimental variable is used. Replication rarely includes an exact duplication of the research it seeks to verify, because the variable of time, if nothing else, has changed. Thus, replications usually change the operational definition of certain variables or procedures in a *planned* way so that generalization to other operational definitions can be tested as well as generalization to other target populations, settings, and time.

Vocabulary

Baseline	Factor
Bias	Factorial design
Blind experiment	First-order interaction
Blocking	Floor effect
Blocking variable	Hawthorne effect
Ceiling effect	History threat
Comparison time-series design	Hypothesis guessing
Compensating equalization of controls	Inadequate explication of constructs
Confounding variable	Independent variable
Constitutive definition	Instrumentation threat
Construct validity	Interaction
Controlled variable	Interactions with selection threats
Demand characteristics	Interaction of testing and treatment
Diffusion of experimental conditions	Internal validity
Double-blind experiment	Intervening variable
Evaluation apprehension	Intrasession history threat
Experimental bias	Limitations of random assignment
Experimenter expectancy	Main effects

Matching

Maturation threat

Mono-method bias

Mono-operation bias

Mortality threat

Multiple-treatment interference

Operational definition

Overlooking interactions

Placebo

Plausible rival hypotheses

Randomized blocks design

Reactivity of measures

Regression threat

Reliability

Replication

Restricted generalizability across constructs

Rivalry and demoralization of controls

Second-order interaction

Selection-history threat

Selection-instrumentation threat

Selection-maturation threat

Selection threat

Single-sample time-series design

Subject protocol

Testing threat

References

1. Cook, T. D., and Campbell, D. T. *Quasi-Experimentation Design and Analysis Issues for Field Settings.* Chicago: Rand McNally, 1979.
2. Campbell, D. T., and Stanley, J. C. *Experimental and Quasi-Experimental Designs for Research.* Chicago: Rand McNally, 1963.
3. Sarason, I. G., Johnson, J. H., and Siegel, J. M. Assessing the impact of life changes: Development of the life experiences survey. *J. Consult. Clin. Psychol.* 46:932, 1978.

5: *Descriptive Designs*

Chapters 3 and 4 have focused on experimental research designs—those which test *causal* hypotheses. This chapter presents descriptive research designs— those used for all other kinds of research. Descriptive designs describe variables, compare groups of subjects (e.g., different diagnoses, compliers and poor compliers, mild and severe disease) on some dependent variable, demonstrate correlations between two or more variables, and even predict behavior on the basis of knowledge about one or more other variables. They cannot test whether *X* causes changes in *Y,* because an independent variable cannot be *manipulated* via random assignment of subjects to experimental and control groups. Some designs do try hard to approximate causality, as when success in nursing school is predicted by previous grade point average (GPA), motivation, and I.Q. This is as far as descriptive designs can go, however. They can never test a hypothesis in which previous GPA, motivation, and I.Q. are said to *cause* success or failure in nursing school, because previous GPA, motivation, and I.Q. can never be randomly assigned to subjects. When descriptive research of this type is **replicated** in different settings, causality is *often* inferred. It is called **implied causality.** In fact, hypotheses tested by nonintervention designs that could only imply causality on the basis of significant differences between groups have had substantial impact on policy and programs. For example, the assumption that cigarette smoking *causes* cancer and lower birth weights has resulted in the warning labels on the package and in many media campaigns. Many individuals have developed careers related to helping people stop smoking. The assumption that adolescents use illegal drugs because their peers use them is part of the reason for school-based drug education programs which focus upon peer group dynamics. The list is endless.

Descriptive research wears many hats. It can be very sophisticated and easily as complex as experimental research. At other times it must be the pathfinder in areas about which little is known. Often it plays a key role in theory development. Before a body of knowledge can be developed and experimental hypotheses be tested, variables and their relationships to other variables must be *described*. Once these observations are made, often via descriptive research although clinical observation also can be utilized, theoretical frameworks (the beginnings of full-fledged theory) are formulated by experts in which causal relationships are hypothesized. Then these are tested via experimental designs if the independent variable can be manipulated. If it cannot, more descriptive designs test hypotheses derived from the theory. Finally, descriptive research often provides very practical data on which are based many decisions related to activities of daily living. For example, survey research results determine our choice of television programs. When a program's ratings as determined by survey research are down, it is taken off the air. Market research into potential new products describes their potential use and acceptance. Upon these research results is based the decision to spend sometimes millions of dollars to bring new consumer goods to the public.

The descriptive research designs can be subdivided into three types of descriptive research which are not mutually exclusive:

1. Survey designs in which variables are described in terms of average response or the percentage of persons choosing each possible response to a question are commonplace, and large firms make millions of dollars each year conducting surveys—mail, door-to-door, or telephone—to assess the public's preference for political candidates, solutions to world or national problems, and so forth. Surveys can range from a few (or even one) simple questions to lengthy questionnaires encompassing scales which measure at the interval level attitudes or personality variables to even more complex designs used as tools for interactive problem solving (e.g., Delphi technique). Many are described in this chapter.

2. Comparative designs compare levels or categories of an independent variable which generally cannot be manipulated experimentally (e.g., gender, religious affiliation, education level, diagnosis) on some dependent (or criterion) variable for which it is hypothesized that differences exist. Sometimes these designs use more than one independent variable, and so interactions, as described in Chapter 4, can be observed. Quite often, comparative designs are incorporated into surveys. However, for simplicity they are treated as a separate group here, because all these designs use comparative statistical tests rather than just the summary statistics typical of a simple survey.

3. Correlation designs assess the extent to which variables are related, such as risk taking and fear of failure among women. When only two variables are of interest, this is known as a simple (or one-way) correlational design. Sometimes several variables are used to predict performance on yet another variable. This is a predictive design. Sometimes relationships between variables are examined over time. This is known as a *cross-lag panel design*. Just as comparative designs can be embedded within surveys, so correlational designs can be embedded within surveys. However, the correlational designs are treated as a separate group here because they use correlational statistical procedures and test, of course, correlational hypotheses.

While the threats to construct validity presented in Chapter 4 pertain to both descriptive and experimental research (as do the threats to external validity presented in Chap. 10 and threats to statistical conclusion validity presented in Chap. 20), the threats to internal validity presented in Chapter 4 are rival hypotheses to observed differences between experimental and control groups and thus pertain primarily to *experimental* research design. Only in some comparative designs would those threats be relevant, for example, when the differential mortality between two comparison groups occurs *after* the groups have been formed or when the manner in which two comparison groups are formed varies drastically, thereby introducing selection as a rival explanation for differences observed between the two groups.

Experimental research *requires* a hypothesis. Descriptive research does not, although hypotheses are certainly appropriate when there is theory or research literature to suggest them. Sometimes there is no such guidance from the existing body of knowledge. In this case, a research question guides the research.

Survey Designs

"Survey" is a catch-all word that can include a variety of designs from the simple to the very complex. The key to a good survey is the procedure used to select a sample of subjects whose responses will be representative of the population to which the results are to be generalized. If the sampling procedure is poor (or the sample is too small), survey results may pertain to only the persons in the sample and not the population whose response the surveyer intended to estimate. Chapter 10 discusses the various sampling procedures in detail, and many of the chapters in Unit VI which present different ways of analyzing data also present a method for determining adequate sample size for research using the particular statistical test being presented.

Simple Survey Design

McGrath and Laliberte [3] surveyed school nurses to assess their level of knowledge about venereal disease. Their mail-out questionnaire asked *demographic* questions (e.g., marital status, number of children, level of education, religious affiliation) and included a 40-item true-false test of knowledge about venereal disease. Their design is shown in Exhibit 5.1. Like the designs in Chapters 3 and 4, the box indicates the sample. Since there were no comparison groups, there is only one box. Here *D* stands for the demographic data gathered, and *K* stands for the knowledge test. The numbers in parentheses indicate the level of measurement. A 1 after *D* indicates nominal level, and 3 after *K* indicates interval level. There are no arrows between variables, because nothing is being compared. Averages, or the percentage of persons answering correctly, are reported instead. Therefore, "Averages" is written above the box to indicate that data are analyzed with summary statistics that yield averages.

This is the simplest and probably most popular form of survey. Designs of this type are not used to imply causality since no comparison groups are involved.

Longitudinal Survey Design

Comparisons are involved in the **longitudinal survey** design shown in Exhibit 5.2. Therefore, "Comparison" is written above the box to indicate that data are to be analyzed via comparison statistical procedures. There is still only one box, because a single sample is used. The variables are paired with arrows between them to indicate that subjects were measured twice, in this example 10 years apart.* This design might be used to assess sexual activity (e.g., kinds of sexual

---

*The design is diagrammed much like the single-group pretest-posttest preexperimental design except that no intervention or independent variable is involved.

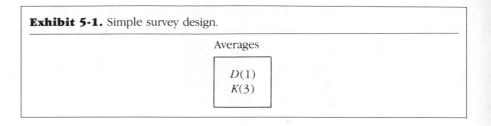

Exhibit 5-1. Simple survey design.

Averages

$$D(1)$$
$$K(3)$$

expression, frequency, satisfaction, orgasmic response, availability of partners, contraceptive practice) among young women 20 years of age and then again 10 years later. In Exhibit 5.2, D stands for **demographic data** measured at the nominal level, and B stands for sexual activity of which some aspects are measured at the nominal, ordinal, and interval levels. The purpose, of course, is to describe their activity and any changes that occur. No attempt at causality would be inferred—only the fact that change had occurred. This design, of course, could be made more complex by adding five more solid-line boxes, each representing an age **cohort** of women at 20, 30, 40, 50, 60, and 70 years of age. Trends over time might be suggested via cross-sectional comparisons from the first measurement period and later supported or amended by additional comparisons (e.g., 20-year-old cohort after 10 years compared with the 30-year-old cohort at inception). Longitudinal changes can be described (if mortality were not too great) and cohorts compared on the basis of change. Again the purpose of this research is descriptive. It describes changes and differences.

This design could be used retrospectively also. For example, a study conducted by this author and others asked 130 women under age 65 who had suffered myocardial infarctions (MIs) at least 6 months earlier about their sexual activity at the current time and before the MIs. Then these two were compared and the changes described. Because the study was in part retrospective and in no way were subjects followed over time (i.e., prospective or longitudinal re-

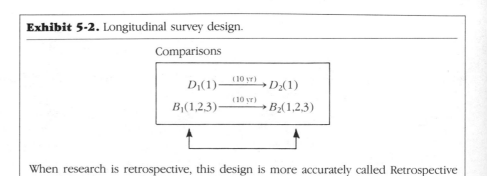

Exhibit 5-2. Longitudinal survey design.

Comparisons

$$D_1(1) \xrightarrow{\text{(10 yr)}} D_2(1)$$
$$B_1(1,2,3) \xrightarrow{\text{(10 yr)}} B_2(1,2,3)$$

When research is retrospective, this design is more accurately called Retrospective Survey Design.

search), the design would more accurately be called a **retrospective survey design.***

Delphi Survey

A more complex survey design, called the **Delphi technique,** was used by Lindeman [2] to assess priorities for clinical nursing research. The Delphi technique is often used for problem solving when face-to-face confrontation in groups would not be productive. Four stages were involved in the Delphi survey of research priorities for nursing, involving over 400 experts as panel members. In *stage 1,* panel members were asked to identify burning questions about the practice of nursing. Then these were subjected to content analysis from which emerged 150 burning questions. Next these were used as a 150-item questionnaire for *stage 2,* in which panel members assessed each item three ways: Is this an area in which nursing should assume primary responsibility? How important, on a scale of 1 to 7, is research on this topic for the profession of nursing? What is the likelihood, on a scale of 1 to 7, of change in patient welfare because of research on this topic? In *stage 3,* the panel was presented with a statistical summary of stage 2 responses, including each individual panel member's response, median for the panel, response range, and middle range (called the *interquartile range,* in which at least 50 percent of responses fell). They were asked to respond to the same 150-item questionnaire and when their response was outside the interquartile range, to make comments. In *stage 4,* panelists again completed the 150-item questionnaire after reviewing the results of stage 3 and a 79-page minority report consisting of the comments from stage 3. Then stage 4 results were reported, since respondents had had two opportunities to revise their responses based on knowledge of what other panelists believed.

The Delphi technique, or modifications of it, has potential for use in situations in which deadlocks are probable in a group meeting or political maneuvering might contaminate results. It also allows participation of more persons without concomitant travel expenses, although the time and work involved for the researchers can be monumental. The four-stage process does offer an opportunity for more accurate results than a one-shot approach does. When this is important, consider using this technique.

Comparative Designs

Descriptive research involves comparisons more often than not. Responses to some questions often are compared on the basis of certain characteristics of subjects, such as gender, age, educational level, capacity for self-care, diagnosis,

---

*You might come up with another name for it that would be even more meaningful to your research situation. That would be fine. These names, or labels, of descriptive designs are not sacred. The labels are designed to *facilitate* communication and mutual understanding, just as are the diagrams shown in the exhibits. They are products of the author's whimsy. Neither should be retained if a researcher gets sidetracked from the generation of knowledge by excessive preoccupation with memorizing the labels and diagrams.

cognitive function, and so on. Various categories of subjects can be compared on the basis of observed behaviors (e.g., frequency of complaints) or characteristics (e.g., nausea) or physical assessments, such as blood levels and electrocardiography. Chapter 4 demonstrates the use of blocking variables. These can be viewed as independent variables which are not manipulated. Comparative designs, by their very nature, use blocking variables as independent variables. If they used only one variable which was manipulated, even if it involved random assignment of just one variable to intact groups, they would be classified as experimental or quasi-experimental designs testing causal hypotheses even though comparative hypotheses were tested as well.

Intact Group Comparison Design

Exhibit 5.3 shows the **intact group comparison design.** The two solid-line boxes represent two levels or categories of an independent variable that are being compared. The letters inside the boxes represent the dependent variables or measures on which the comparisons are based. For example, suppose a group of adolescents coming to a Planned Parenthood clinic are compared on the basis of whether they had a sex education course (the independent variable). The dependent variables include attitude toward premarital sexual activity (A), contraceptive practice (C) for the last 6 months, and knowledge about contraception (K), all measured at the interval level. All willing participants complete a questionnaire which assesses the three dependent variables as well as demographic data and whether subjects had a sex education course. After data are gathered, questionnaires are put into two piles according to whether the respondents had sex education. Then each pile is compared on the other variables. (When computers are used, this sorting is done by the computer as part of your analysis.) Conclusions from this design can be only that differences were found between those with and without sex education. To conclude that sex education *caused* changes in any of the dependent variables, one of the experimental or quasi-experimental designs must be used, since sex education is a variable that can be manipulated. When an independent variable cannot be manipulated, this is the best design possible. As stated earlier, when results are

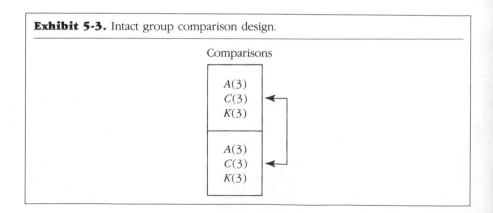

Exhibit 5-3. Intact group comparison design.

Comparisons

$A(3)$
$C(3)$
$K(3)$

$A(3)$
$C(3)$
$K(3)$

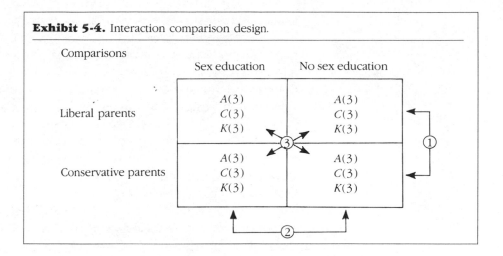

Exhibit 5-4. Interaction comparison design.

replicated over various settings, samples, or operationalizations of the variables, **implied causality** is inferred, although the link is always open to question. Of course, many hypotheses do not even test causality. Instead, comparisons are all that is of interest.

This design can easily become more complex to accommodate greater precision in hypotheses by adding longitudinality or measurement of subjects on two or more occasions. More than two groups or categories of a variable are possible; in fact, they are probable. Two categories are used here and in the following designs only for simplicity.

Interaction Comparisons Design

Just as the experimental designs can incorporate more than one independent variable, so can descriptive designs. The major difference between factorial designs that are experimental and those that are descriptive lies in whether the various independent variables are manipulated. The discussion of factorial designs in Chapter 4 pertains to the **interaction comparisons design** also. It is not repeated here. Exhibit 5.4 is a diagram of a two-independent-variable design. Solid lines separate groups because they are intact. Three comparisons indicate how many comparisons are to be made for *each* dependent variable. If a second independent variable, parental attitudes toward sexuality as perceived by their offspring (i.e., liberal or conservative), were added to our example of an intact group comparison design, it would typify an interaction comparison design, as shown in Exhibit 5.4. To implement this design, completed questionnaires are divided into four piles, each representing one of the solid boxes in the exhibit, for data analysis, and then group averages are compared.

Correlation Designs

The classic example of correlational research is the relationship established between cancer and cigarette smoking. Only implied causality can be inferred from the relationship because experimental design with humans in this instance is not ethically defensible. Instead, experimental designs with animals and numerous replications of correlational and comparative designs with humans have combined to make a very strong case for implied causality. Still other correlational designs do not concern implied causality at all. For example, consider the annual survey of immunization status conducted by the United States Centers for Disease Control. One of their surveys of households assumed representative of the United States population found that the proportion of children between the ages of 1 and 4 years who were vaccinated for polio declined over a 10-year period. The purpose of that research was to describe the association between year and immunization status. Clearly, it was not to determine whether the year caused immunization status or immunization status caused the year.

Four kinds of correlational designs are described in this section. They represent designs appropriate at the introductory or intermediate level of quantitative techniques. Still others, such as path analysis and factor analysis, are available. However, they are beyond the scope of this book.

Simple Correlation Design

A **simple correlation design** is shown in Exhibit 5.5. The single solid-line box represents one group of subjects who are each measured on two variables to test a hypothesis that the two variables are related. For example, a relationship may be hypothesized between knowledge about the side effects of drugs K and adherence to the therapeutic regimen A among hypertensive patients. The nondirectional arrow between the letters representing the variables indicates correlation. "Correlation" rather than "Comparison" is written above the box because correlational statistical procedures are used to analyze data gathered via this design. This design is very common, perhaps because it is so straightforward. It is discussed in greater detail in Chapter 7. When one variable is used to predict another variable, the design is called a **simple prediction design.** When more than one predictor variable is involved, the design becomes the multiple-predictor design shown in Exhibit 5.7 and discussed in the following pages.

Partial Correlation Design

Sometimes intervening variables must be controlled. One such way of doing this involves the **partial correlation design** shown in Exhibit 5.6. In this design the effects due to a third variable, such as age, are removed from the correlation between two other variables. This is known as **partialing out.** The partial correlation describes the relationship between the two variables *after* all the

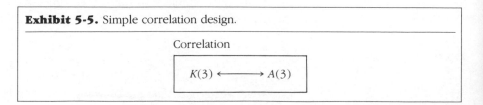

Exhibit 5-5. Simple correlation design.

Correlation

$K(3) \longleftrightarrow A(3)$

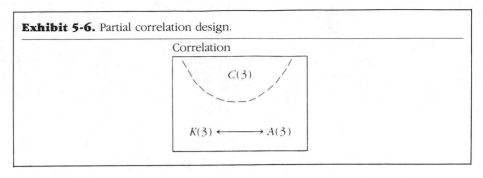

Exhibit 5-6. Partial correlation design.

overlap or factors *each* has in common with the third variable have been removed from analysis.* Chapter 20 describes the uses of and computational procedures involved in partial correlation.

Suppose we did not find a relationship between knowledge about side effects and adherence to the therapeutic regimen among hypertension patients in the simple correlation design. Furthermore, suppose that data snooping revealed great variability in the therapeutic regimens themselves. Some involved only one medication, limited sodium intake, and normal activities of daily living. Others involved concomitant illness, multiple medications taken at different times of day, aerobic exercise, weight loss diets, and some limits placed on activities of daily living. Then we might hypothesize that complexity of the therapeutic regimen was a confounding variable, and if we could remove its influence, our original relationship would be observed, indeed. A partial correlation design is, therefore, appropriate. As shown in Exhibit 5.6, the design is similar to the simple correlation design except that the effects due to complexity of regimen *C* are partialed out, as shown by the broken line around the letter representing the variable to be partialed out.

Multiple-Predictor Design

The **multiple-predictor design,** as shown in Exhibit 5.7, involves predicting values of one variable on the basis of knowledge about a person's score or performance on two or more other variables. Chapter 20 describes the design in detail and presents the computational and computer routines necessary to analyze data from this design. Suppose you wished to test a hypothesis which predicted adherence to the therapeutic regimen *A* among hypertensives on the basis of knowledge about medication side effects *K*, complexity of the regimen *C*, and fear of the debilitating effects of noncompliance *F*. This would be a multiple-predictor design requiring the statistical techniques called multiple regression if adherence were measured at the interval level of measurement and discriminant analysis if it were measured at the nominal level.

Cross-Lag Panel Design

The **cross-lag panel design** involves longitudinality and correlations between variables. In its traditional form it involves six correlations between two vari-

*When the factors only one of the variables has in common with the third variable are partialed out, the design is called a **part correlation design.**

Exhibit 5-7. Multiple-predictor design.

Correlation

$$K(3)$$
$$C(3) \longrightarrow A(3)$$
$$F(3)$$

---

ables measured on two different occasions. Like most correlational designs, it involves a single group of subjects, as indicated by the solid-line box in Exhibit 5.8, which illustrates this design. Billings and Moos [1] studied the relationship between support (family and work) and functioning (physical symptoms and depression) among healthy and alcoholic men and women. For each subgroup (e.g., working healthy women), six questions were asked:

1. Is there a cross-sectional association between family/work support and personal functioning (correlation 1 in Exhibit 5.8)?
2. What is the longitudinal stability of support when controlling for (partialing out) the effects of functioning (correlation 2)?
3. What is the longitudinal stability of functioning when controlling for the effects of support (correlation 3)?
4. Is the individual's initial level of functioning predictive of subsequent levels of support once the preexisting level of support is controlled (correlation 4)?
5. Is the initial level of support predictive of subsequent functioning given the effects of prior functioning and current support (correlation 5)?

Exhibit 5-8. Cross-lag panel design.

Correlations

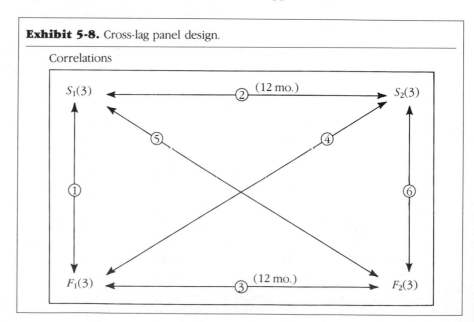

6. What effects do current levels of support have on functioning after controlling for prior levels of both support and functioning (correlation 6)?

As you may have observed, questions 2 through 6 involved partialing out another variable or two, and yet the diagram in Exhibit 5.8 does not show this. Doing so would make the diagram so complex that it would no longer be useful. Therefore, researchers have traditionally used the design as shown.

When independent variables cannot be manipulated and implied causality is of interest, this design is often very useful. Of course, it can continue for several time periods instead of the single one shown in Exhibit 5.8. Recent evidence [4] has demonstrated that multiple-regression statistical analysis (see Chap. 20) is the best approach to data analysis rather than the corrected correlations traditionally associated with cross-lag panel designs. Other variables are controlled with this approach, as specified in the preceding six questions, and greater power (i.e., faith in results) is achieved.

Other Designs

The designs discussed in this chapter presented only an overview of the major approaches to descriptive research. Various combinations of these are possible as well as the addition of more groups or variables to the basic designs. As usual, you must anticipate rival hypotheses and plan their control. A continuing source of ideas for designs is the research literature in your topic area.

Vocabulary

Cohort	Multiple-predictor design
Comparative designs	Part correlation design
Correlation designs	Partial correlation design
Cross-lag panel design	Partialing out
Delphi survey	Replication
Demographic data	Retrospective survey design
Implied causality	Simple correlation design
Intact group comparison design	Simple prediction design
Interaction comparisons design	Survey designs
Longitudinal survey design	Simple survey

References

1. Billings, A. G., and Moos, R. H. Social support and functioning among community and clinical groups: A panel model. *J. Behav. Med.* 5:295, 1982.
2. Lindeman, Carol. *Delphi Survey of Clinical Nursing Research Priorities.* Boulder, Colo.: Western Interstate Commission for Higher Education, 1974.
3. McGrath, P., and Laliberte, E. B. Level of basic venereal disease knowledge among junior and senior high school nurses in Massachusetts: A survey. *Nurs. Res.* 23:31, 1974.
4. Rogosa, D. A critique of cross-lagged correlation. *Psychol. Bull.* 88:245, 1980.

III: *Descriptive Statistics*

This unit presents descriptive statistical procedures as well as some inference (i.e., confidence intervals) when appropriate. Chapter 8 introduces epidemiologic methods as well. Not all the procedures in this unit are necessarily covered at the introductory level. Chapter 6 presents a very comprehensive approach to summarizing data, including data display via tables, graphs, and charts as well as data organization for computer analysis.

Although numerous examples are given throughout this unit, your class may wish to generate your own data set on which to try calculation of the various statistical procedures and development of tables, graphs, and charts. One approach might be to have each class member complete the Likert scale presented in Chapter 2 and also record various demographic characteristics, such as age and proposed specialty area. These data can then be summarized on a coding sheet and used by the entire class.

Do not forget to study the vocabulary words at the end of each chapter. They are important tools for understanding the materials in this unit.

6: *Summarizing Data*

Data can be great fun. We can gather, exchange, manipulate, and graphically display them in all sorts of wonderful ways and use them in a number of fashions. But the central fact of the matter is that data, in and of themselves, are rather meaningless, because they do not explain or cause change. Information does. As true (or altruistic, as opposed to opportunistic) researchers you are interested in explaining or changing the status quo; in other words, you want the results of your research to matter. Therefore, you are (or should be) interested in learning how to summarize data to extract information, and that is what this chapter is all about. We want to discover ways to find out what the data are telling us. Most sets of data can provide some information. If the data are properly gathered, the information may even be useful, and it can be expressed in mathematical language, a mode of expression with good and bad points. Among its advantages are a high level of objectivity, precision, and clarity. Its greatest disadvantage lies in its ability to hide some very poor research behind a brilliant facade. Also, the mere fact that information is expressed in mathematical terms is no guarantee that the information desired has been obtained!

The set of tools that we use to summarize data and extract information from them goes by the collective term *statistics*. A more generalized definition is that statistics is the science of decision making in the presence of uncertainty. This rather global definition is a far cry from the art of constructing charts and tables that formed the wellspring of statistics in its infancy. It is interesting that what we consider to be modern statistics has its origin in two seemingly disparate areas of interest: games of chance and political science. It was through intensive study of games of chance (with obvious rewards for better understanding) that the theories of probability were developed. Probability, which the great eighteenth-century mathematician Pierre Simon de Laplace (1749–1827) observed was at bottom nothing but common sense reduced to calculus, led to the mathematical treatment of errors of measurement and the theory that now forms the foundation of statistics. Also in the eighteenth century interest in the numerical description of political units (e.g., populations, geographic areas, cities, taxes, incomes) led to the development of methods to summarize, or describe, important features of numerical data, mostly by means of tables and charts. The marriage of these two areas of study gave birth to what we have come to know as statistics. No matter how complex the area of inquiry, however, we should keep Laplace's notion in mind—first intuition, then mathematics.

There are two general categories of application of statistics today, *descriptive* and *inferential*. Any kind of data analysis that produces information about the data themselves is considered to be descriptive statistics and is the focus of this chapter. Thus, if someone compiles the necessary information and reports that 2,843 patients were admitted to Mercy Hospital in 1982 and that they spent $3.6 million to get out, the work belongs to the field of descriptive statistics. This also would be the case if the average amount of a Mercy Hospital bill for that year were calculated (3,600,000 ÷ 2,843 = $1,266.27) or if it were observed that the average admission rate for that year was 7.8 patients per day (2,843 ÷ 365), but not if the data were used to predict future admissions, to estimate future revenues, or to make other kinds of generalizations. Such latter efforts belong to the field of inferential statistics. Here the group measured, usually termed the *sample,* is presumed to be a subset of a larger group, the *population,* about which information is sought. Thus, we would use inferential statistics if we wished to predict admission rates at Mercy Hospital in 1986, to compare the effectiveness of two or more different kinds of heart-lung machines, to determine the most effective dose of a new drug, to determine effects of program B, and so forth. Inferential statistics is treated in later chapters. In summary, **descriptive statistics** deals with ways of organizing and summarizing data to obtain information about samples (groups); **inferential statistics** deals with ways to make generalizations from the **sample** about the **population** (larger group) that the sample is believed to represent.

Whereas statistics is a mathematically based science, a *statistic* is a number derived from the manipulation of raw data resulting from a sample of observations (measurements). Thus, the ages of the 20 patients admitted to the intensive care unit of Mercy Hospital last week would be raw data, and the arithmetic average of these ages would be a statistic.

Frequency Distributions

Frequently the sheer bulk of the raw data gathered is overwhelming. Therefore, when dealing with very large sets of numbers, often we can obtain a good overall picture and sufficient information by grouping the data into a number of classes. Consider the plight of a nurse researcher who is studying the earnings of nurses in the United States. Such data are collected by the Bureau of Labor Statistics, and it is possible that they might supply a copy of their raw data. However, the prospect of having to deal with the tens of thousands of figures is not appealing, so our researcher turns to the *Statistical Abstracts of the United States,* which has been published annually by the U.S. Department of Commerce since 1878, in the hopes of finding the data in a more useful form. As a hypothetical example, it might appear in tabular form as in Exhibit 6.1. This kind of table illustrates what is called **frequency distribution.** In a frequency distribution, the data are grouped according to their numerical size, if quantitative, and systematically arranged, say from lowest to highest, as in this example. This would be a typical way to organize **interval and ratio level data** (recall the levels of measurement described in Chapter 2). Not surprisingly, such a grouping is called a **quantitative distribution.** If, however, we are dealing with **nominal level data,** we might group our data into nonnumerical categories. One such **qualitative distribution** is given in Exhibit 6.2. In each case we count the number of times an observation occurs in each class, or category. This is called a **frequency count.**

Essentially four steps are involved in the construction of a quantitative fre-

Exhibit 6-1. Hypothetical salary data for full-time hospital nurses.

Average Hourly Earnings, $	Number of Nurses
Under 9.00	73
9.00– 9.99	100
10.00–10.99	175
11.00–11.99	540
12.00–12.99	1,295
13.00–13.99	2,420
14.00–14.99	3.521
15.00–15.99	3,989
16.00–16.99	3,260
17.00–17.99	1,992
18.00–18.99	1,140
19.00–19.99	612
20.00–20.99	369
21.00–21.99	283
22.00–22.99	174
23.00 and over	97
Total	20,040

quency distribution: (1) We choose the classes into which the data are to be grouped (more about this later). (2) We distribute (tally) the data into the appropriate classes. (3) We count the number of observations in each class. (4) We present the data in a form that displays the information we wish to convey, that is, in such a way that it is usable without making it necessary to check lengthy explanations. The last step is largely a matter of artistic ingenuity, if we assume that labeling is clear and self-explanatory. The second and third steps are purely mechanical (and they are often performed by computer today). The first step, however, requires considerable judgment on the part of the data analyst and so warrants further discussion.

In choosing the classes into which we wish to group the data, we have to make two decisions. First, we must decide on the number of **data classes;** second, we must choose the range of the classes, that is, from where to where each class is

Exhibit 6-2. Hypothetical marriage data for full-time hospital nurses.

Marital Status	Number of Nurses
Single	5,127
Married	9,133
Divorced	4,794
Widowed	986
Total	20,040

to go. These decisions will be based on the nature of the data and the information we seek; or, stated in another way, the ultimate purpose the distribution is to serve. Furthermore, we must keep in mind that our groupings entail a certain loss of information depending on how they are chosen. Referring to Exhibit 6.1, for example, we cannot tell how many nurses averaged exactly $16.50 per hour, we cannot know the lowest average earnings or the highest, nor can we tell how many nurses earn more than $23 per hour. Similarly, we cannot tell from Exhibit 6.2 how many nurses have been divorced more than once or how many remarried after their first spouse died. This loss of information is inevitable; it is the price we must pay for organizing the data in this way. Thus, if we are constructing a frequency distribution to meet a particular need, we simply have to make sure that our classes are chosen appropriately.

There are, however, certain ground rules that constitute good practice in the absence of contravening circumstances. First, it is seldom wise to use fewer than 6 classes or more than 20, but obviously this choice will depend largely on the number of observations that we have to group. We would clearly lose more than we gained if we tried to group 6 observations into 12 data classes; conversely, we probably would give up too much information if we grouped 1,000 observations into two or three data classes. Second, we wish our **data class intervals** to be exhaustive and mutually exclusive. This means that (1) we choose data classes that will accommodate all the data (making sure that the smallest and largest values fall within the data class scheme and that there are no possible holes between data classes into which data can fall) and (2) we make sure that there is one and only one data class into which each data point can go (meaning that we must avoid successive classes that overlap, i.e., which have one or more values in common). Finally, if at all feasible, we make the data classes cover equal ranges of values. Actually, it is desirable to make these ranges (or data class intervals) multiples of some number that facilitates the tally (say, 5, 10, 100, . . .) and makes the display easy to comprehend.

This last ground rule was actually violated in Exhibit 6.1 in that the first and last classes are open, that is, they have no lower and upper bounds, respectively. Some nurses may have worked for nothing and others may have received $100 per hour or more (an equally unlikely prospect). However, if a data set contains a few values that are much smaller or much larger than the rest, the use of **open data classes** (labeled "less than . . . ," ". . . or less," ". . . and over," "more than . . . ," etc.) generally helps simplify the display by reducing the required number of data classes. Depending on the other uses for the data, though, the use of open data classes may make it either difficult or impossible to give certain further descriptions of the data and so should be avoided wherever feasible.

In addition to ensuring that our data classes include the smallest and largest data items in our set, we need to consider the precision of our data in the selection of class intervals, that is, whether they are given to the nearest dollar or to the nearest cent, to the nearest degree or tenth of a degree, or to the nearest hundredth of an ounce or nearest ounce, and so forth. The **data class interval**

Exhibit 6-3. Infant birth weight data.

A. Raw Data (lb)

5.1	7.0	6.2	5.9	6.3	4.2	8.8	6.5	8.4	7.6
6.0	5.9	5.0	6.5	7.2	6.7	7.3	7.6	6.4	5.8
7.2	6.8	7.6	5.7	8.7	6.4	6.2	9.4	7.3	5.4
8.1	5.4	8.1	7.1	5.6	6.0	8.6	6.0	5.8	6.5
6.6	7.6	5.2	5.5	5.8	6.2	5.2	4.0	6.7	7.9
7.5	7.7	6.9	7.3	7.1	8.1	7.6	5.8	5.7	4.5
5.4	9.3	5.3	6.2	5.3	7.3	6.1	9.7	7.2	8.5
4.8	5.0	7.5	5.6	6.7	5.7	6.7	7.7	6.2	6.7
6.0	8.2	6.4	6.7	7.5	6.6	7.8	5.3	7.7	6.1
7.8	6.9	5.4	5.3	5.4	6.8	5.5	6.6	5.7	7.2
7.6	7.2	9.5	7.8	7.7	6.2	6.9	6.8	4.4	5.6
6.4	6.6	7.4	5.4	6.5	7.7	4.5	5.8	6.6	6.9

B. Frequency Distribution

Weight (lb)	Tally	Frequency
4.0–4.9	𝍸 |	6
5.0–5.9	𝍸 𝍸 𝍸 𝍸 𝍸 𝍸 |	31
6.0–6.9	𝍸 𝍸 𝍸 𝍸 𝍸 𝍸 𝍸 ||||	39
7.0–7.9	𝍸 𝍸 𝍸 𝍸 𝍸 𝍸 |	31
8.0–8.9	𝍸 ||||	9
9.0–9.9	||||	4
	Total	120

precision must always equal that of the data if the mutually exclusive rule is to be met. It should not exceed that of the data, however, since then that would give the impression of greater precision than the data warrant.

To illustrate the construction of a frequency distribution, suppose we have access to the birth weights of all infants born in a hospital for a given month. For the month in question, 120 babies were born, and their raw birth weight data are given in Exhibit 6.3a. Although the original data probably were expressed in pounds and ounces, the data that we are given have been expressed to the nearest tenth of a pound. Therefore, this is the precision of the data and should be chosen as the precision for the data class intervals. By observing the data set, we note that the smallest infant weighed 4.0 pounds while the largest infant weighed 9.7 pounds, which establishes the range of the data set. We could use three data classes (4.0–5.9, 6.0–7.9, and 8.0–9.9), but that would be giving up too much information. We could use the 12 classes 4.0–4.4, 4.5–4.9, 5.0–5.4, . . . , 9.5–9.9; another logical choice would be to use the 6 data classes 4.0–4.9, 5.0–5.9, 6.0–6.9, 7.0–7.9, 8.0–8.9, 9.0–9.9. Choosing the last, we perform the actual tally by systematically going through the tabulated raw data and entering a mark for each item falling in a given data class, as shown in Exhibit 6.3b. Finally, we count the number of tallies in each class, the frequency of occurrence, or **data class frequency,** and enter the result in the frequency column. The sum of the class frequencies is equal to the number of items in the **raw data set** (if it does not, we made a mistake and must find our error). The smallest and largest values that can go into any given class are called the **lower** and **upper data class limits,** respectively. In Exhibit 6.3b, 4.0, 5.0, 6.0, 7.0, 8.0, and 9.0 are the lower data class limits of our six classes of the frequency distribution, and 4.9, 5.9, 6.9, 7.9, 8.9, and 9.9 are their upper limits.

Since we are dealing here with birth weights expressed to the nearest tenth of a pound, the first data class actually contains all infants weighing between 3.95 and 4.95 pounds (including 3.95 pounds, which would have been rounded to 4.0 pounds, but not 4.95 pounds, which would have been rounded to 5.0 pounds); the second class contains all those weighing between 4.95 and 5.95 pounds; and so on. These numbers are the **data class boundaries;** that is, they are the "fences" that establish our data classes. And since we do not want any data "sitting on the fence," we must choose these boundaries so that this situation does not occur. We do this by choosing midpoints between the data class limits. Since the data class limits denote the largest and smallest values that can go into any given class, a midpoint between the upper limit of one data class and the lower limit of the next higher data class is just what we want. Thus, the data class boundary between babies weighing 4.0 to 4.9 pounds and those weighing 5.0 to 5.9 pounds is $(4.9 + 5.0)/ 2 = 4.95$ pounds, and as noted earlier, if any baby's actual weight had been 4.95 pounds, it would have been rounded to 5.0 pounds for entry into the data set. This method of determining our data class boundaries ensures that they will be "impossible" values, that is, numbers that cannot possibly occur in our data set. Therefore, any item in our data set can fall into only one data class (remember our mutually exclusive requirement). Clearly the upper boundary of one data class is also the lower boundary of the next.

The difference between the boundaries of a data class is called the *data class interval,* or simply the *interval* of the distribution if all data class intervals are equal. This is the case in Exhibit 6.3b, where the interval is 1.0 (*not* 0.9, as some might guess at first). For open data classes, as in Exhibit 6.1, the data class interval is undefined since the width (or length) of the data class is unbounded. A final term used in connection with the frequency distribution is the data class mark. **Data class marks** are the midpoints of the data class intervals and are obtained by simply averaging the respective upper and lower data class boundaries (i.e., adding them and dividing by 2). Thus, the class marks of the distribution of infant birth weights are 4.45, 5.45, 6.45, 7.45, 8.45, and 9.45.

Frequency distributions can be presented to suit particular needs in two other ways. One way is to convert the frequencies to percentages, which is accomplished by dividing each of the data class frequencies of the distribution by the total number of observations (measurements) and multiplying by 100. If we do this for our infant birth weight data, we obtain the results given in Exhibit 6.4.

Exhibit 6-4. Infant birth weight percentage distribution.

Weight (lb)	Frequency	Percentage
4.0–4.9	6	5
5.0–5.9	31	26
6.0–6.9	39	32
7.0–7.9	31	26
8.0–8.9	9	8
9.0–9.9	4	3
	Total 120	Total 100

Such **percentage distributions** are especially useful if we want to compare two (or more) distributions and the number of items in each raw data set is different. For example, if we want to compare the infant birth weights for one month with those for another month, we convert the frequencies to a percentage distribution and then compare the percentages associated with the various classes for one month with the corresponding percentages for the other month, since it is unlikely that exactly the same number of babies would have been born in each of the two months.

Another popular way in which to present a frequency distribution is to convert it to an "or more," a "more than," an "or less," or a "less than" cumulative distribution. To do this, we simply add the class frequencies, starting at either the lower or higher end, depending on the type of cumulative distribution we seek. For example, using the infant birth weight data in Exhibit 6.3, we can construct the "less than" **cumulative distribution** given in Exhibit 6.5. With cumulative distributions it is even more common to find them expressed as percentages. The values are computed either by dividing each of the cumulative frequencies by the total and multiplying by 100 or by simply summing the percentages (as in Exhibit 6.4) if they have already been calculated. The "less than" cumulative percentage distribution for our infant birth weight data calculated in this manner is also shown in Exhibit 6.5.

Exhibit 6-5. Infant birth weight cumulative distribution.

Weight (lb)	Cumulative Frequency	Cumulative Percentage
Less than 4.0	0	0
Less than 5.0	6	5
Less than 6.0	37	31
Less than 7.0	76	63
Less than 8.0	107	89
Less than 9.0	116	97
Less than 10.0	120	100

D*ata Presentation*

The manner in which we present, or display, the data can have a great bearing on how easy it is to grasp the informational content present. Our choices for data presentation usually are some form of a table, chart, or graph. You are all familiar with tables as a technique for data presentation; we have been using them throughout this chapter without making any big deal about it. The amount of information that one can extract from a purely tabular presentation of data, however, is conditioned by how one has been trained to think and one's experience. A skilled data analyst can gather a fair amount of information by studying the raw infant birth weight data in Exhibit 6.3a. For most of us, however, a tabular presentation such as that in Exhibit 6.4 is much easier to grasp and extract information from.

When we are trying to condense large sets of data into easy-to-digest forms, either for our own use or to convey information to others, graphical forms are preferred to tables. The impact of the visual appeal of charts and graphs should not be overlooked or underestimated. A good rule is that you should use tables to present numbers and pictorial forms to present information. This is especially true for frequency distributions.

Pie Charts

Qualitative distributions, such as that presented in tabular form in Exhibit 6.2, are often presented graphically as **pie charts,** as in Exhibit 6.6. Here a circle is

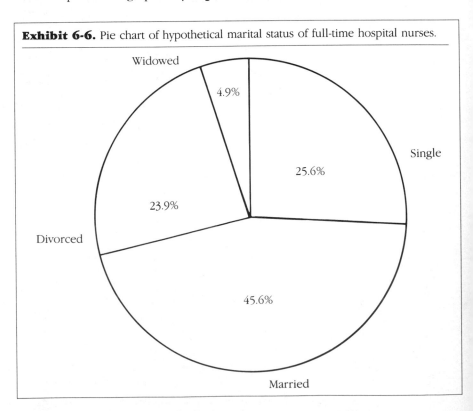

Exhibit 6-6. Pie chart of hypothetical marital status of full-time hospital nurses.

Widowed

4.9%

Single

25.6%

23.9%

Divorced

45.6%

Married

divided into sectors (pie-shaped pieces) which are proportional to the frequencies of the corresponding categories. To construct a pie chart, first we must convert the frequencies to a percentage distribution, as we did for Exhibit 6.4. Thus, for the categorical distribution given in Exhibit 6.2 we find that of the full-time hospital nurses, 25.6 percent are single, 45.6 percent are married, 23.9 percent are divorced, and 4.9 percent are widowed. We now use the fact from plane geometry that there are 360° in a circle; thus, 1 percent of a circle is represented by a sector with a central angle of one-hundredth of 360°, or 3.6°. If we multiply each of our categorical percentages by 3.6 and round to the nearest degree, we obtain 92°, 164°, 86°, and 18° as the central angles of the corresponding four sectors into which we divided the circle in Exhibit 6.6. The visual impact of pie charts can be enhanced by shading, or coloring, the different sectors to create contrast, by giving the whole diagram a three-dimensional effect, or by actually cutting out a piece of the pie to draw attention to a particular category.

Bar Charts

The **bar chart** is another useful way to graphically present frequency distribution data. In a bar chart, the lengths of the bars are proportional to the class frequencies (just as the central angles of the pie chart are). The pie chart data of Exhibit 6.6 are presented in bar chart form in Exhibit 6.7a. As with pie charts, shading, coloring, three-dimensional effects, and other techniques can be used to visually enhance bar charts, with the only real limitation being the imagination and artistic talent of the person preparing the presentation. A simple bar chart of the infant birth weight frequency distribution given in Exhibit 6.3b is shown in Exhibit 6.7b. Note the resemblance of this to the rows of tallies (hash marks) given in Exhibit 6.3. The tallies actually form a somewhat crude bar chart, and so, when you were marking tallies to count frequencies of occurrence within the data classes, you were also constructing a bar chart of sorts.

Histograms

Suppose, now, that we push the bars of Exhibit 6.7b together until they all touch. The result, depicted in Exhibit 6.8, is probably the most common kind of graphical presentation of a frequency distribution, and it is called a **histogram.** Histograms are constructed by representing the class intervals on a horizontal scale and the data class frequencies on a vertical scale and by drawing rectangles whose bases equal the data class intervals and whose heights are determined by the respective data class frequencies. The markings on the horizontal scale can be the data class limits (as in Exhibit 6.8), the data class boundaries, or other key values. This notion of the vertical scale representing the class frequencies in the histogram serves very well to introduce the subject and is correct as long as the class intervals are all equal. In reality, the *area* of each rectangle in the histogram, rather than its height, properly represents the frequency of its respective class. The importance of this distinction becomes clear when you think about a case in which the data class intervals are different. Remember that the frequencies must sum to the total number of raw data items in the set. So must the area

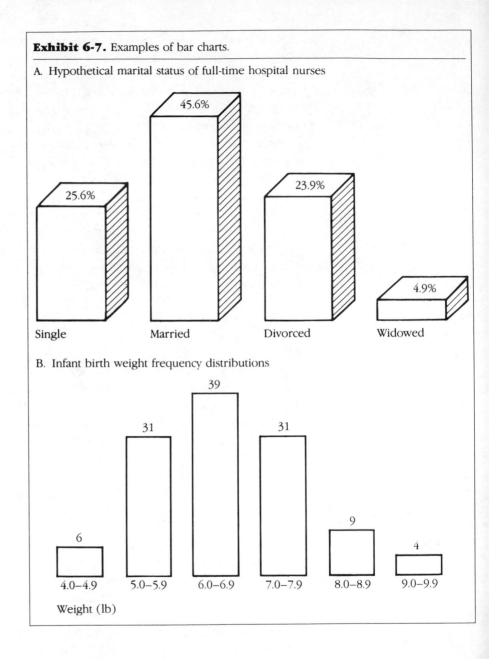

Exhibit 6-7. Examples of bar charts.

A. Hypothetical marital status of full-time hospital nurses

45.6%

25.6%

23.9%

4.9%

Single   Married   Divorced   Widowed

B. Infant birth weight frequency distributions

39

31   31

6

9

4

| 4.0–4.9 | 5.0–5.9 | 6.0–6.9 | 7.0–7.9 | 8.0–8.9 | 9.0–9.9 |

Weight (lb)

under the histogram (the sum of all the rectangles that comprise it). Therefore, if we have a frequency distribution with unequal class intervals, we compute the height of each rectangle by dividing the data class frequency by its respective data class interval and use these heights (multiplied by a suitable scaling factor if we wish) as the vertical scale in constructing our histogram.

The representation of class frequencies by areas is also an essential concept if we want to approximate histograms with smooth curves, that is, to make them

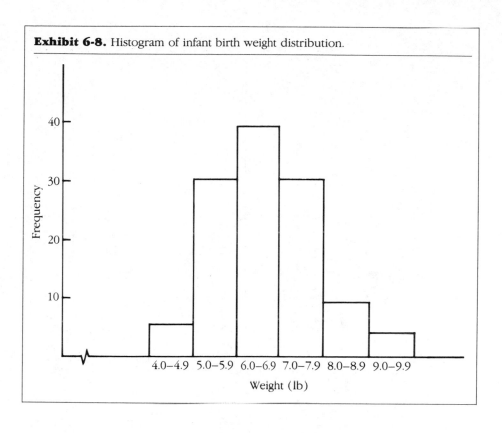

Exhibit 6-8. Histogram of infant birth weight distribution.

less "lumpy." (Reasons for wanting to do this are discussed later.) For instance, if we want to approximate the infant birth weight distribution with a smooth curve as in Exhibit 6.9, we can say that the shaded area under the curve represents the number of babies weighing 7.0 pounds or more. Clearly, this area is approximately equal to the sum of the areas of the corresponding three rectangles.

Frequency Polygons

So far we have spoken only of frequency distributions with respect to histograms, but we could have just as well used **percentage distributions** since the only difference is a vertical scaling factor. We will use percentage values to illustrate another kind of graphical presentation of a distribution known as a **frequency polygon;** an example is shown in Exhibit 6.10 for the birth weight data. Here the class frequencies are plotted at the class marks, and the successive points are joined by straight lines. Although it is not strictly correct, we added a class with a zero frequency at each end of the distribution to "tie down" the graph to the horizontal scale. Note the relationship between the vertical scales of frequency and percentage (percentage = 100/120 × frequency in this case). We note in passing the resemblance of our frequency polygon to the smooth curve approximation to the histogram given in Exhibit 6.9 (more about this later).

We can apply this same plotting technique to the cumulative frequencies (or percentages) with one slight exception, as illustrated in Exhibit 6.11. It stands to

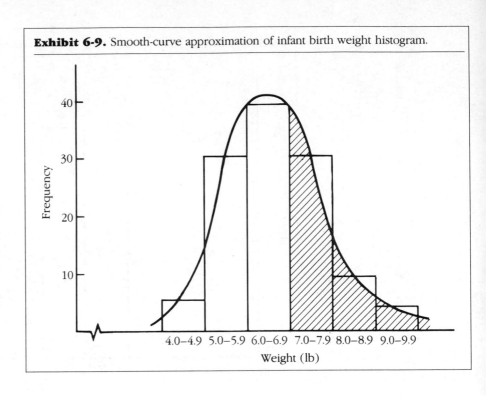

Exhibit 6-9. Smooth-curve approximation of infant birth weight histogram.

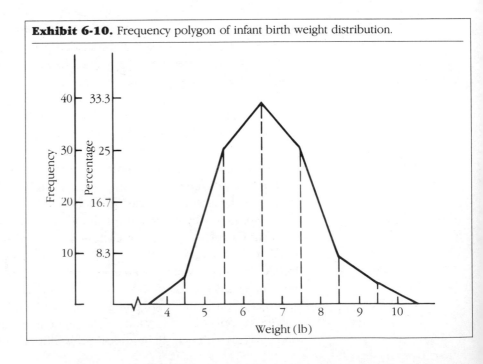

Exhibit 6-10. Frequency polygon of infant birth weight distribution.

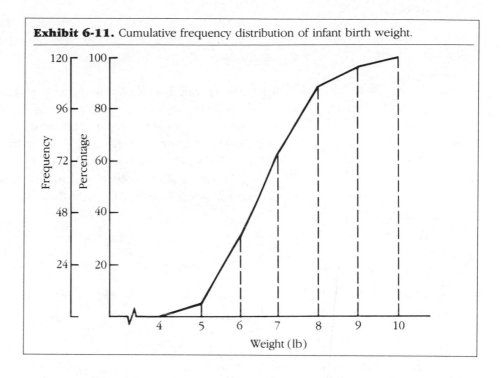

Exhibit 6-11. Cumulative frequency distribution of infant birth weight.

reason that the cumulative frequency corresponding to, say, "less than 7.0 pounds" should be plotted at 7.0 (strictly speaking, it should be plotted at the class boundary 6.95 since "less than 7.0 pounds" actually includes everything up to 6.95 pounds). Such a curve is often referred to as an **ogive.** Remember, it is simply a plot of the accumulating area under the histogram as more and more class intervals are added.

Let us pause at this point to review what we have learned about tables, charts, and graphs as ways to present data. **Tables** present numbers. Tables should be composed artistically and be clear, concise, and self-explanatory. However, since they have no scale of measurement, tables cannot be used to pictorially depict a sense of comparative size, or magnitude. It is up to the viewer to provide this comparative judgment. Still, tables are very useful in research work, and their use in presenting data should not be ignored. If we have a single scale of measurement we wish to graphically portray, we use a **chart.** In the bar charts of Exhibit 6.7, we used a vertical scale to provide a measure of the frequency distribution, but it is important to realize that no horizontal scale was expressed or implied. The width of the bars and their spacing were purely arbitrary. Generally it is good practice, however, to have all bars the same width and to use equal spaces between them. The use of the vertical to provide the measurement scale is also an arbitrary but fairly common practice. The horizontal axis also can be used to provide the measurement scale, and typically this is the case when time is involved. In our pie chart example, the scale used was the number of degrees surrounding the center point (i.e., contained within the circle) and so was neither a horizontal nor a vertical scale. There was, however, only one scale, and this is the essential characteristic of a chart.

Graphs

If we have two scales that we wish to use to provide a visual data display such as the infant birth rates and their cumulative frequency distribution of Exhibit 6.11, what we are using is called a **graph.** A graph has both a horizontal scale (called the **abscissa**) and a vertical scale (called the **ordinate**). See Exhibit 6.12. The choice of scales is rather arbitrary; it is dictated primarily by the desired size of the finished product and, of course, the range of the data. If there are a few data points that are widely separated from the main body of the data set, the involved

Exhibit 6-12. Essential elements of a graph.

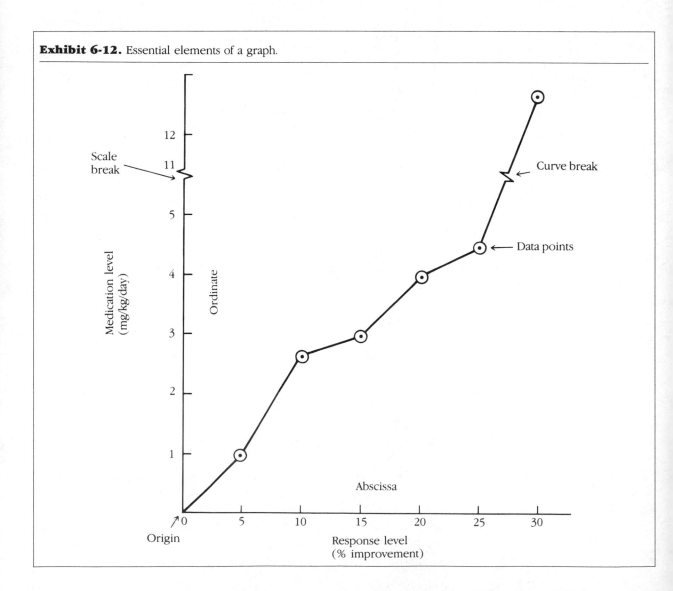

scale (or scales) may be broken to conserve space. This was done in Exhibit 6.11 to indicate that although it is possible for babies to be born weighing less than 4 pounds, there were none in our particular sample. When we deal with interval data, **breaks** are sometimes used to provide a connection to the **origin** (the zero point) when no zero or negative values are in the sample. Breaks also can be used in the scale of charts, but this is not common practice. In a graph the data points frequently are connected by a series of straight lines (as in Exhibits 6.10, 6.11, and 6.12) or by a curve, with the nature of the curve depending on the kind of data we are plotting and the underlying processes or mechanisms (e.g., blood pressure, kinetic response, pharmaceutical efficacy) that gave rise to the data set. Curves are sometimes used to "smooth out" a "lumpy" data set, as in Exhibit 6.9 for example, especially when we suspect that a good portion of the lumpiness may be due to measurement error. Remember, the key feature of a graph is that it has *two* measurement scales. Although in our discussion of tables, charts, and graphs we used frequency distributions as examples, you should not get the impression that this is any kind of a limitation on the use of these data presentation tools. In data summaries, however, it is one of the most common applications.

Contingency Tables

In our discussion of frequency distributions and data presentation, we limited ourselves to single variable **(univariate)** cases such as nurses' salaries, marriage status, infant birth weights, and the like. However, researchers frequently want to deal with situations involving two **(bivariate)** or more **(multivariate)** variables simultaneously. In this chapter we generally limit ourselves to the bivariate case.

Suppose we have access to the following data from nurses who graduated from two universities (say, A and B) and are now working full-time in hospitals: their responses to a questionnaire item asking them to rate the quality of education that they received as good, adequate, or poor; an assessment of their university grades as compared to those of the entire student body expressed as above average, average, or below average; and ratings of their job performance by their supervisor as doing well, doing fair, or doing poorly. What can we do with such a data set to present some information? As one example, consider Exhibit 6.13. Here we can see the distribution of responses about the perceived quality of education by graduate nurses from the two universities. Note that the column totals are fixed; they represent the sizes of the respective samples. The row totals ($186 + 288 = 474$, $100 + 284 = 384$, and $114 + 178 = 292$), however, depend on the response of the individuals and thus are not predetermined. Such a table is called a **contingency table,** or **two-way table.** It is common practice to describe such a table by giving its number of rows and columns. Thus, the table in Exhibit 6.13 is a 3×2 table; in general, a table with m rows and n columns is referred to as an $m \times n$ (or $r \times k$) table. It makes no difference which data go in rows and which in columns, and so Exhibit 6.13 just as easily could have been presented as a 2×3 table. In a similar fashion, we

Exhibit 6-13. Contingency table of quality
of nursing education for two universities.

Quality of Nursing Education	University	
	A	*B*
Good	186	288
Adequate	100	284
Poor	114	178
Totals	400	750

could display the data dealing with the university grade and job performance data as a 3 × 3 contingency table (Exhibit 6.14). Note that in this case both the row and the column totals are response-dependent, and neither is predetermined. Combined, however, the row and column totals must equal the total sample size (356 + 510 + 284 = 440 + 491 + 219 = 1,150).

The analysis of $m \times n$ contingency tables in which the cells are populated by responses is addressed in Chapter 18. For now, we note that it is somewhat difficult to see any trends or gain much information from our two examples, because of the differences in sample size (400 versus 750). As in the discussion of frequency distributions, we can use proportions or percentages (remember, a percentage is simply a proportion multiplied by 100) to help shed a little more light. If we convert the data in Exhibit 6.13 to percentages (by dividing the entries in column A by 400 and those in column B by 750 and then multiplying all the results by 100), we obtain the two-way table in Exhibit 6.15. Note that relatively more (a higher percentage of) students from university A considered their education to be good than from university B, while the percentage of students from university B who considered their education to be only adequate is much greater than that from university A. Of course, the columns in Exhibit 6.15 must now total 100 percent (within roundoff error).

While we lost no information in the univariate case by expressing our results

Exhibit 6.14. Contingency table of nurse
university performance versus job performance.

University Grade Assessment	Supervisor's Rating of Job Performance			
	Doing Well	Doing Fair	Doing Poorly	Totals
Above average	202	102	52	356
Average	170	264	76	510
Below average	68	125	91	284
Totals	440	491	219	—

Exhibit 6-15. Two-way table of quality of nursing education for two universities.

Quality of Nursing Education	University	
	A	B
Good	46%	38%
Adequate	25%	38%
Poor	29%	24%

as percentages, we do lose something in the bivariate case. For this reason, many researchers put both the actual frequency counts and their percentages (the latter usually in parentheses) in their contingency tables. An example for the university performance versus job performance data used to construct Exhibit 6.14 is given in Exhibit 6.16, where the data for the two universities have been *disaggregated.* In calculating the percentages here, we must use the total sample size. This is reasonable since neither the row total nor the column total is predetermined; they depend on the observed responses. Looking at the two

Exhibit 6-16. Contingency tables of nurse university performance versus job performance for two universities.

A. University *A*

University Grade Assessment	Supervisor's Rating of Job Performance			
	Doing Well	Doing Fair	Doing Poorly	Totals
Above average	63 (16%)	20 (5%)	6 (1%)	89 (22%)
Average	103 (26%)	74 (18%)	22 (6%)	199 (50%)
Below average	20 (5%)	59 (15%)	33 (8%)	112 (28%)
Totals	186 (47%)	153 (38%)	61 (15%)	—

B. University *B*

University Grade Assessment	Supervisor's Rating of Job Performance			
	Doing Well	Doing Fair	Doing Poorly	Totals
Above average	139 (19%)	82 (11%)	46 (6%)	267 (36%)
Average	67 (9%)	190 (25%)	54 (7%)	311 (41%)
Below average	48 (6%)	66 (9%)	58 (8%)	172 (23%)
Totals	254 (34%)	338 (45%)	158 (21%)	—

contingency tables of Exhibit 6.16, we observe that nurses with above-average grades seem to do better on the job, nurses with below-average grades tend to do poorly more often than their more scholarly counterparts, and so on. By comparing the contingency tables for the two universities, we can make observations, such as that a proportionally smaller number of nurse graduates from university A are doing poorly on the job than from university B, a higher percentage are doing well on the job, and so on. By making such a side-by-side comparison of two contingency tables, we have left the bivariate world for the multivariate one (actually, trivariate in this instance, since we added a third variable, the university). This topic is treated in a later chapter.

Measures of Central Tendency

The Mean

Although frequency distributions and their related tabular, chart, and graphical displays are useful as tools to help summarize data and present information, they are still rather uneconomical ways of presenting data and do not provide other elements of information that lie buried in the data set. A class of statistical measures that attempts to describe the "center," "middle," or "most typical value" of a set of data is discussed here. Although such measures can be described crudely as "averages," we refer to them as **measures of central tendency.** We put the word "average" in quotes because of its use by laypersons in everyday language—we speak of an average homemaker, a baseball player's batting average, a person's appearance as being average, and so forth. The more precise term is **arithmetic average,** and this is what the statistician calls an **arithmetic mean.**

The Arithmetic Mean

The arithmetic mean, or more simply the mean (we use an appropriate qualifier when we speak of other types of means), of a set of n numbers is their sum divided by n. Thus, if 12 nursing students received test scores of 69, 88, 93, 71, 47, 84, 89, 62, 96, 79, 58, and 84, the mean score is

$$\frac{69 + 88 + 93 + 71 + 47 + 84 + 89 + 62 + 96 + 79 + 58 + 84}{12} = 77$$

We can write a very compact expression (or formula) for calculating the mean, but to do so will require that we represent each data item with a symbol, such as $a, b, c, \ldots$ or $X_1, X_2, X_3, \ldots$ (read "X sub 1," "X sub 2," and so on). This latter type of symbolic notation has a simplistic elegance and convenience and is adopted here. Thus, the expression for the mean can be written as

$$\overline{X} = \frac{X_1 + X_2 + X_3 + \cdots + X_n}{n} \tag{6.1}$$

where we have introduced the symbol $\overline{X}$ (read "X bar") to stand for the mean of the data set and n is the number of data items. We can make our notation more compact if we introduce the mathematical shorthand symbol for summation Σ (capital Greek letter sigma, corresponding to our S) and write

$$\overline{X} = \frac{\sum\limits_{i=1}^{n}}{n} \tag{6.2}$$

Here we understand the subscript i to take on the values $1, 2, \ldots, n,$ and that is what the notation over and under Σ is meant to imply. Since we do not wish to exclude any data items in a set when we calculate the mean, it is common practice to simply drop the subscripts and the range indication and simply write

$$\overline{X} = \frac{\Sigma X}{n} \tag{6.3}$$

Observe, however, that the expressions given by equations 6.1, 6.2, and 6.3 are *all the same.* We are simply adopting a shorthand notation.

The widespread use of the mean as a measure of location when one has interval or ratio level measures (it obviously cannot be used for ordinal or nominal level data, since they lack equal intervals) is not accidental or a matter of custom. If we wish to use a single number to describe an attribute of a whole set of data, it should possess certain desirable properties:

1. It always exists; that is, it can be calculated correctly for any data set.
2. It is unique; that is, for any data set there is one and only one mean.
3. It accounts for the value of each item in the data set.
4. It lends itself to further statistical treatment; for example, the means of several data sets can be combined to produce an **ensemble mean** (sometimes called the **grand mean,** or **mean of means).**
5. It is relatively **robust** in the sense that for sample data it is not generally as strongly affected by chance as some of the other measures of location.

This last property is of special significance when it comes to inferential statistics, discussed in Chapters 15 to 20.

Whether the third property of including all numbers in the set is truly desirable depends on the nature of the data set and the information that we really want to obtain from it. Obviously a single extreme (very large or very small) value in our data set could affect the mean to such an extent that the mean could no longer really represent the data that it is supposed to describe. Suppose, for example, that in our earlier survey of nurses' salaries there was a person who had discovered a cure for cancer but who, rather than sharing it, had chosen to operate a private clinic that delivered (rather than promised) a 100 percent cure rate. That person's income could easily be measured in millions of dollars per year, not quite typical of the income of the "average" nurse, but still a part of the data set. Although the presence of such an extreme data point had no influence when we were concerned with frequency distributions (remember, our data class in that example was open), it could have a profound effect on the mean. Thus, we need to take into account just what we intend to use the mean for. If we want to portray the income of a typical working nurse, the inclusion of such an extreme data point, also called an **outlier,** will clearly produce an incorrect picture. If, however, we wish to speak of the total income received by our sample, we would commit a serious error in omitting it. To illustrate the problem in a more realistic way, suppose that in our earlier example of nurse test scores the ninth value should have been 36 instead of 96. Then the correct mean would have been

$$\frac{69 + 88 + 93 + 71 + 47 + 84 + 89 + 62 + 36 + 79 + 58 + 84}{12} = 72$$

which shows a 5-point difference from the mean calculated earlier.

Given a complete data set, the calculation of the mean is quite easy with formula 6.3. However, what happens when we have only grouped data to work with, as in the infant birth weight frequency data in Exhibit 6.3b? Since many data to which we have access are published in grouped form, this question is not inconsequential. We spoke earlier of the loss of information when data are grouped. So it should come as no surprise that the *exact* mean of a data set cannot be determined after the data have been grouped. Each item loses its identity, and so we know only how many items are in a data class. Nonetheless, a good approximation of the true mean of a data set can be obtained by treating each value in a class as though it equaled the data class mark, namely, the midpoint of the data class. Although some values in the data class will fall below the data class mark, others will exceed it, and (hopefully) all this will "average out." Thus, the 6 birth weight values of the first data class are treated as if they all equaled 4.45, the 31 values of the second class are treated as if they all equaled 5.45, and so on. Then the mean of this frequency distribution can be calculated as follows:

$$\overline{X} = \frac{(6)(4.45) + (31)(5.45) + (39)(6.45) + (31)(7.45) + (9)(8.45) + 4(9.45)}{120}$$

$$= 6.60$$

This is virtually the same as the value 6.62 that we obtain by using formula 6.3 to compute the mean for the entire data set given in Exhibit 6.3a.

To obtain a formula for the mean of grouped data, let us write the class marks as X_j (where j = the number of classes) and denote the corresponding frequencies as f_j. The total in the numerator is the sum of the products of the individual frequencies and class marks, or

$$\sum_{j=1}^{m} f_j X_j = f_1 X_1 + f_2 X_2 + \cdots + f_m X_m$$

and the total in the denominator is simply $\Sigma f_i = n$, the number of observations in the data set (i.e., the sample size). As before, we dispense with the subscripts and write

$$\bar{X} = \frac{\Sigma fX}{n} \tag{6.4}$$

In words, we find the mean of a distribution by first adding the products of each data class mark and its corresponding data class frequency and then dividing this total by the sum of the data class frequencies (i.e., the total number of items grouped).

The Weighted Mean

Although in many situations the simple arithmetic mean provides an adequate representation of the average that we seek to portray, in many others it would be quite misleading to simply average quantities without taking into account in some way their relative importance in the overall picture you are trying to describe (i.e., information you are trying to present). For example, suppose you receive grades of 95, 86, 92, and 89 on four successive 1-hour tests in a particular course, a 67 on the midterm, and a 50 on the final examination. The mean of these test scores is 80 (a solid C) but is meaningless because it does not reflect the relative importance that the instructor assigns to the various examinations. For instance, if the instructor had announced at the beginning of the course that the 1-hour tests would account for 40 percent of the final grade, the midterm for 20 percent, and the final examination for 40 percent, then the average would be

$$\frac{(10)(95) + (10)(86) + (10)(92) + (10)(89) + (20)(69) + (40)(50)}{100} = 70$$

which is 10 points under the simple mean (and at least a letter grade lower). Such an average is called a **weighted mean** because the scores were "averaged" by giving due weight to their relative importance. In general, the weighted mean of a set of n numbers X_i ($X_1, X_2, \ldots, X_n$) whose relative weights are w_i ($w_1, w_2, \ldots, w_n$) is given by

$$\bar{X}_w = \frac{\displaystyle\sum_{i=1}^{n} w_i X_i}{\displaystyle\sum_{i=1}^{n} w_i} = \frac{\Sigma wX}{\Sigma w} \tag{6.5}$$

Note that when the weights are equal, formula 6.5 reduces to formula 6.3, the formula for the arithmetic mean.

As another example of the use of the weighted mean, suppose you are driving to visit your parents and that on the trip you stop at four service stations, buying 21.3 gallons of gas at $1.039 per gallon at the first, 15.7 gallons at $1.099 per gallon at the second, 23.7 gallons at $1.369 at the third, and 16.9 gallons at $1.079 at the fourth. To find the average price paid per gallon, we substitute into formula 6.5 and obtain

$$\bar{X}_w = \frac{(21.3)(1.039) + (15.7)(1.099) + (23.7)(1.369) + (16.9)(1.079)}{21.3 + 15.7 + 23.7 + 16.9}$$

$$= \$1.161$$

We note that in this calculation we actually divided the total amount spent (in dollars) by the total number of gallons of gasoline purchased on the trip, which is obviously the correct way to find the average cost per gallon.

Although the choice of weights in the two preceding examples did not pose any problems, this is not always the case. In many situations the choice of weights is far from obvious (and often the source of much controversy), and this is one of the chief difficulties in the use of the weighted mean in circumstances other than where it can be applied in a straightforward manner.

Some Special Means

Although the arithmetic mean is by far the one that you will use most often, there are some other special means whose use is appropriate under certain circumstances. One is the **geometric mean** $\bar{X}_G$ which, for any set of n positive numbers, is given by the nth root of their product. The geometric mean finds its widest use when we need to average ratios or rates of change, when our data are best described by certain frequency distributions, and in other special instances.

Another special mean is the **harmonic mean** $\bar{X}_H$ which, for any set of n positive numbers, is given by n divided by the sum of the reciprocals of the n numbers. The harmonic mean also is used only in special circumstances. We discuss it further in Unit 6. A fuller discussion of the special means is given in Reference Note 1.

The Median

If we are dealing with situations such as those described earlier in which an extreme datum value gives a very misleading picture, or where a frequency distribution has an open data class, or the data fit certain special frequency distributions, then we are better advised to avoid the mean as a descriptor of the middle, or center, of a data set. One alternative could be the **median.** The median is the 50 percent **quartile,** or the 50th **percentile.** In other words, the median is that value which is as likely to be exceeded as not to be exceeded; to put it another way, the median is a value such that 50 percent of all observations in the data set fall above it and 50 percent fall below it. Thus, the median is the point on the abscissa (horizontal scale) of the histogram (frequency distribution) through which a vertical line exactly dividing the area of the histogram must pass. Like the mean, the median is a number and not necessarily a particular measurement or observation, although in many instances it may be. We use the symbol $\tilde{X}$ (read "X tilde") for the median.

To locate the median, we must *rank-order* our data set; that is, we must arrange the data items from lowest to highest (or vice versa). When there is an *odd* number of data items in the set, the median is the one in the middle. For instance, if the ages of the five patients admitted to the maternity ward yesterday are 18, 22, 23, 29, and 35, the median age is $\tilde{X} = 23$. Although it is easy to visually determine the median in this example because the number of data items was small, a locator rule is helpful for large data sets. If the number of items is odd, the middle value will be item $(n + 1)/2$, counting either from the top or from the bottom (or from the left or from the right). Thus, if we have a data set with 31 items, the median is the value of the $(31 + 1)/2 = 16$th largest item in the rank-ordered set.

If we have an even number of items in the data set, clearly none can be exactly in the middle when they are rank-ordered. In this case, the median is taken to be the average of the two middle values. To illustrate, let us rank-order the 12 nursing student grades used earlier when we discussed the mean (namely, 47, 58, 63, 69, 71, 79, 84, 84, 88, 89, 93, and 96). We use our same locator rule and calculate $(12 + 1)/2 = 6.5$, which is this case tells us that the median lies halfway between the 6th and 7th largest items in the data set (79 and 84). We take the average of these two middle values and find the median to be $\tilde{X} = (79 + 84)/2 = 81.5$. We should not be surprised that this differs somewhat from the mean of 77 that we calculated earlier. Here also we will suppose that the test score of 96 should have been 36 and calculate the median. Our rank-ordered data set is now 36, 47, 58, 62, 69, 72, 79, 84, 84, 88, 89, and 93. Since there are still 12 data items, the *location* of the median has not changed, but the *values* of the 6th and 7th items have. The median now is $\tilde{X} = (72 + 79)/2 = 75.5$, a 6-point drop.

Like the mean, the median possesses certain desirable properties:

1. It always exists; that is, it can be calculated correctly for any data set.
2. It is unique; that is, for any data set there can be only one median.
3. It can generally be found for grouped data, even when there are open classes.
4. It is generally not as strongly affected by extreme values as the mean.
5. It can be used to define the middle of a number of objects, properties, or qualities which do not allow a convenient quantitative description.

As an example of this last property, we could subjectively rank-order a number of nursing courses according to their difficulty and then speak of the middle one as being of "average" difficulty. With respect to the fourth property, consider the data set 1, 2, and 9. Its median is 2, and its mean is 6. If we change the 9 to 99, the median is still 2, but the mean has soared to 51.

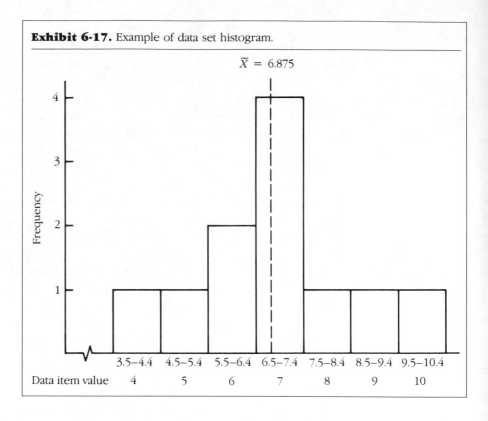

Exhibit 6-17. Example of data set histogram.

We now address the task of calculating the median when the middle value of our data set has a frequency greater than 1. To do this, we have to construct a frequency distribution, and the procedure that we use applies to any grouped data set as well. Let us begin by considering the data set 4, 5, 6, 6, 7, 7, 7, 7, 8, 9, 10. Since there are 11 items, our locator rule tells us that the median would occupy the $(11 + 1)/2 = $ 6th position, whose value is 7. However, there are four data items smaller than 7 and only three data items which are larger, so our concept of the median (namely, a number that exactly divides our data set) suggests that while 7 may be a good *approximation*, the true median should be somewhat less than 7. We can construct a histogram of our data (see Exhibit 6.17). In constructing this histogram, we have used the notion of data class *boundaries* introduced earlier. In particular, we note that the data class boundaries for a data value of 6, for example, are 5.5 and 6.4. To make this clear, we have labeled the data item values in Exhibit 6.17, but this is not standard practice. To locate the line that divides our histogram equally, we first note that the data class intervals are all equal to 1 and that the total area of the histogram is 1 + 1 + 2 + 4 + 1 + 1 + 1 = 11. Then half of the area is 5.5. We could start counting from either end, but let us start at the lower. We have accumulated 1 + 1 + 2 = 4 units of area when we reach the data class in which the median lies. Therefore, we need to take 5.5 − 4 = 1.5 units of area out of this rectangle to

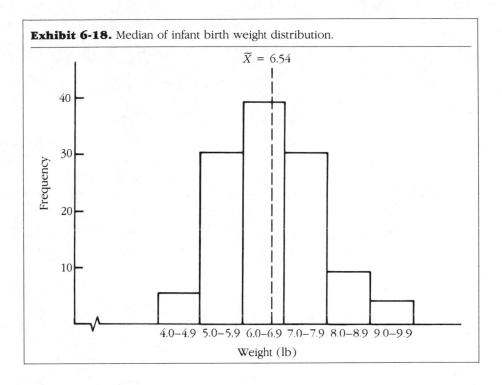

Exhibit 6-18. Median of infant birth weight distribution.

locate our median. Since the area of a rectangle is the product of its base and height, the portion of the base that we must include is 1.5 ÷ 4 = 0.375. We add this to the lower boundary of the data class in which the median falls and obtain $\widetilde{X} = 6.5 + 0.375 = 6.875$, the exact value of the median. We can write a formula to express this procedure if we let L be the lower boundary of the data class into which the median must fall, f its frequency, I its interval, and j the number of items (or remainder of the area) we still have to include after reaching L:

$$\widetilde{X} = L + \frac{j}{f}(I)$$

(6.6)

To illustrate the application of this procedure for determining the median for grouped data, let us consider again the infant birth weight data set of Exhibit 6.3b, the histogram of which is reproduced in Exhibit 6.18. Since $n = 120$ and the data class interval is 1.0, the total area of our histogram is 120 × 1 = 120, and the median will divide it into two areas of 60 each; that is, we want 60 data items to the left of the median and 60 data items to its right. If we begin counting (measuring the area) from the lower end (the left) of the histogram, we find that 6 + 31 = 37 of the values fall into the first two data classes. The next class contains 39 items (i.e., its area is 39), and so must contain the median (37 + 39 = 76 > 60). The median will fall on the 60 − 37 = 23rd item in this data class, and so $L = 5.95, I = 1.0, j = 23$, and $f = 39$. Substituting these values into formula 6.6, we obtain

$$\widetilde{X} = L + \frac{j}{f}(I) = 5.95 + \frac{23}{39}(1.0) = 6.54$$

The Midrange

One other central tendency measure, the **midrange,** is discussed here because it falls in the same conceptual category. The midrange of a data set is simply the average of the lowest and highest values in the set. Its main advantage is that it is very easy to calculate. For the infant birth weight example, the midrange is $(4.0 + 9.7)/2 = 6.85$, which is fairly close to the value of the mean (6.62) and the median (6.54). In the example of the 12 nursing students' grades, the midrange is $(47 + 96)/2 = 71.5$, as compared to the mean of 77 and the median of 81.5.

Other Quantiles

The median belongs to a general class of statistical measures known as **quantiles** (or **fractiles** or **percentiles**), which are defined as values above or below which certain quantities (or fractions or percentages) of the data must fall. They are calculated by using the same general procedure that we used to determine the median. The most common of these are the quartiles, of which there are three. The first, or lower, quartile is such that 25 percent of the data falls below it. Another 25 percent of the data falls between the first quartile and the second, the second quartile being simply the median; and another 25 percent of the data falls between the second and the third quartile. Thus, the third, or upper, quartile is such that 75 percent of the data falls below it (or conversely, only 25 percent of the data falls above it). To calculate the quartiles for the infant birth weight example (see Exhibit 6.3b), we must count $120 \times 0.25 = 30$ data items from the bottom to reach the lower quartile and $120 \times 0.75 = 90$ items to reach the upper quartile. Using formula 6.6 to compute the lower quartile, we have $L = 4.95, j = 30 - 6 = 24, f = 31$, and $I = 1.0$, and so we obtain

$$Q_1 = 4.95 + \frac{24}{31}(1.0) = 5.72$$

In a similar fashion, the upper quartile is

$$Q_3 = 6.95 + \frac{14}{31}(1.0) = 7.40$$

Another popular set of quantiles are the nine **deciles,** which are those points that divide the data into 10 equal groups (or divide the histogram into 10 units of equal area). Thus, 10 percent of the data falls below D_1 (the first, or lower, decile), 10 percent falls between D_1 and $D_2, \ldots$, and 10 percent falls above D_9

(the ninth, or upper, decile). Clearly, the median is also the fifth decile D_5. For the infant birth weight distribution, $L = 7.95, j = (120 \times 0.9) - 107 = 1, f = 8$, and $I = 1.0$, and

$$D_9 = 7.95 + \frac{1}{8}(1.0) = 8.08$$

The upper and lower deciles are important because in all likelihood they will bound any **outliers** (unusually large or small data values) in a given data set. When the data set is extremely large, some researchers simply ignore data above and below the upper and lower deciles (**truncate** the data set) in determining measures of central tendency. This practice is not without controversy, however, and should not be followed without a good understanding of the nature of the features (processes or mechanisms) that the data set is intended to portray.

The Mode

The last popular measure of central tendency we discuss is the **mode.** The mode of a data set is the value that occurs most often. Thus, if more matriculating nursing students are 18 years old than any other age, then 18 is the modal age, or 18 is the mode for this data set. When data are distributed into classes, as is the case with a frequency distribution, the class with the greatest number of data items is called the **modal class.** Obviously, with nominal level data we can have only a modal class. Suppose that of a group of 40 patients, 12 were arthritic, 8 had pneumonia, 6 were diabetic, and 24 were hypertensive. The modal class for this group is hypertensive, since it is the category with the highest frequency. Similarly, in the grouped infant birth weight data given in Exhibit 6.3b, the class which has the limits 6.0 to 6.9 pounds is the modal class—its frequency is greater than that of any other class. The mode or modal class of a data set is determined by visual inspection once the data are arranged into a frequency distribution.

Advantages of the mode (or modal class) as a measure of central tendency include the fact that its determination requires no calculation and that it can be used with nominal level data whereas the median and the mean cannot. The mode also has some definite disadvantages:

1. It is merely a measure of location; its location is not necessarily central.
2. It may not exist.
3. It may not be unique.

This last point deserves further elaboration. A data set with a single mode is said to have a **unimodal** frequency distribution. A group with two modes (or modal classes) is said to have a **bimodal** frequency distribution, and so on. Thus, the data set 1, 2, 2, 2, 2, 3, 4, 4, 5, 6, 6, 6, 6, 7, 8 is bimodal since it has two modes, 2 and 6. Of course, a data set may have more than two modes. The infant

Exhibit 6-19. Allowable central-tendency measures by measurement level.

Measurement Level	Allowable Central Tendency Measure
Nominal data	Modal class
Ordinal data	Modal class, mode, median
Interval data	Modal class, mode, median, mean
Ratio data	Modal class, mode, median, mean

birth weight data set in Exhibit 6.3a has four modes—the weights of 5.4, 6.2, 6.7, and 7.6 pounds all occur 6 times.

Comparison of the Mean, Median, and Mode

The allowable measures of central tendency for the different levels of measurement are shown in Exhibit 6.19. With nominal level data, only the modal class is possible. With ordinal level data, we can use the modal class, the mode, or the median. With interval and ratio level data, we can use any of the measures of central tendency discussed.

Although the advantages and disadvantages of the mean, median, and mode are discussed with each statistic, they are summarized in Exhibit 6.20. Of the three, generally the mean is the most useful when interval or ratio data are involved. One exception occurs when the data set contains one or more extreme, or atypical, observations (i.e., outliers) at either the low end or the high end of the distribution. In such instances (remember the income example), the median is a better choice since, in the presence of outliers, it continues to reflect the middle of the data set and would be more representative of typical values. When you are dealing with ordinal level data, usually the median is the statistic of choice to describe the middle of the data set, although the mode can sometimes provide some useful insights. For example, if there are two modes (or modal classes), the data set may contain two distinct subgroups and a separate analysis of each modal group might be in order. With nominal level data there is no choice other than the modal class.

Exhibit 6-20. Comparison of features of mean, median, and mode.

Mean	Median	Mode
Always exists	Always exists	May not exist
Is unique	Is unique	May not be unique
Accounts for the value of each item	Can be found with open classes	May not indicate the middle
Lends itself to further statistical treatment	Is less strongly affected by extreme values	Is easy to determine
Is robust	Is less robust	

Measures of Variability

Another important characteristic of a data set, in addition to its central tendency, is its **dispersion,** or **variability.** These terms refer to the amount of "spread" in the data. Exhibit 6.21 shows frequency distributions for two data sets (A and B). Each set has the same number of data items (i.e., the areas under their frequency distribution curves are equal), and their central-tendency measures are identical. However, their degree of variability is quite different, with group A being much less variable than group B. It is not difficult to imagine real situations in which this would be the case. The mean ages of those attending a church picnic and those attending a symphony concert might be very nearly the same, but the age composition of the church gathering would presumably be much wider, since attendees could range from babies to grandparents. To more completely describe the data set (i.e., to provide more information about it), we need measures of variability.

Modal Percentages

If we look at the number of data items that the mode represents in relationship to the total sample size, that is, the frequency of the modal class versus n, we can obtain a rough sense of the variability in the data set. The **modal percentage,** defined as the frequency of the modal class divided by the total sample size n with the result multiplied by 100 to yield percent, is such a measure. The higher the modal percentage, the lower the variability. To illustrate, suppose data set C has 60 items, 20 of which fall in the modal class, and data set D has 90 items, 50 of which fall in the modal class. The modal percentage of data set C is $(20 \div 60) \times$

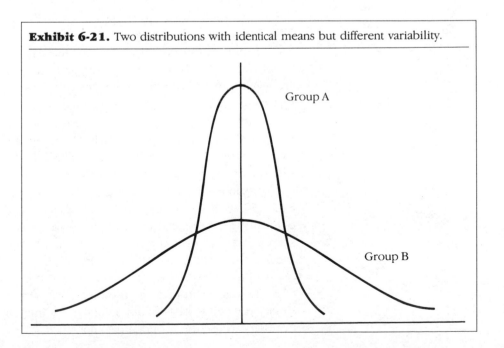

Exhibit 6-21. Two distributions with identical means but different variability.

Group A

Group B

100 = 33 percent while that of data set D is (50 ÷ 90) × 100 = 56 percent, and we would say that data set C has a higher variability than data set D. The modal percentage is very easy to determine and thus has some appeal on this basis alone. Since it is a percentage, comparison with other data sets is simple and straightforward. Finally, if we are dealing with nominal data, the modal percentage is the only practical measure of variability available. Note that while the modal percentage is bounded above by 100 percent (in which case all the data items fell into a single class and there is no variability), it is not bounded below by 0 percent. Since the mode is defined as representing the largest frequency of observations in a distribution, it must contain some items, and so the ratio of the number of data items that the mode represents to the number of items in the entire set must be greater than zero.

Ranges

The Total Range

The total range, commonly called the **range,** is a simple but crude measure of variability. It is simply the difference between the highest and lowest values in the data set. If the highest score on a final examination is 96 and the lowest is 47, the range is 96 − 47 = 49 points. Since the range is based on only two data items and they are the extremes in the group, clearly the range is very sensitive to outliers. Consider what would happen to the above range if the lowest test score had been 23 instead of 47. Another disadvantage of the range as a measure of dispersion is that it really tells us nothing about the extent of variability within the two most extreme data values. The data sets 1, 2, 3, 4, 5, 6, 7, 8, 9 and 1, 5, 5, 5, 5, 5, 5, 5, 9 have the same range (9 − 1 = 8), the same median (5), and the same mean (5), but their degrees of variability are quite different.

The Interquartile Range

We introduced the notion of the quartile earlier. The interquartile range is simply $Q_3 - Q_1$. That is, it is the range of the middle 50 percent of the data (remember that 25 percent of the data falls above Q_3 and 25 percent falls below Q_1). We learned how to calculate the quartiles for grouped data (or for a data set with many repeated values) earlier. Using the values calculated there for the infant birth weight example (namely, Q_3 = 7.40 and Q_1 = 5.72), we see that its interquartile range is 1.68 pounds. To illustrate the determination of the quartiles for an ungrouped data set with few (if any) repeated values, recall our earlier example of 12 nursing students' grades (namely, 47, 58, 62, 69, 71, 79, 84, 84, 88, 89, 93, and 96). Since we have 12 data items, the point at which 25 percent of the distribution is exceeded will lie between the 3rd (0.25 × 12 = 3) and 4th scores. Since in this case Q_1 lies equidistant between them, we calculate their average and write Q_1 = (62 + 69)/2 = 65.5. In a similar fashion, Q_3 will lie between the 9th (0.75 × 12 = 9) and 10th scores and is Q_3 = (88 + 89)/2 = 88.5. The interquartile range is then $Q_3 - Q_1$ = 88.5 − 65.5 = 23. Since the single repeated score (84) did not fall in the immediate vicinity of Q_3, it was not necessary to use the grouped data approach.

The advantage of the interquartile range over the simple range is that by dropping the upper and lower 25 percent of the data, the data set is virtually insensitive to outliers. The smaller the interquartile range on the particular measurement scale of the data set, the lower the variability (or the more "peaked" the distribution). This strength is also a weakness in many instances (data sets without many extreme values), because the interquartile range ignores 50 percent of the data items. Since, like the simple range, it is expressed in terms of the measurement scale of the data, it is difficult to use the interquartile range to compare the variability of data sets with different measurement scales.

Other Measures of Range

One could define a host of other measures of range, such as the interdecile range (D_9 to D_1), based on any of the quantiles. They would offer little overall advantage over the ones already discussed and so are not in common use. Therefore, we do not discuss them further.

Deviations About the Mean

For those data sets that allow the use of the mean (interval or ratio level data), several alternatives that include *all* the data items are available to describe how the observations vary with respect to the mean. We define the **deviation** of an observation as the distance between it and the mean, or more precisely as $X - \bar{X}$. Thus, the deviation is positive for data items that are larger than the mean and negative for data items that are smaller than the mean. By its very definition, the mean is located such that the sum of the deviations is zero. This fundamental fact is illustrated in Exhibit 6.22. Although the sum of $X - \bar{X}$ may not be exactly zero in your calculations owing to rounding error, this is an error (as stated)—the value is precisely zero. Thus, the sum of the deviations is a useless measure.

The Mean Deviation

To avoid the previous difficulty, we could sum the **absolute values** of the deviations, that is, the value irrespective of its algebraic sign and written as $| x |$. Obviously, the sum of absolute values is always positive, and when the sum is divided by the number of items in the data set, the **mean deviation** (MD) is obtained. Mathematically, this can be expressed as

$$MD = \frac{\Sigma | X - \bar{X} |}{n} \qquad (6.7)$$

The interpretation of this value is that it is the average number of measurement units separating any observation from the mean. Thus, for the data given in Exhibit 6.22, the average number of units separating any score from the mean is $MD = 152.67/12 = 12.72$.

Although the mean deviation may have a degree of intuitive meaning as a measure of dispersion that takes the value of every data item into account, the fact that absolute values are not very easily manipulated arithmetically has

Exhibit 6-22. Sum of deviations about the mean for 12 test scores.

X	$X - \bar{X}$	$|X - \bar{X}|$
47	− 29.67	29.67
58	− 18.67	18.67
62	− 14.67	14.67
69	− 7.67	7.67
71	− 5.67	5.67
79	2.33	2.33
84	7.33	7.33
84	7.33	7.33
88	11.33	11.33
89	12.33	12.33
93	16.33	16.33
96	19.33	19.33

$\Sigma X = 920$ $\Sigma(X - \bar{X}) = 0$ $\Sigma |X - \bar{X}| = 152.67$

$\bar{X} = \dfrac{\Sigma X}{n} = 76.67$ $MD = \dfrac{\Sigma |X - \bar{X}|}{n} = 12.72$

caused the mean deviation to be seldom used. Obviously, it has the same units as the measurement scale.

The Sum of Squares

A common ploy to avoid the arithmetic manipulation problems posed by absolute values is to square the values involved. Since the square of either a positive or a negative number is positive, the **sum of squares** (SS) will always be a positive number (and greater than zero). In this context we mean the sum of squares to be the sum of the squared deviations. If we let SS stand for the sum of squares as just defined, we can write

$$SS = \Sigma(X - \bar{X})^2 \tag{6.8}$$

Clearly the sum of squares can range from zero to infinity. The larger the value relative to the measurement scale, the greater the variation in the data set. The fact that SS is a squared value (and dependent on the measurement scale) means that its interpretation usually must be in terms of comparison with the SS of other similar data of interest. Although the sum of squares does not have an immediate intuitive appeal, it is a very valuable and important measure of variation and is used frequently in subsequent chapters. The reason is the fact (which is not proved here) that the sum of the squared deviations about the mean is smaller than the sum of the squared deviations about any other value that might be selected from a given distribution. In mathematic jargon, this is called the *least-squares principle.*

The Variance

Another measure of dispersion that is useful in further statistical analysis is the **variance.** We let V denote the variance; by definition,

$$V = \frac{\Sigma(X - \overline{X})^2}{n} \tag{6.9}$$

Thus, it is the average of the sum of squares. Like the SS, V is a squared value and so lacks an inherent intuitive appeal. Since its value depends on the measurement scale involved, it is difficult to ascribe an absolute meaning to any particular value. But in general, the greater the variance, the greater the dispersion in the data set.

The Standard Deviation

As implied by Reference Note 1, the squaring of a set of scores changes the measurement scale from its original to a relative geometric one. A return to the original can be effected by the reverse operation, namely, taking the square root. We define the standard deviation as the square root of the variance. If we denote it by SD, it can be expressed as

$$SD = \sqrt{V} = \sqrt{\frac{\Sigma(X - \overline{X})^2}{n}} \tag{6.10}$$

The calculation of the standard deviation, although somewhat tedious, is quite straightforward. It is illustrated in Exhibit 6.23 for the example of 12 nursing students' scores. Note that the units of measurement of the standard deviation (unlike those of the variance) are the same as those of the original data set and thus the same as those of the mean.

At this point we must pause and remember that although we are discussing descriptive statistics in this chapter, we are heading toward inferential statistics, which involves making generalizations (from the samples) about the population that the data set is presumed to represent. Although a thorough discussion of the reason is beyond this text or even a reference note, the definition of the standard deviation just given, although precise for the sample, is in a **biased** form when it comes to inference about the population (and the same is true of the variance as introduced earlier). We must replace the value n in equations 6.9 and 6.10 with $n - 1$ if we are to have what, in mathematical terms, are **unbiased,** consistent estimators of the variance and (closely enough for our use) standard deviation of the population from which the sample is drawn. Since this

Exhibit 6-23. Calculation of standard deviation for 12 test scores.

X	$X - \bar{X}$	$(X - \bar{X})^2$
47	−29.67	880.11
58	−18.67	348.44
62	−14.67	215.11
69	−7.67	58.78
71	−5.67	32.11
79	2.33	5.44
84	7.33	53.78
84	7.33	53.78
88	11.33	128.44
89	12.33	152.11
93	16.33	266.78
96	19.33	373.78

$\Sigma X = 920$ $\quad\quad\quad\quad\quad$ SS $= \Sigma(X - \bar{X})^2 = 2{,}568.67$

$$V = \frac{\Sigma(X - \bar{X})^2}{n} = \frac{2{,}568.67}{12} = 214.06$$

$$SD = \sqrt{V} = \sqrt{214.06} = 14.63$$

characteristic is very desirable for future work, we calculate the unbiased variance and standard deviation for any data set as

$$V = \frac{\Sigma(X - \bar{X})^2}{n - 1} \tag{6.11}$$

$$SD = \sqrt{\frac{\Sigma(X - \bar{X})^2}{n - 1}} \tag{6.12}$$

The difference in the unbiased (formula 6.12) and biased (formula 6.10) form of the standard deviation becomes virtually inconsequential for large values of n (say, n greater than 30). In the case of the infant birth weight data given in Exhibit 6.3a, where $n = 120$, the unbiased SD is 1.162 while the biased SD is 1.157.

Just as in the case of the mean discussed earlier, if we are dealing with grouped data, the *exact* value of the sum of squares, the variance, and the standard deviation cannot be determined. Here also, however, a good approximation can be obtained by treating each value in a class as though it equaled the class mark. Again letting f represent the frequency of each individual data class, we can express the respective formulas as

$$SS = \Sigma f(X - \bar{X})^2 \tag{6.13}$$

$$V = \frac{\Sigma f(X - \bar{X})^2}{n - 1} \tag{6.14}$$

$$SD = \sqrt{\frac{\Sigma f(X - \bar{X})^2}{n - 1}} \tag{6.15}$$

The application of these formulas for the grouped set of infant birth weight data given in Exhibit 6.3b is illustrated in Exhibit 6.24. Note that the value of the standard deviation computed in Exhibit 6.24 (1.14) compares very favorably with the exact value computed from the complete data set given in Exhibit 6.3a (1.16).

One problem with the standard deviation as a measure of variability is that it lacks an immediate intuitive meaning. Hopefully, any uneasiness in this regard will be dispelled later when we discuss the normal distribution. For reasons that will become clear then, the standard deviation has become the most popular measure of dispersion for data that allow its use. The interpretation of the standard deviation is that for data sets with comparable means, the greater its value, the greater the variability. For many distributions composed of a large number of observations, the standard deviation is about one-fifth of the range. In the infant birth weight example, one-fifth of the range is $(9.7 - 4.0)/5 = 5.7/5 = 1.15$, which is very close to the value of the standard deviation calculated earlier (1.16). However, for the 12 nursing students' examination scores, one-fifth of the range is $(96 - 47)/5 = 49/5 \approx 10$, while the unbiased standard deviation is 15.3.

Exhibit 6-24. Calculation of the standard deviation for infant birth weights.

X	f	fX	$(X - \bar{X})$	$(X - \bar{X})^2$	$f(X - \bar{X})^2$
4.45	6	26.70	-2.15	4.6225	27.74
5.45	31	168.95	-1.15	1.3225	41.00
6.45	39	251.55	-0.15	0.0225	.88
7.45	31	230.95	0.85	0.7225	22.40
8.45	9	76.05	1.85	3.4225	30.80
9.45	4	37.80	2.85	8.1225	32.49
	$\Sigma f = n = 120$	$\Sigma fX = 792.00$			$\Sigma f(X - \bar{X})^2 = 155.31$

$$\bar{X} = \frac{\Sigma fX}{\Sigma f} = \frac{792}{120} = 6.60$$

$$V = \frac{\Sigma f(X - \bar{X})^2}{n - 1} = \frac{155.31}{119} = 1.31$$

$$SD = \sqrt{V} = \sqrt{\frac{\Sigma(X - \bar{X})^2}{n - 1}} = \sqrt{1.31} = 1.14$$

Exhibit 6-25. Estimating SD from the range for small data sets.

Sample size n		3	4	5	6	7	8	9	10
Divisor	d	1.7	2.0	2.3	2.5	2.7	2.8	3.0	3.0

SD *Range*

To illustrate, consider the following data set:

X	$X - \bar{X}$	$(X - \bar{X})^2$
4	-7.5	56.25
6	-5.5	30.25
16	4.5	20.25
20	8.5	72.25

$\Sigma X = 46$ $\qquad\qquad\qquad\qquad \Sigma(X - \bar{X})^2 = 179$

$$\bar{X} = \frac{46}{4} = 11.5 \qquad\qquad SD = \sqrt{\frac{179}{3}} = 7.7$$

The approximate SD value estimated from the range is

$$SD \approx \frac{20 - 4}{2.0} = 8$$

Thus, this rough rule of thumb is most useful as a check whether a calculated standard deviation is in the right ballpark. If the number of data items n is small, an appropriate divisor d is used instead of 5. This is noted in Exhibit 6.25 with an illustration. By using the small sample range divisor of 3.2 for the examination scores, the approximate value of the SD is $(96 - 47)/3.2 = 15.3$, which happens to be the correct value in this case. The values for the divisor given in Exhibit 6.25 are very closely approximated by $\sqrt{n}$. Thus, for data sets with a small number of items, say 15 or fewer, we can find an approximate value for the standard deviation by using the formula

$$SD \approx \frac{\text{range}}{\sqrt{n}} \qquad\qquad\qquad (6.16)$$

and we avoid having to refer to the table in Exhibit 6.25. Another useful point to note arises from what, in mathematical jargon, is known as Chebyshev's theorem and is the fact that for *any* frequency distribution, *at least* 75 percent of the data items will fall within 2 standard deviations above and below the mean.

We conclude our discussion of the standard deviation by noting that while formulas 6.12 and 6.15 served well to introduce the notion of the unbiased SD

Exhibit 6-26. Calculation of SD for 12 test scores by using computational formula.

X	X^2
47	2,209
58	3,364
62	3,844
69	4,761
71	5,041
79	6,241
84	7,056
84	7,056
88	7,744
89	7,921
93	8,649
96	9,216
$\Sigma X = 920$	$\Sigma X^2 = 73,102$

$$\text{SD} = \sqrt{\frac{\Sigma X^2 - \dfrac{1}{n}(\Sigma X)^2}{n - 1}} = \sqrt{\frac{73,102 - \frac{1}{12}(920)^2}{12 - 1}} = 15.28$$

for ungrouped and grouped data, we can use some algebraic manipulation to convert them to forms that lend themselves more readily to hand calculation:

$$\text{SD} = \sqrt{\frac{\Sigma X^2 - (1/n)(\Sigma X)^2}{n - 1}} \qquad \text{ungrouped data} \qquad (6.17)$$

$$\text{SD} = \sqrt{\frac{\Sigma fX^2 - (1/n)(\Sigma fX)^2}{n - 1}} \qquad \text{grouped data} \qquad (6.18)$$

and are sometimes called the **computational formulas,** as opposed to the **conceptual formulas,** for obvious reasons. Their use is illustrated in Exhibit 6.26, where we repeat the calculation of the SD for our 12 nursing students' test scores.

The Coefficient of Variation

A disadvantage of the standard deviation is that it is expressed in the units of the measurement scale being used, which does not aid in comparison of different data sets. For example, the standard deviation of a set of temperature data is 1°F. We can really tell very little about the amount of variability present because, to do so, we need a sense of the temperature of the object of measurement. If the object of measurement were body temperature, the data set would be more dispersed than if, say, the object of measurement were the boiling point of water. Thus, we would like a measure of variation that accounts for the central tendency of the data set. One such measure, which is increasing in popularity as more and more researchers become accustomed to its use, is the **coefficient of variation** (sometimes called the **relative standard deviation**), which is defined as the standard deviation divided by the mean and is written as CV. Its formula is

$$CV = \frac{SD}{\overline{X}} \qquad\qquad (6.19)$$

Using the coefficient of variation, we can readily compare the dispersion of our nursing students' test score data set with that of the infant birth weight data set. For the former, CV = 15.28/76.67 = 0.20, while for the latter CV = 1.16/6.95 = 0.17. We interpret this to mean that the dispersion of the two data sets is similar, with that of the test scores being a bit larger than that of the birth weights. By contrast, the coefficient of variation of the data set given in Exhibit 6.25 is CV = 7.7/11.5 = 0.76, and its variability is considerably higher than that of either of the two preceding data sets. In addition, some workers multiply the CV as defined above by 100 and thus express it as a percentage.

Comparison of the Standard Deviation, Interquartile Range, and Modal Frequency

All the measures of variability that we have discussed fall into three general categories: the deviations from the mean, the ranges, and the modal frequency. These are directly analogous to the three categories of central-tendency measures—the means, the quantiles, and the modes, or modal classes. The allowable measures of dispersion for the different levels of measurement are shown in Exhibit 6.27. With nominal level data, only the modal frequency is possible. With ordinal level data, we can use the modal frequency or any of the range measures. With interval and ratio level data, we can use any of the measures of dispersion discussed.

Of all the measures of variation discussed, the standard deviation (including its coefficient-of-variation form), the interquartile range, and the modal frequency probably will be most useful. We summarize their features in Exhibit 6.28. Of the three, the standard deviation is by far the most useful when interval or ratio level data are involved. When you are dealing with ordinal level data,

---

Exhibit 6-27. Allowable dispersion measures by measurement level.

Measurement Level	Allowable Dispersion Measure
Nominal data	Modal frequency
Ordinal data	Modal frequency, ranges
Interval data	Modal frequency, ranges, deviations
Ratio data	Modal frequency, ranges, deviations

Exhibit 6-28. Comparison of features of standard deviation, interquartile range, and modal frequency.

Standard Deviation	Interquartile Range	Modal Frequency
Always exists	Always exists	May not exist
Is unique	Is unique	May not be unique
Accounts for the value of each item	Can be found with open classes	Is only a crude indicator
Lends itself to further statistical treatment	Ignores extreme values	Is easy to determine
Is robust	Only uses 50% of the data	Is expressed in percentage
Is expressed in measurement units	Is expressed in measurement units	

either the interquartile range of the modal frequency may be the statistic of choice, depending on the nature of the data. If the frequency distribution is bimodal, the interquartile range probably will be preferred. With nominal level data, there is no choice other than the modal frequency.

Measures of Distribution Shape

Recall the definition of a frequency polygon; it is the class marks of the data classes in the histogram connected by a series of straight lines (see Exhibit 6.10). Now, suppose that we increase our sample size and as a result could increase the number of data classes (i.e., decrease the data class interval). The result would be a greater number of data class marks and, consequently, shorter line segments in the frequency polygon. If we continued this process, we could obtain a very fine-grained frequency polygon, like the one shown in Exhibit 6.29. If we were to continue this process, as our sample size would approach infinity, the data class interval would approach zero, and the frequency polygon would approach a smooth curve. This curve is, in reality, the frequency distribution of the population from which we drew our sample, and by letting our sample approach infinity, what we have really done is sample the entire population. Do not let the idea of an infinite population confuse you. Here, when we speak of a population, we mean all measures of a given variable. For example, suppose that a dependent variable is body temperature and that we have an error-free measurement instrument of unbounded precision. The measurement scale may well be bounded below by 96°F and above by 106°F, but between these limits there are an infinite number of possible readings, since 98.65432...°F is different from 98.65431...°F, and so on. Thus, a finite sample is an approximation of the population from which it is drawn, and this concept is

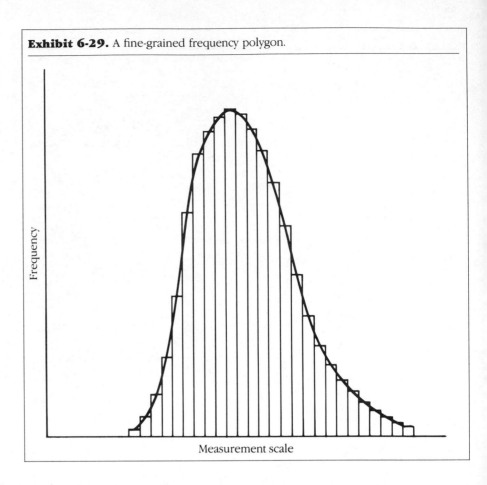

Exhibit 6-29. A fine-grained frequency polygon.

(y-axis label: Frequency)

(x-axis label: Measurement scale)

at the heart of inferential statistics, as discussed in later chapters. Henceforth in this chapter, we use curves to represent our frequency distributions, and it is the shape of these curves that we want to discuss here. While the shapes of distribution curves can vary in an infinite number of ways, we can use some standard terms to describe them. Since the shape of a distribution can yield some very important information about the population that it represents, we need to become familiar with the terms used to describe them.

Symmetry

A **symmetrical** distribution is one for which a line exists such that if the curve on one side of the line were to be rotated through 180°, it would form the other half of the curve (i.e., the left half and the right half of the curves are mirror images). This line is called the **axis of symmetry.** Some examples of symmetrical distributions are given in Exhibit 6.30. We note that the property of symmetry places no other restriction on the shape of the curve. Thus, the distributions in Exhibit 6.30 and c are bimodal, the one in Exhibit 6.30a is unimodal, and the one in Exhibit 6.30d is flat; we could just as easily have included a trimodal

Exhibit 6-30. Some symmetric distribution shapes.

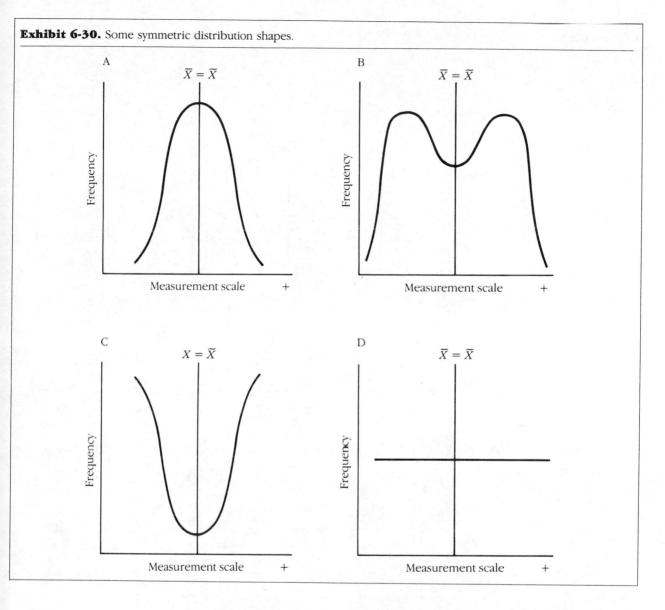

example, and so on, but these should be sufficient to make the point. The property of symmetry can be described mathematically as follows. Let y represent the distance along the measurement scale measured from the axis of symmetry, and call distances to the right of it positive (so that distances to the left are negative). A curve is symmetric if

$$f(+y) = f(-y) \qquad (6.20)$$

That is, if the frequency of a measurement some distance to the right of the axis of symmetry is exactly equal to the frequency of a measurement the same

Exhibit 6-31. Some skewed distribution shapes.

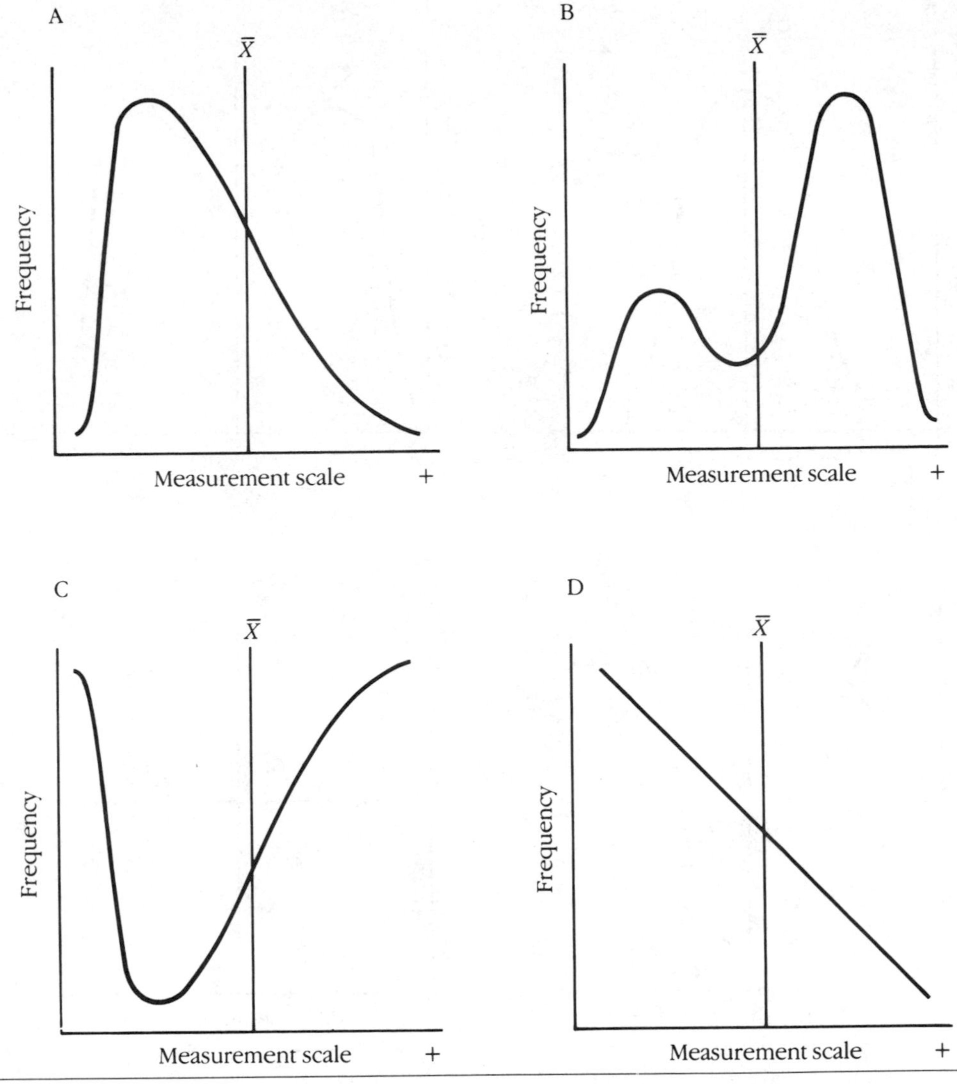

A

B

C

D

distance to the left, we say that the distribution is symmetrical. It is a characteristic (which can be proved mathematically) of a symmetrical distribution that the mean and the median are equal and their location defines the axis of symmetry. However, the converse is not true; that is, just because the mean is equal to the median, it does not necessarily imply that the distribution is symmetrical.

Skewness

If a distribution is not symmetrical, we say that it is skewed. Some examples of **skewed distributions** are given in Exhibit 6.31. Here, also, the distributions in Exhibit 6.31a and d are unimodal, while that depicted in Exhibit 6.31b can be considered bimodal. Mathematically, a curve is skewed **(asymmetrical)** if

$$f(+y) \neq f(-y) \tag{6.21}$$

If the distribution has the property that

$$f(+y) < f(-y) \tag{6.22}$$

which we read to mean that the frequency at some distance above the mean is *less* than the corresponding frequency at the same distance below the mean, then we say that the distribution is **positively skewed,** or that it possesses **positive skewness.** In such a case, the bulk of the data are found at the low end of the measurement scale. Conversely, if the distribution has the property that

$$f(+y) > f(-y) \tag{6.23}$$

which we read to mean that the frequency at some distance above the mean is *greater* than the corresponding frequency at the same distance below the mean, then we say that the distribution is **negatively skewed,** or that it possesses **negative skewness.** In this case, the bulk of the data are found at the high end of the measurement scale. The frequency distributions in Exhibit 6.31a and d are positively skewed, while those in Exhibit 6.31b and c are negatively skewed.

Various measures of **skewness** have been proposed, many of which are attributable to Karl Pearson, who did much of the pioneering work with frequency distribution shapes. The most popular measure of skewness today is derived from the theory of moments (see Reference Note 2) and can be written as

$$\text{Skewness} = \frac{\Sigma(X - \overline{X})^3}{n(\text{SD}^3)} \tag{6.24}$$

We note that since X, $\overline{X}$, and SD all have the same units of measure (dimensions), the expression for skewness given by Equation 6.24 is a pure number; that is, it is **dimensionless,** just like a percentage. For symmetric distributions, the value of the skewness as expressed by formula 6.24 is zero. The measure of skewness is positive for positively skewed distributions and negative for negatively skewed ones. For a positively skewed unimodal distribution, it can be shown that $\overline{X} > \widetilde{X}$ > mode, and for one which is negatively skewed, $\overline{X} < \widetilde{X} <$ mode. These relative locations of the mean, median, and mode for skewed distributions are illustrated in Exhibit 6.32.

Kurtosis

The final measure of the distribution curve shape that we discuss is its **peakedness,** or **kurtosis.** This is related to the relative curvature of the distribution, and examples are given in Exhibit 6.33. You do *not* have to memorize

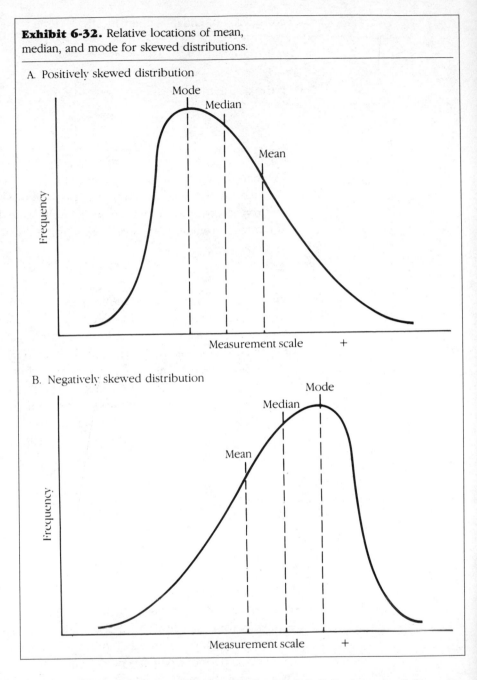

Exhibit 6-32. Relative locations of mean, median, and mode for skewed distributions.

A. Positively skewed distribution

B. Negatively skewed distribution

the jargon (leptokurtic, mesokurtic, and platykurtic). As in the case of skewness, a number of measures of kurtosis have been suggested, but one of the most common ones today is

$$\text{Kurtosis} = \frac{\Sigma(X - \overline{X})^4}{n(\text{SD}^4)} - 3 \qquad (6.25)$$

Exhibit 6-33. Leptokurtic, mesokurtic, and platykurtic distributions.

A. Leptokurtic (peaked) distribution

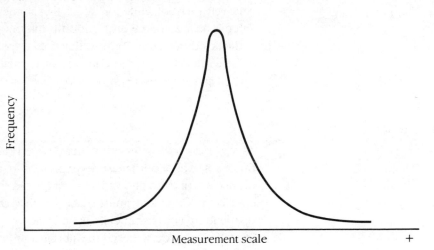

B. Mesokurtic distribution

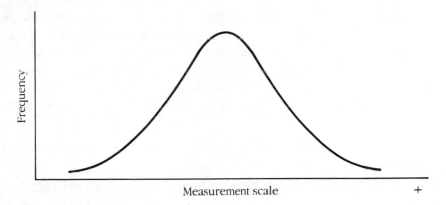

C. Platykurtic (flat) distribution

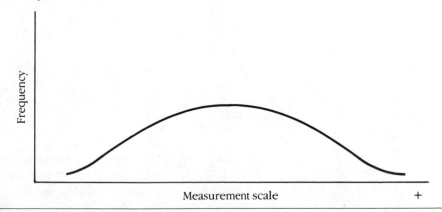

where the biased form of SD is used. Note that this measurement for kurtosis is dimensionless (for the same reason that the measure of skewness was). For kurtosis values as expressed by formula 6.25 that are positive the curve is relatively peaked, while for values that are negative it is relatively flat. When the value is near zero, the distribution is intermediate (mesokurtic). The number 3 is deducted in formula 6.25 so that the kurtosis of a very important distribution, to be discussed later, the Gaussian or normal distribution, will be exactly zero; thus, it can serve as a comparative base for other distributions.

The *z* Score

As you may have guessed, generally we find it advantageous for comparison purposes to have our measures expressed in dimensionless form, that is, as pure numbers. This also allows us to readily see the *relative location* of a particular data item within the entire data set, that is, where it falls in the frequency distribution. For example, if you are told that your score on a particular test was 55, you really know very little about how well you did relatively. You might wonder whether your score is high, low, or average. However, if you know something about the frequency distribution of the scores for this test, you can judge the location of your score in the distribution. Your score of 55 takes on one meaning if the mean for the test is 30 and the standard deviation is 10 and quite a different one if the mean is 60 and the standard deviation is 20.

We can transform a set of scores (values of a data set) into **relative deviates,** or **standardized scores,** by expressing the deviation from the mean $X - \overline{X}$ in terms of standard deviation units. It is often called a **z score:**

$$z = \frac{X - \overline{X}}{\text{SD}} \tag{6.26}$$

Formula 6.26 expresses each score (data item) as a deviation from the mean in standard deviation units. The z scores for the two distributions given previously are

$$z_1 = \frac{55 - 30}{10} = 2.5$$

and

$$z_2 = \frac{55 - 60}{20} = -0.25$$

Thus, in the first instance the score was considerably above average, while in the second it was somewhat below average. In general, a positive z score indicates that the score from which it was calculated falls above the mean, while a negative z score indicates that it falls below the mean. To repeat, you should realize that from its definition as expressed in formula 6.26, the z score represents the deviation from the mean in standard deviation units. Thus, a z score of 1.0 indicates that the corresponding observation falls 1.0 standard deviation units above the mean, a score of -2.5 indicates that it falls 2.5 standard deviation units below the mean, and so on.

As shown in Reference Note 3, the mean of a set of z scores is zero, and its standard deviation is unity (that is, 1). We have merely changed the scale of measurement; we have not altered the frequency of occurrence (i.e., the frequency of a z score is exactly the same as that of the raw score X that it represents). Such a transformation is equivalent to shifting the origin along the X axis to the mean and changing the scale so as to make the standard deviation unity. You should not be skeptical about such "rubber sheet" geometry, because we encountered shifts in origins earlier and you have experienced changes in scale in everyday life. When you change inches to feet, feet to miles, and particularly degrees Fahrenheit to degrees Celsius, you have done the very same thing.

The use of the z score takes on an even greater significance when we discuss the normal distribution, but note that its underlying significance holds for *any* frequency distribution.

The Normal Distribution

As we noted earlier, continuous sample spaces arise whenever we deal with quantitative data that are measured on **continuous scales** (either interval or ratio levels of measurement). This is the case, for example, when we measure the weight of a patient, the time of response to an injection, the amount of nicotine in a cigarette, and so on. Although it is true that we round our answers to the least significant digit justifiable by our measuring instrument (i.e., the nearest whole number or a few decimals), there is a continuum of possible values. This realization led us to suggest earlier that, in the limit, the *possible* histogram for a data set might be better represented by a continuous curve. All the other concepts remain the same, but now, instead of speaking of the areas of rectangles, we speak of the area *under a curve* (more about this later).

Having recalled this concept, there is a continuous frequency distribution with a domain that is all the real numbers and that has assumed prominence among all others (of which, of course, there are an infinite number). This particular distribution was introduced in the thesis of an 18-year-old mathematician named Gauss (1777–1855) and for many years was simply referred to as the **Gaussian distribution.** Today it is more commonly called the **normal distribution.** It arose from the observation that variations among repeated measurements of the same physical quantity displayed a surprising degree of regularity, and it was found that their distribution could be closely approximated by a certain kind of curve—the normal distribution (see Reference Note 5).

There are two key points here. The first is that the term "normal" arises from

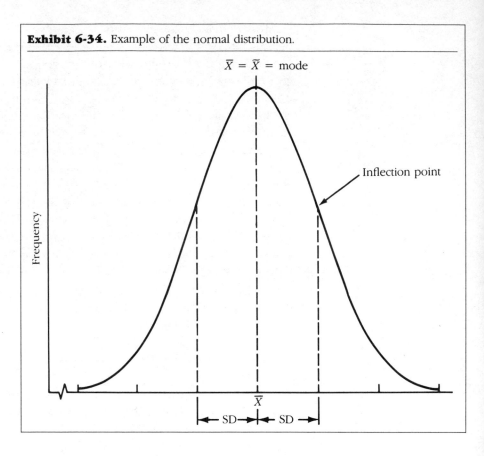

Exhibit 6-34. Example of the normal distribution.

mathematical rather than medical considerations. There is nothing to imply that other types of distribution are abnormal or defective (or even unusual) in any manner. The second point, which really serves to reinforce the first, is that no distribution actually encountered in practice is *exactly* normal, because a true normal distribution is a mathematical construct—an ideal which may be approximated ever so closely but never truly attained. The normal curve is depicted in Exhibit 6.34.

Properties of the Normal Distribution

From its mathematical properties (explained more fully by the formula given in Reference Note 5) and visual inspection of Exhibit 6.34, we note that the normal distribution possesses the following properties:

1. It is symmetrical about its mean.
2. It is unimodal.
3. It is continuous for all values and contains an infinite number of them (i.e., its domain is from $-\infty$ to $+\infty$; therefore, it never quite touches the horizontal axis (i.e., it is *asymptotic* to it).
4. Any interval representing any degree of deviation from the mean is possible.

5. The mean, median, and mode are equal ($\overline{X} = \widetilde{X}$ = mode).
6. Its measures of skewness and kurtosis are zero.
7. "Most" values are near the mean, with their number drastically decreasing at significant deviations from the mean.
8. Its **inflection points** (points where the curvature changes sign) are located 1 standard deviation to either side of the mean.
9. It is a two-parameter distribution; that is, it is completely defined by the values of its mean and standard deviation.

Standardized Normal Distribution

The concept of a **standardized normal distribution** (explained in Reference Note 4) is very important because it allows us to use a single table to obtain the values of *any* normal distribution, given the values of $\overline{X}$ and SD. The standardized normal distribution is expressed in *z* score terms; that is, it has a mean of zero and a standard deviation of unity. Therefore, if we want to find the value of a score *X* in a normal distribution with a mean of 60 and a standard deviation of 10, we simply look up the value associated with a *z* score of $(X - 60)/10$, and this gives us the desired number. [Remember that the *z* score was defined so that $z = (X - \overline{X})/\text{SD}$.] This shift of scale is illustrated in Exhibit 6.35.

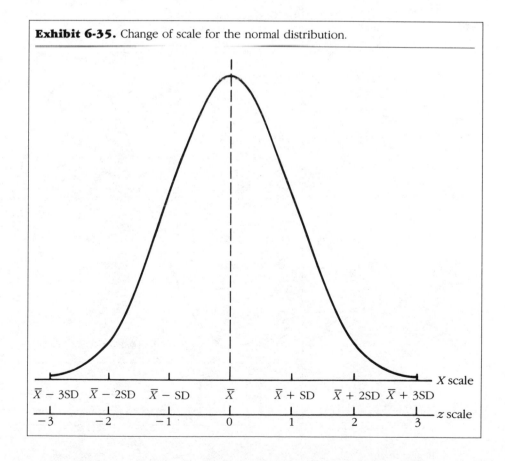

Exhibit 6-35. Change of scale for the normal distribution.

The Area Under the Normal Curve

We made a big point earlier that the *area under* a histogram truly represented the frequency for any particular data class interval. In the same fashion, the *area under the distribution curve* for a particular data interval indicates its frequency. Consider Exhibit 6.36. The proportions of the area under the curve are indicated for intervals of 1 standard deviation. For example, 0.1359 (or 13.59 percent) of the area lies between 1 and 2 standard deviations. We would multiply this value by the total area under the curve if we wanted to express it as a number. If this is considered to be a standardized normal distribution, the values in Exhibit 6.36 would be actual areas, since the total area under the standardized normal distribution is unity (as pointed out in Reference Note 5).

We note from Exhibit 6.36 that $0.3413 + 0.3413 = 0.6816$ of the area (i.e., about 68 percent of the data) falls within ± 1 standard deviation of the mean, that is, within $\overline{X} \pm$ SD. Similarly $0.1359 + 0.3413 + 0.3413 + 0.1359 = 0.9544$, or about 95 percent, of the data falls within ± 2 standard deviations of the mean, and 0.9972 (over 99 percent) of the data falls within 3 standard deviations on either side of the mean.

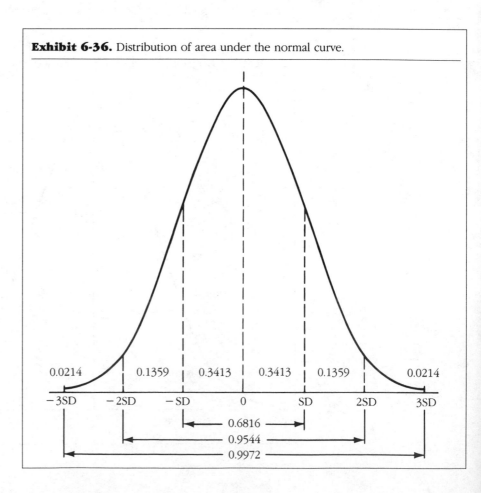

Exhibit 6-36. Distribution of area under the normal curve.

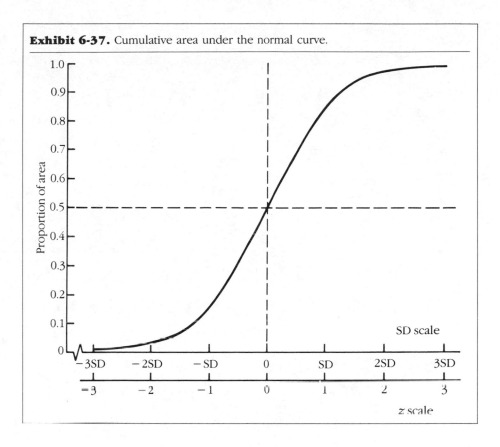

Exhibit 6-37. Cumulative area under the normal curve.

The area under the normal frequency distribution curve can be plotted (remember our earlier discussion of cumulative frequencies) and is shown in Exhibit 6.37. This curve is often referred to as the *normal curve integral,* because a mathematical procedure known as integration is used to determine the area under a curve. This curve also possesses a certain kind of symmetry.

The Use of Tables

The values for the area under the normal curve as measured from the mean are given in terms of z scores in Appendix III, Table B. Because of the symmetry of the normal curve, the values are the same for positive and negative z scores; that is, the area under the normal curve from the mean to some distance to the right is identical to the area under the normal curve from the mean to the same distance to the left (recall Exhibit 6.36). As an example, using Table B, Appendix III, find the area under the normal curve between $z = 0$ and $z = -1.47$. We go down the z column in the table until we reach the first two significant digits (1.4) and then go across that row to pick up the third significant digit (.07) and read .4292 (or about 43 percent) of the area. For the next example, find the area under the normal curve to the *left* of $z = -1.47$. To do this, we use the fact that the mean divides the area under the normal curve exactly in half; that is, 50

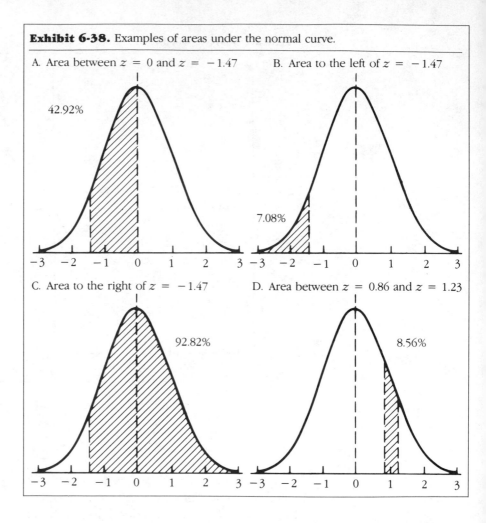

Exhibit 6-38. Examples of areas under the normal curve.

A. Area between $z = 0$ and $z = -1.47$

42.92%

B. Area to the left of $z = -1.47$

7.08%

C. Area to the right of $z = -1.47$

92.82%

D. Area between $z = 0.86$ and $z = 1.23$

8.56%

percent lies to the left and 50 percent lies to the right of the mean. Therefore, since .4292 of the area lies between the mean and $z = -1.47$, $.5000 - .4292 = .0708$ of the area lies to the left of $z = -1.47$. In a similar fashion, the area that lies to the *right* of $z = -1.47$ is $.5000 + .4292 = .9282$. Note that the proportions of the area lying to the left and the right of *any* z score must sum to unity, as do .0708 and .9282. As a final example, find the area under the normal curve between $z = 0.86$ and $z = 1.23$. We go down the z score column in the table to 0.8 and across to .06 and read .3051. We next go down the z score column to 1.2 and across to .03 and read .3907. Since these are the proportional areas from the mean to each z score, we simply take $.3907 - .3051 = .0856$ to obtain the answer. These examples are illustrated in Exhibit 6.38.

In summary, if we want to find the area that lies to the *left* of a given z score, we add the tabulated value to .5000 if z is positive and subtract it from .5000 if z is negative. To find the area that lies to the *right* of a given z score, we simply reverse the process; that is, we subtract the table value from .5000 if z is positive and add it to .5000 if z is negative. To find the area under the normal curve *between* any two given z scores, we subtract their tabulated values if the z scores have the same sign (are either both positive or both negative) and add their tabulated values if one z score is plus and the other is minus. Do not be discouraged if all this seems complicated at first. With a little practice and reference to Exhibit 6.38, it will become clear rather quickly.

As another illustration, suppose you had taken a test (presumably designed to produce a normal distribution of scores) and were told that the class mean was 63, its standard deviation was 10, and your grade was 71. To get a better idea of how well you did in relation to the others in the class, first you would compute your z score as $(71 - 63)/10 = .80$. Going to Table B in Appendix III, you see that the area under the normal curve for $z = .80$ is .2881. Now you know that you did better than about 79 percent of the class, since the area under the normal curve to the left of your z score—the proportion of the class who did more poorly than you—is $.5000 + .2881 = .7881$. However, you also know that around 21 percent of the class outperformed you on this test, since the area to the right of your z score is $.5000 - .2881 = .2119$. Suppose, now, that you wish to find the score of a classmate who, like you, knows about z scores and the normal curve and told you that 40 percent of the class did better than she on this particular test. You realize that she has told you that the area to the right of her z score is .40, and so you subtract this from .5000 to get .1000. You enter the body of the table and see that this value represents a z score between .25 and .26. Since it is closer to .25, you use that value and calculate her grade, using the formula for the z score, $(X - 63)/10 = .25$, to obtain $X = (.25)(10) + 63 = 65.5$. Had you needed to obtain a more accurate value for her z score from the table, you could have used a simple procedure called **interpolation,** which is discussed in Reference Note 2 of Chapter 16, but a higher level of precision was not warranted in this case. The important point here is that you can use the table either way, that is, by using a given tabular value to look up the value of the z score or by looking up a tabular value for a given z score.

Confidence Intervals and Sample Size

When we sample from a population and calculate a mean, often we wish to use this sample mean to estimate the population mean μ [called mu ("mew")]. In so doing, we are departing from the domain of descriptive statistics, strictly speaking, and entering the domain of inferential statistics (more about this in Chapter 15). Of course, we could say that since we took a "representative" sample, its mean and the population mean are the same. We could say that, but very likely we would be *wrong!* It is quite unlikely that if we took another sample (even of the same size) from the same population, we would get exactly the same mean (recall Reference Note 4). Fortunately, there are better ways to get at this problem, but first we need an understanding of the concept of likelihood or **probability.** There are a number of approaches to and definitions of probability, but the one that we introduce is called the *frequency concept of probability*. We speak of the probability of an event as the proportion of the time that this event will occur in the long run, that is, over a large number of trials. Thus, the probability of a uniform coin coming up heads when it is tossed is 0.5, since there are two ways it could land (heads or tails) and we are interested in one of those ways (heads). Now it is quite possible that out of 10 tosses we might have realized 6 heads and 4 tails (which might lead you to conclude that the probability is 6/10 = 0.6), but in the long run—say, after 100 tosses—you might have realized 52 heads and 48 tails, and after 1,000 tosses, 501 heads and 499 tails. Similarly, the probability of any given number (say 3) coming up on the roll of a die is 1/6 = .1666 ... since (if the die is fair) each of the six numbers has an equal likelihood of coming up. We cannot guarantee that we will get exactly one 3 in six rolls of the die; but on average, if we wagered $1 on the number 3 and received $6 each time it came up, we would break even in the long run. Within this context, when we say a given event has a probability of .95, we are saying that it will occur 95 out of 100 times on average. Another way of saying this is that we are 95 percent confident that it will occur.

Confidence Intervals

A second difficulty is associated with simply asserting that the population mean is the same as the sample mean. Such a statement is called a **point estimation** and, being fraught with uncertainty, is seldom used in serious work. Another way of saying this is that, in making such an unqualified statement, there is no way of knowing the accuracy of the estimation. Therefore, researchers usually prefer to establish **confidence limits,** the distance between which we call a **confidence interval** and within which we expect the population statistic (e.g., the mean) will fall a certain percentage of the time in the long run. We use the term "confidence" here to mean *probability,* except that usually we express confidence in percentages. Thus if a given event has a 0.95 probability of occurrence, we say that we are 95 percent *confident* that it will occur, meaning that it will occur 95 times out of 100 on average.

From the earlier discussions in this chapter, clearly our problem of estimating the population mean from the sample mean will involve the distributions involved. Let us assume that our population has an almost normal distribution. We saw earlier that 95 percent of the area of a normal curve fell within 2 standard deviations of the mean (1.96 to be exact) and 99 percent fell within 2.575 standard deviations of the mean. Making use of the fact that the population mean is *about* normally distributed with a *population* standard deviation, called the **standard error,** about equal to the *sample* standard deviation divided by the square root of the size of the sample ($SD/\sqrt{n}$), we can establish confidence intervals around the sample mean (see Reference Note 4 and Chapter 15). The method presented here applies to samples at least as large as 30. For smaller samples see Reference Note 6.

Suppose a mean of 72 in sexual liberalism (where the possible range of scores is from 16 to 96 or 80) was found among 36 nursing students. We wish to estimate the population mean (presumably the population is all nursing students at the school) at a confidence level of 95 percent. Obviously, we need one more piece of information, namely, the standard deviation of the test scores. We could use our range rule (SD is approximately one-fifth of the range) to estimate it and find

$$SD \approx \frac{96 - 16}{5} = 16$$

but we are told that it was calculated to be 17, and so we use that value. We can use Table B in Appendix III to find that 95 percent of the area under the normal curve falls within 1.96 standard deviations of the mean. We then calculate the standard error of the mean:

$$SE = \frac{SD}{\sqrt{n}} = \frac{17}{\sqrt{36}} = \frac{17}{6} = 2.83 \tag{6.27}$$

To obtain our desired 95 percent confidence level, we multiply the standard error by 1.96 and then add it to and subtract it from the mean to obtain the respective upper and lower **confidence limits:**

$(2.83)(1.96) = 5.5468$
$72 + 5.547 = 77.547$ (upper confidence limit)
$72 - 5.547 = 66.453$ (lower confidence limit)

We interpret this to mean that we can be 95 percent certain that the population mean falls between 66 and 78 for this test. That is, 95 percent of the time, $66 < \mu < 78$.

If we want to be 99 percent sure, we find from Table B in Appendix III that 99 percent of the area under the normal curve falls within 2.575 standard deviations of the mean, and we calculate

$(2.83)(2.575) = 7.287$
$72 + 7.287 = 79.287$ (upper confidence limit)
$72 - 7.287 = 64.713$ (lower confidence limit)

We conclude that 99 times out of 100 the population mean will fall between 65 and 79, or, to state it another way, on average only 1 replication out of 100 will fall outside this range.

We can summarize this notion as follows:

$$\bar{X} - z\frac{SD}{\sqrt{n}} < \mu < \bar{X} + z\frac{SD}{\sqrt{n}} \tag{6.28}$$

where z is the z score corresponding to the proportional area under the normal curve equal to one-half our desired confidence level; for example, for a 90 percent confidence level $z = 1.645$, for a 96 percent confidence level $z = 1.9600$, for a 99 percent confidence level $z = 2.575$, and so on. To illustrate the use of formula 6.28, suppose that we are told that, for a sample of 36 subjects, the mean of some measured attribute is $\overline{X} = 7.26$ and the standard deviation is SD $= 1.92$. We are asked to provide an estimate of the mean of the population (that the subjects presumably represent) at the 98 percent confidence level. We first go to Table B in Appendix III and look up the z score corresponding to a proportional area under the normal curve equal to $.98/2 = .4600$. We interpolate to find $z = 1.751$, and substituting into formula 6.28, we obtain

$$7.26 - (1.751)\frac{1.92}{\sqrt{36}} < \mu < 7.26 + (1.751)\frac{1.92}{\sqrt{36}}$$

$$7.26 - .56 < \mu < 7.26 + .56$$

$$6.70 < \mu < 7.82$$

We could state our answer as follows: If we assume that the population is approximately normal, 98 percent of the time its mean will fall between 6.70 and 7.82.

Suppose that on receiving our answer we are told that this confidence interval $(7.82 - 6.70 = 1.12)$ is a little too large, and we were asked what level of confidence we would have if it were only 1.0. Since we know from formula 6.28 that our upper confidence limit is $\overline{X} + (z)$ SD/$\sqrt{n}$ and our lower confidence limit is $\overline{X} - (z)$ SD/$\sqrt{n}$, we take their difference (i.e., upper minus lower) to find an expression for the confidence interval:

$$X + z\frac{SD}{\sqrt{n}} - \left(X - z\frac{SD}{\sqrt{n}}\right) = 2z\frac{SD}{\sqrt{n}}$$

Since we were told that a confidence interval of unity was desired, we substitute our values and obtain

$$2z\frac{(1.92)}{\sqrt{36}} = 1$$

$$z = \frac{6}{(2)(1.92)} = 1.56$$

Referring to Table B in Appendix III, we see that the proportional area under the normal curve corresponding to $z = 1.56$ is $.4406$. Multiplying this value by 2 (we have to account for the area under the other half of the normal curve), we have $.8812$ and can state that we are 88 percent confident that the mean will fall between 6.76 and 7.76. Note how the level of confidence dropped (from 98 to 88 percent) for such a seemingly small narrowing of our confidence limits (i.e., from 6.70 to 6.76 for the lower and from 7.82 to 7.76 for the upper).

Sample Size

To close the circle, let us suppose that the results in the sexual liberalism example were from a pilot test and that we can tolerate as a confidence interval a range of no more than 8 (in the raw score units) for our estimate of the population mean at the 99 percent confidence level. We want to know what the minimum sample size for our research project must be. To answer this, first we assume that the population standard deviation is the same as that of our pilot test. Since we seek confidence limits of $8 \div 2 = 4$ raw score units on either side of (i.e., above and below) the mean, we set this equal to the desired standard error $[(2.575)(SD/\sqrt{n})$ in this case] and obtain

$$\frac{(2.575)(17)}{\sqrt{n}} = 4$$

$$\sqrt{n} = \frac{(2.575)(17)}{4} = 10.9438$$

$$n = 119.77$$

or a sample size of 120 is required. Had we been willing to accept a 95 percent confidence level on our acceptable interval of 8 raw score units, the required sample size would have been

$$\frac{(1.960)(17)}{\sqrt{n}} = 4$$

$$n = \left[\frac{(1.96)(17)}{4}\right]^2 = 69.39$$

or a sample size of 70, showing again the price that we have to pay in sample size for a seemingly small increase in our confidence level.

In general, if we want the estimate of the population mean to be within plus or minus some value (say, k) of the sample $\overline{X}$, we can use the following formula:

$$n = \left[\frac{(z)(SD)}{k}\right]^2 \tag{6.29}$$

where n = required sample size
z = z score corresponding to one-half the confidence level expressed as a proportion
k = one-half the desired confidence interval in raw score units
SD = standard deviation of sample

When you have an estimation of the population standard deviation from the literature or a pilot study, this is a very useful method for determining the required *minimum* sample size for a survey. Again we stress that these are *minimum* sample sizes, i.e., those that would be required if the distribution were *exactly* normal. If it is nearly so, this sample size or one slightly larger should suffice. Similar procedures exist for estimating confidence limits for the population standard deviation, but they are based on more advanced mathematical concepts which are beyond the scope of this book.

Putting It All Together

To sum up much of what has been presented in this chapter so far, assume that you are a student in a class of 36, which is one section out of three of a particular course. All classes are given their final examination on the same day, and you are now anxiously awaiting your final grade. On your second trip to your instructor's office, you find that final grades have still not been posted, but the following are scores for your section:

85	92	64	52	71	86
77	85	75	65	76	77
58	73	87	73	84	65
85	75	79	74	82	72
65	75	68	88	78	67
75	63	98	62	66	83

You quickly copy these and later begin to analyze them. The analysis you might perform is shown in Exhibit 6.39. You decide to use the indicated data classes, recognizing that the class intervals are not exactly equal, but you are in a hurry. Tallying the scores, you obtain the frequency distribution given and decide to work with the grouped data. Using the formulas given in this chapter, you calculate the various measures of central tendency, variability, and shape, as indicated in Exhibit 6.39.

From your results, you know that the frequency distribution of your section's grades is unimodal and symmetrical; that the mean, median, and mode are all equal to 75; and that the measure of skewness is zero (which also told you the distribution was symmetrical) and the measure of kurtosis is very nearly zero (-0.45). You now know that the distribution is very nearly normal.

Knowing that your name is the sixth in the instructor's gradebook for this class, you guess that your score might be 86, which is the sixth one listed if you read across the posted table. You calculate the z score to be $(86 - 75)/10 = 1.1$ and, from Table B in Appendix III, find that since the tabulated value is 0.3643, you did better than about 86 percent of the class—only about 14 percent outperformed you.

Curious as to what the confidence interval of the mean might be for all three

Exhibit 6-39. Summary evaluation of examination scores.

Data Class	Class Mark	f	fx	$X - \bar{X}$	$f(X - \bar{X})^2$	$f(X - \bar{X})^3$	$f(X - \bar{X})^4$
90–100	95	2	190	20	800	32,000	320,000
80–89.9	85	9	765	10	900	81,000	90,000
70–79.9	75	14	1,050	0	0	0	0
60–69.9	65	9	585	−10	900	−81,000	90,000
50–59.9	55	2	110	−20	800	−32,000	320,000
Totals		36	2,700	0	3,400	0	820,000

From either Eq. 6.3 or 6.2 the **mean** is $\bar{X} = \dfrac{\Sigma X}{n} = \dfrac{\Sigma fX}{n} = \dfrac{2,700}{36} = 75$

From Eq. 6.6 the **quartiles** are $Q = L + j(I)/f$ and $Q_1 = 60 + {}^{7}\!/_{9} = 67.8$; the **median** is $\bar{X} = Q_2 = 70 + {}^{7}\!/_{14} = 75$; and $Q_3 = 80 + {}^{20}\!/_{9} = 82.2$.

The **mode** is 75; the **modal class** is $70 - 79.9$.

The **midrange** is $(98 - 52)/2 = 75$.

The **modal percentage** is ${}^{14}\!/_{36}(100) = 39\%$. The **range** is $98 - 52 = 46$.

The **interquartile range** is $82.2 - 67.8 = 14.4$.

From Eq. 6.15 the **standard deviation** is

$$SD = \sqrt{\frac{\Sigma f(X - \bar{X})^2}{n - 1}} = \sqrt{\frac{3,400}{35}} = 9.9$$

while from Eq. 6.18 it is

$$SD = \sqrt{\frac{\Sigma fX^2 - (\Sigma fX)^2/n}{n - 1}} = \sqrt{\frac{206,080 - (2,700)^2/36}{35}} = 9.9$$

The range rule estimate of SD is $(\text{range})/5 = {}^{46}\!/_{5} = 9.2$.

The **coefficient of variation** is $SD/\bar{X} = 9.9/75 = 0.13$.

From Eq. 6.24 the **skewness** is

$$\frac{\Sigma(X - \bar{X})^3}{n(SD)^3} = 0$$

From Eq. 6.25 the **kurtosis** is

$$\frac{\Sigma(X - \bar{X})^4}{n(SD)^4} - 3 = \frac{820,000}{36(9.9)^4} - 3 = -0.59$$

sections (i.e., the population of interest), you decide to calculate it at the 95 percent confidence level, using formula 6.28:

$$75 - 1.96\left(\frac{10}{\sqrt{36}}\right) < \mu < 75 + 1.96\left(\frac{10}{6}\right)$$

$$71.7 < \mu < 78.3$$

and you know that means of the other two sections are likely to fall within this range. About this time, a friend who is in one of the other sections of this same course drops by. On a chance meeting with her instructor, she received her examination and had scored 78; however, she has no other information and is curious as to her class standing. You show her what you have done and point out that you can provide a ballpark estimate based on your confidence limits of the course mean. You use these to estimate the possible range of her z scores, assuming that the standard deviation of her class is not very different from that of yours:

$$\frac{78 - 71.7}{10} = .63 > z > \frac{78 - 78.3}{10} = -.03$$

Since the tabular values for the proportional area under the normal curve are .2357 and .0120, respectively, for these z score limits, you know that it is very unlikely that she did better than 73 percent of the class, but that she very likely did better than half the class (actually around 49 percent). On hearing this, she sighs, knowing that any hope she had of getting an A in the course has gone down the drain. You, however, are not at all surprised when, on the next day when the grades are posted, you see that you received an A. After all, you did learn something about statistics.

Automatic Data Processing

The computer is both a bane and a blessing. We have come a long way from the time when computers filled large rooms; now some hardly fill large briefcases, and their arithmetic power is awesome. Performing calculations at lightning-fast speed (often measured in billionths of a second or less), computers can inundate us with pages of numbers, which may or may not be meaningful, depending on our ability to properly interpret them. They can lull us into a false sense of security, with their results presented to ever so many decimal places, to the point that we may loose sight of the precision (i.e., number of significant digits) of the inputs we gave them. Computers can relieve us of a great deal of computational tedium, but at the same time they can obscure many insights into what the numbers are telling us. As a crude illustration, recall the difference between the *conceptual* and *computational* forms of the expression for calculating the standard deviation. The former, by having you tabulate values of $X - \overline{X}$, gave you a real insight into the distribution that the latter, with its simple ΣX^2 amd $(\Sigma X)^2$, could not.

Today we cannot be afraid of the computer. It is here to stay as a part of our everyday lives. With the current explosion in the personal computer market, soon virtually everyone who needs access to a computer will have it. Even today, there are hand-held computers on the market that will quickly perform every calculation needed in this chapter. The value of a particular z score is only a keystroke away, as is the corresponding proportional area under the normal curve. After raw data are entered, a single keystroke can produce the value of the standard deviation (in either biased or unbiased form), the mean, ΣX^2, and other statistics of interest. What we lose is the heuristic value of tables and the intuitive sense of what is happening (i.e., of nearby values). A point made at the beginning of this chapter was "first intuition, then mathematics," and with the advent of the computer this is even more true.

Statistical Programs

The computer does not bite, (the number of bits to a byte notwithstanding), but it does not think either. It simply does what we tell it to—timelessly, effortlessly, and patiently—right or wrong. Thus, it is up to us to tell it just what we want done. So we must know just what we want to do. The computer will not tell us what should be done; it is up to us to know.

Statistical routines are available for virtually every decent computer on the market today (by decent, we exclude the four-function pocket calculators and arcade-type game devices intended primarily for children). The extent of their capabilities tends to be a function of their price, but price is such a variable scale today that only gross comparisons are meaningful. Virtually all computers, however, are capable of producing the results needed for this chapter. It is not necessary that you know the distinctions among minis, micros, and large mainframes. But you must realize that much labor has gone into the generation of software packages to make the computer do what we want. The term "software" refers to the collection of instructions (commands) that tell a computer what to do.

You are using software when you communicate with a computer in any of the common languages in use today (e.g., BASIC or any of its derivatives, FORTRAN in whatever version, ALGOL, COBAL, PASCAL, or whatever—the list seems endless). Each language was designed with a particular application, or class of applications, in mind. For example, FORTRAN (*FOR*mula *TRAN*slation) has evolved to meet the needs of the scientist and engineer (hence its name), as has ALGOL, a very popular language in Europe. COBAL, on the other hand, has been designed with business applications in mind. Many of these languages, though originally developed for use with large central processing units, have made their way into the small personal computer market, and variations abound. The point is not that you need to become familiar with all the computer languages in order to take advantage of what the computer can offer. But you should be aware that differences abound and that what is written in one language for use on a particular machine may well be totally incompatible for use on another.

It may be intuitively obvious that a program written in a particular language for use on a large mainframe machine probably will not work on a small personal microcomputer, but it is probably not so obvious that a program written for a particular microcomputer may not work on a larger machine (or even another brand of microcomputer). This incompatibility need not bother you unless you are planning to purchase a microcomputer for your own use, as more and more people are doing every day. If this is the case, however, you need to pay particular attention to the *statistical* software capabilities of the machine of interest. For the typical computer user, software availability is legion.

There exist a number of statistical software packages, intended for use on the larger computer systems, that will do virtually everything covered in this book. They go by acronyms such as SPSS, SAS, MIDAS. Despite their seemingly overwhelming capabilities, keep this point in mind: These programs can execute virtually any task, but they can only provide prompts to help you understand how they function—they cannot tell you what you should do. SPSS stands for statistical package for the social sciences, and it is typical of the modern breed. It contains data management routines that allow you to arrange, rearrange, cut, and sort the data in almost any way imaginable. It will print tables of your data in virtually any form, perform all the calculations we have discussed, alert you to missing data, produce contingency tables (together with a complete analysis of them), and so on through a seemingly inexhaustible series of analytical options. It is really an integrated system of computer programs designed primarily for the analysis of social science data. The user need only employ seemingly natural language control statements to have the menus of available options at a fingertip. The programs included allow one to perform all the usual descriptive statistics, frequency distribution analysis, cross-tabulations, and the like, and also to perform correlations for both ordinal and interval level data; examine subpopulations; and carry out the analysis of variance, analysis of covariance, multiple regression, Guttman scaling (all this is covered in subsequent chapters), and other options too numerous to mention. SPSS data management routines can be used to modify data files (either temporarily or permanently); to generate new variables that are combinations of existing variables; to sample, select, or weight specified cases; and so on.

The somewhat extended discussion of the capabilities of SPSS should not be construed as a recommendation of its use over that of its competition. The Statistical Analysis System (SAS) will do most of what SPSS can do and some things it cannot (and vice versa). MIDAS has its adherents, and the argument about which is preferable doubtless will go on for some time (and probably never be completely resolved). It is important to realize that these packages are not static; they are all constantly being improved and upgraded, so much so that often it is difficult for their user manuals to stay up to date.

The use of these grand-scale packages is not without its pitfalls. With such extensive menus of options available, even experienced researchers are tempted to abandon careful consideration as to interactions of theory, hypothesis, and appropriate data analyses and instead simply exercise every available statistical option, substituting the crudest form of empiricism for intelligent forethought. The typical hallmark of an amateur is the production of a printout whose size is measured in inches (or even feet) rather than pages. This problem of overproduction can be solved once one realizes the difficulty of digesting, let alone interpreting, the information in such a mountain of computer output. Of even greater concern, however, is the tendency for these powerful routines to be misused—by both experienced researchers as well as students, who do not understand (or have forgotten) their underlying assumptions or mathematical bases. This is quite understandable, given the widespread availability of such all-encompassing tools and the human fact that "a little knowledge is a dangerous thing." The sad fact is that these "canned procedures" have little ability to distinguish between proper and improper applications. They are essentially blind computational algorithms that apply formulas to whatever data the user inputs. The fact that the results may be meaningless is completely obscured by the orderliness of the output. In some respects, it would be desirable if these all-encompassing statistical packages would administer a test to the would-be user to determine whether the procedure requested were appropriate for the data submitted and the meaning of the statistics to be produced well understood. But even if such checks were programmatic possibilities, their existence would be a bother to the knowledgeable user. The user's manuals of all these widely utilized statistical packages warn against their misuse. Unfortunately, they are not read by many users, and their significance is grasped by even fewer.

Organization of Data for Computer Analysis

Data can be input for computer analysis in innumerable ways. The user's manuals of the machines (or of the extensive data analysis systems just discussed) provide very clear direction as to what will be accepted and how. But regardless of whether one is directly entering data via a keyboard, punching cards, or filling out coding sheets, the notion of "good housekeeping" prevails. That is, the data must be presented in an orderly fashion and in a way that the machine, through the software being employed, can understand. Without considerable "coaching" (i.e., programming), it is difficult for the computer to accept anything but numeric data. In the final analysis, the computer is a binary device that can only distinguish between a 1 and a 0. Thus, it is generally advisable to convert nonnumeric data (e.g., patient's sex, religious preference, psychiatric diagnosis) to a numeric code (e.g., female = 1, male = 2) before entry into the computer. Clearly the nature of the underlying data is not changed at all by the use of such numeric codes.

As far as the actual input of data to the machine is concerned, the most common technique of data coding today uses the 80-column format. This simply means that a maximum of 80 characters (including blanks, spaces, etc.) can be put on a single input line. This is about the same number of characters (including punctuation marks, spaces, etc.) that a 12-pitch typewriter can put on a line while maintaining reasonable margins. An input line may be the number of keystrokes allowed (if data are entered directly) before a return key is struck, the maximum number of characters that can be put on a single card (if data are keypunched), the width of a row on a data coding sheet, the assigned field to a magnetic tape, or whatever. Since computers can read data in a number of ways (e.g., by direct entry, punched cards, punched paper tape, and a variety of magnetic media with tapes and disks being the most common), we really are concerned with data organization rather than actual input mechanics.

We do not elaborate on the administrative requirements for the use of a computer, for example, the user's name, a password perhaps, a job number (so that computer time can be charged appropriately), and the like, since they vary so widely from installation to installation and are of no matter insofar as personal computers are concerned. Here we are interested in the rudiments of data organization for computer analysis, not the nitty-gritty details for a particular application.

The Codebook

Although its name may sound formidable, a **codebook** is the researcher's best friend. It may, in theory, be nothing more than a sheet of paper on which you have written "female = 1, male = 2" and the like or an elaborate bound volume for a particular research study. The codebook serves as a permanent record of how you coded the data [i.e., into which column(s) you put a particular piece of information] and what the codes mean (you may think that you will remember at the time, but you may not later on). An example of a codebook for a hypothetical research project is shown in Exhibit 6.40.

Since you want to keep track of each subject individually, you assign a unique identifier, that is, a number (01, 02, . . . , 99). In this case we assume that you have to deal with fewer than 100 subjects. Otherwise, you would need a larger field (i.e., more columns—three columns would accommodate 999 subjects). You have decided to allocate the first two columns of your 80-column line for this identifier. Since you believe the subject's age might be a factor, you have decided to enter it in the next two columns. Note that the age is that as of the patient's last birthday (in years) and presumably you have no persons over 100 years old in your sample (or else you would need a three-column field). Since you want to distinguish gender, you have used the next column to indicate the sex of the patient. You expect that the marital status of your subjects will be a factor in your research, so you have allocated the next column to those data, and so on.

The point is that the codebook tells you not only what data go in which columns of your 80-column line but also what the number codes (which you have assigned to help make the data machine-readable) mean in terms of the variable involved. Even though you *might* remember a year from now that you entered marital status in column 6 for this particular research study, it is even

Exhibit 6-40. Example of a codebook.

Column(s)	Variables and Their Codes
1– 2	Subject's identification number (1–99)
3– 4	Age at last birthday
5	Sex: Female = 1; male = 2
6	Marital status: single = 1, married = 2, divorced = 3, widowed = 4, living with a significant partner = 5, undetermined = 6
7	Blood type: A positive = 1; A negative = 2; B positive = 3; B negative = 4; AB positive = 5; AB negative = 6; O positive = 7; O negative = 8; not available = 9
8	Psychiatric classification: schizophrenic = 1; manic-depressive = 2; other = 3; not available = 4
9–10	Rank order in terms of likelihood to benefit from therapy: most likely = 01 to least likely = 99
11–12	Scores on depression scale: 36 to 62
13–17	Oral body temperature to nearest 0.1°F (five columns required since one is needed for the decimal place)
18–20	Height to the nearest inch
21–23	Weight to the nearest pound
24–25	Number of previous admissions
26–27	Day of current admission
28–29	Month of current admission
30–31	Year of current admission
⋮	⋮

less likely that you would remember that you used 04 to indicate widowed. Your codebook is a permanent reminder. If you need more than 80 columns to code the data, you can simply use two lines (or more)—but you must tell the computer that you are doing so. Otherwise, the computer would read the second line as a new subject and (probably) give you an error message.

Coding Sheets

Once the researcher has chosen a coding scheme and allocated the columns, typically the next step is to fill out a **coding sheet,** which contains the data for each subject. The use of machine-readable questionnaires obviates the necessity for this step. Lacking such a convenience, you must use available records for each subject and enter data for each subject in the appropriate row and column of the coding sheet. Thus, the data for the first two subjects in your survey might appear as indicated in Exhibit 6.41 (where we have skipped a line to improve legibility).

Using your codebook (Exhibit 6.40), you verify that the first subject (i.e., the

Exhibit 6-41. Example of a coding sheet.

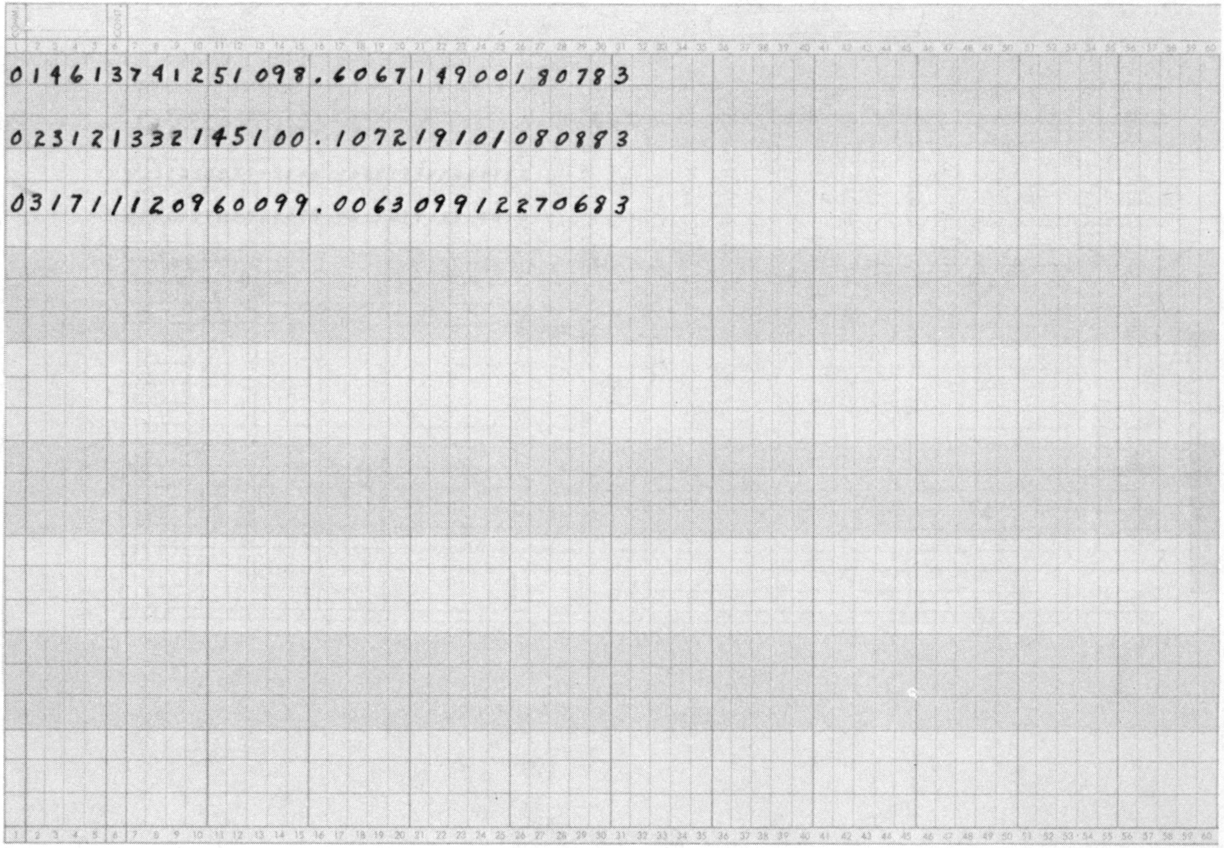

first line) in Exhibit 6.41 is a 46-year-old female who is divorced, has blood type O positive, has no available psychiatric classification, is ranked 12th most likely to benefit from therapy, scored 51 on the depression scale, had a normal oral temperature of 98.6°F, is 67 inches tall, weighs 149 pounds, has no prior admission history, and was admitted on July 18, 1983. Even with all these data, we have not used half of one 80-column line. The compactness that this form of data presentation affords is clear.

Other instructions (the administrative, or housekeeping, ones) have told the computer what data are to be found where. So when you ask it to compute a certain statistic on your data, for example, the mean and standard deviation of the ages of the male patients in the study, it simply does a sort on column 5 (i.e., accepts all data values where the entry in column 5 is a 2 and rejects all others) and performs the requested calculations on the data in columns 3 and 4 for all the patients thus sorted. The marvel is that the machine can present this information almost instantaneously upon receipt of the command. By contrast, no doubt you labored much longer in confirming the results of some earlier examples in this chapter. By so doing, however, you gained valuable insight into what was really happening in the calculation (and hopefully, how certain values affected the final result), something the computer can never give you.

It is fitting that we close this chapter with a rephrasing of what has been its common theme, "first intuition, then mathematics to express it, and finally to the computer to relieve tedium." If this order is reversed, you are in danger of being like the old man who claimed that he had psychic powers. He asserted that he could prove this by placing his fingertips against the end of his aquarium, whereupon all the fish would go to the opposite end. When an intuitive researcher placed a sheet of opaque paper over one end of the aquarium and asked that the demonstration be repeated, on seeing the result, the old man remarked in bewilderment, "It's amazing, my power is blocked by a piece of paper."

Reference Note 1

We can define the *generalized mean* as

$$M_t = \left[\frac{1}{n} \sum_{i=1}^{n} (X_i)^t \right]^{1/t}$$

For the case where $t = 1$, we have the *arithmetic mean*

$$M_1 = \overline{X} = \left[\frac{1}{n} \sum_{i=1}^{n} X_i \right]^1 = \frac{\Sigma X}{n} = \frac{X_1 + X_2 + \cdots + X_n}{n}$$

For the case where $t = -1$, we have the *harmonic mean*

$$M_{-1} = \bar{X}_H = \left[\frac{1}{n} \sum_{i=1}^{n} (X_i)^{-1} \right]^{-1} = \left[\frac{\Sigma 1/X}{n} \right]^{-1} = \frac{n}{1/X_1 + 1/X_2 + \cdots + 1/X_n}$$

In the limit as $t \to 0$, we have the *geometric mean*

$$M_0 = \bar{X}_G = (X_1 X_2 \cdots X_n)^{1/n} = \sqrt[n]{(X_1)(X_2) \cdots (X_n)}$$

By using our formula for the generalized mean, it can be shown that

$$\bar{X}_H \leq \bar{X}_G \leq \bar{X}$$

which, in words, says that the harmonic mean will *always* be equal to or less than the geometric mean which, in turn, will *always* be equal to or less than the arithmetic mean. If we wish to ascribe different weights to the data values, we simply substitute the product $w_i X_i$ for X_i and the sum of the weight for n in the above formulas. Thus the *weighted mean* is

$$\bar{X}_w = \frac{1}{\displaystyle\sum_{i=1}^{n} w_i} \sum_{i=1}^{n} (w_i X_i) = \frac{w_1 X_1 + w_2 X_2 + \cdots + w_n X_n}{w_1 + w_2 + \cdots + w_n}$$

The only other member of the generalized mean family that we discuss here is the root mean square (RMS), which occurs when $t = 2$:

$$M_2 = \text{RMS} = \left[\frac{1}{n} \sum_{i=1}^{n} (X_i)^2 \right]^{1/2} = \sqrt{\frac{(X_1)^2 + (X_2)^2 + \cdots + (X_n)^2}{n}}$$

Reference Note 2

In the description of a frequency distribution, the *r*th moment is defined as

$$\bar{X}^r = \frac{1}{n} \sum_{i=1}^{n} (X_i)^r$$

We note that the first moment is simply the mean:

$$\bar{X}^1 = \bar{X} = \frac{\Sigma X}{n}$$

In a similar fashion, the *moments about the mean* are defined as

$$m_r = \frac{1}{n} \sum_{i=1}^{n} (\bar{X} - X_i)^r$$

We note that $M_1 = 0$ and that

$$m_2 = \frac{1}{n} \sum_{i=1}^{n} (\overline{X} - X_i)^2 = \frac{\Sigma(\overline{X} - X)^2}{n} = SD^2$$

in its biased form. The third moment is related to skewness, with the most common measure of skewness in use today being

$$\text{Skewness} = \frac{m_3}{m_2\sqrt{m_2}} = \frac{(1/n) \Sigma (\overline{X} - X)^3}{[(1/n) \Sigma (\overline{X} - X)^2]^{3/2}} = \frac{\Sigma(\overline{X} - X)^3}{n(SD^3)}$$

and is presented in text as formula 6.24. The fourth moment is related to kurtosis. The most common measure of kurtosis in use today is

$$\text{Kurtosis} = \frac{m^4}{(m_2)^2} - 3 = \frac{(1/n) \Sigma (\overline{X} - X)^4}{[(1/n) \Sigma (\overline{X} - X)^2]^2} - 3 = \frac{\Sigma(\overline{X} - X)^4}{n(SD^4)} - 3$$

and is presented in the text as equation 6.25.

For a given frequency distribution, all values of the moments are expressed in terms of the same measurement unit. Therefore, the measures of skewness and kurtosis just given are dimensionless (i.e., "pure") numbers and are independent of the units of the data set (e.g., centimeters, pounds, minutes, IQ). Thus, if we have the distribution of the heights and weights of a number of patients, the measure of skewness for the height distribution may be directly compared with that for the weight distribution.

Although the entire set of moments for a distribution ordinarily will determine the distribution exactly, the higher moments have relatively little use in elementary applications of statistics. In fact, it is seldom advisable to compute them for sample sizes much less than 100. Nonetheless, it is important for the researcher to know something of the measure of skewness and kurtosis, because they are frequently calculated automatically by some of the packaged statistical computer programs (say, SAS, SPSS).

Reference Note 3

Since, by definition, the mean of *any* set of scores is their sum divided by their number (recall formula 6.3 and Reference Note 1), it follows that

$$\overline{z} = \frac{\Sigma Z}{n} = \frac{1}{n} \Sigma \frac{X - \overline{X}}{SD} = \frac{1}{SD} \Sigma \frac{X - \overline{X}}{n}$$

However, the mean is located so that the sum of the deviations about it is zero (recall Exhibit 6.22). Therefore

$$\overline{z} = \frac{1}{SD} (0) = 0$$

In a similar fashion, the variance of the z scores (from formula 6.9) is

$$V_z = \frac{\Sigma (z - \bar{z})^2}{n} = \frac{\Sigma z^2}{n}$$

But substituting for z from formula 6.26 (and recalling formula 6.9), we have

$$V_z = \frac{\Sigma (X - \bar{X})^2}{n(\mathrm{SD}^2)} = \frac{1}{\mathrm{SD}^2} \Sigma \frac{(X - \bar{X})^2}{n} = \frac{\mathrm{SD}^2}{\mathrm{SD}^2} = 1$$

Since the standard deviation is the square root of the variance by definition (formula 6.10),

$$\mathrm{SD}_z = \sqrt{V_z} = 1$$

which is what we wished to demonstrate.

Reference Note 4
_____

Although the normal distribution arose by observing that it closely represented the distribution of measurement errors (the differences between the values of repeated observations of an object and its true value), its utility goes far beyond that. Within this context, however, you can see why it was called "normal," or expected. This notion also serves to introduce a very powerful mathematical theorem.

Suppose that we have a bowl filled with slips of paper on each of which you have written a two-digit number. These slips of paper are the population, and the numbers on them represent the values of some attribute. We now take a number n of slips of paper from the bowl (a sample of size n) and compute the mean of the numbers written on them. We call this the **sample mean.** We now replace the slips in the bowl and mix them up. Since the bowl must contain a finite number of slips of paper (otherwise, either it would be so large we could not recognize it as a bowl or the slips of paper would be so small we could not read the numbers), this process of replacement is technically necessary to restore the population. We call this process *sampling with replacement.* As a practical matter, sampling with replacement is not really necessary if the population size is quite large compared with the *total* number of samples to be drawn, that is, the product of the sample size n and the number of samplings we intend to make. We repeat this process a large number of times, thus obtaining a large number of sample means, which themselves form a new population. We can construct a histogram for our population of sample means and thus observe its frequency distribution. We could also calculate its standard deviation. This leads us to the following statement of the **Central Limit Theorem:**

For large values of n, the distribution of the sample means is approximately normal.

What is more, by making use of the mathematical equation for the normal population (to be given shortly), it can be shown that if the parent *population* has a finite mean $\overline{X}$ and variance SD^2, then the distribution of the sample means will have a mean $\overline{X}$ and a variance SD^2/n. It is difficult to say just how large n has to be for the Central Limit Theorem to apply. But unless the distribution of the parent population, which need not be normal, is very unusual, n can be relatively small. It would certainly apply when n is 30 or more. If the parent population has a normal distribution, the theorem holds regardless of sample size.

If all this seems a little farfetched, we suggest that you actually conduct the experiment just described. Try it with around 200 slips of paper, and use a sample size not less than 20.

Reference Note 5

The mathematical equation for the normal distribution is

$$f(X) = \frac{1}{SD\sqrt{2\pi}}\, e^{-(X-\overline{X})^2/[2(SD^2)]}$$

where π ($= 3.1415\ldots$) and e ($= 2.7183\ldots$) are well-known mathematical constants and $f(X)$ is the height of the curve above the horizontal axis at any point X. Since the value of X enters into the formula only in a squared form, the distribution is symmetrical (remember that the squares of a negative and positive number are the same). Since the exponent of e (i.e., the power to which it is raised) has a minus sign, the distribution has a single maximum value at $X = \overline{X}$ equal to $1/(SD\sqrt{2\pi})$ and decreases rapidly for $X \neq \overline{X}$. The value of the maximum is determined by SD alone; the value of $\overline{X}$ determines only its location. Since for any X the curve is completely determined by the values of $\overline{X}$ and SD, it is called a two-parameter distribution.

Note that since $\overline{X}$ can assume any finite value and SD can be any finite *positive* number, the normal distribution is actually an infinitely large family of distributions. Thus, in an analogous fashion to the introduction of the z score in text, we can introduce the notion of a *standardized normal distribution*. If we substitute

$$X = (z)(SD) + \overline{X}$$

into our equation for the normal distribution and carry out the necessary algebra, we obtain

$$f(z) = \frac{1}{\sqrt{2\pi}}\, e^{-z^2/2}$$

the mathematical formula for the standardized normal distribution. By comparison of these two formulas, we can see that the standardized normal distribution has a mean of zero and a standard deviation of unity (recall also Reference Note 3). For this reason the notion of the z score and the standardized normal distribution are considered inseparable by some researchers; but as you have learned, such is not truly the case. We close by noting that the area under the standardized normal distribution is exactly unity.

Reference Note 6

When we are dealing with small sample sizes, say n under 30, the discussion in this text about estimating the population mean from the sample mean and, in particular, formulas 6.28 and 6.29, is no longer strictly correct (i.e., the confidence limits so calculated or the estimated required sample size will be somewhat in error, with the error increasing as n gets smaller). For small sample sizes, we *must* assume that the population distribution is nearly normal. Next, we must base our confidence intervals for μ on the *t distribution* (discussed in Chapter 16), which is very similar to the normal distribution. It is symmetrical and has a zero mean (as does the standardized normal distribution), but its shape depends on a parameter of the t distribution called *degrees of freedom*. For our purposes here, the degrees of freedom will be taken to be the sample size n minus 1.

If we use a line of reasoning similar to that used in text leading up to formula 6.28, we have

$$\bar{X} - t_\alpha \frac{\text{SD}}{\sqrt{n}} < \mu < \bar{X} + t_\alpha \frac{\text{SD}}{\sqrt{n}}$$

where $\bar{X}$ = sample mean
t_α = tabulated value of t distribution for $n - 1$ degrees of freedom
α = 100 minus the desired confidence level, divided by 200
SD = sample standard deviation
n = sample size
μ = population mean

Note that this is very similar to formula 6.28, except that the z score is replaced by the value of t_α.

As an illustration, we will use the example in text that led to formula 6.28, namely, the sexual liberalism test results where $n = 25$, $\bar{X} = 72$, SD = 17, and the desired confidence level is 95 percent. We have $\alpha = (100 - 95)/200 = 0.025$, and we look up the value for $t_{0.025}$ for $25 - 1 = 24$ degrees of freedom in Table D, Appendix III. We see that this is 2.0639, and so our formula becomes

$$72 - \frac{(2.0364)(17)}{\sqrt{25}} < \mu < 72 + \frac{(2.0364)(17)}{\sqrt{25}}$$

$$65.1 < \mu < 78.9$$

which is only a slightly larger confidence interval than the one obtained in text, namely,

$$65.3 < \mu < 78.7$$

This relatively small difference (i.e., error arising from the use of formula 6.28) is due to the fact that our sample size of 25 is not much less than our ballpark size of 30. To continue this parallel, if we now increase our desired confidence level to 99 percent, we find that the value of $t_{.005} = 2.7969$, and we have

$$72 - \frac{(2.7969)(17)}{\sqrt{25}} < \mu < 72 + \frac{(2.7969)(17)}{\sqrt{25}}$$

$$62.5 < \mu < 81.5$$

compared with the result obtained by using formula 6.28, namely,

$$63.2 < \mu < 80.8$$

Thus, at this higher confidence level our error is greater but still not too serious.

Suppose, however, that everything else remains the same except our sample size, which we now take to be 6. Since $t_{.025}$ for 5 degrees of freedom is 2.5706, our above expression yields

$$72 = \frac{(2.5706)(17)}{\sqrt{6}} < \mu < 72 + \frac{(2.5706)(17)}{\sqrt{6}}$$

$$54.2 < \mu < 89.8$$

while formula 6.28 would give

$$72 - \frac{(1.96)(17)}{\sqrt{6}} < \mu < 72 + \frac{(1.96)(17)}{\sqrt{6}}$$

$$58.4 < \mu < 85.6$$

For a desired confidence level of 99 percent, we would have from above ($t_{.005} = 4.0321$ for 5 degrees of freedom)

$$72 - \frac{(4.0321)(17)}{\sqrt{6}} < \mu < 72 + \frac{(4.0321)(17)}{\sqrt{6}}$$

$$44.0 < \mu < 100.0$$

while formula 6.28 would give

$$72 - \frac{(2.575)(17)}{\sqrt{6}} < \mu < 72 + \frac{(2.575)(17)}{\sqrt{6}}$$

$$54.1 < \mu < 89.9$$

We note that these latter values obtained by using formula 6.28 at a confidence level of 99 percent are almost exactly the same as the correct ones for a confidence level of only 95 percent. Thus, you can see how serious the error made by incorrectly using formula 6.28 is when we have a small sample.

In a similar fashion, if we wish to have a better estimate of sample size (for $n < 30$) than the one given by formula 6.29, we have

$$n = \left[\frac{t_\alpha(\text{SD})}{k} \right]^2$$

where n = required sample size
t_α = tabulated value of t distribution for $n - 1$ degrees of freedom and α
SD = sample standard deviation
k = one-half the desired confidence interval

Here, however, we have somewhat of a dilemma. We want to use this expression to find the sample size, but we need to know the sample size in order to look up the appropriate value of t. We have to use an iterative approach known as "successive trials and discards" (otherwise called "trial and error"). Let us take the example where we wanted to be 90 percent confident that our estimate of the population mean fell within ± 0.5 of a standard deviation of the mean. Here $\alpha = (100 - 90)/200 = 0.05$ and $k = 0.5(\text{SD})$. We need some place to start, so we use the large-sample estimate obtained in text, namely, 10.8. Since we know that the real value of n is higher than this (or we would not be bothering with an improved estimate), let us try $n = 11$, for which $t_{.05} = 1.8125$ (for $11 - 1 = 10$ degrees of freedom). We have

$$11 = \left[\frac{1.8125(\text{SD})}{.5(\text{SD})} \right]^2 = 13.1$$

Since the equality is not true ($11 \neq 13.1$), our estimate of n is too low. Therefore, let us try $n = 12$, for which $t_{.05} = 1.7959$, and we find

$$12 = \left[\frac{1.7959(\text{SD})}{.5(\text{SD})} \right]^2 = 12.9$$

We are closer but still not there. We next try $n = 13$, for which $t_{.05} = 1.7823$, and we find

$$13 = \left[\frac{1.7823(SD)}{.5(SD)} \right]^2 = 12.71$$

Now we know that the true value of n (assuming a normal distribution, remember) lies somewhere between 12 and 13. Since it is hard to take a fractional sample size, we assert that the correct minimum sample size is 13, not 11 as we obtained from large-sample theory.

Vocabulary

Abscissa	Dispersion
Absolute value	Ensemble mean
Arithmetic mean	Fractile
Asymmetrical	Frequency count
Axis of symmetry	Frequency distribution
Bar chart	Frequency polygon
Biased	Gaussian distribution
Bimodal	Geometric mean
Bivariate	Grand mean
Break	Graph
Chart	Harmonic mean
Codebook	Histogram
Coding sheet	Inferential statistics
Coefficient of variation	Inflection point
Computational formula	Interpolation
Conceptual formula	Interquartile range
Confidence interval	Interval level data
Confidence limit	Kurtosis
Contingency table	Law of large numbers
Continuous scale	Lower data class limit
Data class	Mean deviation
Data class boundary	Mean of means
Data class frequency	Measure of central tendency
Data class interval	Median
Data class interval precision	Midrange
Data class mark	Modal class
Decile	Modal percentage
Descriptive statistics	Mode
Deviation	Multivariate
Dimensionless	Negatively skewed

Negative skewness
Nominal level data
Normal distribution
Ogive
Open data class
Ordinate
Origin
Outlier
Peakedness
Percentage distribution
Percentile
Pie chart
Point estimation
Population
Positively skewed
Positive skewness
Probability
Qualitative distribution
Quantile
Quantitative distribution
Quartile
Range
Ratio level data

Raw data set
Relative deviate
Relative standard deviation
Robust
Sample
Skewed distribution
Skewness
Standard error of the mean
Standardized normal distribution
Standardized score
Sum of squares
Symmetrical
Table
Truncate
Two-way table
Unbiased
Unimodal
Univariate
Upper data class limit
Variability
Variance
Weighted mean
z score

The technique used for measuring the degree, or amount, of relationship between two variables is called *correlation*. It shows the extent to which values of one variable are linked or related to values of another variable. Correlation is a basic concept in research—like the mean and standard deviation. This chapter describes correlation that utilizes only two variables. That is why it is called **bivariate** correlation. Some multivariate correlation procedures, which use three or more variables, are described in Chapter 20.

The uses of bivariate correlation, henceforth called correlation, are many. For example, a researcher may wish to examine the extent to which presurgical anxiety among certain patients is related to postsurgical recovery. Or, in computing the reliability of a measurement instrument, you may wish to determine the extent to which the test and retest total scores are related, which means, in this case, how much they remain the same. Or, in determining the validity of a measurement instrument, you may wish to find out how much your instrument is related (and thus is measuring the same thing) to another longer, more complicated instrument for which good validity was already established.

In research using experimental design, one is concerned about being able to say that the independent or experimental variable *caused* the changes or differences observed in the dependent variable. Thus, you wish to make a *causal* statement. Sometimes, when random assignment is not possible, two intact groups are compared, and you are only able to interpret statistically significant results as a significant difference between the groups. In a simple correlational study, you do not do either of these. Instead, you study the extent to which two variables are related in *one group* of subjects.*

Beware of the popular use of the word "correlation." Laypersons often make statements such as, "Knowledge about breast cancer is correlated with weekly self-examinations." This is not necessarily a correlational statement. Instead, it could be comparative if two groups—those who do weekly self-examinations and those who do not—are compared on the dependent variable, which is knowledge about breast cancer. The statistical computations involved in testing comparative hypotheses are very different from those used to test correlational hypotheses. Therefore, it is important to know this difference. If we wanted to turn this comparative statement into a correlational statement, we would say that the frequency of breast self-examination is related (or correlated) to knowledge about breast cancer. Then we would be dealing with one group of subjects who were measured on two variables—frequency of self-examination during a specified period and knowledge about breast cancer. Recall, in comparative

---

*Of course, it is always possible to lump two intact groups together as one heterogeneous group and then correlate group membership (i.e., to which of the two intact groups each subject belongs) with the dependent variable. With rare exception, if one is statistically significant, the other one will be, too, because comparison and correlation are really two different sides of the *same* coin. Your choice of either a correlation or a comparative approach depends on the purpose of your research—what kind of answers you want.

research, that subjects are divided into at least two groups, based on some cutting point, or categories, of the independent variable, and then the group means on the dependent variable are compared.

Characteristics of Correlation Coefficients

A number of different correlation coefficients exist, and the Pearson product-moment correlation coefficient (labeled r) is the granddaddy of them all. Which coefficient you use depends on the level of measurement for each variable and other characteristics of your data. These are discussed later in the chapter. For example, the Pearson r requires that both variables be measured at the interval level of measurement.

The Pearson r and most other correlation coefficients vary from -1.00 to $+1.00$. The closer a correlation coefficient is to 1 or -1, the stronger is the relationship between the two variables; conversely, the closer it is to zero, the closer it comes to no relationship. If a **positive relationship** occurs, you can say that as one variable increases, the other one increases also. In a **negative relationship,** which is signified with a minus sign before the number, you say that as one variable increases, the other variable decreases.

Descriptive and Inferential Aspects of Correlation

In Chapter 6 we introduced two approaches to statistical treatment of data, *descriptive* and *inferential.* Means, medians, and standard deviations, which are all ways of summarizing many scores or data points, are part of the descriptive approach. So is a correlation coefficient. It describes the relationship between two sets of scores, or values, in which each score in one group can be linked to a single score in the other group. This link is usually a person, because correlations generally describe the strength of relationship between scores on one measure and scores on another measure among a single group of subjects for whom scores are available on both measures. Less often, a correlation describes the relationship between persons who are linked, such as mother and child or father and son, on one variable (e.g., intelligence, blood pressure, or attitudes toward health promotion practices).

Correlational research in which hypotheses must be tested demands more than description, however. It requires knowing whether a correlation is statistically significant, given a designated probability of being wrong, such as 5 or 1 percent. To do this, procedures from inferential statistics must be used—usually the t test or z test. These calculations are explained in Chapter 16. These statistical procedures actually test a hypothesis that the correlation coefficient, the descriptive statistic, is different from zero.

In some research studies using large sample sizes, correlations as low as 0.15 prove to be "significantly different from zero," and so the variables are declared to be significantly related. Whether this small r is practically significant is determined by the situation and your judgment. This same problem exists in the case of experimental research design. That is, because of a large sample size, two groups may be significantly different according to the statistical test applied to your data. If the means (or standard deviations, depending on your purpose) of these groups are not spectacularly different, your practical *so-what* test may deem your results not strong enough to justify introducing the experimental variable into routine nursing practice. This is true with significant correlations also. However, when you do obtain statistically significant results without a corresponding practical significance associated with them, you should consider whether your results may be raising a red flag which indicates *better research needed here*. Perhaps with more accurate and precise measurement instruments, improved research designs, and analyses that control more confounding variables, your results might become practically significant. All other things being equal, the smaller the sample, the lower will be r. In addition, all other things being equal, the smaller the variance or range of either or both variables, the smaller will be r. This is due to the mathematical properties of correlation coefficients.

Symmetrical and Asymmetrical Regression Coefficients

Correlation coefficients can be used for two purposes: to describe the nature (i.e., positive or negative) and magnitude of relationship between two variables and to predict a subject's score or performance on one variable on the basis of his or her score on the other variable. When the nature and magnitude of the relationship are of interest, the coefficient is called a *correlation coefficient*. However, when prediction is of interest, the coefficient is called a **regression coefficient,** in order to easily distinguish the two purposes and more appropriately describe the procedures used in the calculations.

Moreover, regression coefficients are of two types. One is **symmetrical,** meaning that the direction of prediction can be either variable Y predicted by variable X or X predicted by Y. The other kind is called **asymmetrical,** because Y (sometimes referred to as the dependent variable) can be predicted from X (sometimes called the independent variable) but not vice versa. This is because of the manner in which it is computed. Thus it is possible to come up with two different regression coefficients from the same data if, say, you label a variable X in one computation and label it Y in the other. In most asymmetrical coefficients, the average of these two different values equals the value of what a symmetrical coefficient would be for that particular kind of coefficient (e.g., tau). When there really is predictive capability, an asymmetrical coefficient will be slightly larger than a symmetrical one. However, depending on the nature of the measures for the two variables (e.g., level of measurement), asymmetrical measures may not be available.

The Pearson Product-Moment Correlation Coefficient r

In much of the preceding discussion, r has been used to denote a correlation, because r is the most desirable and most common coefficient of all. Its formal name is the *Pearson product-moment correlation coefficient*. It is named for the man who devised it, Pearson. It is called many names in the literature, such as Pearson *r, r,* product-moment coefficient, PMC, PM, PPMC, PPMCC, and so forth. Many of the other kinds of coefficients are special versions of the Pearson *r*. They are attempts to approximate it.

The Pearson *r* is a symmetrical coefficient. When it is used as a regression coefficient, prediction is possible in either direction. It requires that both variables be measured at the interval level.

Interpretation of a Pearson r
Correlation Coefficient

In a correlational research situation, a small additional step is needed before interpreting the number you have computed as the value of *r*. Although simple, this step is usually omitted in research literature, perhaps because the reader is expected to do it. You simply square the correlation *r,* multiply it by 100, and interpret it as the percentage of variance shared by the two variables. This is what they have in common. If an *r* of .85 were found between the number of breast self-examinations in a 6-month period and knowledge about breast cancer, it would *not* mean that the two variables were 85 percent related. To obtain an estimate of how much they overlap, the correlation coefficient must be squared [that is, $(.85)^2 = .7225$] and read as a percentage. Thus, the overlap— **shared variance**—is 72 percent. In other words, if you knew all the factors that explained the frequency of self-examinations and all the factors that explained knowledge about breast cancer, you would find that 72 percent of those factors were common to both variables.

Another way of interpreting an r^2 correlation coefficient is in terms of prediction. If you know a woman's score on knowledge about breast cancer, you know 72 percent of what you need to know to predict the frequency of her breast self-examinations. Since the *r* coefficient is reversible, you can also say that if you know how frequently a woman completes a breast self-examination, then you know 72 percent of what you need to know to predict her score on knowledge about breast cancer.

Exhibit 7.1 presents some correlation coefficients that have been squared and converted to percentages. Note that squaring always reduces the size of *r* except when it is ±1.00. Therefore, do not be misled when the value of the correlation coefficient is presented; the shared variance between the two variables is not as high. A correlation must reach .70 before it accounts for almost half of the variance. The popular rule of thumb for judging correlations is that it is a *strong* correlation when it accounts for half the variance. Correlations of 0.50, which may seem high, actually account for only 25 percent of the shared variance and are considered moderate. Also note that shared variance is influenced only by the magnitude of the correlation and not by whether it is a *plus* or a *minus r*. A good way of remembering the unique relationship between *r* and r^2 is to recall the equally unique relationship between the standard deviation and variance.

There is one situation in which this squaring rule is inappropriate. It is with correlation coefficients describing the reliability of an instrument. Reliability coefficients are interpreted as they are, owing to their definition as the ratio of

Exhibit 7-1. Percentage of variance explained by correlation coefficients.

r	r^2	Percentage of Variance Explained
.95	.9025	90
.90	.8100	81
.85	.7225	72
.80	.6400	64
.75	.5625	56
.70	.4900	49
.65	.4225	42
.60	.3600	36
.55	.3025	30
.50	.2500	25
.45	.2025	20
.40	.1600	16
.35	.1225	12
.30	.0900	9
.25	.0625	6
.20	.0400	4

the true score *variance* to the observed score variance. Thus a reliability of .85 means a shared or stable variance of 85 percent.

A Linear Relationship

In addition to requiring interval level measurement, the Pearson *r* requires the two variables being correlated to be **linearly related.** In fact, it is a measure of *how much* they are linearly related. A linear relationship means that if all data points were plotted on a graph, they would approximate a straight line. The greater they approximate a straight line, the larger the *r*. To better explain this, consider the scatter plot, or scatter diagram.

With the **scatter diagram,** you are making a two-dimensional graph with a vertical and a horizontal axis. One set of scores is plotted on the horizontal *X* axis (usually called the **abscissa**), and the other set is plotted on the vertical *Y* axis (called the **ordinate**). Each subject in your sample is indicated by a dot on the plot. First you move along the *X* axis to your subject's score on variable *X,* and then you move vertically from that point to the subject's score for variable *Y* as marked on the *Y* axis. This is where you put the dot for that subject. Exhibit 7.2 is a hypothetical example of a scatter diagram for a correlational study of the relationship between frequency of breast self-examinations during a 6-month period and knowledge about breast cancer as measured by a 25-item, summated scale, where all correct answers to the **items** (i.e., questions) are counted, or summed, to yield a total score. Subject *A* has a score of 16 on the knowledge measure and a frequency of 14 on self-examination. Similarly, subject *B* has a

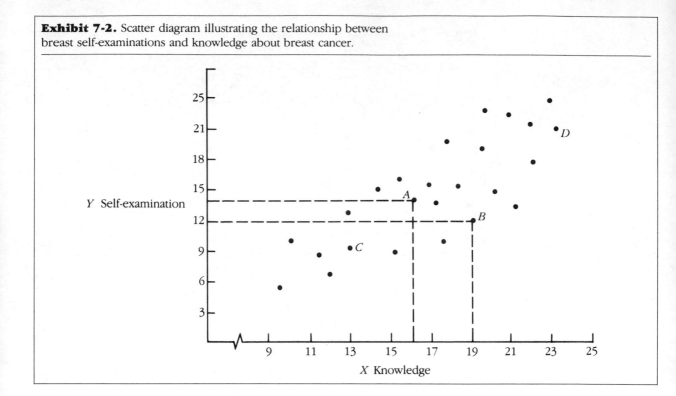

Exhibit 7-2. Scatter diagram illustrating the relationship between breast self-examinations and knowledge about breast cancer.

score of 19 on the knowledge measure and a frequency of 12 on self-examination. What do subjects *C* and *D* have?

The reason for making a scatter diagram is to determine whether the two measures are linearly related, because of this basic assumption of the Pearson *r* coefficient. Examination of Exhibit 7.2 indicates that the data points do resemble a line. If a curved line describes a relationship, then the relationship is said to be **curvilinear,** and a different coefficient, the correlation ratio *eta,* is used. Eta is discussed later and in Chapter 17. Exhibit 7.3 illustrates linear and curvilinear correlations. A line that is passed through the points so as to reflect how they are clustered, or distributed, must be straight when a linear coefficient, like *r,* is used. The Pearson *r,* therefore, is a measure of how much the two variables are linearly related; it tells how close the points are to the line. Look at scatter plot *A* shown in Exhibit 7.3. The line that is drawn through the points is known as the **line of best fit.** It is drawn in a specific way, known as **least squares,** in order to minimize the sum of the squared distances between all points and the line. To repeat, the closer the points are to the line of best fit, the higher *r* will be.

When *r* = 1.00, the scatter diagram is a perfectly straight line, the line of best fit. If you were predicting one score from another, you would always be right. That, however, is dreaming. Correlations are almost always less that 1.00, and so prediction is never 100 percent accurate. Exhibit 7.4 illustrates scatter diagrams

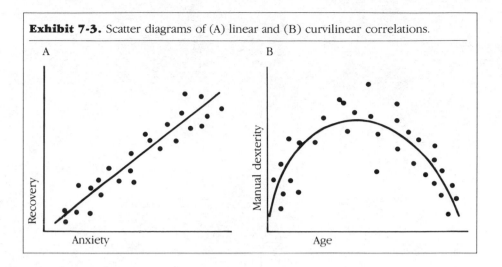

Exhibit 7-3. Scatter diagrams of (A) linear and (B) curvilinear correlations.

for selected values of *r*. As you can observe, the less the cluster of data resembles a straight line, the lower is *r*, until finally it is zero. Also note the difference in appearance between positive and negative relationships.

Draw a straight line through scatter plots *B, C,* and *E* in Exhibit 7.4. By observing distances between the points and your line, you see why *r* is higher in plot *B* and progressively lower in plots *E* and *C*. Where would you draw a line for scatter plot *D?* There are many alternatives. That is why *r* = 0 in that plot.

The line of best fit is used when *r* is utilized for prediction. If you know an individual's score on variable *X,* you can draw a vertical line from that *X* score to the line of best fit, and then from it is drawn a horizontal line to the *Y* axis. The point where the line intersects the *Y* axis is an estimate (or prediction) of the individual's score on variable *Y*. The higher the *r*, the more accurate your estimate will be. More about this and the line of best fit is presented later.

The inferential statistic to determine whether *r* is significantly different from zero requires some assumptions about the frequency distributions of the two groups of scores. Both are assumed to be normal distributions, at least in the population from which they were sampled. They also need to have the property of **homoscedasticity.** That is, all along the line of best fit, there will be about equal scatter of the data points above and below the line. There are special tests of homoscedasticity when a scatter diagram suggests this may be a problem.

When you observe much lower correlations than expected, it is best to draw a scatter diagram. You may be observing a nonlinear relationship. When many data points are being used, it is wise to use a computer program (e.g., SPSS). If a computer is not available and hand-plotting all points is prohibitively time-consuming, you might consider plotting a sample of your data points.

Calculating the Pearson r

There are numerous ways to calculate the Pearson *r*. As in the discussion of the variance and standard deviation in Chapter 6, both a conceptual and a computa-

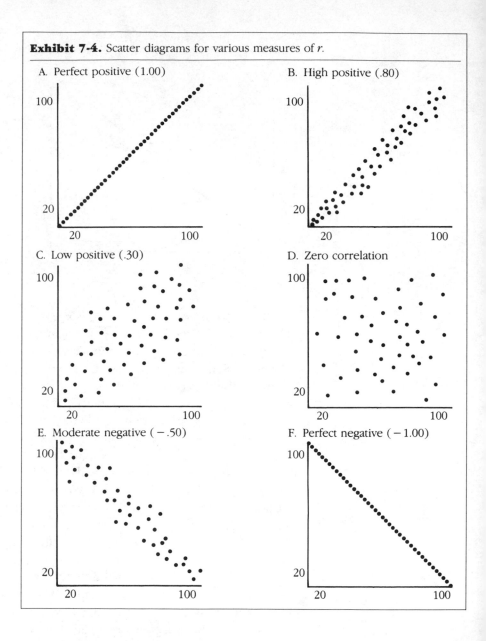

Exhibit 7-4. Scatter diagrams for various measures of *r*.

A. Perfect positive (1.00)

B. High positive (.80)

C. Low positive (.30)

D. Zero correlation

E. Moderate negative (− .50)

F. Perfect negative (− 1.00)

tional formula are presented. The conceptual formula has the advantages of being easier to remember and more clearly presenting what the procedure involves. However, when many subjects are involved, it becomes tedious and vulnerable to human error. Then a computer should be used and one of its computations verified via hand calculation. Simple problems out of textbooks for which answers are already known often are submitted to a computer for this purpose. Then if the computer output agrees with the book, all other calcula-

Exhibit 7-5. Fictitious data for relationship between
mother-daughter attitudes toward contraception ($n = 12$).

Subject Pair	Attitude		Subject Pair	Attitude	
	Mother	Daughter		Mother	Daughter
01	5	1	07	9	8
02	7	3	08	11	9
03	5	4	09	11	10
04	7	5	10	8	10
05	8	6	11	11	11
06	6	6	12	8	11

tions can be done by the computer. If a computer is not available, use the computational formula.

Since computers are becoming so readily available, a fair question is, Why bother learning to compute statistics at all? The same reasoning that says everyone should still learn multiplication tables even though pocket calculators are commonplace says you should know at least the basics. Furthermore, advanced inferential procedures that control or incorporate into analysis numerous confounding and other variables are becoming more common because computers are available to do the calculations. These are all based on basic procedures such as variance, correlation, and z scores. You would not be able to learn enough to understand or use those procedures appropriately without a good familiarity with these basic concepts.

Suppose a researcher correlated mother and daughter attitudes toward contraception by using a 12-item Likert scale (i.e., an item response is chosen from "strongly agree," "agree," "undecided," "disagree," and "strongly disagree"). Since we have no reason to believe that the relationship between mothers' and daughters' attitudes is nonlinear, we assume linearity and generate fictitious data for 12 mother-daughter pairs. These are presented in Exhibit 7.5. Because the mothers and daughters are linked as pairs, a correlation is appropriate. To phrase it in correlation terminology, variable X scores represent mother's attitudes and variable Y scores represent daughter's attitudes. For each (subject) pair, the mother's attitude is X and her daughter's attitude is Y. The pair of scores is *linked* by family membership.

Conceptual Formula

The **conceptual formula** for the Pearson r is

$$r_{XY} = \frac{\Sigma xy}{\sqrt{(\Sigma x^2)(\Sigma y^2)}} \tag{7.1}$$

where r_{XY} = correlation between variables X and Y
  x = **deviation scores** $(X - \bar{X})$ for X
  y = deviation scores $(Y - \bar{Y})$ for Y
  xy = product of a **linked pair** of deviation scores
  Σxy = sum of products for each linked pair of deviation scores (also known as the **sum of cross products)**
  Σx^2 = sum of squared deviation scores for X (also known as the **sum of squares** for X).
  Σy^2 = sum of squared deviation scores for Y (also known as the **sum of squares** for Y)

Exhibit 7.6 presents the organization of data for computing r according to this formula. First, the subject pair numbers are listed (step 1), and then the X and Y scores for each pair are listed (steps 2 and 3). All X scores are summed (step 4) and divided by n to get the mean of X (step 5). Then the same thing is done for the Y scores—they are summed (step 6) and divided by n (step 7). By using the mean which has now been calculated, deviation scores $X - \bar{X}$, denoted as a lowercase x, are calculated (step 8). Each deviation score is squared (step 9), and all these squared deviation scores are summed (step 10). Recall, the result of step 10 is known as the **sum of squares** for X. Next, the same procedures as steps 8 through 10 are followed for Y. The deviation scores for Y are calculated

---

Exhibit 7-6. Data organization for computation of r according to the conceptual formula.

(1) Ss	(2) x	(8) $X - \bar{X} = x$	(9) x^2	(3) Y	(11) $Y - \bar{Y} = y$	(12) y^2	(14) xy
01	5	−3	9	1	−6	36	18
02	7	−1	1	3	−4	16	4
03	5	−3	9	4	−3	9	9
04	7	−1	1	5	−2	4	2
05	8	0	0	6	−1	1	0
06	6	−2	4	6	−1	1	2
07	9	1	1	8	1	1	1
08	11	3	9	9	2	4	6
09	11	3	9	10	3	9	9
10	8	0	0	10	3	9	0
11	11	3	9	11	4	16	12
12	8	0	0	11	4	16	0

(4) $\Sigma X = 96$ (10) $\Sigma x^2 = 52$ (6) $\Sigma Y = 84$ (13) $\Sigma y^2 = 122$ (15) $\Sigma xy = 63$
(5) $\bar{X} = 8$ (16) $V_x = 4.32$ (7) $\bar{Y} = 7$ (18) $V_y = 10.16$
  (17) $SD_x = 2.08$ (19) $SD_y = 3.18$

Note: Numbers in parentheses denote the step in the calculations. Variances were computed with n rather than $n - 1$.

(step 11), squared (step 12), and summed (step 13). Step 13 is known as the **sum of squares** for Y.

Steps 14 and 15 involve calculating the **sum of cross products.** First, for each pair, the deviation scores for X and Y are multiplied, xy (step 14). Then they are summed (step 15). At this point you are ready to use the conceptual formula. However, since you are so close, you may as well calculate the variances (steps 16 and 18) and standard deviations (steps 17 and 19) of X and Y. To do this, the sums of squares Σx^2 and Σy^2 are divided by n or $n - 1$ to yield the variances. The square roots of the variances (steps 17 and 19), then yield the standard deviations. These steps are shown in boxes in Exhibit 7.6 to indicate they are not required for computation of r according to the conceptual formula. The computation, using values from Exhibit 7.6, is

$$r_{XY} = \frac{63}{\sqrt{(52)(122)}} = \frac{63}{\sqrt{6344}} = \frac{63}{79.649} = .79$$

The relationship between mothers' and daughters' attitudes about contraception is strong—62 percent of the variance is shared.

Look at the conceptual formula for r. Note that the denominator can never be a negative number because the sum of squares is never negative. Therefore, the positive or negative direction of the correlation is determined by the numerator, the sum of cross products.

Computational Formula
The **computational formula** for r is

$$r_{XY} = \frac{n(\Sigma XY) - (\Sigma X)(\Sigma Y)}{\sqrt{[n(\Sigma X^2) - (\Sigma X)^2][n(\Sigma Y^2) - (\Sigma Y)^2]}} \tag{7.2}$$

where

$$
\begin{aligned}
r_{XY} &= \text{correlation between variables } X \text{ and } Y \\
n &= \text{number of linked pairs of scores} \\
XY &= \text{product of paired scores } X \text{ and } Y \\
\Sigma X &= \text{sum of all } X \text{ scores} \\
(\Sigma X)^2 &= \text{sum of all } X \text{ scores which is then squared} \\
\Sigma Y &= \text{sum of all } Y \text{ scores} \\
(\Sigma Y)^2 &= \text{sum of all } Y \text{ scores which is then squared} \\
X^2 &= \text{an } X \text{ score squared} \\
\Sigma X^2 &= \text{sum of all squared } X \text{ scores} \\
Y^2 &= \text{a } Y \text{ score squared} \\
\Sigma Y^2 &= \text{sum of all squared } Y \text{ scores}
\end{aligned}
$$

While this formula may seem very formidable, it involves fewer calculations than the conceptual formula. Exhibit 7.7 shows how the data from Exhibit 7.5 can be used to calculate r via this method.

Exhibit 7-7. Computation of r according to the computational formula.

Ss	X	Y	XY	X^2	Y^2
01	5	1	5	25	1
02	7	3	21	49	9
03	5	4	20	25	16
04	7	5	35	49	25
05	8	6	48	64	36
06	6	6	36	36	36
07	9	8	72	81	64
08	11	9	99	121	81
09	11	10	110	121	100
10	8	10	80	64	100
11	11	11	121	121	121
12	8	11	88	64	121

$$\Sigma X = 96 \qquad \Sigma Y = 84 \; \Sigma XY = 735 \; \Sigma X^2 = 820 \; \Sigma Y^2 = 710$$
$$\bar{X} = 8 \qquad \bar{Y} = 7$$
$$(\Sigma X)^2 = 9216 \; (\Sigma Y)^2 = 7056$$

$$r_{XY} = \frac{12(735) - 96(84)}{\sqrt{[12(820) - 9216][12(710) - 7056]}}$$

$$= \frac{8820 - 8064}{\sqrt{(624)(1464)}} = \frac{756}{\sqrt{913,536}} = \frac{756}{955.79} = .79$$

Bivariate Regression

Bivariate regression means predictions using two (hence, *bi*) variables. A person's score on one variable Y is predicted on the basis of her or his score on another variable X. As in the discussion about scatter diagrams, if you know a person's score on X, you locate it on the horizontal axis or abscissa and then draw a perpendicular line from it to the line of best fit. From the point where the perpendicular hits the line of best fit, you draw a second line perpendicular to the vertical axis, or ordinate. The value at the point where your line intersects the vertical axis is the predicted value of Y, denoted as $\hat{Y}$ (called "Y hat"). Sometimes it is denoted Y' "Y prime").

Linear Regression Equation
Following the method of drawing lines on the scatter diagram is actually not a very efficient way to do things, particularly if many scores are to be predicted. There is a better way, based on the formula for a straight line which is also the basic **linear regression equation:**

$$\hat{Y} = a + bX \tag{7.3}$$

where $\hat{Y}$ = predicted value of Y

X = known value of X

a = Y **intercept,** or point on the vertical axis through which line of best fit passes

b = **slope** of line of best fit, or number of units of Y upward (or downward if b is negative) for every unit change in X

When you already know r_{XY}, you can compute the value of a and b with the following formulas*:

$$b = r_{XY}\frac{SD_Y}{SD_X} \quad \text{or} \quad b = \frac{\Sigma xy}{\Sigma x^2} \tag{7.4}$$

$$a = \overline{Y} - b\overline{X} \tag{7.5}$$

Therefore, still using data from Exhibit 7.6, we have

$$b = (.79)\frac{3.18}{2.08} = 1.21$$

$$a = 7 - (1.21)(8) = 7 - 9.68 = -2.68$$

To compare formula 7.3 with prediction via scatter diagram and the line of best fit, refer to Exhibit 7.8. It is a scatter diagram of the data which have been utilized in Exhibits 7.5 through 7.7 to illustrate computation of r. The line of best fit is drawn, and as shown in the calculation of a, it intercepts the Y axis at -2.68. The slope is also 1.21. Perhaps this is shown more easily if, instead of saying the line rises $1.21Y$ units for every unit X, we multiply by 5 and say the line rises the 6.05 (that is, 1.21×5) units of Y for every 5 units of X. As shown by the dotted lines going perpendicular to the Y axis for 5 units of X from A, the intercept, and up perpendicular to the X axis 6.05 units of Y, we arrive at point B, which is on the line of best fit.

The slope b is the same as that from formula 7.4. For a mother with a score of 8, using the line of best fit, we would predict that her daughter had a score of 7. Dotted lines from an X value of 8 to the line of best fit, point C, and then to the Y axis intersect at point 7. Using formula 7.3, we get the same result:

$$\hat{Y} = a + bX = -2.68 + 1.21(8) = 7$$

---

*An alternate formula for b, like the computational formula for r, is

$$b = \frac{n(\Sigma XY) - (\Sigma X)(\Sigma Y)}{n(\Sigma X^2) - (\Sigma X)^2} \tag{7.6}$$

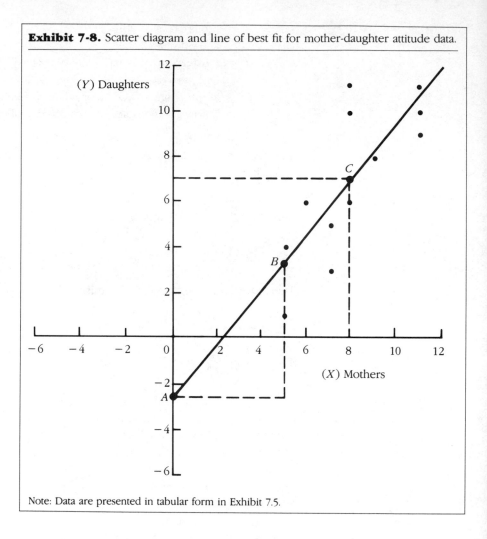

Exhibit 7-8. Scatter diagram and line of best fit for mother-daughter attitude data.

Note: Data are presented in tabular form in Exhibit 7.5.

Error of Estimate

How correct would we be in predicting a daughter's score of 7 based on her mother's score of 8? Once a person's score has been predicted, the discrepancy between it and the actual score is called the **error of estimate** e. Exhibit 7.9 displays predicted Y scores $\hat{Y}$ based on formula 7.3. The discrepancy between the known scores Y and predicted scores $\hat{Y}$ is shown in the column headed e, the error of estimate for each score. These are squared in the next column, headed e^2, and summed to equal 45.67. This is known as the *sum of squared residuals*, or error term. To figure what proportion of the total sum of squares for Y is accounted for by error, we divide 45.67 by Σy^2, or 122. It is 37.4 percent. It is the same, if we allow for errors due to rounding in computation, as the error computed via $1 - r^2$, which is 37.6 percent. These rounding errors (37.4 versus 37.6 percent) are another good reason for using computers where numbers can be carried out for more decimal points than hand calculation can easily use.

Exhibit 7-9. Prediction error for daughter scores from mother scores.

Ss	X	Y	$\hat{Y}$	Errors of Estimate $Y - \hat{Y} = e$	Squared Residuals e^2
01	5	1	3.37	−2.37	5.61
02	7	3	5.79	−2.79	7.78
03	5	4	3.37	0.63	0.40
04	7	5	5.79	0.79	0.62
05	8	6	7.00	−1.00	1.00
06	6	6	4.58	1.42	2.02
07	9	8	8.21	−0.21	0.04
08	11	9	10.63	−1.63	2.66
09	11	10	10.63	−0.63	0.40
10	8	10	7.00	3.00	9.00
11	11	11	10.63	0.37	0.14
12	8	11	7.00	4.00	16.00

$$\Sigma e^2 = 45.67$$

$$\frac{\Sigma e^2}{\Sigma y^2} = \frac{45.67}{122} = 0.374, \text{ or } 37\%$$

Note: $\hat{Y} = -2.68 + 1.21X$.

Looking at our error of 37.5 percent, we see that our prediction is better than chance but not fantastic. If r were larger, the prediction would be more accurate.

Standard Error of Estimate

Now we discuss one last concept about bivariate regression. The **standard error of estimate** SEe is a more useful index of error than $1 - r^2$ because it allows you to gauge how far off a predicted score might be. The standard error of estimate is like the average of all standard deviations (or points above and below the line) for each value of X. In other words, for each value of X, a frequency distribution of the Y points which are paired with that X value is made and its SD computed. Then the standard deviations for each value of X are averaged to yield a mean standard deviation, which is called the standard error of estimate. The formula* is

$$SEe = SD_Y \sqrt{1 - r_{XY}^2} \qquad (7.7)$$

where Y scores are predicted from X scores.

The SEe assumes that the Y distributions for each value of X are *normal* and that the property of *homoscedasticity* is present. Homoscedasticity is harder to

*The name for $\sqrt{1 - r_{XY}^2}$ is the *coefficient of alienation*.

spell and pronounce than it is to understand. Recall it merely refers to approximately equal scatter of points above and below the line of best fit for each value of *X*. Another way of looking at it is that all standard deviations (or the *Y* frequency distribution for each value of *X*) would be *approximately* the same. In bivariate regression these assumptions are usually assumed rather than checked. Instead, when an *r* or prediction turns out dramatically different from what is expected, usually researchers investigate the possibility that these assumptions were violated. In complex advanced procedures correlating many variables (i.e., multivariate statistics), some computer programs automatically check assumptions prior to executing the analysis, since violations can produce very misleading and erroneous results.

Using the formula and our data from Exhibits 7.5 through 7.9, we compute the SEe:

$$SEe = 3.18 \sqrt{1 - .624} = (3.18)(.61) = 1.95$$

Also there is an intuitive way to calculate the SEe by using the data displayed in Exhibit 7.9. Just as the variance of a set of scores is obtained by dividing the sum of squares by $n - 1$ (or n), the variance of errors or residuals can be obtained by dividing the sum of squared residuals e^2 by n. Thus, $45.67/12 = 3.8$. Then, just as the standard deviation of a set of scores is obtained by taking the square root of the variance, the standard error of estimate is obtained by taking the square root of the variance of residuals—$\sqrt{3.8} = 1.95$, the same as formula 7.6.

Now what does 1.95 tell you that the 37.5 percent error variance does not? Recall the normal distribution (see Chapter 6) in which about 68 percent of the scores fall approximately $\pm 1SD$, 95 percent fall approximately $\pm 2SD$, and 99 percent fall approximately $\pm 3SD$. The true values are 1.96SD for 95 percent and 2.58SD for 99 percent. Thus, the standard error can be interpreted and used in the same way as the standard deviation in the preceding statement. Therefore, if we were to predict a daughter's score of 7 on the basis of her mother's score of 8, then 95 percent of the time her real score would be $\pm 1.96SEe$ of her predicted score or somewhere between 3.178 [$= 7 - (1.96)(1.95)$] and 10.822 [$= 7 + (1.96)(1.95)$]. If we wanted to be accurate more often than 95 percent of the time, we would say that 99 percent of the time her score would be within 2.58SEe of her predicted score, or between 1.969 and 12.031. In our example, the tradeoff between increased correctness and the enlarged range within which a daughter's real score would fall would make this prediction a waste of time— even though the *r* of .79 is extremely high relative to most correlations found in behavioral research. That is why most predictions are based on more than one predictor variable in order to reduce error. The procedure is called *multiple regression,* and we introduce it in Chapter 20.

Besides multiple regression, several other correlation procedures are introduced in Chapter 20. Multiple correlation involves correlating two or more variables with another variable, but not in a predictive sense. Partial correlation removes the effects of, or variance due to, a third variable from two variables which are then correlated. Computational procedures for these when three variables are involved are presented, as well as a description of four or more variable cases where computer analysis is more appropriate. This concludes our discussion of the Pearson *r*. As you will notice as you proceed through this book, the Pearson *r* is often mentioned. It, like the mean, standard deviation, variance, and sum of squares for various kinds of deviation scores, is a very basic concept to quantitative research. Moreover, all other correlations are either special versions of *r* or seek to approximate it. Some of the special versions of *r* are becoming obsolete owing to the widespread use of computers. The biserial, for example, was developed to simplify hand computation when one of the variables was **dichotomous** (i.e., had only two values). If you know *r,* the others are easy. Moreover, *r* yields a prediction equation and leads to a standard error of estimate. There are, of course, mathematical statisticians working to develop prediction equations with, say, ordinal level measures. These are still experimental, however, and thus hardly material to be included at the introductory or intermediate level in research methods and statistics.

The Spearman Rank-Order Correlation Coefficient Rho

The Spearman rho is the major backup correlation coefficient used when the requirements of *r* cannot be met or data are too skewed. It is designed for use with ordinal level data. Therefore, if scores are used, they must be converted to ranks as shown in Exhibit 7.10. The data from Exhibit 7.5 (i.e., the mother-daughter attitudes toward contraception) are used in this example. The Spearman rho correlation is computed by using the ranks instead of scores. Sometimes, data are ordinal when gathered. Then this step is not necessary.

The calculation of the Spearman rho statistic is straightforward. Exhibit 7.11 displays the organization of data for this purpose. Steps 1 and 2 show that for each pair, the ranks on variables *X* and *Y* are listed in columns. Then *D,* the difference between the ranks for each pair, is computed (step 3). These are squared (step 4), and the sum of squared differences ΣD^2 is calculated (step 5). Now the formula for rho is used:

$$\text{Rho} = 1 - \frac{6\Sigma D^2}{n(n^2 - 1)} \tag{7.8}$$

where 6 = constant that is always used
D = difference between ranks for each pair
D^2 = squared difference between ranks
ΣD^2 = sum of squared differences between ranks
n = number of pairs

Using the data from Exhibit 7.11, we can calculate the Spearman rho coefficient as follows:

Exhibit 7-10. Method to rank-order scores.

---

1. Rank-order each group of scores from highest to lowest, ignoring to which pair each score belongs.

2. Assign ranks from 1 for the highest score to *n* for the lowest score. When scores are tied, such as 11, 11, and 11, assign the *median* of the ranks they would have received if they had not been tied. For example, the first three scores for mothers should receive ranks of 1, 2, and 3. However, if they are tied at 11, each receives the median of 1, 2, and 3, which is 2.

Mother			Daughter	
Score	Rank		Score	Rank
11	2		11	1.5
11	2		11	1.5
11	2		10	3.5
9	4		10	3.5
8	6		9	5
8	6		8	6
8	6		6	7.5
7	8.5		6	7.5
7	8.5		5	9
6	10		4	10
5	11.5		3	11
5	11.5		1	12

3. Returning to the paired scores, assign each score its appropriate rank based on your calculations in step 2:

Pair	Mother	Daughter	Pair	Mother	Daughter
01	11.5 (5)	12 (1)	07	4 (9)	6 (8)
02	8.5 (7)	11 (3)	08	2 (11)	5 (9)
03	11.5 (5)	10 (4)	09	2 (11)	3.5 (10)
04	8.5 (7)	9 (5)	10	6 (8)	3.5 (10)
05	6 (8)	7.5 (6)	11	2 (11)	1.5 (11)
06	10 (6)	7.5 (6)	12	6 (8)	1.5 (11)

Note: Numbers in parentheses are actual scores.

$$\text{Rho} = 1 - \frac{(6)(59.5)}{12(144 - 1)} = 1 - \frac{.357}{1716} = 1 - .208 = .79$$

The fact that the sum of the *D* values is always zero can be used as a way of checking *D* column values. In our example, rho is the same as *r*. When two variables are normally distributed, rho tends to be either the same or slightly lower (< 2 percent) than *r*. Therefore rho is comparable with *r* as a measure of

Exhibit 7-11. Organization of data for computation of Spearman rho.

Pair	X Ranks (1)	Y Ranks (2)	D (3)	D² (4)
01	11.5	12	−0.5	0.25
02	8.5	11	−2.5	6.25
03	11.5	10	1.5	2.25
04	8.5	9	−0.5	0.25
05	6	7.5	−1.5	2.25
06	10	7.5	2.5	6.25
07	4	6	−2	4.00
08	2	5	−3	9.00
09	2	3.5	−1.5	2.25
10	6	3.5	2.5	6.25
11	2	1.5	0.5	0.25
12	6	1.5	4.5	20.25

$\Sigma D = 0$ (5) $\Sigma D^2 = 59.5$

the strength of relationship. Rho does not possess the mathematical advantages of r (i.e., yield a prediction equation), however. Therefore, it is used only when r cannot be used. The significance of rho is tested via a t test.*

Kendall's tau has been proposed for use with ordinal data and is superior to rho when there are many tied ranks or $n < 10$, as far as testing significance is concerned. In other circumstances tau tends to be lower than rho, sometimes by as much as one-third. Therefore tau is not always comparable to rho or r. For a more detailed discussion see Kendall [1].

Other Correlational Procedures

A host of other correlational procedures are available. Each addresses a specific research purpose and depends on the level of measurement and distribution of the data themselves. Some are discussed in this section, although their computation is not.

Gamma, Yules' Q, Somers' d, and Kendall's Tau†

This family of correlations, which came primarily from the discipline of sociology, is designed for ordinal level measures which have fewer values and so can

---

*The formula is

$$t = \text{rho} \sqrt{\frac{n-2}{1-\text{rho}^2}}$$

See Chapter 16 for a discussion of the t test.

†For a description of computational routines, begin with Kviz and Knafl's *Statistics for Nurses* [2].

Exhibit 7-12. Contingency table for rank-order correlations.

Variable X	Variable Y		
	Negative	Moderate	Positive
Negative	NN (1,1)	NM (1,2)	NP (1,3)
Moderate	MN (2,1)	MM (2,2)	MP (2,3)
Positive	PN (3,1)	PM (3,2)	PP (3,3)

Note: Contingency tables move from lowest to highest with lowest beginning in the upper row and left column and highest in the lowest row and far right column. Lowest, in this example, is based on attitude scores. Numbers in parentheses are the ranks which have been assigned to X and Y, respectively.

be summarized in a contingency table like the one shown in Exhibit 7.12. They differ according to whether they are symmetrical or asymmetrical and whether they can describe negative relationships, the size and shapes of the contingency table to which they can be applied, and their degree of **conservatism** (i.e., the tendency to result in a lower correlation than other methods, thereby, according to one point of view, preventing inflated correlations which lead to erroneous interpretation of results). They are often interpreted as the amount of error in predicting Y that is reduced as a result of knowing X or the amount of variation in Y explained by X. Their computation is more complex than Spearman's rho.

All correlations in this family have the same numerator. Their denominators differ in whether they include pairs of observations whose ranks are **tied** with other pairs. Furthermore, the way in which two pairs of observations can tie varies. Their ranks can be tied on both X and Y or on just one. Consider Exhibit 7.12. All pairs of observations falling within each cell obviously are tied with each other on *both* X and Y. In addition, all pairs in the first row are tied on the X variable because they are all negative attitudes and are assigned a rank of 1. Also similarly tied on X are the observations which fall in the second (rank 2) and third (rank 3) rows. None, however, are also tied on Y. Similarly, pairs within each of the columns are tied with each other on Y (but not on X). As the denominators of these various measures of relationships include more ties, as error, thereby resulting in a larger number as the denominator, the correlation itself becomes smaller, all other things being equal. All these correlations, then, are measures of the magnitude of same- or reverse-order pairs of observations. Each pair is examined in relation to all other pairs, and these results are summed. The proportion of correct calls, the numerator, to all calls, the denominator, is the correlation. When ties are excluded from the denominator, it is smaller, and the resulting measure of association is larger.

Gamma

Goodman and Kruskal's G, usually called *gamma*, is the least conservative measure of association, because it includes no ties in the denominator. Therefore, it can easily be inflated and so is misleading. It is a symmetrical measure whose values can range from -1.00 to $+1.00$. A major disadvantage of gamma is that it will equal ± 1.00 if any cell in a 2×2 table equals zero, regardless of the number of observations in other cells. Therefore, other procedures are used with 2×2 tables.

Yules' *Q*

Yules' Q is a special version of gamma for use with 2×2 tables. Its formula is easier to compute. All the cautions which apply to gamma apply to Yules' Q.

Somers' *d*

Somers' d is an asymmetrical correlation that can range from -1.00 to $+1.00$. Because it is asymmetrical (i.e., designates variables as predictor or criterion), two different vaues of d can result when each of the variables are considered the criterion. Somers' d usually is lower than gamma, because its denominator includes as error the number of pairs that are tied on the dependent or criterion variable (but not those tied on the predictor variable). A symmetrical version is available which is just an average of the two asymmetrical coefficients.

Kendall's tau

Kendall's rank-order correlation coefficient tau is really three symmetric measures which can vary from -1.00 to 1.00. Tau is the most conservative because it considers all tied pairs as error and includes them in the denominator. If any ties are present, and there usually are, tau_a cannot reach a value of 1.00. Therefore it is rarely used. Tau_b excludes from the denominator any pairs that are tied on *both* variables but includes all others. Therefore, it tends to be smaller than Somers' d. However, when the number of ties on X is approximately equal to the number of ties on Y, tau_b is about the same magnitude as Somers' d. A disadvantage of tau_b is that it can never reach 1.00 if the contingency table for which it is computed is not square (say, 2×2, 3×3, 4×4). Therefore, tau_c is used. Tau_c is identical to tau_b in every way except that it includes an adjustment so that a maximum value of 1.00 can be obtained from a rectangular table.

Just how do you select the appropriate measure from this family? First, decide if an asymmetrical measure is appropriate. If so, use Somers' d. If a symmetrical measure is appropriate, your choice is between a gamma or tau correlation. How do you wish to define ties? If you consider them error, use tau; if not, use gamma; if uncertain, use both. One rule of thumb says to use gamma when there are few ties and to use tau when there are many ties.

Eta, Contingency Coefficient, Phi, Cramer's Phi

The correlation ratio, or *eta*, is the commonly used measure of relationships that are not linear. One variable is interval level while the other is considered nominal. This is discussed further in Chapter 17.

The contingency coefficient *C,* phi, and Cramer's phi are a family of measures used with nominal level data summarized in a contingency table. These are discussed in Chapter 18.

Vocabulary

Abscissa	Line of best fit
Asymmetrical coefficient	Linked pair
Bivariate correlation	Negative correlation
Conceptual formula	Ordinate
Computational formula	Positive correlation
Conservatism	Regression coefficient
Deviation scores	Scatter diagram
Dichotomous variable	Shared variance
Error of estimate	Slope
Homoscedasticity	Standard error of estimate
Intercept	Sum of cross products
Items	Sum of squares
Least squares	Symmetrical coefficient
Linearly related	Tied observations
Linear regression equation	

References

1. Kendall, M. G. *Rank Correlation Methods.* London: Griffin, 1948.
2. Kviz, F. J., and Knafl, K. H. *Statistics for Nurses: An Introductory Text.* Boston: Little, Brown, 1980.

8: *Epidemiologic Methods*

Peggy Parks

Epidemiology is the investigation of the distribution and causes of diseases in a *population* [1]. Currently, epidemiologic methods are employed to investigate both health and illness including the biologic, psychological, social, and physical aspects of human functioning. There are parallels between the clinical process used by health professionals and epidemiology. Epidemiology studies and treats populations as the health professions study and treat clients—through assessment, planning, treatment, and evaluation. For both epidemiology and the health professions, one goal is to prevent illness and maintain health, but the unit of interest for epidemiology is a population whereas for the health professions it is the client. One way epidemiology can complement the clinical process is to provide information about a population which can be used to improve services for clients. For example, school nurses who know that venereal disease is a significantly greater problem among students in one high school than in another can plan programs and allocate resources to address this need. Epidemiologic methods can be used to monitor the health of a population receiving clinical services and to provide contextual information about clients.

Basic Assumption

A basic assumption of epidemiology is that disease is an interaction of three factors: **agent, host,** and **environment** [1, 3]. The host is the person who is afflicted with the disease. For investigatory purposes, the host is considered holistically. Age, sex, race, level of income, history of disease, and behavior are examples of host variables that may be studied. The agent is the source of the disease. Examples are infectious agents such as bacteria, chemical agents such as poisons, and nutritive elements. And the environment is the place and circumstances under which the disease occurs and includes physical, biologic, and socioeconomic variables. An example of the environment in a study of rape is the unlighted streets in a nightclub district. This triad—agent, host, and environment—must be considered when an epidemiologic study is planned.

Knowledge about the existence of a health problem and about how it is related to host, agent, and environment provides contextual information for planning clinical intervention for individuals in the population. For example, nurses could recommend the modification of an environmental factor for clients whose host characteristics place them at risk for a specific disease. Health professionals can, with the aid of a few basic statistics, locate or generate information about populations which will be helpful when they plan interventions for clients.

Basic Statistic: Rate

A basic statistic used in epidemiologic methods is the **rate.** A rate is composed of a numerator and a denominator and is multiplied by a constant C such as 100, 1,000, or 10,000:

$$\frac{\text{Frequency of events occurring over specified time frame}}{\text{Number of people at risk over specified time frame}} \times C$$

The result is the rate of occurrences over a specified time period per X number of people. Rates are used instead of frequencies, which are employed in descriptive statistics, because they facilitate comparisons in groups having an unequal number of members or different host characteristics. For example, let us assume that there were 50 heart attacks (frequency) among the professional employees of the First Federal Bank during the past calendar year and 5 heart attacks among the professional employees at the Home State Bank during the same year. When the frequency of heart attacks in the two groups is compared, the First Federal Bank employees seem to have a more serious health problem than the Home State Bank employees. If a rate were used instead, a different conclusion would be reached. For each group, the number of employees must be determined. Then the rate of heart attacks is calculated for the First Federal Bank:

$$\frac{\text{Number of heart attacks in 1983}}{\text{Number of professional employees in 1983}} \times 100 = \frac{50}{1,000} \times 100 = 5$$

The same procedure is conducted for the Home State Bank:

$$\frac{\text{Number of heart attacks in 1983}}{\text{Number of professional employees in 1983}} \times 100 = \frac{5}{100} = 5$$

When the rates, 5 and 5, are compared instead of the frequencies, 50 and 5, there is no difference in the groups with respect to this health problem.

A second example illustrates the usefulness of a rate when the groups have different host characteristics. Let us assume that there are 50 heart attacks among the professional employees of the First National Bank during the past calendar year and 15 heart attacks among professional employees of the School of Nursing during the same year. The School of Nursing employees are predominately female, and the bank employees are predominately male. The host variable, sex, is important to consider because it is associated with heart disease. The hypothetical data are displayed in Exhibit 8.1. When the rate of heart attacks for each group is calculated, regardless of sex (a host characteristic), the two values are the same. These rates are displayed in Exhibit 8.2. When the rate of heart attacks for each group is calculated for males and females separately, a different conclusion is reached. These rates are also displayed in Exhibit 8.2. The rates for males in the two groups are different, and the rates for females in the two groups are different. For male employees, the health problem appears more serious in the School of Nursing, but for females it seems more serious in the bank.

Given the usefulness of rates for epidemiologic methods, an investigator must have data for both a numerator and a denominator. When nurses are using these methods, sometimes it is easy to obtain information about the number of people afflicted with a disease, but difficult to obtain information on the number of people at risk. One contributing factor to this difficulty is that the data for each part of the rate may be stored in separate places. For example, nurses interested

Exhibit 8-1. Number of employees with heart attack in 1983

	Number of employees with heart attack in 1983	Number of employees in 1983
First National Bank		
Males	24	800
Females	26	200
Total	50	1,000
School of Nursing		
Males	7	50
Females	8	250
Total	15	300

Exhibit 8-2. Rate of heart attacks in 1983

Rate of Heart Attacks in 1983
First National Bank

$$\frac{50}{1,000} \times 100 = 5$$

School of Nursing

$$\frac{15}{300} \times 100 = 5$$

Rate of Heart Attacks for Males and Females in 1983
Males

First National Bank: $\frac{24}{800} \times 100 = 3$

School of Nursing: $\frac{7}{50} \times 100 = 14$

Females

First National Bank: $\frac{26}{200} \times 100 = 13$

School of Nursing: $\frac{8}{250} \times 100 = 3$

in child abuse among 0- to 12-year-olds might have to obtain the reported number of abuse cases from the city department of social services and the number of children 0 to 12 years old who reside in the city from the department of census. Even when data for both the numerator and the denominator are located within the same institution, they may be in different offices or departments. For example, nurses interested in low-birth-weight infants might obtain data on the numerator (the number of low-birth-weight infants born) from pediatrics and on the denominator (the number of live births) from obstetrics. In this case, the nurses probably work for pediatrics and have easier access to data for the numerator than for the denominator. It is possible, however, that the medical records department compiles a registry with statistics of births which includes data for both the numerator and denominator. When epidemiologic methods are used, the investigators should always ask, Can data for the numerator and denominator be obtained from *one* source? If not, where can accurate information for each be obtained?

Death Rates

Mortality, or death rate (the terms are used synonymously) is commonly used in epidemiologic studies. In general, the numerator consists of the number of people dying and the denominator of the number of people exposed to the risk of dying. This number is multiplied by a constant C, such as 1,000 or 10,000. In addition, the rate is specified for a time frame, usually 1 year. Conventionally, the number of people exposed to the risk of dying is estimated by using the population census at midyear [3, 5]. There are several variations of death rate which provide different types of information.

Crude Death Rate

The **crude death rate** represents the proportion of the population dying in a 1-year period. The calculation of this rate is displayed in Exhibit 8.3. The crude death rate for Baltimore City in 1979 was 11.1 per 1,000 population. It was calculated by dividing the number of deaths, 9,262, by the population at midyear, 837,760, and multiplying by 1,000. This death rate is called crude because it incorporates information about the number of people dying and the composition of the population in an unspecified manner.

Specific Death Rate: Age

Specific death rates are variations of the crude death rate and have the advantage of allowing the investigator to isolate subgroups or diseases in the population and examine these death rates separately. For example, if there is a large proportion of elderly people in the population, the crude death rate will be relatively high because of death from old age. This rate does not necessarily indicate a significant health problem. The investigator could calculate death rates *specific to age* to determine whether rates are unusually high for people not dying from old age. The Baltimore City health department reports age-specific death rates for the following groups: under one, 1 to 4, 5 to 14, 15 to 24, 25 to 34, 35 to 44, 45

Exhibit 8-3. Crude death rate.

$$\frac{\text{All recorded deaths in one calendar year}}{\text{Population at midyear}} \times 1,000 = \frac{9,262}{837,760} \times 1,000 = 0.011055 \times 1,000 = 11.055$$

Exhibit 8-4. Age-specific death rate for Baltimore City [5].

$$\frac{\text{All recorded deaths of 65- to 74-year-olds in 1979}}{\text{Population of 65- to 74-year-olds at midyear}} \times 1,000 = \frac{1,054}{36,250} \times 1,000 = 0.0290758 \times 1,000 = 29.08$$

---

to 54, 55 to 64, 65 to 74, 75 to 84, and 85 years and over [5]. The calculation of the age-specific death rate is displayed in Exhibit 8.4.

Specific Death Rates: Sex, Race, or Cause

A procedure similar to that for calculating the age-specific death rate is used to ascertain sex- or race-specific rates. Death rates specific to cause are also used for comparisons and the determination of major health problems in a population. An investigator might be interested in the death rate from malignant neoplasms and from major cardiovascular disease. Exhibit 8.5 displays specific rate calculations according to cause. The variable, for example, cause of death, that separates the rates determines the type of rate that is calculated. The most common use of specific death rates is the combination of variables that allows the characteristics of the population to be examined separately from the cause of death. For example, cause-specific death rates could be calculated for races. In 1979, the suicide rate per 100,000 people in Baltimore City was 18.25 for whites and 7.05 for nonwhites [5].

Infant Death Rate

A special case of age-specific death rates is the infant death rate. Conventionally, the denominator is the number of births for the specified year instead of the number of infants at midyear [2, 5]. See Exhibit 8.6. The infant death rate for Baltimore City in 1979 was 19.11. There were 233 infant deaths and 12,193 live births [5]. Unlike the case of other age-specific death rates, it is possible for an infant to be represented in the numerator but not in the denominator. For

---

Exhibit 8-5. Cause-specific death rates per 100,000 in Baltimore City, 1979 [5].

Formula: $\dfrac{\text{Number of deaths in 1979 from a specified disease}}{\text{Population in 1979}} \times 100,000$

Malignant neoplasms:

$$\frac{2,083}{837,760} \times 100,000 = 248.63$$

Major cardiovascular diseases:

$$\frac{4,323}{837,760} \times 100,000 = 516.01$$

Exhibit 8-6. Infant death rate.

$$\frac{\text{Number of infant deaths in a specified year}}{\text{Number of live births in a specified year}} \times 100$$

example, a 9-month-old who died in February 1983 was not born in 1983. Infant death rates are further specified by age of the infant (neonatal, postnatal, perinatal). The denominator for all these rates is the number of live births. Death rates are usually higher for the neonatal period (0 to 27 days) than for the postnatal period (28 days to 1 year).

Adjusted Death Rates

After specific death rates are determined, they may be adjusted so that two populations can be compared. For example, an investigator wants to compare the death rates for two Maryland cities in 1983 and has the age-specific death rates for both. The hypothetical data and the formula are displayed in Exhibit 8.7. The rates for children and adults cannot simply be averaged because the proportions of adults and children in the populations are not equal. The age distribution in both cities for 1983 was approximately one-third children and two-thirds adults. To determine one death rate for each city that takes into account the population age distribution, the formula is applied:

Age-adjusted rate for city A $= 8(\frac{1}{3}) + 10(\frac{2}{3}) = 9.3$

Age-adjusted rate for city B $= 5(\frac{1}{3}) + 13(\frac{2}{3}) = 10.3$

This technique gives greater weight to the death rate of the group that is proportionally the larger (in this example, adults). Even though the death rate for children was higher in city A, the age-adjusted rate for city B was higher because there is a greater proportion of adults in the populations of both cities and the death rate for adults in city B was higher than for city A. If the age distribution

Exhibit 8-7. Age-specific death rates per 1,000.

	Age	
City	Children 0 to 18	Adults 19 and older
A	8	10
B	5	13

Age-adjusted death rate for city $= Pa + Pb + \ldots + Pn$
where $Pa = $ (death rate for persons in group a) (proportion of the group in the city population)
Note: The groups are mutually exclusive and exhaustive and in this example are $a = $ children and $b = $ adults.

Exhibit 8-8. Case fatality rate.

$$\frac{\text{Number of deaths due to a specified disease in a specified year}}{\text{Number of cases of a specified disease in a specified year}} \times 100$$

---

for city B were one-fourth children and three-fourths adults, the calculation of the adjusted rate for city B would be

$$5(\tfrac{1}{4}) + 13(\tfrac{3}{4}) = 11$$

This same principle and formula can be applied for adjusted rates specific to factors other than age, such as race or sex.

Case Fatality Rate

All death rates discussed thus far have used the number of people in the population as the denominator. They provide information about the probability of dying if people have a specific disease. Whether people die from disease can be dependent on host and environment characteristics. For example, children between the ages of 5 and 14 years may be less likely to die from diarrhea than newborns. The formula for case fatality rate is displayed in Exhibit 8.8. For example, the case fatality rate for encephalitis in Baltimore City in 1978 was 14. The number of deaths was one and the number of cases was seven [4]. Case fatality rates for several diseases can be compared to determine their **potency** for killing. In addition, case fatality rates for one disease can be compared for several populations to discover host or environment variables that might contribute to the potency. For example, the case fatality rate for a disease in a developing country may be higher than in an industrialized one. Better nutritional status, in this instance, may be related to the lower potency of the disease in the industrialized nation.

Proportionate Death Ratio

One final statistic is useful for determining the leading causes of death in a population. This is a ratio rather than a rate. Recall that a ratio is a simple fraction. In the proportionate death ratio, the denominator is the number of deaths due to all causes and the numerator is the number of deaths due to specific causes. The formula is displayed in Exhibit 8.9. For example, the proportionate death ratio for accidents in Baltimore City in 1979 was 5.25:

$$\frac{486}{9262} \times 100 = 5.25$$

There were 486 deaths from accidents and 9,262 total deaths [5]. Five percent is a

Exhibit 8-9. Proportionate death rate.

$$\frac{\text{Number of deaths due to a specified cause in a specified year}}{\text{Number of deaths in the population in a specified year}} \times 100$$

small proportion of 100 percent, and therefore accidents were not a leading cause of death that year.

Morbidity

Morbidity measures the relative existence of disease in a population. Incidence rates and prevalence rates are two commonly used types of morbidity statistics. Rates for two or more different diseases in a population can be compared. In addition, rates for a specific disease can be compared for two or more different populations.

Incidence Rates

The incidence rate provides information about the appearance of new cases of a disease in a specified time frame. It is the probability that people in a population will become afflicted with a disease. The formula is displayed in Exhibit 8.10. For example, health care professionals are interested in the incidence of measles in two elementary schools which are located in different census tracts. The hypothetical data are displayed in Exhibit 8.11. The incidence in school A is $\%_{125}$ = 0.06, or 6 percent. The incidence in school B is $\frac{1}{350}$ = 0.003, or 0.3 percent. The knowledge that the incidence was higher in school A could lead to the decision that immunization efforts in the well-child clinics of that census tract should be accelerated. Although 6 percent seems low, it may indicate that many more than 6 percent of the children are not immunized.

Prevalence Rates

The prevalence rate provides information about the existence of all cases of disease, old or new, in a specified time frame. It is the probability of people in a population being afflicted with a disease. The formula for prevalence is displayed in Exhibit 8.12. The specified time may span months or a year (**period prevalence**) or may be theoretically only one "instant" (**point prevalence**). Prevalence can be a useful rate if the disease or condition is chronic and requires special services to the afflicted persons. For example, special techniques may be needed to provide deaf (chronic condition) persons with health information. If, for example, the state health department in Kansas is conducting a health infor-

Exhibit 8-10. Incidence rate.

$$\frac{\text{Number of new cases of a specified disease in a specified time}}{\text{Number in the population}}$$

Exhibit 8-11. Number of reported cases of measles in 1983

School	Number of Cases	Number of Students Enrolled
A	8	125
B	1	350

mation program, knowledge of the prevalence of deafness as well as the environmental characteristics of the counties could help in the design of special techniques to reach the deaf. Hypothetical data for prevalence of deafness in three counties of Kansas are displayed in Exhibit 8.13. The prevalence in Ford, Johnson, and Sedgwick counties is 0.004, 0.006, and 0.001, respectively. Ford is rural and sparsely populated, Johnson is suburban, and Sedgwick is industrial. The proportion of deaf persons who are provided health information should be similar to their proportion in the county population. If a particular industry in Sedgwick County is a major employer of deaf persons, corporations or unions can be helpful in the health education effort. People who are afflicted with a condition having a small prevalence rate can be neglected in health programs, which results in failure to prevent or detect conditions in addition to the handicap.

Both incidence and prevalence are useful types of morbidity rates, and sometimes it is difficult to know which one to use. Two generalizations can be helpful in reaching this decision. Prevalence is affected by the number of new cases and by the duration of old cases. If a disease persists after its appearance, such as tuberculosis, and there are relatively few new cases, then prevalence rates may be more informative than incidence rates. Prevalence rates help in planning services and the allocation of resources to meet the needs of afflicted people within a large population. Incidence rates, however, may be more informative when health professionals are searching for causes or correlates of infectious diseases of short duration. Comparisons of incidence rates for two or more populations with different host or environment characteristics may provide clues to factors that influence the risk of disease.

Birthrates

The *birthrate* is the proportion of births in the population. The formula for the **crude birthrate** is

$$\frac{\text{Number of live births in a specified year}}{\text{Population at midyear}} \times 1,000$$

Exhibit 8-12. Prevalence.

$$\frac{\text{Number of cases of a specified disease in a specified time}}{\text{Number in the population}}$$

Exhibit 8-13. Hypothetical data for number of deaf adults in Kansas.

County	Number of Cases	Number of Residents
Ford	100	24,115
Johnson	1,500	268,157
Sedgwick	500	365,431

For example, the crude birthrate for Baltimore City in 1979 was 14.55 per 1,000 people. There were 12,193 live births, and the population was 837,760 [5]. Birthrates specific to factors such as age and race also may be calculated and are called **fertility rates.** For example, the fertility rate for 10- to 14-year-old females in Baltimore City in 1979 was 3.40, and that for 15- to 19-year-old females was 74.47 [5]. These rates are calculated by using the number of births to mothers of a specified age as the numerator and the number of females in the population who are the specified age as the denominator. Then the result is multiplied by 1,000. Knowledge of the fertility rate and of the number of 15- to 19-year-olds could lead to the decision to create a special high school for teenage mothers.

With respect to all the rates discussed, an important concept is that specific rates provide more information about potential health problems in a population than do crude rates. Resources always will be limited by the number of personnel and money for programs. Discovering where health problems are concentrated is necessary to help distribute services where they are most needed. Health professionals should select characteristics that define the clients they serve and use these for specific rates. For example, age- and race-specific fertility and abortion rates would help determine where family planning services are needed most.

Death rates, morbidity, and birthrates are the basic statistics used by health professionals to generate information about the populations they serve. These, however, should not be the only ones employed. The basic concepts of rates and ratios should be applied to specific issues by health professionals in each clinical specialty.

Z *Tests for Proportions*

In the previous discussion of rates, we noted the importance of comparisons. For example, the incidence of measles in school A was 0.06 compared with the incidence in school B, which was 0.003. Sometimes it is not sufficient to conclude that there is a difference between the rates, because this could be due to chance factors. Therefore, inferential statistics can be used to determine whether there is a **significant difference** between the two rates. This is a multiple-step process which begins with formulating a research and a null hypothesis and ends with either supporting the **research hypothesis** or failing to reject the

null hypothesis. We discuss two types of Z tests which are appropriate for some types of rates, the Z test for the significance of a proportion and the Z test for two independent proportions.

Z Test for Significance of a
Proportion

A research hypothesis that states a difference between an observed and an expected proportion is appropriate for this Z test of proportions. If it states that the observed proportion will be larger or smaller, the hypothesis is directional. An example is that the proportion of immunized children is larger than .98. If the research hypothesis does not state whether the proportion will be larger or smaller, it is nondirectional. An example is that the proportion of immunized children is different from .98. In both cases, .98 is the expected proportion.

Two pieces of information are needed for this test. The first is a proportion consisting of a numerator and a denominator, which are data about a designated group. The total number of people in the group is the denominator, and this should be 30 or larger in order to apply the Z test. The number of people in the group who meet a specific criterion is the numerator. For example, the proportion of students passing the R.N. board examinations from a specific school is $^{298}/_{300}$, or 300 students took the tests (denominator) and 298 passed (numerator). Another example is the proportion of pregnant women in clinic Z who attended prenatal classes in 1983, which is $^{50}/_{150}$; or 150 pregnant women were treated in clinic Z (denominator) and 50 attended classes (numerator). The second piece of information needed is a proportion against which to compare the data. This can be a theoretical standard, previously obtained knowledge about a population, or chance (.50). Examples of theoretical standards are (1) 95 percent of the students must pass tests for a school to be accredited, (2) 98 percent of school-age children should be immunized, and (3) 100 percent of the adolescents should receive a passing grade on a test of contraceptive knowledge.

Consider the following example in which the Z test for the significance of a proportion can be used. A health maintenance organization (HMO) located in a large metropolitan area offers obstetric and gynecologic services. Nurses working in this area began a program to teach all patients about breast self-examination. Teaching was conducted when clients were in the clinic for routine physical examinations. Two years after continuous operation of the program, the nurses wanted an index of their effectiveness. They failed to assess the level of patient knowledge of self-examination prior to implementing the program, so they could not compare this to current knowledge. Instead, they used information found in a recently published descriptive study of women similar in social and demographic characteristics to their clients. The authors of the investigation reported the proportion of women who had not received health teaching and who were able to correctly perform breast self-examination was .20, which was used by the nurses as their expected proportion. Similar techniques for determining correctness were used for both samples.

The research hypothesis in this instance is that the proportion of patients able

---

Exhibit 8-14. Formula for the Z test for the significance of a proportion.

$$Z = \frac{p - P}{\sqrt{P(1 - P)/N}}$$

p = obtained proportion
P = expected proportion
N = number of people in the sample

Computation of Z:

$$Z = \frac{0.30 - 0.20}{\sqrt{0.20(1 - 0.20)/100}} = \frac{0.10}{\sqrt{0.20(0.80)/100}} = \frac{0.10}{\sqrt{0.16/100}} = \frac{0.10}{\sqrt{0.0016}} = \frac{0.10}{0.04} = 2.50$$

---

to correctly perform a breast self-examination is higher than .20 (directional). Correspondingly, the null hypothesis is that the proportion of patients able to correctly perform a breast self-examination is not different from .20.

Data collection began 2 years after the program was initiated. The sample consisted of the first 100 clients who came to the clinic. Each client was asked to perform a breast self-examination and was placed in one of two categories: (1) able to correctly perform it or (2) unable to correctly perform it. Thirty clients were in the first category. The obtained proportion for the Z test is $30/100$. The expected proportion against which this is compared, .20, is the one obtained from published data. The formula for the Z test statistic and the computation are displayed in Exhibit 8.14. For this example, $p = 30/100 = .30, P = .20$, and $N = 100$.

If the research hypothesis is nondirectional, then the Z statistic is significant if it is larger than 1.96 when you tolerate a five percent chance of drawing the wrong conclusion. If only a 1 percent chance of incorrectly supporting the research hypothesis is tolerable, the Z statistic must be larger than 2.58. Similarly, if the research hypothesis is directional, the Z statistic is significant if it is larger than 1.64 for a 5 percent chance error and significant if it is larger than 2.32 for a 1 percent chance error. For this example, 2.50 is larger than 1.64, and so the research hypothesis is supported. The proportion of clients able to correctly perform a breast self-examination was higher than the proportion of similar women reported in the literature to be able to perform it who did not receive teaching.

It is very tempting for the nurses to conclude that the level of ability in clients enrolled in the HMO resulted from their educational program. The results of the Z test, however, are only one small piece of evidence to support the possibility that this conclusion is valid. Because of the limitations of this research design, there are rival explanations to this statement. Some possibilities are that the patients sampled 2 years after the implementation of the program were new patients who did not receive the intervention, that patients who were able to correctly perform the examination learned it from a source other than the clinic, that the level of knowledge was always higher than the comparison sample, and that there was a difference between clinic and comparison samples on an unmeasured variable which explains the Z test results. If the nurses had planned the evaluation prior to the implementation of the program, these pitfalls could have been avoided. Even with the limitations of the design, the nurses acquired some information from their investigation, and their expenditure of time and effort was minimal since data collection was incorporated into routine clinic visits. Analysis of data took only a few minutes with a hand calculator. The nurses know that the breast self-examination ability in their clients is above the level recently reported in the literature for women not exposed to a teaching program. They know that there is still "room for improvement" in their population, and they may employ an experimental design to test the effectiveness of a revised educational program.

Z Test for Difference Between Two Independent Proportions

A research hypothesis that states a difference between proportion *A* and proportion *B* is appropriate for this Z test. If it states that one of the proportions is larger or smaller, it is a directional hypothesis. One example is that the proportion of graduating seniors from nursing school A passing the R.N. board examinations is larger than the proportion of graduating seniors from nursing school B passing the R.N. board examinations. If the research hypothesis does not state which proportion is larger (or smaller), it is nondirectional. An example is that there is a difference between nursing school A and nursing school B in the proportion of graduating seniors passing the R.N. board examinations.

For the previously discussed Z test, data from only one group were needed, but data from two independent groups are required for this Z test. The label *independent* means that people or events cannot be counted as belonging in both groups being considered. The denominators of each proportion are the number of people in each group (30 or more are needed), such as the number of graduating seniors. The numerators are the number of people in each group who meet a specific criterion, such as passing the R.N. board examinations.

Consider the following example in which the Z test for difference between two independent proportions can be used. Public health officials were concerned about the level of immunizations in a large metropolitan area, and the issue had received publicity in the local newspapers. Both a health maintenance organization and a continuity clinic in one of the major medical centers were located in the same health district of the city. Prevention was one of the major claims of the HMO, and immunizations had been cited as one of their features in a recent drive to recruit members. They also claimed that "other facilities" in the area might not place enough importance on this. Nurses in the continuity clinic, who paid diligent attention to immunizations, decided to investigate this claim.

The research hypothesis in this instance is that the proportion of 3- to 5-year-olds with complete immunizations in the HMO is different from that in the continuity clinic (nondirectional). Correspondingly, the null hypothesis is that there is no difference between the proportions of 3- to 5-year-olds with complete immunizations in the HMO and in the continuity clinic.

Medical records were the source of data. A sample of 400 children between the ages of 3 and 5 was selected from the membership of the HMO. According to their records, 300 of the 400 had complete immunizations. A sample of 200 children between the ages of 3 and 5 was selected from the membership of the continuity clinic. According to their records, 160 of the 200 had complete immunizations. The sampling technique for the two groups was the same. The two proportions were

HMO: $300/400$ = .75   Continuity clinic: $160/200$ = .80

The formula for the *Z* test statistic and the computation are displayed in Exhibit 8.15.

The same rules for determining the significance of the previously discussed *Z* test apply for this *Z* test. Recall that for a nondirectional research hypothesis, the *Z* statistic is significant if it is larger than 1.96 when a 5 percent chance of incorrectly supporting it is tolerated. For this example the *Z* test statistic, 1.35, is smaller than 1.96 and so is not significant. When the *Z* test statistic is not significant, investigators may make two conclusions: (1) the null hypothesis cannot be rejected, and (2) the research hypothesis cannot be accepted. The minus sign before the 1.35 simply indicates that the second proportion in the formula was smaller (although not *significantly*) than the first. Thus the nurses conclude that they cannot reject the hypothesis of no difference in immunizations between the HMO and continuity clinic.

It is very tempting for the nurses to conclude that the HMO does not pay more diligent attention to this preventive measure than the continuity clinic. First, this is not a correct statement because it is based on the assumption that the nurses accepted the null hypothesis (P_{HMO} = P_{CC}). The null hypothesis can never be accepted. Therefore, they can conclude only that the data do not support the statement of differences between the HMO and continuity clinic and do not support the rejection of no differences. The failure to detect immunization differences between the HMO and continuity clinic may be due to the "real" absence of one or may be due to other factors imposed by the limitations of this research design. The host characteristics of the two groups may be different, and perhaps these account for the lack of significant difference in immunized children. Perhaps patients in the continuity clinic receive health care from many places at the same time, while patients in the HMO receive health care from only one place. If this is true, it is possible that the continuity clinic patients received their immunizations from some place other than that clinic. The clinic could be paying very little attention to this preventive health practice and still have patients who are immunized. Even with the limitations of the design, the nurses acquired information about their population. They know the level of immuniza-

Exhibit 8-15. Formula for the Z test for differences between two independent proportions.

$$Z = \frac{P_1 - P_2}{\sqrt{p(1-p)/N_1 + p(1-p)/N_2}}$$

P_1 = obtained proportion for group 1
P_2 = obtained proportion for group 2
N_1 = number of people in group 1
N_2 = number of people in group 2

$$p = \frac{N_1 P_1 + N_2 P_2}{N_1 + N_2}$$

Computation of Z:

P_1 = Health Maintenance Organization (HMO): $\dfrac{300}{400}$ = 0.75

P_2 = Continuity clinic: $\dfrac{160}{200}$ = 0.80

N_1 = HMO sample = 400
N_2 = Continuity clinic sample = 200

$$p = \frac{400(0.75) + 200(0.80)}{400 + 200} = \frac{300 + 160}{600} = \frac{460}{600} = 0.77$$

Inserting the numbers into the formula, we calculate the Z statistic:

$$Z = \frac{0.75 - 0.80}{\sqrt{0.77(1-0.77)/400 + 0.77(1-0.77)/200}} = \frac{-0.05}{\sqrt{0.77(0.23)/400 + 0.77(0.23)/200}}$$

$$= \frac{-0.05}{\sqrt{0.18/400 + 0.18/200}} = \frac{-0.05}{\sqrt{0.00045 + 0.00090}}$$

$$= \frac{-0.05}{\sqrt{0.00135}} = \frac{-0.05}{0.037}$$

$$= -1.35$$

tions among their 3- to 5-year-old patients, and they have important data with which to confront claims of HMO advertising.

Data Sources

Data for the statistics just discussed may be obtained from many sources. Major sources are local and state departments of public health. Birth and death certificates are registered in the municipality of occurrence. Information from them is summarized and sent to state and federal governments. Large metropolitan areas issue yearly reports of vital statistics. If the specific question is not addressed in the report, a special request for the data may be made, usually to a bureau of biostatistics. Blank copies of birth and death certificates allow investigators to know the variables on which data are available.

A very important source of data which is needed for the application of epidemiologic methods is the nurses' record-keeping system. The most advanced systems available are computerized ones into which data about each client are entered and accessed through visual display terminals. Information about host, environment, disease, and treatment can be entered in a comparable manner for each person. This system, for example, could contain data on the number of diagnosed cases of venereal disease among 15- to 19-year-olds and the number of 15- to 19-year-olds in the clinic population. A rate could be compared to an expected rate for the general population of 15- to 19-year-olds or to the rate for adults in the clinic population. When these computerized systems are not readily available, health care professionals should not be discouraged from the systematic use of important information. Medical records are valuable sources of data, even though obtaining the information is time-consuming. If a research question is posed and data can be collected in a prospective manner, a record-keeping system can be set up and used. In the example of venereal disease among 15- to 19-year-olds, an index card could be made for each person in the age range who received health care from the facility in a specified time frame, and these could be kept in a file box, indexed by I.D. number. Clinicians could keep their own files of diagnosed cases of venereal disease and I.D. number. At the end of the year, the incidence of venereal disease could be quickly calculated.

Summary

Epidemiologic methods can be used by health care professionals to provide information about the health status of their clients. Rates of occurrences over a particular time period for a specified number of people are statistics which aid this process. Death rates, morbidity rates, and birthrates are the basic ones, but rates that are specific to special clinical problems (for example, abortion rate) are employed also. Some statistics are available to health care professionals from public sources (for example, state or city health departments), and others must be computed from data in the clinical site. Remember that the basic statistics, rates and ratios, simply consist of a numerator and a denominator for which data are easy to obtain.

A basic assumption of epidemiology is that illness or health in a population is the combination of host (characteristics of individuals), environment (circumstances of occurrence), and agent (source of occurrence). Knowledge about the transaction of these three factors provides clues about variables to change to facilitate health care for individuals. Rates or ratios can be determined for specific environment, host, and agent characteristics and compared by using the *Z* test for proportions. The challenge for health care professionals is to identify rates that are relevant to the population served (for example, the elderly in a specific county), to locate sources of existing statistics, to set up systems for collection of new data, and to use this knowledge to plan programs and to enhance clinical practice.

Vocabulary

Adjusted death rate	Infant death rate
Agent	Morbidity
Case fatality rate	Null hypothesis
Crude birthrate	Period prevalence rate
Crude death rate	Point prevalence rate
Environment	Potency
Epidemiology	Proportionate death ratio
Fertility rate	Research hypothesis
Host	Significant difference
Incidence rate	Specific death rate

References

1. Friedman, G. D. *Primer of Epidemiology.* New York: McGraw-Hill, 1974.
2. Heshmat, M. Y., and Herson, J. *Introduction to Epidemiology and Biostatistics.* New York: MSS Information Corporation, 1974.
3. Morton, R. F., and Hebel, J. R. *A Study Guide to Epidemiology and Biostatistics.* Baltimore: University Park Press, 1979.
4. *Vital Statistics, 1978, Baltimore, Maryland.* Baltimore City Health Department, Bureau of Biostatistcs, 1980.
5. *Vital Statistics, 1979, Baltimore, Maryland.* Baltimore City Health Department, Bureau of Biostatistics, 1982.

IV: *Sampling*

In this short unit we discuss some very important aspects of research—your selection and interaction with the subjects of research. While this unit focuses on human subjects, most of the principles presented apply to nonhuman subjects as well. The material in Chapter 9 has been changing rapidly. Therefore, it is important to check with your human subjects review committee for the latest regulations before embarking on a project.

In addition to the usual exercise with vocabulary words, select a recent issue of a nursing research journal. For each research study reported, read the abstract and then skim the article to identify how subjects gave informed consent, in what ways their rights were protected, the sampling technique used, and to whom results were generalized. Do you believe these were the best procedures available for this research situation? What threats to external validity appear to be present?

9: *Ethical Considerations for Research with Human Subjects*

As knowledgeable participants, nurses need also to become informed about various legal parameters affecting practitioner-client relationships. With respect to human rights, legal accountability focuses upon evidence that the professional practitioner or researcher has not failed his/her responsibility by either intentionally or unintentionally withholding relevant information that might have altered the patient or subject's decision. Knowledge about the changing scope of nursing responsibility and the emerging ethical issues affecting all practitioners in health care today is a necessary requirement for professional nursing practice in which accountability for the protection of human rights of consumers is accepted.
American Nurses' Association [1]

Research subjects have the right to freedom from intrinsic risk of injury and the right to privacy and dignity. As a consequence of participating in some studies, an individual may be exposed to the possibility of injury, including physical, psychological, or social. This means that a subject is at **risk.** It is the researcher's responsibility to determine whether risk is potentially present and, if so, to predict its extent in comparison to the potential **benefit** in knowledge to be gained and clinical benefits to patient subjects. When risk is present, if the benefits sufficiently outweigh the risks to justify pursuit of the research, a prospective subject must be given all relevant information prior to participation.

In studies where side effects including physical injury may result, the researcher must inform subjects about the extent to which his or her institution will be responsible, for both immediate and long-term care. If only acute, immediate, and essential treatment is available, it should be stated. If financial compensation is not available but medical treatment excluding hospitalization costs is provided free of charge, this must be stated.

In addition, any proposed study should not withhold from any subject or group of subjects treatments (i.e., educational or health services) which have been established as necessary and appropriate. Research studies also must be designed to maintain the **confidentiality** of information obtained, **anonymity** of subjects, and protection from misuse of the findings. The data provided by subjects must not be used in any way that could adversely affect them as individuals or as members of any group of which they are a part.

Finally, research subjects have the right to exercise free choice to participate or not to participate in research without undue inducement of any kind of force, fraud, deceit, duress, or other form of coercion. The following, excerpted from the code of Federal Regulations and ADA guidelines, are the basic elements of **informed consent:**

1. A fair explanation of the procedures to be followed and their purposes, including identification of any procedures which are experimental and the time involved in participation

2. A description of any attendant discomforts and risks, invasion of privacy, or threat to dignity reasonably to be expected
3. A description of any benefits reasonably to be expected
4. A disclosure of any appropriate alternate procedures that might be advantageous for the subject
5. A description of the methods used to protect anonymity and/or to ensure confidentiality (e.g., code numbers)
6. An offer to answer any inquiries concerning the procedures
7. An instruction that the person is free to withdraw consent and discontinue participation in the project or activity at any time without jeopardy or prejudice to the subject including his/her care

Special attention, moreover, should be given to studies of subjects who are a dependent population such as prisoners, residents or clients in institutions for the mentally ill and mentally retarded, children, military personnel, and any others who may be vulnerable to **coercion** as a result of their relationship to the researcher or administrative authority. Consent forms, when used, should be kept for 3 years following termination of participation. These, too, must be protected with respect to confidentiality. Exhibit 9.1 presents an example of a **consent form.**

Exhibit 9-1. Example of consent form.

This is to certify that I, _____, agree to participate in the stress management project conducted by Elizabeth Rankin, R.N., Ph.D., and Margaret McEntee, R.N., M.S. I have heard the explanation of the program and have read the attached description. My participation is voluntary, and I may withdraw at any time without jeopardizing my future at the University of Maryland School of Nursing. I have had the opportunity to ask questions and have received satisfactory responses. I know that I may ask further questions, should they arise, at any time.

I agree to abide by the expectations of the study. I agree to accept and support the norm of group confidentiality, and I will not discuss the activities of the group or its members outside the group sessions. I understand that all data pertaining to my participating in the project will be identified by code number and that the data and my identity will remain confidential unless I submit a written request for release of specific information.

Signature of Subject: _____

Signature of Witness: _____

Date: _____

Institutional Review Boards

With the passage of the National Research Act in July 1974, a mechanism was provided under which research proposals would be reviewed from the standpoint of protection of human participants in proposed research. This was in response to numerous violations, primarily in biomedical research (see reference note 1). As a result of that act, in all institutions receiving U.S. Department of Health, Education, and Welfare (HEW) funds, all research utilizing human subjects was reviewed and approved by an **institutional review board (IRB)** prior to implementation. The institutions, moreover, then submitted to HEW certification to that effect. The act also established the National Commission for the Protection of Human Subjects to develop guidelines, criteria, definitions, and mechanisms required to implement the act. During the 6 years following the Commission's inception, almost all research was reviewed, regardless of whether it posed risk. IRBs were flooded with work, and many questioned this practice. Finally, in January 1981, the Commission issued new guidelines excusing from review most research that poses no risk. These and some more recent amendments are shown in Exhibit 9.2. In addition, over the same period of years, the commission clarified the definitions of research risk and the nature of consent in various research settings. The clarifications in effect as of 1983 are presented in this chapter.

Research Versus Practice

Research, not practice, is subject to the ethical considerations of the 1974 act and its subsequent clarifications. Therefore, the distinction between research and practice has been the subject of debate, especially when an activity evaluates the effect of a medical therapy. In *The Belmont Report* [2], the Commission concluded that a clinician's departing significantly from standard or accepted practice in the treatment of a patient did not automatically place it in the category of research. Instead, they considered this the purview of medical practice committees who would, in most cases, insist that a major innovation be incorporated into a formal research project. However, when an entire activity including practice components was evaluated, then it was considered research [8].

Risk

Initially, HEW viewed virtually all research subjects as being at risk, without distinguishing between harm and inconvenience. Therefore, the Commission developed the concept of **minimal risk.** By this is meant the "probability and magnitude of physical or psychological harm that is normally encountered in the daily lives, or in the routine medical or psychological examination, of healthy subjects" [8]. Thus, only when risk to subjects is substantially beyond this definition is a subject considered at risk.

Exhibit 9-2. Research qualifying for exemption or expedited IRB review.

1. All research involving human subjects which is supported by HHS funds *and* does not qualify for exemption from coverage must be reviewed. The guidelines no longer extend to research not supported by HHS funds. However, institutions must submit a statement of principles for protecting the rights and welfare of human subjects of any research regardless of funding source.

2. Exempt from coverage is most social, economic, and educational research in which the only involvement of human subjects will be in one or more of the following categories:

   a. Research conducted in established or commonly accepted educational settings, involving normal educational practices.

   b. Research involving the use of educational tests (cognitive, diagnostic, aptitude, achievement) *if* information taken from these sources is recorded in such a manner that subjects cannot be identified directly or through identifiers or code numbers linked to the subjects.

   *c. Research involving survey or interview procedures, *except* where *all* of the following conditions exist:

      (1) Responses are recorded in such a manner that the human subjects can be identified directly or through identifiers, or code numbers, linked to the subjects.

      (2) The subject's responses, if they became known outside the research, could reasonably place the subject at risk of criminal or civil liability or be damaging to the subject's financial standing or employability.

      (3) The research deals with sensitive aspects of the subject's own behavior, such as illegal conduct, drug use, sexual behavior, or use of alcohol.

   All research involving survey or interview procedures is exempt, without exception, when the respondents are elected or appointed public officials or candidates for public office.

   *d. Research involving the observation (including observation by participants) of public behavior *except* where *all* of the following conditions exist:

      (1) Observations are recorded in such a manner that the human subjects can be identified, directly or through identifiers or code numbers linked to the subjects.

      (2) The observations recorded about the individual, if they became known outside the research, could place the subject at risk of criminal or civil liability or be damaging to the subject's financial standing or employability

      (3) The research deals with sensitive aspects of the subject's own behavior such as illegal conduct, drug use, sexual behavior, or use of alcohol.

   e. Research involving the collection or study of existing data, documents, records, pathological specimens, or diagnostic specimens, if these sources are publicly available or if the information is recorded by the investigator in such a manner that subjects cannot be identified, directly or through identifiers linked to subjects.

   f. Unless specifically required by statute, research and demonstration projects which are conducted by or subject to the approval of the U.S. Department of Health and Human Services and which study, evaluate, or otherwise examine:

      (1) programs under the Social Security Act or other public benefit or service programs,

(2) procedures for obtaining benefits or services under those programs,

(3) possible changes in or alternatives to those programs or procedures, or

(4) possible changes in methods or levels of payment for benefits or services under those programs.

3. *Expedited* review (by committee chairperson or designated members) for the following research involving no more than minimal risk is authorized:

   a. Collection of: hair and nail clippings, in a nondisfiguring manner; deciduous teeth; and permanent teeth if patient care indicates a need for extraction.

   b. Collection of excreta and external secretions including sweat, uncannulated saliva, placenta removed at delivery, and amniotic fluid at the time of rupture of the membrane prior to or during labor.

   c. Recording of data from subjects 18 years of age or older using noninvasive procedures routinely employed in clinical practice. This includes the use of physical sensors that are applied either to the surface of the body or at a distance and do not involve input of matter or significant amounts of energy into the subject or an invasion of the subject's privacy. It also includes such procedures as weighing, testing sensory acuity, electrocardiography, electroencephalography, thermography, detection of naturally occurring radioactivity, diagnostic echography, and electroetinography. It does not include exposure to electromagnetic radiation outside the visible range (for example, x-rays, microwaves).

   d. Collection of blood samples by venipuncture, in amounts not exceeding 450 milliliters in an eight-week period and no more often than two times per week, from subjects 18 years of age or older and who are in good health and not pregnant.

   e. Collection of both supra- and subgingival dental plaque and calculus, provided the procedure is not more invasive than routine prophylactic scaling of the teeth and the process is accomplished in accordance with accepted prophylactic techniques.

   f. Voice recordings made for research purposes such as investigations of speech defects.

   g. Moderate exercise by healthy volunteers.

   h. The study of existing data, documents, records, pathological specimens, or diagnostic specimens.

   i. Research on individual or group behavior or characteristics of individuals, such as studies of perception, cognition, game theory, or test development, where the investigator does not manipulate subjects' behavior and research will not involve stress to subjects.

   j. Research on drugs or devices for which an investigational new drug exemption or investigational device exemption is not required.

4. Research involving pregnant women, fetuses, human in vitro fertilization, and prisoners is subject to additional rules and regulations. Please consult the Code of Federal Regulations, 45CFR46, November 16, 1978, subparts B and C.

Excerpted from the *Federal Register* of January 26, 1981 [4], these changes are in response to the recommendations of (1) the National Commission for Protection of Human Subjects of Biomedical and Behavioral Research, (2) the President's Commission for the Study of Ethical Problems in Medicine and Biomedical and Behavioral Research, and (3) public comment. They are intended to decrease costs and delays in implementing research.
*Not exempt when research subjects are children [5].

Informed Consent and Consent Forms

The purpose of informed consent is to allow subjects to make free choices. If risk is involved, subjects must know about these risks. However, documenting consent on a consent form protects the investigator and his or her institution, not the subject, against legal liability. In fact, in some circumstances signed consent forms can be detrimental to subjects in terms of violation of privacy and confidentiality. Therefore, the Commission recommends IRB waiver-of-consent forms when (1) the existence of signed consent form would place subjects at risk (e.g., as a member of a known group surveyed about sensitive topics) or (2) the research presents no more than minimal risk and involves no procedures for which written consent is normally required.

In addition, the Commission has pointed out other studies in which informed consent may not be necessary. These include studies of documents, records, or pathologic specimens when the benefits of the research justify the invasion of a subject's privacy (and when confidentiality, of course, is maintained). Also included are studies of public behavior that have scientific merit and in which there is not more than minimal risk or minimal chance of embarrassment to subjects [8]. The 1981 regulation [3], moreover, specified that some or all *elements* of informed consent could be waived by an IRB when (1) no more than minimal risk was involved, (2) a waiver would not affect the rights and welfare of subjects, and (3) the research could not be carried out without the waiver and, when appropriate, the subjects could be given additional information after participation.

These clarifications represent significant departures from research review practices in the late 1970s. They will, of course, make behavioral research, which ordinarily involves no more than minimal risk, easier to conduct in terms of red tape. However, it may take some time before individual institutions bring their current requirements in line with them. Moreover, the 1981 regulations clearly indicate that institutions are entitled to adopt any *additional procedures they deem appropriate*. Thus, you must investigate those regulations that prevail at your institution.

Finally, the 1981 regulations do not address the nature of informed consent for research which is exempt from IRB review. You are therefore advised to obtain informed consent in exempt research as well, except perhaps in the two situations (i.e., records and public behavior) previously identified. There are, of course, situations in which a complete explanation of the research can bias results. When no more than minimal risk exists and all other safeguards are present, researchers withhold details which can then be presented in a debriefing session after data are gathered. When you are in doubt about how to proceed, consult the IRB chairperson of your institution—even if your research is exempt. The IRB is there to help you as well as to protect research subjects. Exhibit 9.3 presents a set of ethical principles for conduct of research activities which are used by most investigators conducting behavioral research and should help to clarify the investigator's responsibilities.

Exhibit 9-3. Ethical principles for the conduct of research activities.

1. In planning a study, the investigator has the responsibility to make a careful evaluation of its ethical acceptability, taking into account the following additional principles for research with human beings. To the extent that this appraisal, weighing scientific and humane values, suggests a compromise of any principle, the investigator incurs an increasingly serious obligation to seek ethical advice and to observe stringent safeguards to protect the rights of the human research participants.

2. Responsibility for the establishment and maintenance of acceptable ethical practice in research always remains with the individual investigator. The investigator is also responsible for the ethical treatment of research participants by collaborators, assistants, students, and employees, all of whom, however, incur parallel obligations.

3. Ethical practice requires the investigator to inform the participant of all features of the research that might reasonably be expected to influence willingness to participate and to explain all other aspects of the research about which the participant inquires. Failure to make full disclosure imposes additional force to the investigator's abiding responsibility to protect the welfare and dignity of the research participant.

4. Openness and honesty are essential characteristics of the relationship between investigator and research participant. When the methodologic requirements of a study necessitate concealment or deception, the investigator is required to ensure as soon as possible the participant's understanding of the reasons for this action and of a sufficient justification for the procedures employed.

5. Ethical practice requires the investigator to respect the individual's freedom to decline to participate in or to withdraw from research. The obligation to protect this freedom requires special vigilance when the investigator is in a position of power over the participant, as, for example, when the participant is a student, client, employee, or otherwise is in a dual relationship with the investigator.

6. Ethically acceptable research begins with the establishment of a clear and fair agreement between the investigator and the research participant that clarifies the responsibilities of each. The investigator has the obligation to honor all promises and commitments included in that agreement.

7. The ethical investigator protects participants from physical and mental discomfort, harm, and danger. If a risk of such consequences exists, the investigator is required to inform the participant of that fact, secure consent before proceeding, and take all possible measures to minimize distress. A research procedure must not be used if it is likely to cause serious or lasting harm to a participant.

8. After the data are collected, the investigator provides the participant with information about the nature of the study to remove any misconceptions that might have arisen. Where scientific or human values justify delaying or withholding information, the investigator has a special responsibility to assure that there are no damaging consequences for the participant.

9. When research procedures may result in undesirable consequences for the individual participant, the investigator has the responsibility to detect and remove or correct these consequences including, where relevant, long-term aftereffects.

10. Information obtained about the individual research participants during the course of an investigation is confidential unless otherwise agreed. This possibility, to-

gether with the plans for protecting confidentiality, should be explained to the participants as part of the procedure for obtaining informed consent.

11. A researcher using animals in research adheres to the provisions of the Rules Regarding Animals, drawn by the Committee on Precautions and Standards in Animal Experimentation and adopted by the American Psychological Association.

12. Investigations of human participants using drugs should be conducted only in such settings as clinics, hospitals, or research facilities maintaining appropriate safeguards for the participants.

Reprinted with permission [3].

Anonymity Versus Confidentiality

Anonymity and confidentiality are often confused. **Anonymity** prevails when a subject's identity can never be linked to her or his responses. In most cases, this means that subjects' names were never recorded. However, when subjects' identities can be linked to their individual responses, the researcher must keep this linkage confidential or secret. **Confidentiality** is usually maintained by use of code numbers. The instrument or data sheet on which responses were recorded typically has only a code number as an identifier. This is used in data analysis to link pretest and posttest scores, for example. The name of the person and his or her code number are filed in a separate, locked place accessible to only the researcher and very few others with a "need to know." As soon as the need for knowing the identity of the person for each code number has passed, such as when all follow-up measures have been made, usually the list is destroyed. This is not true for questionnaires or data forms themselves, however. These are usually retained for at least 5 years to enable checking of coding accuracy and for use by other researchers.

Additional Protections for Children

Additional safeguards for children who may not fully understand the implications of their participation in research were published in March 1983 [5]. These regulations define children as "persons who have not attained the legal age for consent to treatments or procedures involved in the research, under the applicable law of the jurisdiction in which the research will be conducted." In essence, IRBs are instructed to review research involving children to ensure (1) an adequate **risk-benefit ratio** regarding the **scientific merit** of the research and (2) adequate provision for (informed) **assent** of children *and* (informed) **permission** of parents or guardians. The regulations, hardly the most clearly written document on record, exempt from review most social, economic, and educational research in which the only involvement of children as subjects is in

1. Research conducted in established or commonly accepted educational settings involving normal educational practices

2. Research involving the use of educational tests
3. Research involving the observation of public behavior (unless the researcher is a **participant-observer**)
4. Research involving the collection or study of existing data, documents, records, or specimens

All other research involving children requires IRB review. This includes two categories of research that are exempt when subjects are adults: research involving survey or interview procedures and observations of public behavior when the researcher is a participant-observer. Children may not be capable of recognizing that their responses to questions on sensitive issues could be potentially damaging to themselves or others, and so IRB review determines whether the rights and welfare of children are protected. Similarly, when children are involved in observation research where the investigator is also participating in the activities being observed, they may not have the capability to determine whether to participate.

The IRB can determine when a child's assent and/or parent's permission can be waived. The permission of only one of the parents is sufficient for research when no more than minimal risk is involved or when more than minimal risk presents the prospects of direct benefit to the individual subjects that is at least equal to that presented by available alternative approaches. With these two categories of research, sometimes a child's assent can be waived by the IRB, which can also determine alternate mechanisms for assent/permission under unusual circumstances. When in doubt, always consult your IRB.

Emergence of Review Committees

The original IRBs began operating with few guidelines and a public outcry based on new abuses uncovered and publicized monthly. As an example, reference note 1 presents summaries of a series of seven articles that appeared in the Washington, D.C. newspapers during a 6-month period. They include the U.S. Army LSD experiments, extraordinary pressures put on prison inmates to participate in research, the discovery that much of medical research utilized poor or minority populations unable to refuse, and so forth.

In this climate, then, it is no wonder that committees regulating research sprang up almost overnight and those in existence tightened their belts and became even more cautious of what research they approved. There were, in some cases, review committees to review other review committees. Although the incidents provoking regulation have been precipitated by medical research, often involving drugs and new treatments of disease, the psychological risks to research subjects became of major concern also. People questioned whether the research was worthwhile enough to justify use of a subject's time to complete a questionnaire. And the people making those decisions often were not familiar with the nature of behavioral research and so were not very supportive. Nursing research, over 90 percent of which posed absolutely no risk to research subjects, began to have a hard time getting approval. So did psychology, sociology, social work, behavioral medicine, education, and other disciplines whose focus was behavioral rather than medical and whose research rarely posed risks to subjects. In response, an additional tier of regulatory committees sprang up which were self-regulating: a discipline or profession regulating itself. A research proposal already approved by peers fared better with the formal IRB mandated by HEW.

In *Nursing Outlook,* Hodgman [7] described the review process involved when a researcher wished to study patients in a Boston area hospital. The division of nursing services had set up a review committee to screen proposals and, if approved, submit them to an ad hoc committee which decided whether to submit them to the overall hospital review board. This could occur after a researcher's own review processes within her own institution. While the benefits of such scrutiny can be many in terms of improved design, the research review process as it was practiced in the late 1970s and into the early 1980s, for nurses in particular, added weeks and sometimes months to the planning process and considerable extra effort and expense, since the various review committees, often as not, had different guidelines and requirements for proposals, which in turn required revisions and sometimes new proposals at various stages along the way. Some committees even wanted complete literature reviews to determine whether the researcher knew her content area—a long way, indeed, from descriptions of how subjects would be solicited and treated in connection with the research. Hodgman concluded that because of the time constraints imposed by review, it was impractical for faculty to expect students to conduct clinical research as part of the curriculum, and she defended her institution's position as appropriate. As a result of activity like this in many locations, nursing, which badly needed clinical research, closed its doors to it in terms of providing opportunities for students to do it. Students were therefore encouraged to do research outside the clinical setting, thus promulgating what nursing leaders had hoped to change.

From the previously described flurry of regulators have emerged fairly clear guidelines regarding the rights of research subjects. The American Nurses Association (ANA) issued a position paper in 1975 describing these as they pertained to nursing research and added a very important dimension involving nursing staff in clinical settings who might be expected to help carry out the research. Informed consent and the right to refuse participation were extended to them. If nurses were expected to routinely help out with research, that had to be spelled out as a condition of employment from the beginning. Moreover, the guidelines strongly urge that if nurses are to participate in research reviewed by an IRB, then there should be nurse members of the IRB.

Two Kinds of Review Committees

Basically, there are now two kinds of review committees. The first is the IRB mandated for all Health and Human Services (HHS, formerly HEW) funded research that falls outside the categories described in Exhibit 9.2. The second kind of review committee is unique to the setting in which it functions, and its demands beyond protection of the human rights of research subjects will vary. Some agencies, moreover, have none of this type of committee at all. Where they exist, these committees are primarily watchdogs for the institutions they serve, in order to guarantee that there is not an undo amount of research conducted at any given time and the research that is approved for implementation is good-quality research. Therefore, many such committees have the power to allow or deny access to clinical settings. These decisions are sometimes political, and some require that the researcher or her coresearcher be a member of the institution's staff. When you are contemplating research, it certainly behooves you to investigate the particular channels and requirements for access to a given agency. (Nurses, unfortunately, are often more demanding of other nurses wishing to do research than are other professionals within their professions or even nurses of other professions.) If the requirements appear achievable or negotiable, then it is essential that quality research be proposed via a quality research proposal. Development of such a proposal is worthwhile even when it is not mandated, because it requires greater thoughtfulness and attention to detail which, in turn, cannot help but strengthen a research design.

Another version of this second kind of review committee exists within some academic institutions. Peer review within the department, primarily for quality control, although often masked behind more lofty titles, is required for faculty and students regardless of the IRB status of the research and prior to review by the IRB or any agency review committees.

A new era is now beginning in which ideally the review committee can be viewed as a helper and supporter of your research. For a researcher working alone, the committee is invaluable as a source for advice, feedback, and guidance about the research. If the review committee can be approached openly with a willingness to consider its suggestions, good relationships and research can result. A review committee, however, has a responsibility to not mettle in areas beyond its expertise. If questions arise, suitable experts should be consulted before demands are made for, say, changes in design or measurement instruments for the purpose of improving the research. But if sampling procedures or administration of the experimental variable interferes with the normal functioning of an agency, the committee and researcher should meet to negotiate changes that are less disruptive of the agency but maintain the integrity of the research. After all, the agency must weigh the advances in knowledge gained by research against any inconvenience in delivery of good patient care.

Rights of Researchers

Except for the ANA guidelines [1] which address the right to informed consent for nurses expected to help conduct research, little attention has been given to

> **Exhibit 9-4.** Common ethical and human relations
> mistakes made by researchers in clinical settings.
> ──
> 1. Researcher does not follow proper channels in setting up a study in a health agency.
> 2. Researcher is not prepared to adequately answer questions likely to be asked by administrators of the institutions in which the research is proposed.
> 3. Researcher weakens the research design by making changes for the administrative convenience of the clinical setting or whimsy of review committee members who are not expert in the research area.
> 4. Researcher establishes good rapport and then loses it by failing to maintain good ongoing communication with those in the clinical setting.
> 5. Researcher uses poor measures or design or inadequate sample that cannot be defended to critics of the research.
> 6. Researcher does not follow correct procedures for obtaining informed consent from parents and/or subjects.
> 7. Researcher does not adequately safeguard the confidentiality of research data.
> 8. Researcher does not adequately debrief research subjects.

the researchers themselves. Certainly they as a discipline group deserved representation on committees reviewing their research. This was also foreseen and advocated in the ANA guidelines. There are several others areas in which researchers have a right to expect respect. First, the committee review process should be approached by committee members with a positive (i.e., helpful) rather than adversary philosophy. Second, the committee should be knowledgeable in the content area of research or obtain such expertise via consultations before demanding design changes for the sole purpose of improving the research. Third, researchers should be protected from undue red tape and expense as a result of the review process. Last, researchers deserve freedom from sabotage and unnecessary explanations in the clinical setting once data gathering begins. As agents of their institutions, the second type of review committee (non-IRB) should be willing, prior to implementation of the research, to make these committments to researchers working in their setting or else point out those areas in which commitments or assurances cannot be made.

No list of rules or rights can ensure clear sailing for a research project. Much is dependent on a researcher's interpersonal skills. Exhibit 9.4 lists the most common errors made by researchers in clinical settings. Hopefully, they will help prevent similar errors in your research.

No doubt, other rules and regulations regarding research with human subjects will appear and disappear. It is important to keep up with most recent developments. However, if you use common sense and are always concerned about the welfare of your research subjects, you should have no problem.

Reference Note 1

The following are a series of abridged or paraphrased excerpts from Washington, D.C. newspapers over only a 6-month period in 1975–1976, more than a year after the Research Act which brought research under review in order to prevent the blatant violations of the past. Not all articles appearing during that time are cited:

DRUG TEST ERRORS ADMITTED, Bill Richards, *The Washington Post,* September 9, 1975:

The Army acknowledged yesterday that it apparently violated military guidelines and professional medical ethics and safety procedures in a number of its drug experiments on thousands of human volunteers between 1953 and 1969.

. . . Army researchers failed to follow guidelines issued in 1953 . . . which ordered the appropriate military branch secretary to authorize in writing his approval of experimental research on human volunteers. . . . Despite tests involving dozens of substances from alcohol to powerful hallucinogens, . . . there is no evidence of requests for approval after 1958–9 until 1969.

. . . About 1500 persons were given LSD and last month the Army said it was trying to locate all of its LSD test subjects for medical and psychological testing. . . . There may be others who took the drug who are not known . . . records have either been destroyed or mislaid.

Thirteen contracts were funded by the Army with private research facilities for tests of drugs that induce hallucinations or delirium . . . what information is available does not show that research subjects were always told details about the substances they were being given.

The former civilian director of a testing program for the Army is alleged to have said most of the research reports sent in by outside contractors were "useless" and "not worth reading."

PROBE TOLD INMATES PRESSURED ON EXPERIMENTS, Bill Richards, *The Washington Post,* September 30, 1975:

. . . Regulating factors such as "informed consent," which are required during experimentation on civilian populations outside prisons, sometimes are lacking during programs inside prison walls because of pressures on prisoners to participate.

A former inmate who was recently released said he allowed himself to be given malaria, typhoid fever, and shigella while he was in prison to raise money to fight for an appeal of his conviction, . . . Such luxuries as airconditioning, adequate heating in winter, television, and extra money are used to lure prisoners into research programs. . . most prisoners believe they will get extra time off their sentences if they take part in the experiments . . .

Another inmate said that although they were promised they could leave the program whenever they wanted, it often took weeks before requests to get out were heeded.

SAFEGUARDS ON MEDICAL RESEARCH ON HUMANS URGED, Victor Cahn, *The Washington Post,* January 9, 1976:

There are no precise figures, but one study estimates that 80% of all research is done on minorities and the poor . . . Addressing the first National Minority Conference on Human Experimentation, M. Carl Holman, president of the National Urban Coalition stated that . . . minorities have become deeply suspicious of researchers as a result of a long series of research atrocities like the federal study that denied treatment to black syphilis patients at Tuskegee, Alabama.

EXPERIMENTS ON HUMANS QUESTIONED, Christine Russell, *The Washington Star,* February 1, 1976:

The studies conducted on the attitudes and practices in the total range of experimentation with human subjects included a national mail survey of nearly 300 biomedical research institutions and intensive interviews of 350 individual investigators at 2 medical institutions.

. . . Most researchers were strict in balancing risks against benefits. The permissive researchers who were more willing to accept an unsatisfactory risk-benefit ratio tended to be the extreme, mass producer scientists, competing for recognition among their peers . . . and also unrewarded competent scientists.

Of more than 400 projects reviewed, half posed no risk at all. But in 18%. . . the risk was not adequately counter-balanced by benefits . . . Less favorable experiments were twice as likely to involve largely poorer patients—those in hospital wards and clinics.

Barber, the researcher, concluded that the abuses "can be traced to defects in the training of physicians and in the screening and monitoring of research by review committees."

ON REACHING THE END OF AN ODYSSEY THROUGH BUREAUCRACY, Lawrence Stern, *The Washington Post,* February 20, 1976:

. . . In an executive order on U.S. intelligence activities, President Ford said the CIA could no longer conduct drug experiments on human subjects unless it followed "the guidelines issued by the National Commission for the Protection of Human Subjects for Biomedical and Behavioral Research."

Thereupon, this reporter tried to locate the Commission via the telephone book, a perusal of the Congressional Directory Index and calls to Nessen at the White House and the office of the White House Counselor. No one knew where to locate it. Finally, the next day another reporter declared, "I can't believe that neither you nor the White House were aware of the Commission. They have just had public hearings." They are part of NIH.

. . . the temporary two year legislative charter expires soon unless an amendment by Kennedy to extend its life passes in this session of Congress . . . Because it is now part of President Ford's intelligence reorganization, "we are obviously going to have to support the Kennedy amendment," said an informed White House official after he, too, succeeded in unraveling the mystery of the Commission's identity.

18 INJECTED IN 1945 PLUTONIUM TESTING, George C. Wilson, *The Washington Post,* February 22, 1976:

The government (ERDA) injected plutonium into 18 people from 1945 to 1947 in an experiment aimed at determining what the poisonous, radioactive substance would do to workers manufacturing the atomic bomb. . . . Only one of the 18 knew what the injection was. The subjects ranged in age from 4 to 68 and were all believed suffering from terminal illnesses. Three are still alive.

. . . records on the experiment are so unclear that it is not known how subjects were selected and it is possible that more than one of the 18 was told the truth about the injections.

PRISONERS X-RAYED IN STERILITY TEST, George C. Wilson, *The Washington Post,* February 28, 1976.

The Atomic Energy Commission in the 1960's beamed x-rays into the testicles of 131 state prisoners to learn whether heavy radiation made them sterile. The prisoners (and their wives) gave written consent, and men underwent vasectomies after the radiation had damaged their reproductive systems to the point they could have fathered deformed children.

. . . There is no evidence the radiation provoked cancer. . . . The federal government is not certain because no follow-up check has been made. An ERDA spokesman said the agency wants to do a follow-up study but that state authorities and some of the prisoners are reluctant to cooperate because of possible embarassment.

Vocabulary

Anonymity

Benefit

Child's assent

Coercion

Confidentiality

Consent form

Informed consent

Institutional review board (IRB)

Minimal risk

Parental permission

Participant-observer

Risk

Risk-benefit ratio

Scientific merit

References

1. American Nurses' Association Commission of Nursing Research. *Human Rights Guidelines for Nurses in Clinical and Other Research.* Kansas City, Mo.: American Nurses Association, Publication No. 0-46, 1-11, 1975.
2. Commission for the Protection of Human Subjects for Biomedical and Behavioral Research. *The Belmont Report: Ethical Principles and Guidelines for the Protection of Human Subjects of Research.* Washington: DHEW, Publication No. (05) 78-0012, 1978.
3. Committee on Scientific and Professional Ethics and Conduct of the American Psychological Association. Ethical standards of psychologists. *APA Monitor* 8:22, 1977.
4. Department of Health and Human Services (DHHS). Final regulations amending basic HHS policy for the protection of human research subjects. *Fed. Reg.* 46:8366, January 26, 1981.
5. Department of Health and Human Services (DHHS). Children involved as subjects in research: Additional protections. *Fed. Reg.* 48:9814, March 8, 1983.
6. Department of Health, Education, and Welfare (DHEW). Code of federal regulations and certain other related laws and regulations on use of human subjects. Washington: *PRR Reports,* No. 45-CFR-46, November 16, 1978; *Fed. Reg.* 43:515, November 3, 1978.
7. Hodgman, E. C. Student research in service agencies. *Nurs. Outlook* 26:558, September 1978.
8. Levine, R. J. Clarifying the Concepts of Research Ethics. Hastings Center Report, June 1979.

10: *Sampling Techniques*

Eleanor Reiff-Ross

The impetus behind the drive for research in nursing and health behavior is to describe the universe and its phenomena, to understand it, and ultimately, to control it. This trilogy of goals, common to all research, can be implemented through generalizations or principles that describe or apply to categories of people, events, places, or phenomena. The application of principles such as Pasteur's germ theory of disease allows us some control over morbidity rates with infected populations. Such advances in accretions to human knowledge form the building blocks of science. These accretions may be gained via data from repeated trials of experiments with humans or inanimate objects. The data from repeated trials, called **replications,** are synthesized into **generalizations.** The rationale behind replications of an experiment is the search for valid generalizations that permit wide application. More often, the wider the application is, the more useful is the generalization. It would be of limited advantage if the germ theory of disease were applicable only to the Basque peoples of the Pyrenees. It would be helpful to the Basques, but not to the remainder of the world.

Certainly not all potential contributions to science are in the polished form of a principle or generalization. While working on a medical unit with cardiac patients, you might observe that those patients who ingest large quantities of cooked or raw onions with their meals seem to be recovering faster than other patients. Should you make a beeline to the head dietician and strongly recommend onions for cardiac patients? And if so, should it be for some cardiac patients or all cardiac patients? Can you reliably make the generalization that onions contribute to patient cardiac recovery? You may have inadvertently picked up an enormously important effect that needs to be tested in subsequent research before there can be any consideration of clinical implementation of this potential generalization.

Health care professionals are uniquely confronted with research possibilities from which generalizations may follow and significant contributions to science emerge. For example, as a nursing student desirous of a wide base of experience before opting for a specialty area, you might decide to attempt a part-time job in a halfway house for female alcoholics. After awhile, you become sensitized to interpersonal problems between the clients and their mothers. On Mother's Day a large number of the female clients disparage the need for a day to honor mothers. On later occasions you overhear negative comments about some mothers and vilifications of others. Do all female alcoholics hate their mothers? Have you discovered an important factor in the psychological constellation of female alcoholics? What do you need to do specifically to test your hunch and generalize your findings to female alcoholics and not just the women in your halfway house?

External Validity

Another procedure advised in doing quantitative research is probability sampling of data. These procedures feature *random sampling* and then *random assignment of subjects* to different experimental groups. Randomization procedures allow you to say what chance, or probability, each unit in your study had of being included in your research. In addition, randomization procedures enable you to estimate the amount of error in the sample data and thus the degree of bias in your data. Randomization procedures are the preferred method of selecting samples. When a design has these features, it is characterized as possessing **external validity,** or generalizability of its findings. External validity is the extent to which results of a research study can be applied or generalized to other persons, settings, and times. Although the sampling procedures in this chapter focus on how subjects become members of a sample, the same principles can be applied to the sampling of settings and times—the other considerations of external validity. In fact, some procedures incorporate sampling of settings as well as subjects.

The external validity of a design is also threatened by attributes of the design other than random sampling procedures. Many threats to external validity in a research design have been identified. Among the most important are these:

1. The effect of *measurement* on subjects, especially the **pretesting effect,** may alter the subjects so that they no longer are typical of the population. If you plan to assess knowledge of colorectal cancer in an automotive plant prior to presenting a talk on it, the questionnaire itself may elevate anxiety levels to the point where workers screen out the substance of your talk. Or it might serve as a source of information to the workers. Either way, they are no longer typical of the population to which you wish to make generalizations.

2. The **Hawthorne effect** occurs when your experimental *and* control or comparison group subjects behave differently from their customary way because they are in a study. You are investigating maternal verbal stimulations of neonates with primiparous mothers, and the mothers put on a show with their babies just because you are there to record the interactions.

3. Another threat to the external validity of a design, one that is even more subtle than the previous two, is the **experimenter effect.** It results from some unintended communications by researchers to all subjects of the hypotheses about experimental effects. It can be countered by **double-blind experiments** in which the researchers and the subjects are unaware of which group is receiving the experimental variable and which the control.

4. **Population validity** involves generalizing to a **target population** (e.g., all women over age 40) from a sample selected from a **study population** (e.g., women over 40 at three work sites in four cities). Even if the sampling procedure was adequately precise, is the study population representative of the target population? In what ways? Population validity can be subdivided into two categories. The first, **interaction of setting and experiment,** can

threaten external validity when subjects from one setting, such as a hospital, are used in research that is generalized to subjects in other settings, such as outpatient clinics. Would effects found on a university campus be generalizable to factory populations? The second category, **interaction of selection and experiment,** involves generalizing from those willing to participate in research (e.g., volunteers, exhibitionists, do-gooders, hypochondriacs) or those with certain characteristics (e.g., race, socioeconomic status, sex, age, personality) to others who may not possess these very same characteristics.

5. Finally, the **interaction of history and experiment** involves generalizing results obtained in one period of time to other periods in history or the future. Replications over time or a literature review that reveals similar results found in other time periods counteracts this threat.

Definition of Sampling Terms

Most attitudes, decisions, and behaviors of people are derived from awareness of selected information. Rarely are we lucky enough to have all the facts; and even when we do, there is the possibility of misinformation attached to the data we do have. Typically our purpose is to use selected information to make a generalization about a wider class of phenomena. Such a selection is called a **sample.** The sample represents a part of the whole.

Sampling Unit and Element

The smallest and most fundamental unit of a sample is the **element.** Occasionally there are **sampling units** as well as elements. Sampling units contain a set of elements. In the example of female halfway houses, you might have wondered whether the phenomenon of mother derogation was specific to certain halfway houses rather than to one client. Could it be that the staff fostered those feelings? Possibly the negative reactions to mothers are not characteristic of female clients in other halfway houses for alcoholics. If such were your thinking, you would want to investigate different halfway houses; then the houses would be your sampling units with the female clients constituting the elements.

Population and Sample

If you were an R.N. student applying to a graduate school of nursing in the United States, you could prepare a list of *all* United States graduate schools of nursing. Those schools would constitute a **population** of nursing schools. Would you apply to each one? You could. But it is costly in time, effort, and money. Most probably you would apply to a portion of all the schools, a **sample.** Maybe you would choose to apply to a selection of the graduate nursing schools in your geographic area, or to a selection of some highly rated graduate schools in the country, or to those graduate nursing schools whose tuition was fairly congruent to your pocketbook's capacity. Thus you would be applying to a sample of all United States graduate nursing schools.

Parameter and Statistic

From your list of all United States graduate nursing schools, you could compute the mean tuition. This would constitute a **parameter,** or value derived from measuring population data. If you considered graduate nursing schools located only in the Baltimore-Washington area and computed a mean tuition for those schools, from which to estimate the national mean, that Baltimore mean would be called a **statistic,** because only sample data were used in its calculation to estimate the value of the parameter, the mean population tuition. You would be using a sample to learn the mean national tuition. In so doing you can never absolutely know the accuracy of your statistic, although you can compute confidence intervals around your statistic within which the parameter can be expected to fall in, say, 95 or 99 percent of such instances (see Chapter 6).

Target Population and Study Population

The realities of research often (but not always) require a distinction between two kinds of populations. The population to which you hope to generalize the results of research is the **target population.** The population from which your actual sample is drawn is a **study population.** In the female halfway house example, all the clients in residence at a given time at two specific halfway houses comprise the study population. The target population is all possible female halfway house residents. If you are interested in making generalizations to a target population of all female halfway houses, there are several further considerations. Do you intend to include all halfway houses in the Eastern Seaboard? Do you want to include all female halfway houses of a specified age **cohort,** for example, 20 to 50 years? Are you interested in all United States halfway houses? You are the one who defines your *target* population. Once you have done so, you will need to examine your study population to judge how well it represents your *target* population. This judgment is basic to generalizing findings from the study population to the target population. Does your study population reflect the proportions of the target population in which you are interested? If the target population is characterized by a 35 percent morbidity rate of tuberculosis in which the median income is $7,500 and the ethnic composition is 10 percent Caucasian, 65 percent black, and 25 percent Oriental, your study population should reflect a similar profile if you are to generalize your results to the target population.

Why Sample?

Suppose you have just received a legacy. The money you have been waiting for has finally arrived, so you have tuition funds for graduate school. You have only one day to apply for admission. You cannot possibly apply to all graduate schools. If you do, you will lose a semester or even possibly a year. Besides, there are two graduate schools you respect and would be delighted to attend. Also, you find that filling out application forms can be tiresome, and although you have a new legacy, costs are involved in application and you want to economize wherever possible. Sampling is the answer.

It often surprises students that while we have to consider possible sampling inaccuracies or sampling errors, we also have to consider errors involved in using the entire population. The reason is that any time we assess people, places, or things for the purpose of data collection, we are liable to **measurement error.** In effect, we always run a risk of measurement error regardless of the sampling procedures used to collect the data. (Measurement error attributable to instrumentation is discussed in Chapter 4.) Measurement error is a threat to both the internal and external validity of a design. Should you, as a researcher, elect to utilize an entire target population in lieu of a representative sample, you might be introducing error anyway, depending on the method used to collect data. For example, when personal interview techniques are used to collect data, interviewers need to be hired, trained, and evaluated to standardize their performances. A small corps of well-trained interviewers may be more effective, more accurate, and cheaper than a larger corps of mediocre or poorly trained interviewers. With the target population as the sample, there are greater opportunities for errors of measurement to accumulate and, of course, to contaminate the data. Time and money are usually important considerations in planning and implementing a research design. It takes longer and costs more to train 1,000 data collectors than 100. With a set time frame, the probability is that the 100 data collectors will be better trained than the 1,000. With a fixed budget, greater selectivity of data collectors is possible because the 100 can be paid more than the 1,000.

Probability Sampling

There are several approaches to sampling. They may be divided into **probability** and **nonprobability** sampling. The goals of samplers are representativeness, freedom from bias in selection, and thus generalizability to the target population. A sample is defined as a probability sample when the probability of each unit's inclusion is equal. The index of probability ranges from 1 to 0.00, where 1 is certainty of inclusion and 0.00 is absence of inclusion. There are various methods for probability sampling; each starts with a definition of the target population and study population to be sampled.

Using a Table of Random Numbers

Let us assume you are a non-U.S. resident interested in applying to four baccalaureate education nursing schools along the Atlantic Coast from Massachusetts to Virginia. You acquire a list of such schools and then number them, beginning with 1. See Exhibit 10.1. This is known as a **prelisting.** The most highly recommended method for sampling from a prelisting uses a table of random numbers, which you will find in Appendix III. You can start at any point in the table and move up-down, down-up, or diagonally; but once you have started, you must proceed systematically in the direction chosen.

The list in Exhibit 10.2 is part of a table of random digits. You decide to start with the first value at the top of the extreme left column in Exhibit 10.2. The first

Exhibit 10-1. Mid-Atlantic baccalaureate nursing schools along the United States coast.

Connecticut
(01) Fairfield University   (02) Southern Connecticut State College   (03) University of Bridgeport   (04) University of Connecticut   (05) Western Connecticut State College   (06) Yale University

Delaware
(07) University of Delaware

District of Columbia
(08) American University   (09) Catholic University of America   (10) Georgetown University   (11) Howard Universtiy

Maryland
(12) Columbia Union College   (13) Towson State University   (14) University of Maryland

Massachusetts
(15) Boston College   (16) Boston University   (17) Fitchburg State College   (18) Northeastern University   (19) Salem State College   (20) Simmons College   (21) Southeastern Massachusetts University   (22) University of Lowell   (23) University of Massachusetts

New Jersey
(24) Fairleigh Dickinson University   (25) Rutgers, The State University, Newark   (26) Rutgers, The State University, Camden   (27) Seton Hill University   (28) Trenton State College   (29) William Paterson College

New York
(30) Adelphi University   (31) Alfred University   (32) The City College of the City University of New York   (33) Columbia University   (34) D'Youville College   (35) Hartwick College   (36) Herbert H. Lehman College of the City University of New York   (37) Hunter College   (38) Keuka College   (39) Long Island University   (40) Molloy College   (41) Mount Saint Mary College   (42) New York University   (43) Niagara University   (44) Roberts Wesleyan College   (45) Russell Sage College   (46) Skidmore College   (47) State University of New York College of Arts and Sciences   (48) State University of New York at Binghamton   (49) State University of New York at Buffalo   (50) State University of New York Downstate Medical Center   (51) State University of New York at Stony Brook   (52) Syracuse University   (53) University of Rochester   (54) Wagner College

Rhode Island
(55) Rhode Island University   (56) Salve Regina College   (57) University of Rhode Island

Virginia
(58) Eastern Mennonite College   (59) George Mason University   (60) Hampton Institute   (61) Old Dominion University   (62) Radford College   (63) University of Virginia   (64) Virginia Commonwealth University

Exhibit 10-2. Table of random digits.			
66	07	06	84
91	76	06	24
04	98	03	72
21	04	14	91
12	01	66	86

random digit is 66. But your total sample size is 64. Go on. The next random digit is number 91. Again, there is no number 91 on your prelist, and you press on. The third random digit is 04. Aha! That is your first sampling unit, the University of Connecticut. Your next selection is 21, which is Southeastern Massachusetts University. Fine. Digit 12 follows, and it is Columbia Union College in Maryland. Digit 07 is next in sequential order. It is the University of Delaware. You then apply to the four schools for admission.

Selection of schools for admission, nursing or otherwise, is not typically done this way by United States resident citizens. However, in the absence of any qualifying information whatsoever, this approach is feasible. This is called simple random sampling.

Simple Random Sampling

In **simple random sampling** every unit of the study population has an equal and independent chance of selection. In selecting four baccalaureate nursing institutions, the sampling procedure was simple random sampling, and it involved using a table of random digits. Other procedures to control for bias in selection do exist, such as rotation of units in a drum or huge bowl. However, this may contribute to bias when elements cling in masses to a side of the drum or bowl. Use of a table of random digits controls best for bias, or error, in sampling. In the example of choosing four baccalaureate institutions, we were interested in only those on the Atlantic Coast. Had we been interested in locations throughout the United States, our prelisting job could have been formidable. You can readily see that "simple" random sampling can be quite a misnomer, depending on the task at hand.

Systematic Sampling

A second type of sampling is **systematic sampling.** It requires calculation of an interval width and a random start. You can use a prelist or just natural ordering (e.g., the order patients arrive at an emergency room). First, you decide on your sample size and then proceed by dividing this number into the size of the study population. The answer, or quotient, is your interval width (IW):

$$IW = \frac{\text{total number of units in population}}{\text{number of units needed for sample}} \qquad (10.1)$$

Systematic sampling is a rare bird. It can float in either of two classifications of sampling, probability and nonprobability, depending on how you handle your *first* selection. If your first sampling element is made via a table of random numbers, the procedure falls in the probability group of sampling. All you need, then, is to add your interval width to your first pick, and you have your second selection. You continue this way until finished.

Let us assume you need a sample of 100 and your study population contains 1,000 units. First you calculate your **interval width.** It is 1,000 divided by 100, or 10. A random start can be any number between 1 and 10. By random selection the first inclusion happens to be 09. Your second inclusion is 9 plus 10, or 19. The third is 19 plus 10, or 29, and so on. Why is the first inclusion selected randomly? At the onset, using a random start should give all subjects an equal chance of being selected. However, sometimes even this yields a biased sample. Let us consider that we are engaged in a study to measure student attitudes toward the school nurse in a specific school. The student names are listed so that males alternate with females; the odd numbers are males, and the even numbers are females. Probability systematic sampling will bias your sample; either all males or all females. Thus, look carefully to see whether a prelist or natural ordering has any possible bias or **cyclic effect** which could invalidate your sample even though you utilize a **random start.** A cyclic effect could result in overselection of some types of units to the detriment of other types. For example, if you are sampling from a list of patients admitted daily to a community mental health center for a week and it happens to be Christmas week, it is possible the alcoholism unit would have heavier than usual admissions. Your sample might have a disproportionate number of alcoholics. To modify the bias, you could randomly select within each interval width. However, then you might just as well use simple random sampling. Probability systematic samples are easy to use and conserve both time and energy. However, they are generally inappropriate for lists with cyclic effects. Generally probability systematic sampling yields comparable precision to simple random sampling.

Stratified Random Sampling

A researcher investigating student attitudes in a certain school toward the school nurse would have been well advised to use **stratified random sampling,** which ensures inclusion of components of a population at a fixed ratio to each other, such as half males and half females. Let us assume a sample size of 100 has been chosen. If the appropriate gender ratio in the school is 1 to 1, or half males and half females, the sample should include 50 males and 50 females. Then all that needs to be done is to record the first appropriate 50 digits from a table of random numbers for males and repeat the process for females.

In the example that focused on selecting nursing schools from the list presented in Exhibit 10.1, suppose a student wished to apply to one school in *each* state. She would need to use stratified random sampling. Having first *stratified* the prelisted schools according to state, as shown in Exhibit 10.1, she would use simple random sampling of the schools within each state to select the one to which she would apply. Another version of stratified random sampling would occur if she decided to sample 20 percent of the schools, with a minimum of one, in each state. In this case, she would be applying to more schools in the state of New York than in, say, Maryland. She would be using a proportionate rather than a disproportionate sample.

Cluster Sampling (Multistage)   **Cluster sampling** is also known as a multistage sampling because it involves taking samples in stages, from the more general to the more detailed unit. It is particularly useful when widely dispersed geographic areas are to be sampled by personal interview or contact. To illustrate, you are interested in evaluating pediatric patient care in hospitals throughout the United States and you need a representative sample of patients. It is a staggering, if not impossible, job to compile patient lists to make a simple random or systematic selection. With cluster sampling, the job is manageable. You simply sample the hospitals and then randomly sample only patients within the hospitals selected. The patients comprise a cluster. It certainly is easier to get a list of hospitals than a list of patients in the United States.

When there are large clusters of unequal size, such as hospitals whose bed capacities differ, additional procedures need to be followed. One approach is first to determine hospital size, in terms of bed capacity, number of annual discharges, or mean daily census. Then you can calculate a mean size for the hospitals and divide each hospital by that mean size. The resulting quotient will indicate how many times each hospital should be prelisted before you take your first sample. If the mean hospital size is 100 beds and University Hospital in Madison, Wisconsin, has 500, put University Hospital on your prelist five times. Large hospitals have, by this procedure, greater chances of inclusion in the first round than smaller hospitals. Next you sample patients, and equal numbers of patients are sampled from each hospital selected from the prelist. This technique is cluster sampling with probability proportionate to size.

Let us look at another use for cluster sampling. You are considering additional training as a primary care nurse practitioner but are not sure there is widespread public acceptance of the role. You recently became involved with a Southern Regional Educational Board (SREB) research team, and they think it would be useful to appraise national opinion. How can you go about it most efficiently by using personal-interview techniques? (Of course, with mailed questionnaires you would not be limited to using cluster sampling. Nor would you be limited to cluster sampling were national WATS lines used for telephone interviewing unless your research design included visual behavior cues.) Your first task in cluster sampling might be to randomly sample 10 of the 50 states, using simple random sampling. You then list all the cities, possibly defined as containing 5 million inhabitants or more, in the 10 randomly selected states and randomly sample a predetermined number of the cities, possibly again 10. For each of the 10 cities you list the census tracts. As a possible last step, you randomly sample 10 census tracts in each city. This process may be repeated for blocks and wind up with households where your interviewing takes place.

A problem with cluster sampling is that as the geographic unit becomes smaller, the clusters become more homogeneous, or similar, regarding a particular variable. The households of a number of blocks of downtown Baltimore might be racially black, socioeconomically comparable, and attitudinally similar. To interview them might yield nonrepresentative data and provide a threat to external validity. But as clusters increase in size, suggesting larger geographic areas, so do the cost factors.

Throughout this chapter we have been aware that while we can usually anticipate some **sampling error,** the object is to have as representative a sample as possible with as little sampling error as possible. Recall that even when the unlikely event of accessibility and availability of the population obtains, increased measurement error may accompany it. Catch 22. The name of the game is generalizability. We want to be able to extrapolate our findings beyond the sample to the target population. When we cannot do so because our sample is biased or too small, even with probability sampling techniques, we incur the risk of threatening the external validity of the design. While probability sampling techniques *tend* to control better for nonrepresentativeness, often nonprobability sampling is all that can be done. Practically speaking, the opportunity to use random sampling procedures occurs infrequently. Nonprobability procedures also may have advantages over probability procedures in lower cost and greater administrative convenience; they often compare favorably with probability sampling in precision of estimates.

Nonprobability Sampling

There are four types of nonprobability samples. For each type, the probabilities of inclusion in the sample are not equal or known in advance of selection, and in some cases may equal zero. When the probability equals 0, there is no way the unit can be included in the sample. What can you say about the resulting sample? Is it representative? Why not? What about sampling error? Is it known?

Convenience Sampling

The simplest and most commonly used for the four types is the **convenience,** or accidental, sample. It is obtained by including in the sample whatever elements happen to be available or are convenient to use. Let us assume you are a middle-aged male, and before enrolling in a given nursing school, you want to learn how much (if any) attention is given by the school to the educational needs of older students. You approach the first 10 middle-aged students you see and talk to them. In effect, you have chosen to address the first 10 people who conveniently crossed your path. Thus a convenience, or accidental, sample is one in which the elements of the study population are haphazardly selected.

Quota Sampling

Now let us assume you recognize that an institution in which approximately 90 percent are female and 10 percent male may differentiate between males and females to the disadvantage of males. Instead of speaking to the first 10 middle-aged students you meet, you decide one must be a male and the remainder must be female. This is **quota sampling.** It involves the imposition of a criterion on your haphazard sampling procedures.

Quota sampling can be very sophisticated. When you are studying two kinds of intervention or need two groups, you can predetermine a set of criteria, or characteristics, you want common to both groups prior to the intervention. This is called **matched pairs,** and pairs of patients can be selected because they share age, education, diagnosis, sex, or any other variable intrinsic to your research design. It may be superior to stratified sampling in that by careful attention to important variables in matching your subjects, you may have cut more finely the sampling error or bias of your sample than is possible with probability procedures. To the extent that the sample represents the target population, generalizability of findings may follow.

Purposive Sampling

It could happen that you already have a middle-aged male friend whom you consider a reliable observer. You may rate him as typical of middle-aged male students. What do you do? You confer with him. This is **purposive sampling.** A sample is selected because the researcher judges it to represent a whole set of predetermined criteria or one predetermined criterion. Another example could be the election of the University of Maryland's shock trauma unit for intensive study since you consider it illustrative of the highest quality trauma unit in the United States today.

Systematic Sampling

The final type of nonprobability sample is **systematic sampling.** The first element chosen here is selected arbitrarily rather than randomly. In the baccalaureate example associated with the discussion of simple random sampling (Exhibit 10.1), the first step was to prelist all the baccalaureate institutions in the desired areas, and the second step was to determine the sample size. That was easy since you were going to contact 4 institutions out of a total of 64. Systematic sampling offers a clear advantage over simple random selection whenever the study sample contains long lists of units and the sample size is large. In this example the sample size was small (4), and so simple random procedures were followed. But had we decided to use systematic sampling, the next step would have been to determine the interval width, $64/4 = 16$. In nonprobability systematic sampling, you do not have a random start. Your first pick is the IW number on your prelist, or item 16. The next three are 32, 48, and 64.

Had you opted for systematic sampling, the four institutions would have been 16, Boston University; 32, The City College of the City University of New York; 48, State University of New York at Binghamton; and 64, Virginia Commonwealth University. Not only are these a different sample from the units selected by simple random sampling, but also this procedure resulted in two inclusions of a New York State nursing institution. The situation can be remedied by opting for another sampling procedure or by continuing to the next element on the prelist before invoking the interval width.

Vocabulary

Cluster sampling	Population validity
Cohort	Prelisting
Convenience sampling	Pretesting effect
Cyclic effect	Probability sampling
Double-blind experiment	Purposive sampling
Element	Quota sampling
Experimenter effect	Random effect
External validity	Replications
Generalizations	Sample
Hawthorne effect	Sampling error
Interaction of history and experiment	Samping unit
Interaction of selection and experiment	Simple random sampling
Interaction of setting and experiment	Statistic
Interval width	Stratified random sampling
Matched pairs	Study population
Measurement error	Systematic sampling
Nonprobability sampling	Table of random numbers
Parameter	Target population

V: *Measurement*

This unit includes four chapters that focus on measurement—how variables are operationally defined (i.e., assigned a number) and how this measure is evaluated. Chapter 11 encourages multiple measures of a dependent variable, called multimodal measurement, and organizes the various ways of operationalizing variables into three modes: self-report, behavioral observation, and physical assessment. It begins by presenting common sources of measurement error and then discusses each kind of measure in terms of its potential for these kinds of errors and how they are assessed. Chapters 12 and 13 present more advanced procedures for using and evaluating a particular instrument in a given research situation. Finally, Chapter 14 presents an overview of questionnaire design, because we almost always are called upon to gather some basic information via this technique at some time in our lives. This is different from development of an interval level test or scale, however, which is an advanced procedure often requiring several years from beginning to readiness for research—which is not the same as completion.

The basic vocabulary words at the end of the chapters provide a good guide for comprehending the material. In addition, you might review articles in a recent nursing research journal to determine how variables were operationally defined and whether the authors present adequate evidence that error was minimized. How might the operational definitions be improved? What additional evidence would you like? Finally, try your hand at designing a questionnaire to assess preferences for associate degree, diploma, or baccalaureate graduates among directors of nursing, as well as their opinions about internships and their reasons for both. How could you maximize your response rate? How would you insure that your sample was representative? What additional variables should be considered in order to account for responses?

One of the most challenging and yet most vulnerable (to error) aspects of the research process is the **operational definition** or **quantification** of the variables being studied. The choice of an appropriate measure is a complex process, and it usually involves selecting from several ways to operationally define or assign a number to a given variable. Sometimes, considering the research setting and circumstances, the best way to proceed is clear; however, most of the time it is not. It then becomes a matter of researcher judgment—your judgment. Knowing your **measurement smorgasboard,** all the options available to you for operationally defining a variable, is the first step in making a good selection. That is what this chapter is all about.

Researchers have been exceptionally creative in meeting the challenges of quantifying variables. For example, students at the University of Arizona, under the guidance of their professor, combed through samples of daily refuse from 5,000 Tucson households as part of a 6-year federal grant to analyze America's eating habits. Among other things, they found that 15 percent of food purchased is wasted (not counting that put in kitchen garbage disposals), amounting to an annual waste of $12 million in Tucson and $11 billion nationally. During shortages of particular foods, even more is wasted—presumably because of hoarding and subsequent spoilage. Interestingly, when these results were compared with those of personal interviews, residents at all income levels underreported the amount of beer they drank and overreported the amount of milk used.

As another example, observers have noticed that health professionals and even parents spend less time with fatally ill children as their conditions become worse. Researchers at San Diego State University and Children's Hospital of Los Angeles wondered about the children themselves and whether they felt increasingly isolated and left alone to work out their fears and concerns. Therefore, as part of a larger study, they attempted to measure the children's sense of isolation in an **unobtrusive** (or nonreactive) way by using a scale model of a hospital room, with four appropriately-sized adult dolls representing a doctor, nurse, mother, father, and a small doll lying in bed. Twenty-five children with leukemia and twenty-five others with chronic but not fatal illness were asked to tell a story about a friend who was sick in the hospital by placing the figures in the room. Next they were asked to place the figures where they would like the people to be. Fatally ill children placed the four figures further away from the bed than did the chronically ill and children hospitalized more than once did also. When asked to put the figures where they wanted them to be, the dying continued to put them further away, thereby leading the researchers to conclude that fatally ill children not only perceive a growing psychological distance from those around them but also prefer it that way.

Still other researchers have used, among other measures, the number of daily pain medication requests as an operational definition of pain or the number of visitors (or amount of time spent with family members) as an operational definition of social support for hospitalized patients. The possibilities are endless, although, of course, each also carries with it a set of limitations that may make the measure unreliable or invalid. That is why it is essential that you consider the whole measurement smorgasbord for a variable before choosing those you will use in your research. The best source of ideas, as usual, is the research literature and theory related to the topic about which you are conducting research. Do not overlook or underestimate your own creative ability, either.

A *Measurement Smorgasbord*

We often hear that patients experiencing stress may not stabilize as quickly. Nursing actions are routinely designed to reduce the negative impact of stress. But what is meant by the term *stress?* Is it environmental stress as measured by the Holmes–Rahe *Recent Life Events Scale* [28] or its more recent modifications (e.g., Sarasan [54])? In these, events like divorce, a large mortgage, death in the family, and even a vacation accumulate points that yield a total stress score. When the stress score exceeds a certain amount, the individual is considered at risk.* More recently, the *Hassles and Uplifts* scales [12, 32] have been developed and found to correlate with both psychological and somatic symptoms. On the other hand, in defining patient stress, is stress as measured by these scales being substituted for a similar but different variable—*anxiety,* such as that measured by the Spielberger et al. *State-Trait Anxiety* scales [56] or the Zuckerman *Affect Adjective Check List* [60]? These scales focus on internal feelings. In the case of the Zuckerman scale, subjects check from a list of 61 adjectives—like friendly, frightened, or furious—all those that describe how they feel at the moment. Then again, why not just ask the patients if they feel stressed or anxious?

Often there are reasons why any of the foregoing measures might not be appropriate—patients' perceptions may be inaccurate, or they may over- or underestimate their own anxiety. They may fear giving an accurate report if they believe it makes them appear, for example, unmanly or socially unacceptable. They may want to protect loved ones from the truth about how they really feel. Therefore, if patient self-reports seem inappropriate, perhaps observations by a health care provider would be more accurate. Checklists have been used on which nurses check observed behaviors such as hand tremors, verbal dysfluencies, sweaty palms, or lack of eye contact. However, it is known that some very anxious persons show no observable symptoms at all.

Some nurse researchers believe that physiological measures of stress are more objective. Chapman [6] used as physiological measures of patients' stress response increased plasma nonesterified fatty acids and decreased blood eosinophils, although in that study the data may have been confounded by effects due to the surgery itself. Others have used, for example, radial pulse count (e.g., Johnson, Kirchhoff & Endress [31]). Numerous other physiological

---

*The original work based on Holmes–Rahe's *Recent Life Events Scale* has received criticism, even from its authors. See Cohen [8] and others.

measures have been used to operationalize stress (e.g., changes in blood pressure, plethysmograph wavelength height, volume of palmar sweat, 24-hour urine), and each has had limitations as well as strengths.

The choices are indeed many. In this example of the measurement smorgasbord for the variable of stress, measures may involve patients reporting (1) events in their environment that are *assumed* to cause stress or (2) feelings they perceive internally that, again, are *assumed* to be inclusive of a cluster of feelings representing stress (perhaps better labeled distress or anxiety). Other measures involve (3) observation and recording of patient behaviors *assumed* to be associated with stress, and (4) physiological measures also *assumed* associated with a stress experience. Selection of the appropriate measures involves discovery of measures known to be sensitive to the independent variables included in your research. As usual, a review of the research literature related to the variables you wish to study is mandatory. How have other researchers measured the dependent variable? With what independent variables has the measure demonstrated change or correlation? Measures already used in related research are best, because your research can more easily be integrated into the existing body of knowledge. If you are uncertain about the quality of these preexisting measures, consider using the measures in combination with other, better (although new to this type of research) measures.

Multimodal Measurement

One of the problems associated with the preceding measurement examples of patient stress is that we were not sure that the same kind of stress or anxiety, if any, was being measured by each example. Therefore, some were probably better than others. Some measures might correlate to other variables, and other measures would not. Even when we are measuring a variable that is more precisely defined than stress, different measures of that same variable are usually not well correlated, and, as often as not, one measure might prove significant in demonstrating group differences while other measures would not. This is due in part to the fact that the measures are **indirect.** A ruler could be used to measure a person's height because we can easily *see* height; however, we can never *see* anxiety in its entirety and thus there is no easy ruler available for use. Instead, we use various **indicators** and some are better than others. Some are more sensitive to experimental settings and some work better with certain individuals. The phenomenon that involves some measures of a variable being sensitive to differences or change when other measures of the same variable are not is called **response fractionation** (or **response desynchronization**). Although this is not a new phenomenon, it is now receiving increased attention [25]. The major impact of response fractionation is an emerging emphasis on **multimodal measurement.** If a research variable can be measured in a variety of ways, multimodal measurement occurs when several measures instead of just one are selected for use in research study. Moreover, whenever possible (and it not always possible), we select measures to include at least one from each of the three major **modes of measurement: self-report, behavioral observation,** and **physical assessment.** These three modes of measurement will be discussed in detail in the following pages.

Reliability and Validity

In Chapter 2, reliability and validity of tests and measures were introduced and defined. Chapter 13 goes into even greater discussion about the various kinds of reliability and validity and presents methods for inferring them. To review and elaborate a little further, all measures must be reliable. This refers to consistency of measurement. Assuming your weight has not changed, a weight scale used to measure your weight would yield the same number on two separate occasions. This is reliability. If two separate scales are used on the same occasion, they should also yield the same number. This is also reliability. The first is an example of **test-retest reliability** (or, when the measure is a behavioral observation, **intrarater reliability**—if the comparison is between two observations of the same event made on separate occasions by the same observer or rater). The second corresponds to **alternate forms reliability** (or **interrater reliability**—if the comparison is between two raters or observers of the same event). A third form of reliability is known as **internal consistency** or **scale homogeneity.** It describes how well all the test **items** (called questions by lay persons) measure the same variable. Internal consistency is also called **split-half reliability** because, when computers are not available for statistical analysis, a test can be divided into two halves, (e.g., odd-numbered items versus even-numbered items or randomly), two scores computed by adding item responses from each of the halves separately, the scores for each half correlated using the Pearson product moment coefficient presented in Chapter 7, and the resulting correlation coefficient adjusted upward by a special formula (i.e., the Spearman Brown) in order to make up for the fact that there were only half as many items contributing to the scores as there would be when the test is actually used. The rationale behind split-half is that if all items relate to the same variable, total scores for the two halves should be highly correlated.

Thus, there are three kinds of reliability. They can all be represented by correlation coefficients of one sort or another. Reliabilities of .80 are considered adequate for research (sometimes even .60 or .50 is permissible when there are few items). However, reliability of .90 is a bare minimum for measures used for clinical diagnosis of individual patients, particularly when the measure will affect their care.

Validity refers to evidence that the **instrument** (test or observation) actually measures what it purports to measure. Questions of validity are questions of what may correctly be inferred from a test score. It is important to note that validity itself must be inferred, not measured. Therefore, although a series of correlation coefficients might be presented as evidence to infer validity, you must judge the quality or adequacy of the evidence as it relates to your research setting. Validity is never proved once and for all.

Reliability is a basic requirement for validity. Once a measure is considered reliable, it becomes necessary to make sure it is measuring what you think it measures. As with reliability, there are three major kinds of validity evidence. Unlike reliability, it cannot always be indicated by a correlation coefficient, and two types have many subcategories within them. A fourth kind of validity, **face validity,** refers to whether or not a measure *looks* as if it will measure what is purported, and this is really no kind of validity at all.

Chapter 13 details the many subcategories of validity and also describes how evidence can be gathered. The three major types of validity are described here in very general terms:

1. **Content validity** refers to the fact that the items comprising the measure represent a reasonable sampling of all possible items or behaviors that make up the domain being measured. Experts in the content area are often called upon to analyze the items to see if they adequately represent not only the content universe or domain but also the correct proportions.

2. **Criterion-related validity** seeks to establish that the measure correlates to another criterion. Persons who are known to be anxious (e.g., students prior to a difficult examination) would be expected to have high scores on an anxiety scale. Groups known to possess or not to possess the characteristics being measured would be the criterion. If the purpose is prediction of performance, subjects' performance at some future time would be predicted by test scores and then, at the later time, predictions would be compared with what actually occurs.

3. **Construct validity** begins when the investigator formulates hypotheses, based on theory, about characteristics of those who have high scores on a test (compared to those with low scores) and then tests them. The measure can be a dependent variable in some hypotheses and an independent variable in others. Evidence of construct validity is not established within a single study.

Sensitivity and Appropriateness

Although sensitivity and appropriateness are just plain commonsense qualities that must be possessed by a good measure, they are now and then overlooked. **Sensitivity** refers to the capability of detecting changes or differences when they do occur. Variations in sensitivity are one of the two plausible explanations for response fractionation, which was mentioned previously and used as the rationale for multimodal measurement. Some fear-reduction research, for example, has shown that changes in subjective feelings are not necessarily accompanied by changes in *elevated* heart rate. Heart rate, therefore, may not be sensitive enough to demonstrate change as a result of some interventions—particularly if it is observed immediately after administration of the experimental variable. In the mental health field, new physiological correlates of schizophrenia and depression are emerging owing to the improved sensitivity in blood chemistry measurement. Researchers using the *Rorschach Ink Blot Test* are finding unique response patterns that detect sexual abuse among children, although the test was not intended for this use. Finally, administration of the *Stanford-Binet Intelligence Test* was long thought to measure only intelligence; however, psychometricians have detected patterns of response that correlate with various psychological characteristics in children.

Researchers could conclude no differences or changes and discontinue pursuit of their research efforts when, in reality, their failure to support their hypotheses is due to the poor sensitivity of their measures. Therefore, it is essential to investigate the sensitivity of a measure. There is a way to ascertain the sensitivity of a measure you wish to use. It involves reviewing the research literature (again!) in which the measure was used to determine situations in which it was sensitive. If it has been shown effective in research situations similar to yours, you need not proceed further. If is has not, then you should pilot test the measure under conditions similar to your research. For example, if you are investigating an objective checklist purported to measure pain among patients undergoing physical therapy for low back pain, but you intend to use it among surgical patients (or even burn patients), you might administer the instrument to no fewer than 10 surgical patients known to be experiencing pain and no fewer than 10 who are not. If there is a reasonably large difference between these two groups, the instrument may be sufficiently sensitive. If not, find another measure. If none exists, the first step in your research may have to be instrument development.

Appropriateness refers to whether or not the measure can be used for your particular target population. Reliability, validity, and sensitivity data must, of course, use subjects similar to your target population. The further these data deviate from this, the more suspect is your measure for the use you intend. Beyond this, *appropriateness* refers to the extent to which the target population can meet the demands of the instrument, such as understanding and following the directions and having the physical stamina and motivation to complete the measure. If a measure is inappropriate, you could be measuring, for example, reading ability or vocabulary level instead of the research variable.

Reactivity

When a pencil and paper test is used as a measure, it is usually not 100 percent reliable or valid. If a midterm exam yields an .83 reliability coefficient, the difference between it and 1 (unity) is attributed to measurement error. Thus, $1 - .83$ or 17 percent of the variance of scores on the midterm is due to measurement error. **Measurement error** is created by all random events and things that adversely affect a person's true response to a test or measure. A commotion in the hall, excessive heat in the test administration room, headache or other illness, hunger or fatigue, and even hostile test administrators are potential causes of measurement error. The sources of possible measurement error associated with the measures themselves are known as a measure's **reactivity.** Does the operational definition process itself cause a research subject to behave in ways different from those in which he would if another, less obvious operational definition were used? The very presence of an interviewer may cause a respondent to answer in a way that makes him appear more socially desirable. An anxious patient may fear retribution if health care is evaluated negatively by him. The mere presence of elaborate mechanical apparatus may create artificial physiological readings. The possibilities are endless. All can never be completely controlled; however, use of multimodal measurement, careful selection of measures, and documentation regarding the presence or absence of anticipated reactivity can greatly improve the operational definition process.

Like the many threats to the internal validity of experimental designs that have been isolated from among all other possible confounding variables, several sources of reactivity can be named and described. Some overlap with the threats to internal, external, and construct validity presented in Chapters 4 and 10. Do not be concerned about this. The lists are designed as guides to stimulate your thinking and not as inviolate laws carved in stone.

1. Examiner or observer bias is present when subjects respond to overt or covert behavior or characteristics of the test administrators or interviewers. For example, male examiners have been found to elicit more personality (Rorschach) responses from female than male clients [21, 26], while this cross-sex discrimination was not evidenced by female examiners. Verbal reinforcement and examiner warmth have also been found to influence personality assessment [20, 27]. Examiners may also see what they want to see. **Expectancy,** the examiner/observer's anticipated findings, can influence measurement results. This is particularly a problem when a researcher performs in a dual role as both the experimenter (conducting or administering the experimental variable) and examiner/observer (measuring the dependent variable). Research in the area of expectancy is contradictory; however, in situations in which its presence is possible and resources are adequate, (1) **double-blind** designs are used in which neither the subjects nor the experimenter knows who is in the experimental or control/placebo groups and/or (2) the experimenter and examiner roles are separated.

2. Demand characteristics refer to situations in which subjects who know the hypotheses and expectations of the research respond in accordance with the expectations. Repeated measures, behavioral observations in which subjects know they are observed, and self-report measures are especially vulnerable. In fact, the very nature of informed consent to participate and use of volunteer subjects increases the likelihood that demand characteristics are present.

3. Procedural artifacts include a variety of influences due to the manner in which data are gathered, such as use of tape recorders, the presence of observers, and self-monitoring. The presence of live observers can be a stimulus for parents to engage in special activities with their children, for example, thereby creating more parent–child interactions than would normally occur. Numerous researchers [14, 59] have found that observation procedures can affect measurement. However, reactive effects do not always occur, and it is therefore important to estimate the probability of these effects in your unique research setting. Another area of possible concern may be the "instructional set" communicated as a result of self-monitoring. It is known, for example, that self-monitoring was associated with a reduction in gasoline consumption by college students [17]. It has also been associated in varying degrees with frequency of drug ingestion [23], school performance [34], and other dependent variables. On the other hand, other studies have reported minimal or no reactive effects from self-monitoring [24]. To repeat, estimate reactive effects in your setting and, if the probability of reactivity is high, use other measurement approaches in addition to or in place of the reactive measures. Try to assess the extent of reactivity by, for example, using an additional control group that is not exposed to the specific measure in question but is administered all others.

4. Impression management and faking needs little elaboration. Subjects may give only socially desirable responses or may simply guess at answers.

5. Subject response bias involves a tendency either to be agreeable or to be disagreeable in general. That is why most true–false and Likert format items are **flipped,** half worded so the correct response is true and half worded so the correct reponse is false. Similarly, some subjects tend to either *strongly* agree or *strongly* disagree while others tend to either *somewhat* agree or *somewhat* disagree.

There are numerous other factors that could produce reactivity and thus measurement error. Many are unique to a specific research setting. It is important to anticipate these and take steps to control or measure their effects. It is a waste of time to argue about whether your particular source of error should be classified as a demand characteristic or procedural artifact. Like other lists presented in this book, these categories are often products of the author's whimsy and ways of organizing for research, and they could be replaced by your own system once you become immersed in the unique characteristics of research in your area of interest.

There is a family of measures known as unobtrusive or **nonreactive.** These, like the earlier example of garbage analysis in Tucson, successfully avoid errors associated with reactivity. However, they often introduce other questions concerning validity. In addition, unobtrusive or nonreactive measures are not always available for use in the operationalization of health research variables.

Primary and Secondary Data Sources

The data source, primary or secondary, is another issue to be considered. Does the experimenter herself take a subject's blood pressure (thus using a **primary source**—the subject) or is the patient's medical record used to extract blood pressure readings recorded by others (a **secondary source**). Additional error is usually present when secondary sources are used, and its magnitude should be estimated before the data source is used.

Direct and Indirect Measures

Another issue to consider when examining an operational definition involves whether it is a direct or indirect measure of a research variable. A rule or tape measure used to determine body measurements (e.g., waist or wrist) or a scale used to determine weight is a **direct measure**—although you must presume accurate scales and rulers for both. Demographic variables, such as age, sex, and income, determined by observation or interview, are generally considered direct measures of concrete variables. The number of days hospitalized, the number of pain medications requested, and whether or not a patient is ambulatory are direct measures of days hospitalized, pain medications utilized, and ambulation, although data sources for all three may be secondary if medical charts are used. However, if a research variable, severity of myocardial infarction, is operationalized as number of days hospitalized, the measure is then indirect. Similarly, the number of pain medication requests is an **indirect measure** of the research variable *pain*. A large variety of projective personality tests, such as the Rorschach, are indirect measures. Other indirect measures that are often incorrectly considered direct include most scales and objective personality tests, such as the *Minnesota Multiphasic Personality Inventory* (MMPI) and *California Psychological Inventory* (CPI).

When measurement is indirect, you must insist on evidence to support its validity. Is it really measuring the research variable? Some research studies [47] have compared both indirect personality tests and direct-report data (e.g., responses to "How do you feel?") with independent criteria like peer ratings, grades, and laboratory tasks and found that direct reports are often equal or superior to the indirect measurement techniques interpreted and scored by clinical experts. This makes it imperative that you know your indirect measures are valid.

Modes of Measurement

It seems appropriate to research in nursing and health to use as modes of measurement (1) self report, (2) behavioral observation, and (3) physical assessment. Patients do indeed give self-reports of their health and other matters, and nurses do observe their behavior and conduct certain physical assessments.

However, it is important to emphasize that these modes are not mutually exclusive nor are they the only way to organize the many methods for quantifying variables. Neither are the strategies presented within each of the three modes necessarily unique to that particular mode. The record review, for example, could be included as a part of any of the three modes but is considered in this book as part of behavioral observations, because it shares many of the same problems as do other strategies in that group. As mentioned repeatedly throughout this book, do not waste time classifying measures into the three modes used in this text. Concentrate instead on the strengths and weaknesses of measures themselves. The three modes presented are a beginning. You may very well evolve your own modes or organizational scheme once you have become expert in your area of interest.

In keeping with current trends toward multimodal assessment to control response fractionation better, a variable measured by self-report, behavioral observation, and physical assessment, or any two of these, may yield more significant findings. Examination of the correlations of these to each other and, in some circumstances, to other criteria will do much to enhance construct validity and the current state of affairs regarding measurement. Your final decision, however, must reflect the appropriateness of multimodal measurement to your research study and a cost-benefit analysis in terms of dollars and the time and energy requirements demanded of your research subjects and you, the researcher.

Self-Report

Self-report includes a large variety of tests and scales, both standardized and research; card sorts; questionnaires and interviews that may have embedded within them tests and scales; diaries and records kept by subjects as part of self-monitoring; direct reports by subjects; computer-assisted assessment; and various combinations of these, including simulations. They all share a common data source: the subject's verbalization, sometimes written, which is often but not always a response to some question or stimulus provided by the researcher. This mode or group of measures is especially vulnerable to reactivity. Because of this, many of the tests and scales, and some of the other measures to a less extent, try to disguise their true purpose. Many also present a series of questions intended to represent all aspects of the research variable rather than a single question. When this occurs, it is especially important to insist on reliability and validity data, particularly correlations to measures from the behavioral observation and physical assessment modes. Although self-report measures are often used correctly as the sole dependent variable measures in many research studies, there are many other research studies that would benefit from multimodal measurement.

Standardized Tests

This category of interval level self-report measures could be considered a fourth mode of measurement—mental assessment. However, because many of the tests in this category have not been a major area of concern in nursing research and are likely to remain so because they require a psychologist trained in psychometric assessment to interpret them, it is subsumed within the self-report mode. These tests do, after all, require subjects to "self-report" by responding to a series of multiple choice questions or other stimuli. They are all considered indirect measures because what is being measured, such as dependency, assertiveness, and other personality traits, is not readily apparent.

Standardized tests include a variety of personality, intelligence, achievement, and aptitude tests such as the *Minnesota Multiphasic Personality Inventory* (MMPI), *California Personality Inventory* (CPI), *Tennessee Self Concept* (TSC), *Scholastic Aptitude Test* (SAT), *Stanford-Binet* and *Wechsler Intelligence Tests, General Aptitude Test Battery* (GATB), *Graduate Record Exam* (GRE), and many others. Standardized tests fall, roughly, into one of two groups. The aforementioned tests all share the characteristic of being **objective** or **nonprojective.** That is, they can be scored by computer or answer key. The results of scoring a subject's responses by several different researchers would be the same. As a group they might be compared to a multiple choice final examination in a research methods course, as opposed to an essay examination. The other group of standardized tests, **projective** tests, could be compared to the essay examination, and they include such tests as the Rorschach *Ink Blot Tests, Thematic Apperception Test* (TAT), sentence completion tests, figure drawing, and so forth. The Rorschach consists of a series of designs that resemble inkblots and a subject tells what she or he sees in the blots. The TAT consists of a series of pictures showing persons engaged in different activities and a subject tells a story to describe the persons and activities. There are usually several different ways to score projective tests, depending on the purpose for testing. They generally involve personality assessment, particularly deviations from normal, or assessment of cognitive impairment. They are **subjective** in nature and could very well result in two scorers coming up with different results. Extensive training and practice are required to administer and score this group of standardized tests. For nurse researchers, it requires additional course work and weeks of supervised practice, because this is not usually part of nursing curriculum. Projective tests are therefore rarely used in nursing research. Although projective tests may tend to carry mystical properties akin to mind reading and reading the future among the general public, they are the subject of heated debate among professionals who seem to polarize either as proponents or detractors of their worth and ultimate usefulness.

Many of the standardized tests are available to only psychologists, and others are limited even more. Often they must be returned to their publishers or distributors for scoring. Most standardized tests, both projective and nonprojective, are best used by nurses who have a psychologist available as a consultant to assist in interpreting results. This is absolutely necessary when feedback is to be given to a research subject about the results of her or his tests. It is ethically indefensible to do otherwise. If group data are to be reported and no individual assessments made, it is not as necessary as long as the test manual gives you enough information to intelligently interpret your results.

Standardized tests have been years in development and have reliability and validity data established for use with many different populations. They also have average responses (means and standard deviations) found in populations like nurses, housewives, lawyers, laborers, physical therapists, ministers, women in general, adolescents, various ethnic groups, college graduates, and so forth. This enables clinical diagnoses of an individual by comparing her or his profile of scores with those of the group with which she or he can be identified. This is known as **norm-referenced testing.** Scores from this approach are at the interval level of measurement and yield information about the amount or level of knowledge, dependency, self-esteem, and so forth possessed by an individual or group of individuals. These scores can be compared with either appropriate **norms** or each other (experimental group mean versus control group mean).

As opposed to norm-referenced, another type of test is rising in popularity, although it does not share the wide application of normative tests. This is known as **criterion-referenced testing.** It is an either-or, pass-fail approach in which a specified set of target behaviors (or items sampling a content area) are designated, and, when these are mastered, the subject is considered proficient in that area. This approach enjoys popularity among those charged with assessing, for example, clinical skills among nursing or medical students. Proponents of this approach argue that assessing the *amount* of skill or knowledge beyond a criterion point of competence is irrelevant and also questionable, owing to the inability of test developers to reach the ratio level of measurement and the numerous errors possible with any type of self-report measure. In fact, some question the interval level properties of scales and tests, arguing that they are only ordinal—a belief not shared by the majority of researchers or reflected in the research literature, however. In the opinion of the author, norm-referenced are more appropriate than criterion-referenced tests for research, because they are likely to be more sensitive to experimental manipulations. Even small changes or differences may be recorded. There is certainly more opportunity to measure greater variability among a group of individuals, and therefore it may be easier to reach statistical significance. You must decide, therefore, what is practically significant in your research setting. If slight reductions in patient anxiety are important and cost effective, then by all means use norm-referenced measurement. If the reduction must be accompanied by certain criterion behaviors such as self-care, cooperativeness, and lack of disturbance, then criterion measurement of only these behaviors might be more appropriate. When testing theory, small changes may be of interest and norm-referenced testing may be the appropriate choice. If all of the preceding are of interest, then use both kinds of testing. When using standardized tests this dilemma is unlikely to occur, because at present these measures are almost always norm-referenced.

Research Scales and Tests*

This category includes all measures that have not made it to the "big time" of standardized tests. This category includes many would-be standardized tests that are still being developed, although some **instrument credentialing** data are available. Others are not intended for the wide use to which standardized scales and tests are applied, and they remain in this category as very fine instruments for use in research. As a rule of thumb, standardized tests are considered appropriate for clinical diagnosis of individuals, while research tests may or may not be. Beware of wasting time and energy trying to classify specific instruments as either standardized or research. It really does not matter. The important questions that must be addressed are the appropriateness and quality of the reliability, validity, and normative or criterion data presented—the instrument's credentials.

Research scales and tests can be either projective (subjective) or nonprojective (objective), and special training including supervised practice is necessary when using projective tests. It is important that the data supporting use of a projective test include agreement among several scorers and agreement between two separate scorings of the same test by the same scorer. Like standardized tests, research tests can be norm-referenced or criterion-referenced. All can be reactive and result in various kinds of measurement error. The more items included on a scale, the less chance there is for error. When dichotomous responses are used (e.g., true-false, multiple choice with one correct answer), 30 items are usually the minimum needed to achieve adequate reliability coefficients of around .80. When multipoint responses are used (e.g., Likert scale), sometimes as few as 15 items per scale can be used. Increasing these numbers, of course, can reduce the likelihood of error. Then, however, you must consider the added time and energy burden of longer scales that is placed on both research subjects and researchers.

Nonprojective standardized tests are usually made up of a series of subscales, each measuring a single concept or construct. Some even include a lie scale, which attempts to capture data regarding test reactivity. They can therefore become very long and require several hours to complete. The MMPI, for example, requires 3 to 5 hours. Research scales, similarly, can be quite lengthy, although those measuring only one construct are often short and require only a few minutes to complete. It often happens that a researcher wishes to use only one or two subscales of a larger test with ten or more subscales. The conservative approach in the past has been to administer the entire test and use only those scales of interest, under the assumption that the test credentials (e.g.,

---

*Scales and *tests* are used interchangeably in most settings. However, for the purist, **test** generally refers to items for which there are correct or appropriate responses and **scale** refers to attitudinal measures attempting to assess strength or the amount of an attitude. Most personality tests have appropriate responses (usually, "Yes, I'm like that") to certain items that, when the appropriate responses are summed, denote the intensity of a characteristic such as assertiveness or dependence. The use of the term *scale* is often less threatening to research subjects. In this book, these terms are used interchangeably.

reliability, validity, norms) were valid and "counted" only when research data were gathered under the same conditions of administration that prevailed when the data for the test credentials were gathered. This is true in theory, but in actual practice many researchers administer only the scales of interest, citing ethical concerns about gathering unnecessary data from research subjects. Because articles reporting research rarely indicate which approach to test administration was used, it is difficult to estimate how widespread is the practice of administering only scales of interest. Reporting reliability and validity data based on your research sample can certainly make the practice more defensible.

Chapter 12 describes many types of scales according to how they are scored. Please refer to it if, when reviewing the literature on your topic, you encounter an instrument in an unfamiliar format. Do not ever use an instrument in your research unless you know how to score it and what the high and low scores mean. Try out the **scoring procedure** to see how long it takes and whether it makes sense. Estimate how long scoring all your research instruments will take. Many of the articles reporting the results of research that include copies of the research scales or tests do not report the scoring procedure. Make sure you write to the author for the method of scoring and permission to use the instrument well in advance of data collection.

When selecting a standardized or research scale it is especially important, also, to look at each item and even complete the scale yourself. This is often overlooked in the quest for measures with good credentials and could mean disaster. As you are going through the items for the first time, remember your first impressions (e.g., difficult vocabulary, ambiguous or embarrassing questions). Write down your impressions if necessary. The first impression is usually your most accurate. Imagine how your research subjects would react. Instruments with outstanding credentials could still fail this evaluation, and, if so, either the instrument must be modified or another one must be selected.

If modifications are made, remember to (1) keep items simple and easy to understand (e.g., avoid double negatives: I do not believe there is no reason to hope) and (2) include only one idea per item (e.g., wrong: Hope is a basic need of all humans, because without it there is little chance for survival in difficult circumstances which are beyond our control and therefore in God's hands.) Make only those changes that are absolutely necessary. Item writing is an art and good ones that hold up over repeated testing situations are difficult to compose. Just as it is impossible to give a recipe for painting a masterpiece or composing a symphony, there really is no checklist for item writing (or modifying) that can give you all you need to know. You must use creativity and your own judgment. When a scale is modified, it becomes, essentially, a new instrument for which new credentials must be developed. Unless modifications are severe, this can usually be accomplished by reporting a reliability coefficient based on your sample data, content validity by involving a few experts in review of the new version of the test, and evidence for one other kind of validity. Depending on your research situation, construct validity may be appropriate if other measures are being used. If modifications are severe, pilot testing may be necessary along with some of the procedures described in Chapter 13.

Finally, the circumstances under which a scale or test was intended to be administered must be examined. Tests designed to be administered under controlled conditions that include time limits and no discussion of item responses could hardly be sent home with subjects for completion and return at a later date. Sometimes group testing is inappropriate when subjects can observe the responses of others.

Card Sort

Sometimes, for a variety of reasons, it is necessary to modify the traditional pencil and paper format for scaling or measuring a research variable. For example, in a study [2] of sexually deviant arousing scenes, a series of scenes was developed and each was then typed on individual index cards. Subjects were given the cards and five envelopes, labeled from 1 to 5 to correspond with *no arousal, little arousal, fair amount, much,* and *very much,* and instructed to read each card and place it in the most appropriate envelope. The card sort is a flexible technique that can be modified for use in many settings in which, say, the sensitivity of the topic makes other approaches too reactive or there is a probability of increased missing data. Moreover, sometimes, due to concerns about subject literacy, pictures (e.g., action scenes, persons with special characteristics) are substituted for typed narrations of scenes on the cards. Envelopes may need to be coded by color or pictures. This technique is especially useful in cross-cultural research or research with children.

Questionnaires

The most widely used instruments in nursing research, and also in behavioral research, are **questionnaires.** They are a marvelous means for getting a large amount of information from a large number of people quickly and cheaply. They have the advantage of being able to offer complete anonymity to subjects. They vary considerably in content and method of administration. Because of their widespread use, either by themselves or in conjunction with other modes of measurement, a separate chapter (Chap. 14) in this book is devoted to questionnaire development. This discussion, therefore, provides only an overview of this approach to the quantification of variables.

At the very least, questionnaires solicit pertinent demographic data such as age, sex, ethnic identification, income, education, occupation, and so forth. They often include survey questions eliciting opinions about, for example, waiting times in outpatient clinics, medical insurance coverage, or conditions in the workplace. They may ask questions about the respondent's behavior or experiences such as frequency of well baby clinic visits, satisfaction with care, compliance with various aspects of the therapeutic regimen, or frequency and nature of sexual activity. The list of possibilities is endless and depends on the purpose of the research. Many questionnaires, in addition, have embedded within them tests or scales that measure knowledge of and attitudes about variables of interest. Sometimes research scales assessing various personality traits are included. The final product, then, includes all self-report measures of interest at that point in time and should flow together into a unified whole, appearing as a single questionnaire whenever possible, rather than as a handful of four or five separate tests.* This appearance of wholeness enhances the likelihood of not only a good response rate but also completed rather than partially completed questionnaires. In addition, it is often appropriate to use the less threatening term **opinionnaire** instead of the term *questionnaire,* which as often as not suggests that it has *correct* answers.

The methods of administration range from one-to-one contact to group administrations to mail-out questionnaires. The likelihood of participation increases with one-to-one contact, although care must be taken to protect anonymity (if appropriate) and confidentiality. You must also guard against subject coercion to participate. One way of doing this is to allow return of questionnaires, completed and blank (for those who cannot say no but really do not wish to participate), to a locked slotted box or via mail. This practice, of course, decreases the response rate (and the researcher's bank account, if postage is provided). Envelopes for completed questionnaires may need to be provided to encourage return to a drop box which is not locked. Group administration, especially if questionnaires are collected afterward, yields a high response rate and makes the most of the researcher's time. It also creates less opportunity for variations in explanations and directions—a possible threat to the construct validity of the research. If multiple administrations are given, care must be taken to avoid changes in procedure that could affect results. Sometimes for questionnaire administration among experimenters, a form of *interrater* reliability is appropriate. You should, at the very least, keep a diary recording deviations from the planned procedures and other unexpected events that occur during the various administrations. On rare occasions, events such as these have accounted for unusual and unexpected research findings. On others, the documentation has justified exclusion from data analysis of responses gathered when these unusual conditions prevailed.

In addition to one-to-one, group, and multiple administrations, many researchers use mail-out questionnaires that include stamped, self-addressed envelopes for returning the completed forms. This, of course, is more expensive. A much larger and possibly more varied sample can be achieved, although response rates are generally lower. As a rule of thumb, a 50 percent response is to be expected. If a follow-up second mailing is used, you are doing well to bring in half of those still out. A third mailing generally yields slightly less than half of those remaining. A good way to save money and account for more persons is to ask those not wishing to participate to return (in the stamped self-addressed envelope provided) their blank questionnaire. In so doing, you can

*Some researchers call this type of questionnaire a *composite questionnaire.*

tell them that they will avoid future solicitations. This approach, of course, requires use of code numbers, so that you send follow-ups to only those who have not responded. **Confidentiality** can still be maintained because the names associated with each code number are kept locked and in the care of the researcher or a designated neutral person. When **anonymity** is essential, follow-up must include all people on the mailing list with instructions to disregard if the individual has already responded.

Writing cover letters for mail-out questionnaires is an art. They should be as short and as clear as possible in explaining the purpose of the research and what is expected of participants (including time requirements). It is helpful to include how the research will benefit society and, if appropriate, the participant. If you are using code numbers, explain how they will be used to maintain confidentiality. Be sure to actually ask the recipient to participate, preferably toward the beginning of the letter. We are constantly amazed at how many researchers forget to do so. Finally, using institutional letterhead and mentioning the name of your professor or mentor as the supervisor of your project (with permissions, of course) give added clout to the request and generally bring in a few participants who might otherwise have declined. This added clout is even more important when the subject matter is sensitive (e.g., sexuality, euthanasia, alcohol or drug use). When your letter is as good as you can make it, have it reviewed by several other researchers. Their comments and feedback will bring needed improvements that will, in turn, increase your return rate.

There are, of course, disadvantages to the use of questionnaires. Respondents may misinterpret questions or not follow directions. Others may skip entire sections, especially when more than 25 minutes are required for completion. Respondents must be literate. Sometimes someone other than the subject you solicited completes the form. When one person is filling out a form designed to represent an institution, bias occurs depending on who actually completes the form. Researchers in one mail survey, for example, solicited the opinions of directors of nursing. They found out later that in several instances the directors had given the questionnaires to staff members to complete, because they wished to support the research but had no time to give to it. In this case, it was detected because the occupation of the respondent was requested (as a check) and the nondirector responses were discarded. The major drawbacks to questionnaires, however, involve whether or not the nonparticipants are different in other ways from the participants (thereby creating problems in generalizing results) and the absence of an opportunity to probe in-depth or otherwise clarify certain issues and variables related to the research. The latter is addressed when using the interview techniques and the former is a problem of varying magnitude in all research for which informed consent by participants is required.

Interview

The **interview** is similar to the questionnaire in most respects. The major difference is that participants are asked questions by the interviewer instead of just reading them from the printed page. There is, therefore, greater opportunity to probe and clarify questions, and this results in nearly complete data from all subjects. Interviews are the preferred approach with sensitive topics with subjects who cannot read or otherwise respond to a questionnaire, or when all items must be completed. They are more costly, running between $25 and $100 each when interviewer time and travel expenses are paid. Most home-visit interviews run for a minimum of 30 to 60 minutes with additional time required if subjects offer snacks or extraneous (although often valuable) information. Two to three home-visit interviews can make a very busy day. A few more interviews can be completed each day if they are all conducted in the same location, like an outpatient clinic.

Nearly all interviews use an **interview schedule,** which is a written document listing the questions to be asked and providing space for the interviewer to record the subject's responses. Responses are usually recorded as they are given rather than afterward when the interviewer must depend on his or her memory. Some interviewers use tape recorders in order to avoid recording responses during the interview, because they believe it jeopardizes rapport and eye contact. They also like the security of being able to "look up" answers that need clarifying. Tape recorders, of course, require the permission of subjects, preferably written. They may also inhibit responses, especially at the beginning of the interview. A major drawback to the use of recorders in this instance involves doubling the time the researcher must devote to data gathering. In our experience, the use of tape recorders for this purpose is rarely justified. We have found, moreover, that after the first few interviews, interviewers no longer use the tapes because they are indeed too time consuming.

A special version of the interview is the **telephone interview.** This involves asking questions over the telephone instead of face to face. Its advantage in terms of time and travel is obvious, because the transportation time and expenses associated with face-to-face interviews are eliminated. The telephone interview is usually shorter and more focused—even when the same interview schedule is used. However, when an interview is expected to take more than 30 to 60 minutes, it is desirable to use a face-to-face approach, because it allows the interviewer greater latitude in maintaining participant motivation. The telephone interview, of course, is often a necessary step prior to making an appointment for a face-to-face interview. When this is done, it is particularly helpful to note reasons for nonparticipation. When accumulated, these reasons can illuminate the shadowy area surrounding generalizing from a sample of volunteers to a target population made up of both volunteers and nonvolunteers. The telephone interview is also useful when subjects from many geographic areas are desired and as a follow-up procedure in longitudinal research after an initial face-to-face interview. It does eliminate as potential subjects all those who do not have telephones and, in most cases, those with unlisted numbers. Also, sometimes people are wary of answering questions from a stranger over the telephone.

It is essential that the interviewers be trained. Just as the age, sex, race, and appearance of the interviewer can produce reactivity, the manner in which questions are asked and clarified can influence whether and how a subject responds. Entire books are written about the principles of good interviewing; this discussion therefore can present only some of the major areas of concern. Interviewers must present a neat appearance and be as much like respondents in demographic characteristics as possible. They must be friendly, courteous, encouraging, punctual, and accept all responses without disapproval, approval, or surprise. Using a conversational tone rather than just reading questions is appropriate, and questions should follow the wording of the interview schedule. If the subject does not understand a question, it should be repeated as originally worded rather than making extensive departures from the schedule. The extent to which departures from the schedule are permitted should be thoroughly understood during **training sessions** in which interviewers **role play** interviewing and being interviewed in order to gain greater familiarity with the schedule and how the subjects might feel.* For complex questions or answers, consider rewording during training sessions. If they must remain, it sometimes helps, if subjects can read, to give them a card with the question and/or response alternatives printed on it. Sometimes subjects respond with questions or "I don't know" or irrelevant comments. The interviewer generally pauses to indicate more is needed and if nothing is forthcoming, repeats the question. If the same response is received, the interviewer must gently probe with nondirective or neutral comments like "Could you explain that some more?" or "Anything else?" **Probing** must in no way hint at the nature of a response desired or otherwise influence it. Sometimes it is necessary to come back to the question later (if in training sessions this option was approved). The ability to establish a rapport in which subjects eagerly give candid responses and to use nondirective probes are the critical skills that all interviewers must possess. When the interview is completed, subjects should feel good about the experience and be willing to repeat it.

When interview schedules are complex or lengthy and more than one interviewer is being used, it is important to establish the sameness of their interviews. This can usually be done by having two interviewers interview several of the same people. In large-scale surveys in which many interviewers are employed, it is sometimes necessary to **verify the interviews** to document that all interviews did indeed occur. There have been instances in large surveys when

---

*Role playing for interviewers, even those who are experienced, is essential. When many interviewers are involved, begin with one individual role playing the interviewer and one playing the subject. The rest of the group watches and makes comments. Continue (sometimes over several sessions) until each interviewer has played both roles at least twice. Have some role play difficult subjects. It is important to get this practice. It is also particularly important to have role played a subject, in order to gain insight, understanding, and greater empathy for this role. Sometimes interviewer reliability will be established in these training sessions, also. When only one individual is involved, solicit a colleague to join in role playing sessions.

interviewers made up fictitious responses to interview schedules in order to avoid the work of actually conducting them. Large surveys, therefore, will randomly select around 10 percent of the completed interviews submitted and telephone subjects to ask whether the interview occurred. Sometimes a random subsample of these interviews, or all of the 10 percent, are repeated by a different interviewer and the responses are compared to the original data.

Like the questionnaire, the interview can have questions whose responses are closed-ended or open-ended. **Closed-ended responses** are like multiple choice, yes–no, or Likert scale statements. The subject merely selects one of the response alternatives that is offered. **Open-ended** responses are like answers to an essay examination. A question is asked and the subject responds with whatever comes to mind. The advantages of closed-ended responses is the ease with which results can be tabulated and the knowledge that all possible responses have been considered before one is chosen. The disadvantage (and therefore an advantage of open-ended) is that some responses may have been overlooked by the researcher and thus never be presented as options, thereby dangerously biasing results. Sometimes, a category of "other" can be added in order to capture this information. Unfortunately, because such an alternative would not be presented to all subjects, the researcher never knows how often that alternative might have been chosen had all subjects been given the opportunity.

One of the advantages of an interview is the capability of receiving unexpected responses or more in-depth responses to questions than are usually forthcoming from questionnaires, in which probing cannot occur. For this reason, interviews often include some open-ended responses, which interviewers record almost verbatim or in a manner strictly prescribed during training sessions. During data analysis these responses are treated in a special way, using a technique called content analysis.

Content analysis involves converting all open-ended answers into categories of a structured format (called a **framework),** in which the frequency of responses in each category is reported. First, a framework of all possible responses is made (based on review of all the responses). Then the responses are read again, classified as fitting into one or more categories of the framework, and the classification recorded. When all responses have been classified, the number in each category is summed and that frequency reported. For example, perhaps 100 patients who had dropped out of treatment (for at least 2 years) at a clinic for hypertensives were telephoned and asked why they had done so. Of the 100, 69 were located and their reasons listed. Next, all 69 responses were reviewed and each new (unique) reason listed. This then becomes the basis for the framework. The researchers then review and refine the framework, generally deleting and combining reasons. Finally, each response is read, classified, and noted on a **tally sheet.** When all responses have been classified into categories, the tally sheet is used to determine how often each reason was given.

This, then, is the data or content analysis of that response. In all probability there will be between 5 and 10 reasons cited by at least 80 to 90 percent of the respondents. These would be reported separately and all other reasons combined into an "other" category. Speculation about the 31 patients not located (e.g., deceased, moved) might add categories, depending on the purpose of the research.

Content analysis can take many forms and become very complex. In the interview, it usually involves analysis according to content. However, there are other research situations in which the analysis might take the form of various feelings or attitudes expressed. For example, advertisements in medical journals have been analyzed in terms of how women versus men and older versus younger persons were depicted (e.g., strong and in control versus sick and dependent). Anecdotal notes that are part of the medical chart are sources of data for numerous studies. As another example, best-selling books (several for each year) might be analyzed for changing (or unchanging) role stereotyping of nurses. In this case, each reference toward nurses in the entire book is numbered for future classification after a framework is developed. Raters who do the classification when frameworks are complex must receive intensive training, and the research findings must report the percentage of rater agreement in classifying.

In summary, questionnaires are cheaper, can reach larger numbers of subjects more quickly, provide anonymity when necessary, and are not vulnerable to reactivity due to the interviewer. Nevertheless, interviews have some clear advantages in terms of fewer unanswered questions, probing and protection from confusing or misinterpreted questions, reaching individuals who cannot answer questionnaires (e.g., illiterates, young children, the blind, or the very ill) and additional data produced through observation. You can be sure that questions were answered in the intended order and by the intended subject. Moreover, greater depth of response is achieved from persons who dislike writing out lengthy replies.

Because of the relative costs in time and money, researchers often use a combination of the questionnaire and interview techniques in their research. For example, the first phase of a study might use an interview technique with open-ended questions for say, 25 to 30 subjects. Based on content analysis of responses, a closed-end questionnaire might be developed and pilot tested with 25 new subjects. After the revisions suggested by pilot testing, mass distribution of the questionnaire to hundreds would then complete data gathering. Or the reverse could occur. Mass distribution of questionnaires, including a form to complete if subjects are willing to participate in future research, occurs. From those willing to continue as participants, a subsample, random or based on certain characteristics measured by the questionnaire, is then selected for more in-depth interviews or case studies, or subjects might participate in self-monitoring.

Self-monitoring

Self-monitoring involves having research subjects keep diaries or records of specified behaviors over a period of time. Research in patient compliance to various therapeutic regimens often uses this approach in order to provide data that indicates continuous or repeated compliance over time. Although there are drawbacks associated with this approach, the less reactive laboratory analysis of blood for tracer substances associated with ingestion of prescribed drugs also has drawbacks. It can (1) be done only at larger intervals such as clinic visits and (2) give a misleading positive reading for compliance if the drug was only taken a day or two before. Rankin and McIntee [49], in an intriguing research study concerned with reducing stress among nursing students, used a self-monitoring checklist, an abridged version of which is shown as Exhibit 11-1. The stress diary checklist was developed from content analysis of handwritten, free-form diaries kept by pilot study subjects who reported them as excessively time consuming and urged development of the checklist. Events were categorized into general school or work experiences (18 events), academic (23 events), clinical (26 events), organization related (10 events), living arrangement (5 events), health related (32 events), personal (41 events), and other (events to be inserted). In all, 155 events are listed. Subjects complete the checklist daily by placing, in the column for that day, numbers from 3 (extremely positive) to −3 (extremely negative) opposite all events which have occurred. The researchers calculate 3 daily scores—total number of events, total positive events, and total negative events—as well as weekly totals. At its present stage of development,* the *McIntee–Rankin Stress Diary,* although lengthy, shows promise as an instrument for use with numerous nursing studies. It certainly provides a good model whereby other variables might also be self-monitored. One limitation of this approach appears when data are analyzed. A complex time series approach may be required. In addition, daily measures may not be comparable because life events vary over time and the variation, like the number and nature of test items varying from one administration to another, acts as a confounding variable. In other words, the *reliability* of daily events is low. Ways to control this are by (1) comparing change (or difference) scores from pretest or Day 1 to posttest or Day 20 for at least two groups, like experimental and control, or (2) using analysis of covariance. In addition, accuracy rather than classical reliability is assessed by comparison of known events (e.g., exams, vacations) with whether or not they are reported, since the purpose of both is estimation of the amount of error present. This brings up a very important point. Just as you should know how to score an instrument before you use it, so should you know how your data can be analyzed before it is gathered. For the novice researcher, your

---

*At the time the book went to press, the Rankin and McIntee research was still in progress. Note that multimodal measurement of dependent variables from each of the three modes was used in their research.

mentor or instructor will help with this. (There is nothing so sad as a researcher who has spent many hours of many days gathering data that cannot test her research hypotheses.)

Self-monitoring was also the basis for another nursing research study in which Hoskins [30] examined the relationships among level of activation, body temperature, and interpersonal conflict. During the midweek days of Tuesday, Wednesday, and Thursday for 2 consecutive weeks, 16 husband–wife dyads recorded their body temperatures each waking hour, completed one of 12 alternate forms of a level of activation checklist (with nine items) four times daily, and completed one of two alternate forms of the *Interpersonal Conflict Scale* (with 45 items) twice daily. To minimize error, subjects were thoroughly briefed on procedures and also given written instructions. They were trained to use an IVAC electronic thermocouple thermometer, gave return demonstrations, and were contacted at the end of the first day of data collection to provide an opportunity to answer questions and clarify problem areas. After the first 3 days of data collection, completed data forms were collected and new forms issued for the last 3 days. At the end of the 6 days of the data collection period, couples were debriefed and allowed to compare husband–wife responses, because they were asked not to do so before. Although none of the hypotheses were supported, Hoskins' work provides another intriguing model on which to build future research, particularly since she presents no evidence to indicate that the self-monitoring was reactive.

When subjects monitor their own behaviors they must be given very specific instructions about what and when to record. Every effort must be made to standardize these procedures in order to get greater accuracy in monitoring. Often researchers, like Rankin and McIntee [49], provide checklists or forms to complete. When doing so, you must take extreme care to give neutral instructions that do not influence how subjects respond.

The greatest disadvantage to self-monitoring involves its reactivity. The very fact that an individual is monitoring and recording certain behaviors could cause a change in the behaviors, even in the absence of any intervention. For example, McFall [42] unobtrusively monitored smoking base rates of two groups of subjects prior to asking them to self-monitor under one of two conditions. One group recorded instances of smoking and the other recorded instances of nonsmoking. The researchers found that when compared to their base rates, the group who monitored instances of smoking actually increased their rate while the group who monitored nonsmoking decreased. One approach to investigating possible reactivity involves obtaining baseline data before an intervention to assess the presence of systematic increases or decreases in behavior. These would indicate reactivity. Once baseline data stop systematically increasing or decreasing and become stable, you could proceed with your intervention and look for changes in this new stabilized baseline. Another approach would use a third group to act as a type of control group, which would do everything the

Exhibit 11-1. Abridged McIntee-Rankin
Nursing Education Experiences Record (NEER).

Life Experiences: Each day of the week that you are in the project, indicate which of the events on this list occurred and the impact it had. Use the following scale to record the impact of each occurrence in the appropriate date column.

Extremely Positive	Moderately Positive	Slightly Positive	No Impact	Somewhat Negative	Moderately Negative	Extremely Negative	
+3	+2	+1	0	−1	−2	−3	
				Dates			

Events							
A. General school/work experience							
Starting new rotation							
Job interview							
Lose job							
Not living up to your own expectations							
B. Academic events							
Listening to a boring lecture/presentation							
Failing exam							
Receiving/giving passing grade on term paper							
Having work criticized by authority figure							
C. Clinical events							
Extending into a new clinical area							
Doing/correcting care plans (or equivalent)							
Having clinical assignments changed/ changing clinical assignments							
Caring for/working with a student with a dying client							

D. Organization-related events							
Too many meetings							
Being late for a meeting							
Change in work organization							
Having to take on a leadership role							

E. Living arrangement events							
Disagreement with roommate(s)							
Changing roommate(s)							
Search for living accommodations							
Moving into new accommodations							

F. Health-related events							
Feeling physically/mentally fatigued							
Feeling alone/isolated							
Minor illness: Self							
Significant other							
Major illness: Self							
Significant other							

G. Being in debt							
Trying to help a friend in crisis							
Locking self out of room/house/car							
Waiting for other people							

H. Other (be specific)							

Reprinted with permission [49].

others did except self-monitor. Some research, such as that involving only one measure, does not lend itself to this approach. However, most research that uses multimodal measurement can do so.

Direct Reports

Direct reports are just what the name implies. If you want to know how much pain a patient is experiencing, you simply ask him and use his response as your measure. Major advantages of direct report are its simplicity, inherent validity, and the absence of complex interpretation of scales based upon similarly complex theory. On the other hand, faking, impression management, and conformity to experimental demands are all possible. Direct report is enhanced when repeated measures are made, and it is used as part of multimodal measurement. Direct report is often incorporated into the self-monitoring approach.

Computer-Assisted Measurement

The emerging area of **computer-assisted measurement** promises more extensive and in-depth measurement without the accompanying one-to-one time involvement of the researcher. Various combinations of scales and questionnaire items can be combined and individually administered to assure that all questions are answered, while at the same time reducing the amount of reactivity usually associated with interviews.* Moreover, computers can be programmed to skip automatically whole groups of questions depending on responses to other items, thereby saving time for subjects. They can also explain a question by automatically rewording it so that all subjects receive identical clarification. The one-to-one advantage of interviews combines with the less costly questionnaire. Although the probing and behavioral observation advantages of the interview are absent, some modified probing can be built in as a response to inappropriate answers.

Computer-assisted assessment systems usually have subjects seated in front of a console with a screen (i.e., similar to a television screen) on which questions or stimuli are presented by a computer. Subjects respond using a keyboard (i.e., similar to a typewriter) to give yes–no, multiple choice, or even short essay answers, and subsequent stimuli are presented as a function of each subject's responses. The advantage of computer-assisted assessment is its use of an **interactive decision tree** with paths selected according to the responses of individual subjects. When this advantage is not used, computer-assisted measurement may not be appropriate in terms of the costs of programming and computer time. This is a new area, and more research is needed in order to know its true usefulness. It appears to be appropriate in patient education and continuing education programs involving large numbers of people learning

*Lucas et al [39] concluded that computer interviews produced more valid data than psychiatric interviews of alcohol ingestion among alcoholics. Subjects also considered the computer interview as a very acceptable form of measurement.

essentially the same material. Keep your eye on developments in the arena that may be adapted for use in research.

Others

There remain a few other techniques or categories that can be classified as part of the self-report mode. These include, among others, combining or weighting of response alternatives and simulations.

Combining or **weighting of response alternatives,** also known as a **composite score,** is best explained through use of an example. Aston [1] wished to have an interval level score for contraceptive practice in her study of adolescent females, their attitudes, behaviors, and knowledge. It was reasoned that the effectiveness of the contraceptive used could be multiplied by the frequency with which it was used (which varied from 1 for nonuse to 5 for use every time). Both of these questions and possible responses were included on her questionnaire. A high contraceptive practice score would indicate that effective contraception was often practiced. However, weights were needed for each of the contraceptive methods or combination of the methods. Exhibit 11.2 lists these methods and the weights that were found in the literature [55] and given by two physician/sex therapists. The first column gives the exact figure or range of figures and the second column gives the weight used in her research. As you can surmise, there is some researcher judgment required in determining the final weights. As long as you have a rationale for what you do, it is within your prerogatives as the researcher to make these decisions. In the Ashton study, an interesting fact emerged as the contraceptive practice score was studied further. Frequency of use was always *all the time* for the IUD, and, if not *all the time* for oral contraception, it was coded as *not at all,* because the pill cannot be effective when taken only occasionally. Combining, weighting, or both can often yield interval level scores from nominal level data gathered via questionnaire or interview. There are numerous possibilities in nursing, such as frequency of pain medication multiplied by the kind of medication as weighted according to potency by experts. These scores, of course, need validation prior to widespread use.

Another technique is **simulation measurement.** Again, it is best explained with an example. Damrosch [11] described in a short paragraph a woman who had been raped. Nursing students were then asked to respond to a series of items that assessed their attitudes toward the woman. Half of the (randomly assigned) subjects received a description in which the woman had taken proper precautions, such as locking her car and parking under a streetlight. The other half received a slightly altered description, in which the woman parked on a dark street and did not lock her car. Findings were that the nursing students were much more positive toward the woman who took adequate precautions. Thus, perceived carelessness *caused* less positive attitudes. In this study, the measurement instrument was also the experimental variable. Therefore, we call it simulation measurement. Damrosch [10] has used this same approach in

Exhibit 11-2. Percent of effectiveness of contraceptive method.

Method	Experts/Literature	Weight
Oral contraceptive	99.7–99.9	100
IUD		
Copper 7	98.6	98
Lippes loop	97–98	98
Diaphragm	96–97	97
Condoms and foam combined	95	95
Foam or suppositories	92–94	93
Condoms	90	90
Coitus interruptus	80	80
Rhythm	50	50

Used with permission by Ashton [1].

research on sexuality among the elderly in which the traditional stereotype of nurses' not approving of this activity was exploded. It is a particularly useful technique when attitudes are of interest and a researcher wishes to experimentally control variables toward which attitudes are being assessed. It can test causal hypotheses involving variables like sex and age, which are not usually amenable to manipulation by a researcher.

Behavioral Observation

The second mode of measurement, behavioral observation, also involves tradeoffs and choices. You cannot possibly record all that you observe. In research, you are not usually interested in everything that is observed anyway. You are interested in a sample of all possible observations. What is observed, of course, depends on the variable(s) being measured. Sometimes it is fairly straightforward, such as the amount of time a nurse spends touching a patient during an **observation period.** In this case an observer merely depresses the button of a mechanical device during the times when touching occurs. If, however, a number of variables are being observed at the same time, the **observation code** (i.e., the specific behaviors to be recorded) becomes much more complex. The possibilities, as usual, are unlimited. In this discussion, what is observed is usually referred to as a behavior. This is for the sake of convenience. In actuality, variables that are not behaviors could also be observed—such as smells, sounds, characteristics, appearance, even texture or feel.

   Behavioral observation, as the term implies, involves observing research subjects (or, in a broader sense, the objects of research). Generally, the observation or measure consists of recording the occurrence of one or more behaviors during a specified period of time. The frequency of occurrence for each variable is then determined by adding all single occurrences that were recorded. This is the number that is then attached to the variable (as its quantification) and used in data analysis. Sometimes, in addition to the frequency of occurrence, researchers will study the sequence of occurrence among several variables. For example, they may record, in the order they occur, a series of naturally occurring nurse behaviors and patient responses to these behaviors. This type of behavioral observation is much more complex in recording and analysis and well beyond the scope of this book.

Behavioral observation can be conducted obtrusively or unobtrusively. In the former case, subjects are aware that they are being observed, because they can actually see the observer. They often forget they are being observed, however, when they become absorbed in the activities around them. The observer may be sitting quietly to the side of a room recording events, or the observer may in fact be a video camera or audio tape recorder placed either obtrusively or unobtrusively in the room. Each of these kinds of observations has associated with it varying kinds and amounts of reactivity and measurement error as well as cost.

The major advantage of behavioral observation as a mode of measurement for operationally defining research variables is that the best way to study behavior is actually to observe it. The question of content validity is no longer as critical, although the issue of measurement error must be considered if the observation procedure is reactive. Recently published research studies indicate that, although reactivity can affect observation data, it does not always do so. Numerous factors determine the occurrence and degree of reactivity. They include (1) the obtrusiveness of the observation procedure itself, (2) the sensitivity of the variables under study (e g , sexual and antisocial behaviors), (3) biases or expectancies of subjects, (4) characteristics of the observers or method of recording (e.g., complicated machinery can create fear, which in turn can change performance), (5) previous experiences of subjects with the observation procedures, (6) subject age, and (7) instructions given to subjects prior to observation.

Nursing effectiveness, for example, is best measured by observation. Most other measures of nursing effectiveness are indirect and based on an *assumed* link between a measure or index and actual nursing effectiveness, thereby introducing, via this link, increased probabilities for error. Patient response to removal of sutures or bandages, noise associated with night-shift staff talking at the nurses' station, territoriality among hospitalized geriatric patients, and many other topics of nursing research are appropriate for measurement by observation. However, scientific observation as contrasted to routine observation by clinicians involves more than the general skills developed by health care professionals. Scientific observation must be objective, systematic, and clearly defined. This is discussed in greater detail in the following pages.

In some studies, observation measures have turned out to be better than self-report measures. For example, nursing observations made of (1) talking, (2) smiling and (3) motor activity were found in one study [58] to predict post-hospitalization adjustment more accurately than did either of two self-report measures. In this study nursing assistants made 16 behavioral ratings each day, one each half hour, between the hours of 8:00 a.m. and 4:00 p.m., on a presence or absence basis. Interobserver agreement averaged 96 percent for each of the three behavioral categories.

Behavioral observation is not new to nurses in research settings. For example, nurses have acted as observers in numerous research studies of hospitalized psychiatric patients. In one [38], members of the nursing staff interviewed patients for 10 minutes four times daily after having been trained in appropriate topics of conversation to use if it was necessary to initiate conversation. During conversations, nurses surreptitiously monitored with a stopwatch the amount of time spent in rational conversation. When delusional talk was made, the stopwatch was stopped. Nurses maintained the flow of conversation by acknowledging patient comments every 15 seconds by nodding their heads or saying 'humm-mmm," "sound good," and so forth. If patients were silent for 30 seconds or more, nurses prompted conversation according to plan. A percentage of time engaged in delusional talk for each session was the quantification yielded in this study where observer agreement ranged from 75 to 95 percent with a mean of 82 percent. In another study of schizophrenic withdrawal [37], the nursing staff tried to initiate short casual chats with patients 18 times per day. Using the number of refusals to participate as the dependent variable, the researchers found differences between those receiving the drug trifluoperazine (Stelazine) and those receiving a placebo. A correlation with rate of rational speech was also found. In yet another study, this one of patients with handwashing compulsions [44], the researchers constructed an observation device to record the frequency of handwashing episodes. They used a "washing pen," consisting of a 6 × 8 foot wooden board with a gate, which enclosed the wash basin in the patient's room and allowed activation of a recorder that marked the frequency of handwashing on a 24-hour basis. Interestingly, nurses' reports of handwashing correlated 96 percent with the frequency obtained by the mechanical device.

There are books and articles that misleadingly present as the advantages of observation (1) the ability to gather large quantities of data with ease and the facts that (2) subjects do not need to be recruited and therefore are always available in great abundance, (3) observation techniques are relatively inexpensive to employ, (4) data recording (and coding) instruments are more simple to develop than lengthy questionnaires, (5) observing can be stopped or begun at any time, and (6) because recording occurs as behavior occurs, bias due to recall error is eliminated. In some research settings one or more of these advantages might prevail. However, in many they do not. For example, (1) when you gather large amounts of data via, say, audio recording, you must then subject your tapes to content analysis. Content analysis requires, on the average, at least twice as much time as it takes to listen to all tape recordings which have been made. (2) In many research settings, subjects must give informed consent and thus must be recruited. (3) When one-to-one observations occur, costs are the same as for interviews, and (4) good recording instruments, which involve a number of variables, require not only great care in development but also great care in use. Of course, if the behavior is, for example, the number of times a call light is turned on during a given time interval, it is indeed easier than a lengthy questionnaire because recording involves only hashmarks on a note pad, the instrument. Finally, (5) time intervals when a behavior is observed are very important to the rigor of behavioral observation, and (6) there are occasions, albeit rare, when observations must be recorded after they occur. Therefore, do not be deceived into believing behavioral observation to be a quick and easy approach to measurement. It requires the same planning and rigor that self-report measures demand. Sadly, many naive researchers learn this lesson the hard way, when they complete their data gathering and wonder how then to make sense out of the 100 hours of tape they are left with as data.

A number of factors that need careful consideration when behavioral observation is used in research are presented in the following pages. These include obtrusiveness, specification of behaviors being observed, the various available coding devices, observation periods and time sampling to determine just when observations will occur, and observation conditions (i.e., naturalistic, laboratory or analog, video or audio tape, and record reviews). Finally, observer training and clarification of the difference between observer reliability and accuracy is discussed.

Obtrusiveness

It is well known that persons behave differently when they know they are observed. Therefore, to avoid this reactivity and associated error, researchers often resort to unobtrusive or nonreactive measures. The investigation of eating habits via analysis of Tucson garbage was an unobtrusive measure. The "subject" or sampling element in that research, of course, was a household of people rather than just one person. Another interesting approach was used by LeBow, Goldberg, and Collins [36] to observe and record eating behaviors of obese and nonobese persons in a restaurant. The observer, who had been trained by use of videotapes, was seated inconspicuously in a corner of the restaurant. With a tape recorder hidden in a briefcase and the microphone concealed from view, the observer made signals into the microphone to record foods eaten and eating behaviors. For example, taking a bite of hamburger was recorded by clicking a stop watch, eating a french fry was recorded by scratching the surface of the microphone, and chewing was signaled by tapping the microphone. When it is not necessary to obtain informed consent from research subjects, the possibility of unobtrusive measurement is present. However, when subjects know they are being observed their behavior may change. Several approaches can be used to minimize the obtrusiveness of a measure. First, observations may begin after a 30- to 60-minute **adaption period,** during which subjects think they are being observed (but are not), become accustomed to it, relax, and often forget about the observations as they become more involved in the activities under scrutiny. Even when subjects wear recording devices that are difficult to forget (e.g., actometers, biomotometers), an adaption period greatly reduces reactivity.

A second approach involves use of a **participant observer** (e.g., mother, spouse, nurse, teacher) rather than someone who is an outsider or clearly labeled as a researcher. Although the final word is not yet in, current methodology research results indicate that, for example, parents can be trained as participant observers to achieve data highly correlated with outside observers [9]. Not only is reactivity effectively minimized, but also reduced are the time and cost constraints of measurement in family settings.

Finally, when an obtrusive, nonparticipant observer must be used, carefully planned multimodal measurement can provide an indication of the degree of reactivity as well as evidence for criterion-related validity.

Specification of Behaviors

The observation code, or behaviors to be observed, must be as specific as possible. In the beginning phases of development, broad categories of behavior may be examined and some general definitions for these categories set up. As pilot testing occurs, specific behaviors are selected as targets and their definitions narrowed and made more specific in order to avoid overlapping categories. Hart, *et al* [22] defined crying behavior in a child so it could easily be distinguished from whining and screaming. Elements of time and distance were incorporated to lend precision. Thus, a sound with a duration of at least 5 seconds heard within a 50-foot radius was required before it could be recorded as "crying." In another study [15], eye contact in couples seated side by side was defined as a looking response that was preceded by a head turn of at least a 45-degree angle toward the partner with eyes focused between the top of the head and chin. Smiling was defined as, in most cases, requiring a crease to appear in the subject's cheek, usually but not always with teeth showing. Both looking and smiling were recorded as occurring if they lasted at least 10 seconds. To repeat, the definition for each category must be very specific and not overlap with any other category.

The number of categories included in an observation code depends on the purpose of the research and is limited by the maximum number of categories with which an observer can work accurately. Most trained observers can handle 10 to 15 categories easily and some can go well beyond that number. To observe hyperactive and nonhyperactive children in classroom settings, Campbell, Endman, and Bernfeld [4] used six categories of child behavior and three categories of teacher behavior. On the other hand, Marston *et al* [40] used four categories for eating patterns to observe obese and nonobese individuals. These included (1) such extraneous responses as looking at food or using a napkin, (2) counts of chews per bite, (3) frequency of bites, and (4) typical size of mouthfuls on a five-point scale. Each category was defined carefully to avoid confusion. Clarity of definitions and the absolute necessity to avoid overlap of categories may be best emphasized with yet another example. Graffam [19] developed a checklist of eight categories including three for patient distress and five for nurse response. In her directions for use of the instrument, Graffam included actual examples that occurred during pilot testing. For example, one category, "evaluation of complaint," was first described in general terms as a nurse's attempt to ascertain that distress was indeed present and the nature and severity of it. Each subcategory or alternative was then further defined. "Distress confirmed" was defined as "The nurse may ask the patient, 'Do you have pain?' 'Are you nauseated?' She may affirm, 'You do have pain?' " This alternative was clearly distinguished from "Further data sought in questions" which was defined as "The nurse asks questions of the patient in order to help determine the intensity and location of distress. She may ask, 'Where does it hurt?' or 'You have a lot of pain?' "

Unclear definition of the observation code, of course, results in low reliability. Different observers will tend to select different categories in which to classify observed behaviors. The percentage of agreement will be low. If the observation code is vague enough, even the same observer categorizing the same behavior on two different occasions (e.g., video tape at 1-month intervals) will not agree with herself. Therefore, it is not at all unusual to have, as in standardized or many research scales and tests, extensive directions and definitions for use that are considerably longer than the observation code. Sometimes they are presented in an **observer's manual** along with reliability, validity, and normative data.

In addition to detailed descriptions of the behaviors being observed, it is often necessary to be just as specific about who is being observed. For example, Chamorro, *et al* [5] developed and used the Premature Infant Activity Schedule (PIAS), an adaptation of an observation code instrument developed by Reingold [52]. Seven categories of variables were included, with the number of alternatives for each ranging from two to twenty. One such category was "caretaking activities." For this not only did each alternative need specification (e.g., "talks" referred to the caretaker's laughing, talking, crying, or making other vocal sounds to or with a person other than the infant while caring for the infant), but also it became necessary to specify how a nurse could be considered the caretaker. In this study, therefore, the caretaker was considered any adult other than the observer who was able to see, hear, and carry out caretaking activities as specified. The caretaker could be in an adjoining room but with clear visibility, access to the infant, or both. Thus a nurse in an adjoining room who looked at and observed the infant would be considered the caretaker while a nurse in the same room who was in no way watching the infant would not be considered the caretaker for the observation period.

When selecting behaviors (and subjects) to be observed, researchers generally try to sample from all possible behaviors (or subjects). However, now and then only certain behaviors are of interest, such as self-care or disruptive behaviors. When only these are observed and coded, there is a danger of distortion, because no data are gathered to indicate the percentage of, say, self-care or disruptive behaviors as compared with all other behaviors that occur during the same time interval. Great care must be taken in situations such as these when results are interpreted or explained.

Finally, some discussion must be devoted to **unstructured observation.** By this is meant the approach used by anthropologists, sociologists, and others engaged in qualitative ethnographic research. The researcher usually acts as a participant observer and keeps a daily log and field notes. Rarely can these notes be made as events occur. Therefore, they may be subject to observer bias (in selecting which behaviors to record), errors in recall, and observer influence on the events themselves. Proponents of this approach argue that data of this type have richness and depth that are lacking with the traditional quantification/ statistical methods. However, unstructured observation is very dependent on the interpersonal and observational talent and skills of the observer, much more than with structured observation. It requires the talent of a detective or playwright and is quite uncommon. Success in this area requires first a knowledge of quantitative methods and then additional training combined with this talent. It is clearly a methodology whose implementation is beyond the scope of this book. Many mistakenly view it as easier than quantitative methods and therefore eschew learning quantitative approaches in favor of a case study or ethnographic approach. The results are usually disappointing and often embarrassing, because the rigor and objectivity inherent in quantitative methods is never learned and transferred to unstructured observation. Deviation from an unknown (i.e., quantitative methods) is often ignorance, not enlightenment. Do not make that mistake.

Observation Period

In addition to specifying who and what will be observed, just when the observation will occur must be determined. If you wish to observe self-care activities of patients, you would probably not select the night shift. Beyond this, you would determine whether continuous, time sampling, or event observations were appropriate.

Continuous observation is what the term implies. Subjects are observed continuously during a time period, such as the day shift. If the target behaviors are not too numerous or complex, this is a good approach. However, it can result in observer overload and fatigue, which in turn lead to distortions and errors in observations. At the very least, observations may be lost owing to possible inattention while the observer is recording other behaviors. Therefore, **time sampling** over a large time period is often used. For example, Chamorro, *et al* [5], in their study of premature infant behavior, used 1 second for observing and 19 seconds to record for a total time of 10 minutes (or 30 observations) followed by a five-minute rest period. In all, there were 120 observations an hour, 3 per minute during each 10-minute observation period.

When time sampling is used, of course, it is important that the sample be representative of the "population" of all behaviors that occur naturally or continuously. To assure this, Chamorro, *et al* compared time sampling to continuous observations and found a median of 90 percent agreement, which is within acceptable limits. In order to make this comparison, they were unable to use all categories included in the observation code, because to do so resulted in overload for the observers who were doing the continuous observations. Thus, a clear advantage of time sampling over continuous observation is the possibility of more categories or complexity within the observation code.

Just as it is often desirable (but not always necessary) to demonstrate that time sampling and continuous observation results agree, it is also important to provide a rationale for selection of a specific time period out of all other possible time periods. It is rarely necessary, however to demonstrate it empirically by gathering data during various time periods.

Time sampling can also use random rather than systematic sampling of a time period. In this case, it is still important to specify how long the observation will be before recording begins. When random time sampling is used, researchers generally use a small beeper that signals when the observer should start looking and when she may stop. Use of beepers or other devices when time sampling is systematic is also recommended, particularly when agreement between two observers is sought. Often, when video or audio recordings are being coded, visual or audio signals are superimposed on the tapes to avoid errors and poor interrater reliability due to comparison of different time samples.

Besides continuous observation and time sampling, a third approach, **event observations,** is possible. In this approach, all events of interest that occur during a specified time period, whenever and for however long an event occurs, are observed. The times when events are not occurring are used for recording or rest. During the event, observation is continuous. Graffam [19] used this approach in her study of nurse response to the patient in distress. Each event, recall, began with the initiation of a complaint and ended when the nurse's response was concluded. Events not observed in their entirety were not included. Observations were made over a 5-month period and included all days in the week and the time period between 5:00 a.m. and 10:00 p.m. Nurses were observed for an average of 3 or 4 hours and never for more than 6 events.

There are rare circumstances in which the target events do not occur very often. This necessitates long periods of fruitless observation. Therefore, researchers often train participant observers, such as parents or roommates, to do the observing. Sometimes an event is artificially precipitated or simulated in a laboratory setting. Although these approaches are valid if executed properly, they are less desirable and often more vulnerable to error. If they are the only observation approaches available, the research would certainly benefit from multimodal measurement.

Coding Devices

The distinction between observation (i.e., looking) and coding is sometimes overlooked. When time sampling is used, the distinction between these two

Exhibit 11-3. Abridged PIAS checklist.

Caretaker Activities	1	2	3	4	5	6	7	8	9	28	29	30	Total
Looks at face													
Talks													
Talks to infant													
Supports in isolette													
Holds													
Puts infant down													
Caresses face													
Infant Activities													
Eyes open													
Eyes closed													
Hand-mouth contact													
Vocalizes													
Cries													

This checklist was constructed based on the Chamorro et al. [5] article describing their research. It may not represent what was actually used.

observer activities is clear. However, when an observer uses a video camera to record behaviors, the resulting videotape records only the target behaviors. It is not the observation (i.e., looking). The researcher-observer has merely introduced an additional step, a nonhuman observer, into the research. The resulting videotape must then be observed again and coded. Coding involves quantification of the data so that statistical analysis can occur.

The most popular coding devices in nursing research are **checklists** and rating scales of various sorts. Ultimately these resemble the framework used in content analysis and can vary as greatly in complexity. Exhibit 11.3 presents a hypothetical and abridged PIAS checklist based on information provided in the Chamorro *et al* [5] article. This checklist provides for the 30 observations that occur during a 10-minute observation period. Ideally, via open-air earphones a beeper would signal the beginning of each 1-second observation period or, rather than just a tone signal, a number corresponding to the coding column might be given. As a result of training, observers should have a feel for how long the 1-second observation period lasts. Then, eyes down, looking at the checklist, the observer would merely check all observed behaviors in the column appropriate to the observation period. At the next signal, the observer would look up for 1 second and then look down to code what was observed. This would continue for 10 minutes (30 observations), at which time the observer would have a 5-minute rest period to stretch, get a drink of water, put a new checklist on her clipboard, and otherwise prepare for the next 10-minute observing/coding period. This would continue until the required number of observations had been coded. Note that each checklist has a column for totals to aid in quick tabulation of data.

Another approach to coding was used by Downs and Fitzpatrick [13] for the assessment of body position and motor activity. The observation code, which was originally developed by two students for a research course and later modified by the researchers, uses symbols for coding body position (e.g., O— means lying down, ♀ means kneeling) and the intensity of body movement. The symbols are then recorded on a grid sheet on which each vertical line denotes a 15-second interval during the 5-minute continuous observation period. Frequencies can then be tabulated from the coding sheets. This approach uses less paper than Exhibit 11.3, although the absence of cues for observers may invite errors. It also provides for coding the intensity of body movements (e.g., − means minimally active, + means very active). Intensity, of course, can also be recorded with a checklist format by substituting numbers or symbols for check marks.

There are numerous checklists, rating scales, and coding schemes possible for use as pencil and paper coding devices. The best way to locate those appropriate for your research is, as usual, to consult the research literature relating to your topic area and keep abreast of developments in general by regularly reading journals reporting the results of health related research.

There are also many mechanical devices available to nurses for recording and coding observations. They include some devices that actually bypass human observers, such as actometers for measuring activity levels. Others, a series of pocket, computer-type storage devices that have been recently marketed, have capabilities to store, retrieve, and analyze data. In effect, these can actually replace the pencil and paper checklist by having observers code directly into them. Furthermore, they can also be programmed to go on to analyze data and present results. The problems associated with mechanical devices are present, of course, as is human error associated with observing, coding, and programming. However, these new developments should be carefully watched and used whenever appropriate if they can make data gathering and coding easier and faster.

Lawson, Daum, and Turbewitz [35] used an innovative assortment of observation devices in their investigation of environmental stimulation levels in neonatal intensive care units (ICUs). In one study, observers measured light levels with Gossen Lunasix light meters and coded frequencies with which children were handled by staff. Separate coding of speech and nonspeech sounds both inside and outside the room were made. Sounds were also tape recorded by use of microphones in each infant isolette, adjusted for each observer's auditory sensitivity, and then compared with observer coding of speech and nonspeech sounds. In a second study these observations were repeated and an additional dependent variable added: sound pressure level as generated with Bruel and Kjaer precision sound level meters. The researchers reported differences between grower rooms and ICUs and, of course, have developed a creative methodology for both environmental assessment of stimulation levels in neonatal hospital environments and validation of observer codes.

Observation Conditions

Naturalistic. Up to this point the discussion about behavioral observation has primarily centered around **naturalistic** conditions, or, to phrase it another way, **field research.** That is, observations have occurred in the natural environment of subjects. This certainly contributes to greater content validity, particularly if reactivity due to the observer can be minimized.

Analog. Sometimes, however, it is more appropriate to use **laboratory** or **analog settings.** Analog assessment occurs when the target behaviors are observed in environments different from the environment in which the behavior occurs. Usually they occur in clinic or laboratory rooms specially equipped for unobtrusive visual and auditory monitoring (e.g., one-way mirrors). Analog or laboratory settings allow researchers to exercise greater control over extraneous variables while allowing more efficient use of time and finances than is often possible in naturalistic settings. A major assumption of analog assessment, of course, is that observed behaviors are *analogous* to, correlate with, or predict behavior in the natural environment. A number of variables have been investigated via many studies that use analog settings—parent–child interaction, child behavior, marital interaction, fear and anxiety, sleep skills, and ingestive behavior.

An interesting analog measure of assertiveness, the *Behavioral Assertiveness Test* (BAT), which could serve as a model for measurement to predict such nursing variables as stress reaction, coping, and patient compliance, was developed by Eisler, Miller, and Herson [16]. The BAT consists of 14 videotaped interpersonal situations requiring an assertive response by the patient. Seated next to a female role player who helps to prompt a response, subjects hear via intercom from an adjoining room descriptions of a series of interpersonal encounters. For example:

Narrator: You're in a restaurant with some friends. You order a very rare steak. The waitress brings to the table a steak that is so well done it looks burned. *Female Role Playing Waitress:* I hope you enjoyed your dinner, Sir.

Videotapes of responses to each of the encounters are later viewed and coded according to an observation code that includes duration of looking, smiles, duration of reply, latency of response, loudness of speech, fluency of speech, compliance context, requests for new behavior, affect, and overall assertiveness. Observer agreement is usually 90 percent.

Films, Audio and Video Recordings. Recordings of various types are being used more often to record (not code) observations. Although the recordings still must then be observed and coded, they enable coding of more behaviors sometimes via multiple observations and checking the accuracy of coding. Numerous techniques, moreover, have been developed to superimpose signals on the tapes in order to facilitate time sampling. The major drawback to recordings besides additional time for coding is the possibility of reactivity. The literature on this is unclear, however. Some researchers have found that subjects behave differently when being recorded and others have found no differences. As with live observers, the use of an adaption period and multimodal measurement are useful in minimizing or assessing reactivity. One other danger is present, particularly with visual recordings. The camera itself is limited in what it can record. If the interaction among several subjects is being observed, for instance, the recording could miss some of the target behaviors.

Records and Existing Documents. Sometimes it is not possible to observe subjects directly. Instead, secondary sources, such as medical records, are used. In most cases, reactivity is no longer a concern. However, the accuracy, regularity, and objectivity of data must be investigated. It is limited, of course, by the observation skills of the person who entered the recording. In nursing research, medical records are often used to extract various kinds of data including behavioral observations. Before embarking on a study dependent on medical records as a data source, it is advisable to conduct a pilot study to ascertain the extent of missing data and to devise a plan for handling it. If too much information is unsuitable for inclusion in your research, another approach should be found. If data are adequate, a coding device such as a checklist should be developed to facilitate data extraction, coding, and analysis. Often, particularly with anecdotes describing observations, some of the principles of content analysis are employed to develop the coding device.

Observer Training. Like interviewers, observers must be given numerous opportunities to practice before they observe and code behavior in an actual situation. They should achieve at least 80 percent agreement during practice trials, although this may vary depending on the length and complexity of the observation code. Chapter 13 describes the computational steps for calculating observer agreement. Familiarity with the coding device and any other recording instruments (e.g., stopwatches and other timing devices) definitely increases accuracy and reliability.

Training sessions typically include role playing in which one observer plays the subject. This has the advantage that sessions can stop for questions and discussion during early stages of training. By playing the subject, the observer is also able to develop a greater feel for the subject's experience, thereby enhancing empathy. When appropriate, video or audio tape recorders can also be used. Lastly, pilot testing occurs whereby an observer gains practice in the actual research setting with someone just like a real subject. When two or more observers are involved, observer agreement is calculated until it is at least 80 percent for complex or lengthy codes and higher for more simple ones. Furthermore, if at all financially possible, several tapes or films similar to the research setting should be procured for use in computing periodically intraobserver agreement (i.e., the same observer at two different times) in order to guard against changes in the way an observer works over time.

Even when the investigator who designed the study does all or most of the observations, training and practice is still necessary. Someone may have to be brought in to participate in role playing even though he or she will not observe in the actual research. Sometimes consultants who are specialists in measurement by behavioral observation are available to assist. If you are new to this type of measurement and the observation code is lengthy or complex, the consultant fee is generally well worth it.*

Not only is extensive teaching required to achieve acceptable levels of agreement between observers, but also continued monitoring is necessary to maintain acceptable levels. In fact, observer agreement has been found to drop substantially (e.g., 25 percent in two studies) when observers did not know their agreement was being monitored [50, 51, 53]. In addition, underestimates of target behaviors were made by observers who did not know they were being monitored. This phenomenon, known as **observer drift,** must be considered in research that extends over a period of time. Spot checks are, of course, better than no checks. However, they may not be sufficient to maintain high levels of agreement when observation is daily and continues over several weeks. A solution suggested for this involves recording on tape or film all observations and then showing them to observers for coding in random order. When this is impractical, recording over time a sample from each observation period can estimate the degree of observer drift present. In conclusion, the importance of observer agreement, reliability, both among observers and over time, cannot be emphasized too strongly. It deserves the same precision in monitoring that the observation code of target behaviors requires in terms of definition.

Accuracy versus Reliability

When high observer agreement, hence reliability, is achieved, the natural conclusion is that the observations must also be accurate. This is usually a valid assumption when trained observers use a very well-defined observation code. However, high reliability as an indicator of accuracy is an *assumption* and not a fact. This was clearly illustrated in a study conducted by Wahler and Leske [57].

---

*Consultant fees, as a rule, are never below $300 a day and can range upwards to $1,000 per day. Minimum fee is generally $150 for single session of a half day or less.

In their research, six children engaged in silent reading were videotaped over 15 sessions. One of the children was coached to exhibit distractible behaviors in amounts varying from 15 percent to 75 percent on each of the tapes. Two groups of untrained observers were shown the tapes in and out of sequence order. One group (called the subjective group) rated the child's distractibility on a scale from 1 to 7, on which 7 was highly distractible. The second group (the objective group) did the same but were allowed to keep tallies of specific behaviors in order to make their 1 to 7 assessments. The group that did not keep tallies had greater agreement or reliability. However, the group that kept tallies was more accurate. Although further research in this area is needed, it is apparent that without training and objective coding devices, the assumption that high agreement, or reliability, indicates accuracy is questionable.

Physical Assessment

The third and last mode of measurement is **physical assessment.** It can include blood pressure, height and weight, body temperature, electrocardiogram (ECG) readings, various urinalyses, numerous blood analyses, and a myriad of measures based on readings from stethoscopes, bronchoscopes, radiographic measures, and others. They are, so to speak, the heart and blood of the medical chart. Moreover, many are computerized. Many of these measures are already available and need only be extracted from patient charts. Physical assessment has been underused in nursing research, in spite of the fact that when used concurrently with self-report and behavioral observation of the *same variable* as an approach to health research, the research becomes more unique and precise.

The three modes have been used together in a limited number of studies. From these has emerged strong support for physical measures of research variables, particularly because they are often more sensitive to experimental interventions and correlates than are self-report and observation measures. This is due in part to response fractionation. Physical measures themselves can also vary in sensitivity, often owing to timing. For example, heart rate or electroencephalogram (EEG) patterns may demonstrate significant changes within 1 second following a mild stimulus, while diastolic blood pressure may not demonstrate a significant change until minutes and somtimes hours following an intense stimulus. Adaption (return to normal or baseline) rates also vary. Thus it is important that you know how and when the various types of measures change in the presence of other variables prior to actually using them. As a rule, the following factors should be considered when you are selecting physical assessment measures for research:

1. It cannot be assumed that one or even two measures can yield an index of generalized or overall physiological functioning.
2. Multiple measures should be taken whenever feasible.
3. Measures should be selected only after careful consideration of expected effects of the experimental variable or changes in other variables.

4. Some measures are more sensitive to change than others and this should be considered.
5. The underlying physiological mechanisms that are to be represented by the measure must be understood prior to selection.

Extensive study of the literature describing the use of a potential measure as well as discussion with experts in the use of the measure is necessary before final selection. Ideas for potential measures, of course, come from the literature in your topic and related areas.

The number of possibilities for physical assessment in nursing research is too extensive to itemize, let alone describe in this chapter. Many have already been covered in other health care courses. Some, as you know from your clinical experiences and courses, can require whole books to explain. To provide an overview in this book, they are organized into three groups, again not mutually exclusive nor particularly inviolate—you may come up with another way to organize them if you wish.

Observation Measures

Measures in this group include those that can be directly observed by the researcher and health care provider. They include variables like edema, voiding, vomiting, cyanosis, delirium, fainting, bleeding, and so forth. Usually they are coded as either present or absent, although in some cases, such as bleeding or vomiting, estimates of quantity might be expected of the clinician or researcher. Principles relating to behavioral observations are appropriate to this group of measures.

Chemical and Microbiologic Measures

Measures in this group include blood, tissue, and urine laboratory analyses and cultures grown from various body substances (e.g., throat or fecal cultures). In most cases, the actual analysis is done by other professionals even though the researcher may well have taken the specimen. Errors from getting the specimen, its transportation and care, or its analysis in the laboratory are possible. This group is rarely subject to reactivity.

Mechanical and Quasi-Mechanical Measures

Temperature, blood pressure, weight, and height are variables that are measured by mechanical and quasi-mechanical devices. Also included here are ECG readings, x-rays, EEGs, and so forth. Depending on her area of specialty, a nurse will be able to operate a number of the mechanical devices that yield, sometimes only after analysis of output, measures of a large variety of physical variables. In a few cases, nurses have designed and built mechanical devices to measure physical variables. However, engineers usually do this and other medical professionals just learn to operate the devices and make minor repairs and adjustments in order to keep the machines working. As in any other measure, it is essential to know the possible sources of error associated with each machine or interpretation of its output and to take steps to ensure that the chances for error and machine breakdowns are minimized.

Training for Use of a Physical Assessment Device

If you wish to use a physical assessment measure with which you are not normally expected to be familiar, especially if it involves a machine rather than a laboratory blood test, join forces with people who know all about it. They can be found through their research reports in journals (first choice) or investigation of what is going on in the rest of your college or university—particularly the medical school or sometimes a health psychology department. Once you have found your person, try to negotiate a (1) coresearcher position in which you will coauthor publication of the research you work on or (2) researcher–consultant relationship in which you do your own research and the specialist advises and teaches you. When you do not have grant funds to pay consultants, some specialists are hesitant to help you, although in most university settings faculty are generally eager to serve on a thesis committee (and/or copublish) in return for these services. Do not settle for a helper–lackey role unless all else fails. If everything fails, learn as much as you can while in your helper role and then write an article for a journal describing the measure and how to use it. If you are nervous about your document, have your "boss" review it in return for second (not first) authorship. His or her name as an author may help it be published. With your article as a credential, apply for a small grant to rent or buy your equipment and pay your "boss" as a consultant. Make sure his or her job description describes what is expected, particularly authorship credits. You are now in the driver's seat.

Distortion and Reactivity in Physical Assessment

Although many consider physical assessment more objective than the other two modes of measurement, there is still the possibility of distortion or just plain error associated with its use by untrained or poorly motivated clinicians. Therefore, the skill and reputation of the individuals providing the assessment must be demonstrated and, sometimes, documented in the report of research results as well as any mechanical problems that occurred and how they were dealt with.

It seems unlikely (although possible) that physiological responses could be subject to conscious distortion by subjects. However, the biofeedback literature is now presenting evidence that highly sophisticated and trained subjects would have the capacity to control willfully some physiological responses. There is greater possibility of reactivity due to the manner in which the measurement is taken. Being attached with electrodes and other lead wires to monitoring machines can easily result in reactivity. As an extreme example, Freund, Sedlacek, and Knob [18] in research with male sexual deviates, using Freund's penile plethysmograph as a measure of the dependent variable, found that the instrument itself stimulated the penis, and therefore a lengthy adaption period was needed before a stable **baseline** measure was possible. Moreover, other researchers have found that penile circumference stabilizes at a level of 5 percent to 10 percent greater than the initial baseline after arousal, and therefore it is often necessary to establish new baselines after each arousal if repeated independent variables are to be used in the same session. This rather extreme example demonstrates the need to become very familiar with the idiosyncracies of the assessment procedures you are employing prior to beginning to gather research data. In a nursing research example of reactivity, Mills, *et al* [45] found that the frequency of ectopic beats (as recorded by ECGs read out on a central console remote ink writing brush recorder and measured by a Lansing ECG ruler) changed significantly when a nurse palpated the pulse. They concluded that autonomic responses to human contact can alter the rate of ectopic impulse generation. In this study, the subjects, all coronary care unit patients, were free of human interactions for 3 minutes preceding the palpation in order to establish a baseline, palpated for 1 minute, and then again free of human interactions to establish a return to baseline.

The very fact that an adaption period works to minimize reactivity in most cases brings up another possible concern. This is the phenomenon called **habituation.** In some research settings, the galvanic skin response (GSR), a popular measure in behavioral research, has been known to diminish in size when it was repeated at short intervals within a session and sometimes when used only daily [48]. Then again, in other research settings, GSR has been found to hold up over many months of repeated measures [2]. You must investigate and consider, at least, the possibility that your independent variable's effectiveness could be interacting with habituation to your measure. In self-report terminology this is called **practice effect.**

Another source of error, just as with the other modes of measurement, can be due to the effects of the experimenter. Although it is less likely to occur in the physical assessment mode, it is nevertheless a possibility. Consider again, an example from sex research. Chapman, Chapman, and Brelje [7] compared the effects of using two different kinds of experimenters, one who was an aloof, businesslike graduate student and the other who was a casual, outgoing undergraduate, on the pupillary dilation of undergraduate males to slides of nude and partially dressed men and women and control scenes. The males shown slides by the casual experimenter had greater dilation to pictures of women than men, while those shown slides by the businesslike experimenter had equal dilation for both male and female slides. The researchers concluded that different ways of interacting with subjects can produce different pupillary responses, and they added the alarming comment that if the two experimenters had worked in different laboratories, they would have reported contradictory findings. That is something to think about, especially in areas in which research results conflict.

Other intervening variables are also possible. An individual's response to the same stimulus can vary depending upon positive or negative affect. This is particularly a concern in sexual arousal research. The use of multimodal measurement that elicits self-report of affect may be very important in documenting intervening or confounding variables, and the statistical analysis can then include this to advantage rather than have the dependent measures simply cancel each other out. Closely related to this is the fact that very early in life individuals develop unique psychophysiological response systems to stress. Some subjects are GSR responders, some are heart rate responders, some are (increased) blood pressure responders, and yet others are (increased) respiratory responders. This can create problems when group comparisons are made. Therefore, when appropriate to the research topic and especially during pilot testing, several physiological systems might be monitored concurrently to determine the most sensitive indices. If there is a single piece of advice to come from this chapter, it is to be very, very familiar with your operational definitions. This can be accomplished by returning to the literature to review research in which your measures were used (even if not on your topic), talking or corresponding with researchers experienced in their use, and getting hands-on experience by working with one of those experienced researchers or conducting an unhurried pilot test.

Accuracy and Precision

Rather than concerns about the concepts of reliability and validity as defined for application in the self-report and behavioral observation modes, the concerns about the chemical, microbiologic, mechanical, and quasi-mechanical subgroups of the physical assessment mode of measurement are for their accuracy and precision. Because machines are built to measure variables that have already been defined and are known, validity is assumed; instead, the instrument developer concentrates on the accuracy and precision with which his machine or laboratory procedure measures this known physical phenomenon. The exception to this occurs when a physical assessment measure, such as that for blood pressure, is used to operationalize an abstract variable like anxiety instead of the physical phenomenon for which it was intended. The measure becomes indirect, and then we must be concerned about validity, particularly criterion and construct validity. We need data to support use of blood pressure level as a measure of anxiety.

The term **accuracy** is used to refer to the "closeness" of the machine's reading to the true value of the object of measurement. Thus, if a temperature measuring device (say a thermometer) is used to determine the temperature of an open pot of boiling water at sea level and it reads 100°C, we would say that it is accurate, while if it reads 112°C, we would say that it is inaccurate. The process of adjusting the machine's reading to achieve the desired level of accuracy is called **calibration.** Although some measuring devices (e.g., an oral thermometer) cannot readily be adjusted, tests to determine their accuracy are still commonly referred to as calibration tests. In order to perform a calibration, it is necessary to have an object of measurement (actually several, to cover the measurement range of interest) whose true value is known; such an object is called a **standard.** There are innumerable types of standards. For many years, the standard for length was a special alloy metal bar with two carefully inscribed marks on it. Similarly, there are special weights used to calibrate laboratory balances, there are atomic clocks used to calibrate time measurement devices, there are regulated power supplies to provide a known voltage, and so on. The National Bureau of Standards (NBS) of the United States Department of Commerce is the developer and custodian of standards in this country. They provide standards to regional laboratories who may, in turn, provide standards to others, including instrument manufacturers. Thus, a particular manufacturer may state that his machine left the factory with a calibration performed with NBS-traceable standards. A manufacture may typically state that his device has an accuracy of 11 percent of the **reading** (i.e., the actual value or number observed), or 12 percent of **full scale** (i.e., the highest value that can be observed). To illustrate the difference between these two forms of expression, consider the speedometer in a car. Typically, the maximum value is 85 miles per hour, and this is what is meant by full scale. The position of the indicator needle (your speed at the time) is the reading. Thus, if the accuracy claim for the speedometer is ± 3 percent of full scale, it means that it will only indicate the *true* speed within ± 2.5 (85 $\times$ 0.03) miles per hour, no matter how fast you are going. If your actual speed were 20 miles per hour, the possible error would be ± 12.5 (2.5 $\div$ 20) percent. On the other hand, if the accuracy claim is expressed as ± 3 percent of the reading, at 20 miles per hour you would know your true speed within ± 0.6 (20 $\times$ 0.03) miles per hour.

The term **precision** refers to the number of significant digits in the reading of the machine. Thus, a voltage reading of 12.362 is said to be more precise than a reading of 12.4. Precision is closely related to the *repeatability* of the measuring device in question. In fact, manufacturers often use the terms precision and repeatability interchangeably. If a series of repeated measurements are taken of a **stationary** (i.e., unchanging over time) **measurand** (i.e., variable), the precision of the device may be considered to be those digits that are the same for each reading after rounding. To illustrate this notion of precision, suppose the voltmeter mentioned above is used to measure the voltage from a regulated power supply set to output exactly 12 volts. Six readings are taken, and the values are 11.9986, 11.9953, 12.0017, 12.0021, 11.9964, and 12.0039. Because the least significant digits (the last one in each reading) are all different, we drop them by rounding the readings off to five significant digits and obtain 11.999, 11.995, 12.002, 12.002, 11.996, and 12.040. The least significant digits of this set are still different, so we repeat the process to obtain 12.00, 12.00, 12.00, 12.00, 12.00, and 12.00. We conclude that this device has a precision of four significant figures (at least for readings in the vicinity of 12 volts). More typically, however, a manufacturer's precision claim for his machine is expressed as a repeatability of ± 0.5 percent of the *reading,* ± 1 percent of *full scale,* and so on. The precision claims for most devices are generally better than those for accuracy. For example, a manufacturer may state that his machine is accurate to within ± 1

percent of full scale and repeatable to within ±0.25 percent of full scale.

The errors inherent in the machine-associated portion of the measurement process can be broken down into two categories: systematic and random. **Systematic errors** always have the same sign and reflect a bias in the reading. The bias may be a constant, as would result from a zero offset (e.g., labeling error) for example, or may vary with the magnitude of the measurement, and not necessarily in a linear fashion. Systematic errors affect the accuracy of the device, and the calibration process is intended to reduce them to tolerable limits. Random errors, on the other hand, are as likely to be positive or negative because, by definition, they contain no bias. Random errors affect the precision of the device and are usually associated with some aspect of its design. Calibration can do nothing about random errors.

There is a strong analogy between accuracy and precision and the statistical measures of central tendency and variability, with accuracy associated with the concept of the mean and precision associated with the concept of the standard deviation. Consider the illustrations presented in Exhibit 11.4. The data are the values of measurements taken of a stationary measurand; their frequency distributions are the plots given in Exhibit 11.4. In each case a vertical line is used to indicate the true value of the object of measurement. In the first case (Exhibit 11.4a) the device can not be considered very accurate because the mean of its frequency distribution is considerably distant from the true value, and it is not very precise as reflected in the wide spread (high variance) of its frequency distribution. In the second case (Exhibit 11.4b) the device is accurate (the mean of its frequency distribution is the true value) but is still not very precise. In the third case (Exhibit 11.4c) the device is very precise (the standard deviation of its frequency distribution is quite low), but it is still inaccurate because the mean of its frequency distribution is some distance from the true value (i.e., it is biased). The last case (Exhibit 11.4d) illustrates what all manufacturer's strive for, a device that is both accurate and precise.

Accuracy, calibration, standards, and precision apply to analytic laboratory determinations (e.g., blood glucose, ketoacidosis) as well. These are also affected by systematic and random errors as are *all* measures. In fact, if the accuracy and precision of laboratory analysis were more often checked, we would insist on replications before major clinical interventions were instituted.

This chapter has presented a number of considerations related to selection of appropriate measures for use in your research. Multimodal measurement has been stressed. The myriad of possibilities for measures were reviewed according to three modes of measurement: self-report, behavioral observation, and physical assessment. These focus on three possible approaches to measuring a variable associated with human research subjects. This organization into three modes is not engraved in stone. It could be that some researchers will add a fourth mode, ecological assessment, which refers to environmental factors surrounding research subjects including significant others, noise level, air quality,

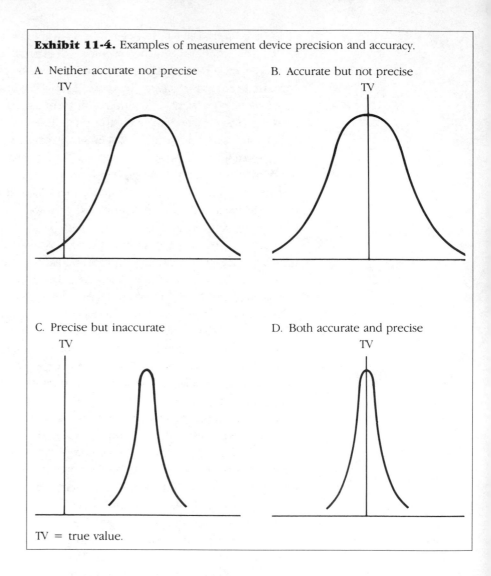

Exhibit 11-4. Examples of measurement device precision and accuracy.

A. Neither accurate nor precise

B. Accurate but not precise

C. Precise but inaccurate

D. Both accurate and precise

TV = true value.

and so forth. If it simplifies your research, do so. On the other hand, ecologic variables are generally measured by one or more of the three modes that have already been presented. This chapter concludes with additional examples of measures used in a series of nursing research studies. None used multimodal measurement of a single variable because it is a relatively new approach to research. The following studies do use measures from all modes, however.

1. Meyer and Morris [43] developed a comprehensive nursing intervention program that included 6 months of home bedrest for 26 patients with acute congestive heart failure who also had alcoholic cardiomyopathy. Aggressive nursing intervention significantly reversed the condition in most patients, apparent also after a 1-year follow-up with continuing close medical and nursing support. Variables in this study included number of episodes of congestive heart failure requiring hospitalization, clinical condition assessed according to stages of cardiomyopathy, and compliance to the program.

2. In an experimental study, McCorkle [41] supported the effectiveness of touch as nonverbal communication with seriously ill patients. Four instruments were used to measure variables. The *Interaction Behavior Worksheet* included four categories of behavioral observation: facial expression, body movements, eye contact, and general response. The Bales *Interaction Process Analysis* was used to code verbal responses (which were tape recorded). An interview elicited patient perception of whether or not the nurse was interested in him or her. Finally, ECG changes in heart rate and rhythm were assessed.

3. Brown and Bloom [3] found that the nurse practitioner's intervention was effective, when patients complied with her suggestions, in reducing sociological stress and blood pressure. Variables included blood pressure and patient report of compliance and stressful life events. Nurse ratings of patient stress as high, medium, or low correlated well with a modified version of the Holmes–Rahe *Stressful Life Events Scale.*

4. Kergis, Woolsey, and Sullivan [33] successfully predicted infant Apgar scores from maternal stress up to 6 months prior to the second trimester, past pregnancy symptoms during first and third trimesters, and illness-proneness ($R =$ .90). Stress combined with past pregnancy symptoms was the strongest predictor. Predictors were measured by means of a single questionnaire, the UTAH, administered during the second or third trimester to 51 pregnant women.

5. Minckley [46] found no difference in the quality of recovery between 60 corrective hip surgery patients who experienced prolonged indefinite presurgical waiting on their day of surgery and those who had early definite scheduling—when patients were convinced the surgery would relieve pain and restore function, and patients were similar in (1) coping characteristics as measured by the Epstein–Fenz *Repression-Sensitization Scale,* (2) blood pressure, (3) pulse rate, (4) finger pulse wave height, (5) palmar sweat volume, and (6) mood. The recovery criteria, developed by the researcher and shown as Exhibit 11.5, provide a model for use in other nursing studies. For each of 14 postoperative days, using a binary system of scoring in which a 1 indicated that the criterion was obtained and a 0 that it was not, each patient's performance was ratioed to the total possible score for the 17 criteria. The resulting daily total score was usually a fraction, although it could be as high as 1. No scores were given for bowel function until the first bowel movement after surgery or for urination until catheters were removed or patients voided without medication. Thereafter, it was assumed. Data sources to indicate achievement of recovery criteria were the surgical staff's progress notes in charts, nursing notes, verbal reports of nursing or medical personnel, patient report, and behavioral observation by the researcher. Verbal statements required validation by statements in the patient's

Exhibit 11-5. Minckley's 17 recovery criteria for elective-surgery patients.

1. *Deep-breathe.* The demonstrated ability of the patient to expand the chest by deep inhalation on command while awake during the 24 hours after surgery. Substantiation of satisfactory respiration was determined from the medical and nursing records, or, if inhalation therapy was used, by the termination of inhalation therapy by doctor's order.

2. *Cough.* The ability to cough two or three times on command while awake during the 24 hours after surgery.

3. *Blow balloon.* The ability to blow up a balloon to the size of a grapefruit on command while awake during the 24 hours after surgery.

4. *Isometrics.* To be able to use the bed trapeze provided to lift buttocks and to perform in-bed exercises ordered (described in illustrated material given to and practiced by the patient the day before surgery) in the 24 hours after surgery.

5. *Nausea.* To be without nausea following surgery.

6. *Vomiting.* To be without vomiting following surgery.

7. *Fever.* To be without fever (by oral temperature) above 37.9°C (100.2°F) following surgery.

8. *Urinate.* To be able to urinate without catheterization or cholinergic medication following surgery.

9. *Defecate.* To be able to defecate without need for enema after surgery.

10. *Sleep.* To be able to sleep at night with no more than one medication dose as ordered for sleep. A recorded second dose of sleep medication in one night was determined a "sleepless night."

11. *Diet.* To resume the normal preoperative diet following surgery. A prescribed diet different from the diet on admission defined failure to resume a normal diet, in addition to inability to eat.

12. *Complications.* To be without unusual complications requiring special medication or therapy following surgery (i.e., conditions that did not exist before surgery). Examples of such complications are thrombophlebitis of extremities necessitating application of hot packs and/or anticoagulant medication, or blisters on buttocks or thighs requiring ointment application.

13. *Dangle legs.* To be able to dangle legs over the side of the bed on the fifth postoperative day.

14. *Sit in chair.* To be able to sit in a chair 15 to 30 minutes on the sixth postoperative day.

15. *Use walker.* To be able to use the walker for ambulation on the seventh postoperative day.

16. *Pool and physical therapy.* To be able to begin pool and dry-land exercise therapy on the tenth postoperative day.

17. *Crutches.* To begin to use crutches on the tenth postoperative day.

From Minckley [46]. This material is copyrighted by the American Journal of Nursing Company and is reproduced with the Company's permission.

chart. A perspiration meter mechanical device was especially designed for this study.

Vocabulary

Accuracy	Instrument credentialing
Adaption period	Instrument sensitivity
Alternate forms reliability	Interactive decision tree
Anonymity	Internal consistency reliability
Baseline	Interrater reliability
Behavioral observation mode	Interview
Calibration	Interview schedule
Card sort	Interview verification
Checklist	Intrarater reliability
Closed-ended response	Item
Coding device	Laboratory or analog setting
Composite score	Measurement error
Computer-assisted measurement	Measurement smorgasbord
Confidentiality	Modes of measurement
Construct validity	Multimodal measurement
Content analysis	Naturalistic observations
Content analysis framework	Nonreactive measure
Content validity	Norm-referenced testing
Continuous observation	Objective tests (nonprojective)
Criterion-referenced testing	Observation code
Criterion-related validity	Observation period
Demand characteristics	Observer drift
Direct measure	Observer's manual
Direct report	Open-ended response
Distortion in physical assessment	Operational definition
Double-blind	Opinionnaire
Ethnographic research	Participant observer
Event observations	Physical assessment mode
Examiner or observer bias	Practice effect
Expectancy	Precision
Face validity	Primary source
Field research	Probing
Flipped items	Procedural artifacts
Habituation	Projective tests (subjective)
Impression management and faking	Quantification
Indicator	Questionnaire
Indirect measure	Random error
Instrument	Reactivity
Instrument appropriateness	Response desynchronization

Response fractionation	Standardized tests
Role playing	Stationary measurand
Scale homogeneity	Subject response bias
Score	Systematic error
Scoring procedure	Tally sheet
Secondary source	Telephone interview
Self-monitoring	Test
Self-report mode	Test–retest reliability
Simulation measurement	Time sampling
Specification of behavior	Training sessions
Split-half reliability	Unobtrusive measure
Standard	Unstructured observation

References

1. Ashton, R. S. Teenage girl's knowledge and attitudes of reproduction, sexual activity, and the utilization of contraception. University of Maryland Master's Thesis, 1981.
2. Barlow, D. H., Leitenberg, H., and Agras, W. S. Experimental control of sexual deviation through manipulation of the noxious scene in covert sensitization. *J. Abnorm. Psychol.* 74:596, 1969.
3. Brown, E., and Bloom, J. R. The nurse practitioner and hypertension control: A pilot study. *Evaluation and the Health Professions* 1:87, 1979.
4. Campbell, S. B., Endman, M. W., and Bernfeld, G. A. Three-year follow-up of hyperactive preschoolers into elementary school. *J. Child Psychol. Psychiatry* 18:239, 1977.
5. Chamorro, I. L., et al. Development of an instrument to measure premature infant behavior and caretaker activities: Time-sampling methodology. *Nurs. Res.* 22:300, 1973.
6. Chapman, J. Effects of different nursing approaches upon selected postoperative responses of male herniorrhaphy patients. In F. Downs and M. Newman (eds.), *A Source Book of Nursing Research,* 2nd ed. Philadelphia: Davis, 1977.
7. Chapman, L. J., Chapman, J. P., and Brebje, T. Influences of the experimenter on pupillary dilation to sexually provocative pictures. *J. Abnorm. Psychol.* 74:396, 1969.
8. Cohen, F. Personality, stress, and the development of physical illness. In G. C. Stone, F. Cohen, and N. E. Adler, (eds.) *Health Psychology.* San Francisco: Jossey-Bass, 1979.
9. Colette, G., and Harris, S. L. Behavior modification in the home: Siblings as behavior modifiers, parents as observers. *J. Abnorm. Psychol.* 5:21, 1977.
10. Damrosch, S. P. Nursing students' attitudes toward sexually active older persons. *Nurs. Res.* 31:252, 1982.
11. Damrosch, S. P. How nursing students' reactions to rape victims are affected by a perceived act of carelessness. *Nurs. Res.* 30:168, 1981.
12. DeLongis, A., et al. Relationship of daily hassles, uplifts, and major life events to health status. *Health Psychol.* 1:119, 1982.
13. Downs, F. S., and Fitzpatrick, J. J. Preliminary investigation of the reliability and validity of a tool for the assessment of body position and motor activity. *Nurs. Res.* 25:404, 1976.
14. Dubey, D. R., et al. Reactions of children and teachers to classroom observers: A series of controlled investigations. *Behav. Ther.* 8:887, 1977.
15. Eisler, R. M., Herson, M., and Agras, W. S. Videotape: A method for the controlled observation of non-verbal interpersonal behavior. *Behav. Ther.* 4:420, 1973.

16. Eisler, R. M., Miller, P. M., and Herson, M. Components of assertive behavior. *J. Clin. Psychol.* 29:295, 1973.

17. Foxx, R. M., and Hake, D. F. Gasoline conservation: A procedure for measuring and reducing the driving of college students. *J. Appl. Behav. Anal.* 10:61, 1977.

18. Freund, K., Sedlacek, F., and Knob, K. A simple transducer for mechanical plethysmography of the male genital. *J. Exp. Anal. Behav.* 8:169, 1965.

19. Graffam, S. R. Nurse response to the patient in distress—Development of an instrument. *Nurs. Res.* 19:331, 1970.

20. Hamilton, R. G., and Robertson, M. H. Examiner influence on the Holtzman Inkblot Technique. *J. Projective Techniques Pers. Assess.* 30:553, 1966.

21. Harris, S., and Masling, J. Examiner sex, subject sex, and Rorschach productivity. *J. Consult. Clin. Psychol.* 34:60, 1970.

22. Hart, B. M., et al. Effects of social reinforcements on operant crying. *J. Exp. Child Psychol.* 1:145, 1964.

23. Hay, R. R., Hay, W. M., and Angle, H. V. The reactivity of self-recording: A case report of a drug abuser. *Behav. Ther.* 8:1004, 1977.

24. Haynes, S. N. *Principles of Behavior Assessment.* New York: Halstead Press, 1978.

25. Haynes, S. N., and Wilson, C. C. *Behavioral Assessment.* San Francisco: Jossey-Bass, 1979.

26. Hersen, M. Sexual aspects of Rorschach administration. *J. Projective Techniques Pers. Assess.* 34:104, 1970.

27. Herson, M., and Greaves, S. T. Rorschach productivity as related to verbal reinforcement. *J. Pers. Assess.* 35:436, 1971.

28. Holmes, T. H., and Rahe, R. H. The social readjustment rating scale. *J. Psychosom. Res.* 4:189, 1967.

29. Hoskins, C. N. Level of activation, body temperature, and interpersonal conflict in family relationships. *Nurs. Res.* 28:154, 1979.

30. Hoskins, C., et al. Social chronobiology: Circadian activation, rhythms of married couples. *Psychol. Rep.* 45:607, 1979.

31. Johnson, J., Kirchoff, K., and Endress, M. P. Altering children's distress behavior during orthopedic cast removal. *Nurs. Res.* 24:404, 1975.

32. Kanner, A. D., et al. Comparison of two modes of stress management: Daily hassles and uplifts versus major life events. *J. Behav. Med.* 4:1, 1981.

33. Kergis, C. A., Woolsey, D. B., and Sullivan, J. J. Predicting infant apgar scores. *Nurs. Res.* 26:439, 1977.

34. Kirschenbaum, D. S., and Karoly, P. When self-regulation fails: Tests of some preliminary hypotheses. *J. Consult. Clin. Psychol.* 45:1116, 1977.

35. Lawson, K., Daum, C., and Turkewitz, G. Environmental characteristics of a neonatal intensive care unit. *Child Dev.* 48:1633, 1977.

36. LeBow, M. D., Goldberg, P. A., and Collins, A. Eating behavior of overweight and nonoverweight persons in the natural environment. *J. Consult. Clin. Psychol.* 45:1204, 1977.

37. Liberman, R. P., et al. Research design for analyzing drug–environment–behavior interactions. *J. Nerv. Ment. Dis.* 156:432, 1973.

38. Liberman, R. P., et al. Reducing delusional speech in chronic paranoid schizophrenics. *J. Appl. Behav. Anal.* 6:57, 1973.

39. Lucus, R. W., et al. Psychiatrists and a computer as interrogators of patients with alcohol-related illness: a comparison. *Br. J. Psychiatry* 131:160, 1977.

40. Marston, A., et al. In vivo observation of the eating behaviors of obese and nonobese subjects. *J. Consult. Clin. Psychol.* 45:335, 1977.

41. McCorkle, R. Effects of touch on seriously ill patients. *Nurs. Res.* 23:125, 1974.

42. McFall, R. M. Effects of self-monitoring on normal smoking behavior. *J. Consult. Clin. Psychol.* 35:135, 1972.
43. Meyer, R. M. S., and Morris, D. T. Alcoholic cardiomyapathy: A nursing approach. *Nurs. Res.* 26:422, 1977.
44. Mills, H. L., et al. Compulsive rituals treated by response prevention: An experimental analysis. *Arch. Gen. Psychiatry* 28:524, 1973.
45. Mills, M. E., et al. Effect of pulse palpitation on cardiac arrhythmia in coronary care patients. *Nurs. Res.* 25:378, 1976.
46. Minckley, B. B. Physiologic and psychologic responses of elective surgical patients: Early definite or late indefinite scheduling of surgical procedure. *Nurs. Res.* 23:392, 1974.
47. Mischel, W. Direct versus indirect personality assessment: Evidence and implications. *J. Consult. Clin. Psychol.* 38:319, 1972.
48. Montague, J. D., and Colis, E. M. Mechanism and measurement of the galvanic skin response. *Psychol. Bull.* 65:261, 1966.
49. Rankin, E., and McIntee, M. Stress management as a health technique. Paper Presented at the Northeast Regional Conference of the National League for Nursing, 1981.
50. Reid, J. B. Reliability assessment of observation data: A possible methodological problem. *Child Dev.* 41:1143, 1970.
51. Reid, J. B., and DeMaster, B. The efficacy of the spot-check procedure in maintaining the reliability of data collected by observers in quasi-natural settings: Two pilot studies. *Oregon Res. Bull.* 12(8), 1972.
52. Reingold, H. L. The measurement of maternal care. *Child Devel.* 31:566, 1960.
53. Romancyzk, R. G., et al. Measuring the reliability of observation data: a reactive process. *J. Appl. Behav. Anal.* 6:175, 1973.
54. Sarason, I. G., Johnson, J. H., and Siegel, J. M. Assessing the impact of life changes: Development of the life experiences survey. *J. Consult. Clin. Psychol.* 46:932, 1978.
55. Sciarra, J. J. (ed.) *Gynecology and Obstetrics.* Hagerstown, Md.: Harper & Row, 1980. Vol. 1.
56. Spielberger, C. D., Gorsuch, R. L., and Lushene, R. E. *The State-Trait Inventory.* Palo Alto, Calif.: Consulting Psychologists Press, 1970.
57. Wahler, R. G., and Leske, G. Accurate and inaccurate observer summary reports: Reinforcement theory interpretation and investigation. *J. Nerv. Ment. Dis.* 156:386, 1973.
58. Williams, J. G., Barlow, D. H., and Agras, W. S. Behavioral measurement of severe depression. *Arch. Gen. Psychiatry* 27:330, 1972.
59. Zegiob, L. E., and Forehand, R. Parent–child interactions: Observer effects and social class differences. *Behav. Ther.* 9:118, 1978.
60. Zuckerman, M. The development of the affect adjective check list for the measurement of anxiety. *J. Consult. Psychol.* 24:457, 1960.

12: *Scoring*

Suppose that, as a parent, you received a report from your child's elementary school stating that Johnny was not working up to his ability. According to his teacher, his deviation IQ score on the Stanford-Binet 2 years ago was 125 and his stanines last year on a national scholastic and aptitude test were 8, 9, and 8 for verbal, quantitative, and nonverbal respectively. However, he is working at a low C level in school. Moreover, recent national achievement tests placed him in the 80th percentile. His teacher says something must be done to improve his performance so that it more adequately reflects his abilities. What is his teacher talking about? Do you know what these numbers mean? This is the objective of this chapter.

Let us consider another example. Suppose, as a researcher, you must interpret the following scores for a subject in your stress reduction study:

Blood pressure	160/110
Checklist of agitated behaviors	40
Paired adjectives checklist	26
Self report on a Likert scale of 1 to 5	3
Memory test for digits	23

Do you know whether or not this subject is stressed? How were the numbers figured? You have a good idea of what the blood pressure "scores" mean, because you are a professional who happens to use this measure as part of your practice. However, others in professions not related to health might not know the meaning of even this number.

Finally, what if you were handed a questionnaire embedded within which were four research scales designed to measure four different personality characteristics. Could you calculate a score for each personality characteristic? If so, would you know what it means? What could you do with it? Is there method to this madness? Are there theories or rules to guide us? Yes, we always have rules and theory to guide us when we calculate scores. If you do not have them for an instrument that other researchers in your topic area have used and that you therefore wish to use in your research, get them or do not use the instrument. *Never* use a test or scale without first knowing how its author intended it to be scored. Reliability and validity data for the scale are based on the author's scoring method and are invalid if a different method is used. Sometimes **scoring stencils** or **answer keys** are required, particularly with most standardized tests, because a subject's responses to items are often compared with a known standard (or the correct answer). In these cases, only when responses match the standard are they included in the total score. In the case of projective tests, training is required to analyze and score responses. This chapter is meant as only an overview of scoring. Those wishing still more information after reading this chapter are referred to some of the more comprehensive works in this area [1, 2, 6, 9, 12, 17].

Basically, quantitative research involves assigning numbers to subjects according to rules, which are usually formulae or equations. When these numbers are at the interval/ratio level of measurement, these numbers are called **scores.** Scores tell how much of a variable is characteristic of a research subject at the time measurement occurs. In this chapter, we focus primarily on tests and scales from the self-report mode of measurement. The same rules that pertain to these can be applied to most measures in the behavioral observation and physical assessment modes as well.

Definition of a Score

An **observed score** is the number we compute according to the rules for scoring a specific instrument and assign to an individual. Furthermore, an observed score is made up of two parts: a true score and an error score. A **true score** represents the actual amount of the variable "possessed" by an individual. The closer it is to the observed score, the higher the reliability of a measure. Unfortunately, when we measure constructs (as opposed to physical phenomena with known standards), we can never know what the true score is. This is because of measurement error, which was discussed at length in Chapter 11. The amount of error associated with a person's observed score is known as the **error score.** We are never absolutely sure what this is, either. However, we are able to estimate it when we compute a reliability coefficient, and this is one reason why computing reliability is so important.

The amount of error variance in a set of scores is estimated by subtracting the reliability coefficient from unity (i.e., 1). Thus, if a test has a .83 reliability coefficient, (1.00 − .83) or 17 percent of the variance of the test scores can be considered to be due to error. Chapter 13 presents the standard error of measurement fomula which uses the reliability of a test and its standard deviation to compute a standard error (SE) for use in placing confidence intervals around a corrected observed score. Depending on the confidence level you select (e.g., 95 percent or 99 percent probability of being correct), the intervals are calculated and form boundaries within which an individual's true score can be expected to fall at the confidence level you have selected. Thus, although we often cannot know what a person's true score is, we do have some tools with which we can estimate it by using our observed score.

Scoring Considerations

Before we consider some of the ways tests and scales can be scored, there are three distinctions relating to how scores are computed or interpreted that must be explored. The first deals with **ipsative testing,** or forced choice. Typically, ipsative measures present two or more statements or alternatives from which a respondent must select one choice. Usually it involves selecting an alternative that represents that which is most or least like the respondent or that which the respondent finds most or least interesting or enjoyable, because this approach to measurement is used in tests of personality, interests, aptitudes, and so on—

tests that contain many subscales. A problem arises when none or many of the alternatives are appropriate. The respondent must still select only one. Thus, some alternatives may be chosen that only weakly (if at all) represent an individual and others would not be selected (although they were more appropriate than the weak one) simply because they were paired with even more appropriate choices. Scores on ipsative measures are not interpreted the same as are others; therefore, although they represent a **relative intensity** for the various subscales on a test, they do not yield an **absolute magnitude** for each scale. A person with intense interest in several areas represented by subscales could appear similar to a more phlegmatic person with only passing interest in those same areas. A person with intense interests in several areas could have the intense interests cancel one another out, while another person, who is generally indifferent and with a somewhat greater interest in only one area, could appear extremely interested in that one area. Thus, the frame of reference with ipsative measures is the individual rather than a normative sample. When ipsative scores are compared to norms it must be done very, very carefully if at all. Nevertheless, ipsative measures are often very appropriate to the purpose of the research or theory being tested. For example, research comparing personalities of various kinds of nurses (e.g., psychiatric, medical–surgical) has often used the Edwards Personal Preference Schedule (EPPS) [5]. The EPPS is based on the personality theory of manifest needs proposed by Murray and his associates of the Harvard Psychological Clinic. Edwards selected 15 of these needs for his test. Whether or not it measures these needs is no concern here (see reviews in Buros [4] and others [1, 2]). The major point here is that the EPPS was designed to control the effects of one of the major response sets, social desirability. Edwards's research had already shown a high correlation between the rated social desirability of an item and the probability of endorsement of that item. His research had therefore cast doubt on most self-report measures of personality. Therefore, he reasoned that the best way to control for social desirability was to force a respondent to choose from two equally desirable or undesirable alternatives, each measuring different traits. Confronted with alternatives having the same rated social desirability, a subject will be forced to focus on the trait content rather than desirability. In this case ipsative measurement was used to control a probable confounding variable in self-report personality measurement—responding in a socially desirable way.

The second consideration in scoring relates to how scores are interpreted, although it affects how items are developed and tests constructed as well. It was introduced in Chapter 11. This involves the distinction between norm-referenced and criterion-referenced testing. Recall **norm-referenced testing** involves comparing the performance of a subject or group of subjects with the performance of others. Most standardized tests are this type. In fact, most measures used in research *at this time* are of this type. **Criterion-referenced testing** involves comparing an individual's performance against a pass-fail standard. This manner of testing, or a combination of it and norm-referenced, is increasing in popularity for tests of achievement—particularly with the widespread use of computers. However, it is not widely used in research and therefore is not covered as completely as norm-referenced measurement in this book. Norm-referenced measurement compares an individual's performance with a *well-defined* group of other persons; criterion-referenced measurement compares an individual with a *well-defined* content domain. Martuza [9] presents a good discussion of criterion-referenced testing.

A last consideration about scoring involves the distinction between a raw score and a derived score. A **raw score** is the number calculated according to the scoring rules for a specific measure. Sometimes the number is useful by itself (e.g., weight in pounds, number of correct answers), but most of the time it is not. It must be interpreted by comparing it to **norms,** that give a range of scores that are "normal" for well-defined subgroups (e.g., women, lawyers, accountants, schizophrenics). Furthermore, raw scores are often converted to **derived scores,** like the z score presented in Chapter 6. In this way, individual scores within a group can be compared to others in the group. They can also be compared to a person's scores on other tests if they have also been converted to similar derived scores. The various kinds of derived scores are presented later in the chapter.

Raw Score Calculations

There are basically two kinds of raw score calculations. Although they are called by various names, we will consider them as content scores and attitude scores. **Content scores** involve comparing a person's responses with responses predetermined to be ideal because they are either correct answers or typical responses for persons who have certain personality characteristics, interests, aptitudes, and so forth. **Attitude scores,** on the other hand, have no predetermined ideal response. An individual simply responds on a given scale (e.g., Likert) or selects from a series of choices, each having certain values that are then summed according to a set of rules. The purpose is to spread out subjects on an interval level continuum according to their attitudes, perceptions, or beliefs about a given variable.

Content Scores

There are basically two kinds of content scores. One kind includes measures of personality, interests, aptitudes, and the like for which the standards against which a person's responses are compared are those that are typical of a well-defined group, like leaders who are assertive, persons exhibiting dependency, anxious persons, those with an internal locus of control, risk takers, and so forth. If a person's responses are similar to those of the well-defined subgroup, then the person's raw score will be high and when compared to norms will lead to the conclusion that the individual is assertive, not anxious, a risk taker, and so forth. Tests and scales of this kind are usually scored by computer or with hand scoring stencils that are placed over an answer sheet. Each subscale stencil is marked with small see-through windows revealing a subject's response to the items of that particular subscale. If the appropriate response was selected, it is observed through the window for that item. The number of appropriate responses is counted and this becomes a person's raw score for that subscale. Usually it is plotted on a profile sheet that is designed to include normative data. Sometimes, the raw score is converted to another score or modified in some other way. The precise rules for the test and scales in this group are given in their **test manuals.** They should be clearly understood *before* the test is used in a research setting. Some tests and scales in this group are ipsative.

The other kind of tests in the content scales category are those for which there are *correct* answers. This groups includes a wide variety of standardized tests that measure performance, intelligence, and achievement. They are generally administered under controlled circumstances and the answer key restricted to only a few professionals, sometimes only a bonded computer scoring service. Researcher developed tests of knowledge are also in this group. Tests are true-false, multiple choice, matching, sentence completion, fill in the blank, or essay. Generally, scoring involves counting the number of correct responses. This number then becomes the raw score. Sometimes a correction for guessing is used in an attempt to reduce error and move the true score closer to the observed score. One of the more common formulas used for this purpose is as follows:

$$S = R - \frac{W}{A - 1} \tag{12.1}$$

where R = the number of items correct
W = the number of items incorrect
A = the number of response alternatives for each item

If an individual had 53 correct and 7 wrong on a multiple choice test on which each question **stem** had 4 **response alternatives**, his score would be

$$S = 53 - \frac{7}{4 - 1} = 53 - \frac{7}{3} = 53 - 2.33 = 50.66$$

If the test were true-false, however, his score would be lower:

$$S = 53 - \frac{7}{2 - 1} = 53 - 7 = 46$$

This is because the extra response alternatives make the multiple choice test harder and less vulnerable to guessing.

In addition to scoring via counting the number correct or using a guessing correction formula, in rare circumstances items are weighted in order to give greater importance to some questions. This approach should be used with care, because it is difficult to determine valid weights. Moreover, raw scores from many weighting schemes have been found to correlate highly with total scores based on the *number* of correct items, ignoring their weights. Most criterion-referenced measures are found among this group of content scores with correct answers.

Attitude Scores

Test and scales that fall into the category of **attitude scores** do not have a standard or correct answer against which a person's response is compared. Therefore, they obviously cannot test knowledge, performance, or achievement. Instead, they measure attitudes, beliefs, and perceptions about things. The scoring rules for these measures are also known as **scaling** rules, because each technique attempts to place on a continuum scale an individual's attitudes toward something. One end of the continuum is negative or lower or less and the other end is positive or higher or more. These measures are usually norm-referenced. Five classical kinds of scales will be discussed: Likert, *Q* sort, semantic differential, Thurstone, and Guttman.

Likert Scales

Likert scales [8] were introduced in Chapter 2. Please refer to it. An example is shown in Exhibit 2.3. Recall, Likert scales ask a subject to respond to a statement with one of the following:

ordinal

Strongly agree	Agree	Undecided	Disagree	Strongly disagree
1	2	3	4	5

Sometimes the undecided category is deleted; sometimes "somewhat agree" and "somewhat disagree" are added. There are cases where the following is used:

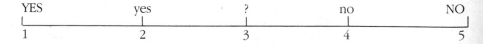

YES	yes	?	no	NO
1	2	3	4	5

It is especially useful with children and semiliterate individuals. Another approach uses pictures depicting, for example, action scenes from the target attitude, which are then sorted into piles labeled, "YES," "yes," "?," "no," or "NO." Characteristics of the ideal nurse might be used for this purpose where each picture depicts one characteristic described in the literature. At this point, one more modification could be made by limiting the number of responses in each of the five categories. The scaling procedure is then known as a *Q* sort.

Q Sort

The procedure for scoring **card sorts** can sometimes become very complex when the cards no longer represent items as they are depicted on a Likert scale, and responses can no longer be anywhere from, say, 1 to 5, for each card. For example, a special version of the card sort, called the **Q sort,** has been used to measure self concept. The cards must be sorted into piles for which a given number of cards has been predetermined, so that the piles approximate a normal distribution. As an example, suppose 60 cards representing 6 subscales of self concept (e.g., physical self, social (friendship) self, emotional self, intellectual self, community self, and family self), each with 10 pictures, is sorted into 9 piles as follows:

Very much like me								Not like me at all
2 cards	3 cards	6 cards	11 cards	16 cards	11 cards	6 cards	3 cards	2 cards
Score: (9)	(8)	(7)	(6)	(5)	(4)	(3)	(2)	(1)

The measure has become ipsative by forcing a given number of cards into each point on the scale. Each card is scored with the number in parentheses and the values of cards in each of the subscales is summed. The result is six subscale scores that represent the *relative* importance to an individual's self concept of the six subscales. Three such subscale **profiles** are shown in Exhibit 12.1. In this fictitious example, let us assume that profiles falling within the shaded area are "normal." When subscale scores are outside the area, an individual has an excessive preoccupation with one or two areas to the neglect of others and might therefore benefit from an intervention designed to change this. The theory behind such an interpretation, of course, would have to concern relationships between the constructs represented by the six subscales rather than their absolute values. Because of the ipsativity of the measure, two individuals could appear similar on the basis of their profiles and yet be very different in terms of the absolute values of the subscales. In fact, the absolute value of one person's highest subscale might be less than the absolute value of another person's lowest subscale.

The Q sort as presented in our example could also be considered as a content score with other measures of personality if the standard against which responses are measured could be construed to be the shaded area of Exhibit 12.1. Then again, since there is no standard against which responses to *each* card are compared, perhaps the Q sort is an attitude score. It really does not matter. As emphasized throughout this book, categories designed to help us organize various kinds of things (in this case scoring rules) are rarely mutually exclusive. Moreover, time spent trying to classify into categories rather than understanding basic concepts is rarely time spent wisely.

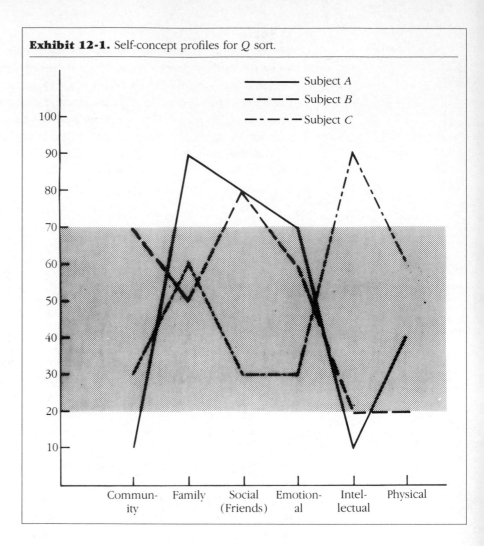

Exhibit 12-1. Self-concept profiles for *Q* sort.

Q sorts have been used to measure a variety of things. For example, in intensive investigations of personality, persons have re-sorted the same set of cards with different frames of reference like ideal self, or as they apply to different people like mother, father, spouse, sibling, or offspring. They have also sorted the cards as they apply to different settings, such as job, home, and social settings. Scores for the various sorts have then been compared. Before you use a Q sort, be sure you know how it is scored and, even more important, what meaning you can attach to the score(s) once you have it.

Semantic Differential

The semantic differential is a procedure to measure the connotations of a given concept or construct for an individual. Concepts can be people (e.g., nurse, father), places (e.g., school, hospital), things (e.g., aspirin, automobiles, dis-

Exhibit 12-2. Semantic differential scale.

Hospital

(E)	1. Pleasant							✓	Unpleasant
*(E)	2. Bad						✓		Good
*(A)	3. Passive						✓		Active
*(P)	4. Weak						✓		Strong
(P)	5. Deep			✓					Shallow
(A)	6. Fast		✓						Slow
(E)	7. Beautiful			✓					Ugly
*(P)	8. Small						✓		Large
*(A)	9. Dull						✓		Sharp

Scoring Scale   (1) : (2) : (3) : (4) : (5) : (6) : (7)

*Bipolar adjective pair has been flipped (i.e., reversed).

interval

eases), abstractions (e.g., democracy) and just about anything else a researcher can come up with. Each concept is then assessed by a series of bipolar adjectives usually separated by a 7 point graphic scale, as shown in Exhibit 12.2. Three, five, and nine point scales are used less often (although 5 point scales have been found more suitable for children). The number of bipolar adjectives pairs used for each concept varies from 9 to 20.

This technique was originally developed by Osgood and his associates [13] as a tool for research on the psychology of meaning. Their research revealed that the 50 bipolar adjective pairs they were using could be grouped into 3 major factors or categories: those which were *evaluative,* measuring such things as good–bad, valuable–worthless, and clean–dirty; those which assessed *potency,* such as strong–weak, large–small, and heavy–light; and those which described *activity*, such as active–passive, fast–slow, and sharp–dull. These have remained the major subscales (with evaluation the most popular) used by subsequent researchers although Osgood himself believed at least 7 or 8 were possible. Nunally [11] in his study of attitudes toward mental disorders found a factor he called *understandability* which consisted of adjective pairs like predictable–unpredictable, understandable–mysterious, familiar–strange, and simple–complicated. Osgood's original 50 scales (i.e., adjective pairs) do not, of course, exhaust all possibilities and other researchers have added other pairs that seemed more appropriate to the concept being investigated. Then again, obvious relevancy of an adjective pair to the concept it reflects has not always been found to be necessary (e.g., sweet–sour is as good as beautiful–ugly for the concept of a motel). As a rule, though, the original 50 adjective pairs provide ample flexibility, and moreover, their known association with one of the three factors makes computation of subscales easier.

Semantic differential scales are scored similarly to Likert scales. Although "item" responses for both could range from -2, to -1, to 0, to 1, to 2; or from -3 to 3; most researchers prefer to keep responses as positive numbers and therefore they use scales of 1 to 5, 1 to 7, 1 to 9, and so forth. In Exhibit 12.2 semantic differential scales of bipolar adjective pairs are used to score attitudes toward a hospital. The pairs represent the three traditional subscales. Like Likert scales some adjective pairs are **flipped** (i.e., reversed) to prevent response bias. These are shown by an asterisk. Preceding the number of each scale is a letter in parentheses that represents the subscale to which it belongs: evaluation (E), potency (P), and activity (A). The scale values for each response are shown at the bottom of the Exhibit and labeled "scoring scale." These, of course, would not be included on an actual instrument. They are shown here as an aid to understanding this technique.

To score, responses are summed after flipping (via a constant number that is one more than the value of the highest response or $7 + 1 = 8$) the designated items:

$$E = 7 + (8 - 6) + 4 = 13$$

Similarly,

$$A = (8 - 6) + 3 + (8 - 6) = 7$$
$$P = (8 - 6) + 3 + (8 - 6) = 7$$

Subscale scores for E, A, and P can vary from 3 to 21, where a higher score is more negative (e.g., bad, passive, weak). The responses in Exhibit 12.2 are somewhat more positive than negative toward hospitals in terms of the **possible range of scores.** However, to find further meaning in these raw scores, we must have norms or other persons with whom these scores can be compared.

Thurstone Scales

As we have said, attitude scales are designed to provide a quantitative measure of a person's position on a continuum from low to high. Thurstone [14, 15, 16] adapted psychophysical methods to the measurement of attitudes in what was an important milestone in attitude scale construction in the late 1920s. Since then this method has been known as a Thurstone scale, although recently some researchers have modified it somewhat and called it the *method of equally appearing intervals.* When a person responds to a Thurstone scale, he is usually asked to mark all statements with which he agrees. (More recently, some respondents have been told to select a certain number of statements that *best* represent his or her attitudes.) An individual's score is then computed by summing the weights (usually from 1 to 11) associated with each of the statements selected.

In order to understand a Thurstone scale, we must explore how values are associated with each statement. In developing the scale for measuring attitudes toward the church [16], Thurstone and associates developed a list of 130 carefully edited short statements that seemed to range from extremely favorable to neutral to extremely unfavorable. They then asked 300 judges to sort the statements into 11 piles, ranging from extremely favorable to neutral to extremely unfavorable. This sorting procedure has come to be called the *method of equally appearing intervals,* although the judges in the landmark study were not actually told the intervals between piles were to appear equal. Judges were asked to not indicate their own attitudes but instead only to classify the statements. Judge classifications were then combined and the medians and interquartile range (see Chapter 6) for each computed. The interquartile range was used as a measure of ambiguity, because a large value indicated greater variability among the judges in classifying statements. Those items with high Qs were eliminated from the final scale. The statements were also checked for *irrelevance* by asking subjects to mark only items with which they agreed. Finally, items were selected to have median values that were distributed across the range of possible weights. Thus, the median value for each item is its weight. If the item is selected, its weight is used to compute the total score.

More recently, researchers [6] used the mean and the SD of judges' ratings as an index of ambiguity. They also instruct judges to (1) disregard their own attitudes and biases and (2) consider the subjective distance between intervals as equal. The Thurstone method remains an important tool in many research settings, although the effects of judge bias or attitude remain a threat. It is also much more difficult to develop and has not been shown to be appreciably more accurate than, say, a Likert scale.

Guttman Scales

A final type of attitude scale is used infrequently, perhaps because it has limited applications and is difficult to develop. The Guttman scale or Guttman scalogram analysis [7] involves selecting items in terms of increasing extremeness of the attitude. That is, the first item might be agreed to by all, the next agreed to by those with moderate attitudes, and the final item by those with extreme attitudes. If a scale is operating correctly, a respondent who endorses an extreme item will endorse those items that are less extreme also and not endorse any items that are even more extreme. It is therefore more an analytic technique for determining whether an existing set of items meets the requirements of a particular scale.

For example, consider the following statements, which might be expected to measure attitudes toward glaucoma testing:

1. Free glaucoma tests might be beneficial to the state.
2. It would be beneficial for the state to offer free glaucoma tests.
3. Free glaucoma tests would be the best thing for the state.

If you agree with item 3, you should agree with items 1 and 2. If you agree with item 2, you should agree with item 1 but not 3. If you agree with item 1, you would not agree with items 2 and 3. A respondent receives the highest scale value to which he or she agreed (i.e., 1, 2, or 3).

If reversals occur (e.g., a respondent selecting 3 but not 2), the scale homogeneity in regard to that attitude is in doubt. The amount of reversals, or errors, can be computed via the **index of reproducibility.** It is computed as follows:

$$R = 1 - \frac{\text{Total errors}}{(\text{Total responses})\,(\text{Number of items})}\,(100) \qquad (12.2)$$

Thus, if among 50 respondents, 6 chose 2 but not 1, and 2 chose 3 but not 1 or 2, the total number of errors would be $(6 \times 1) + (2 \times 2)$ or 10. Using the formula, we compute the index of reproducibility:

$$R = 1 - \frac{10}{50 \times 3}\,(100) = 1 - \frac{10}{150}\,(100) = (1 - .07)\,(100) = (.93)\,(100) = 93\%$$

The index of reproducibility ranges from 0 to 1. Experts disagree on the acceptable level. Some say 85 percent and others demand 90 percent. In our example, the error is within acceptable bounds.

Interpreting Raw Scores

There are, basically, two ways in which meaning is given to raw scores. In the first, the raw score is used and simply compared against a known standard or norm. In the second, the raw score is converted to a **derived score,** either as a standardized score (e.g., the z score presented in Chap. 6), a percentile, or a developmental score (e.g., age, grade in school). Derived scores serve a dual purpose. First, they indicate a person's relative standing in the normative sample and therefore allow assessment of high performance in reference to others. Second, they provide a means for comparing scores for an individual on several different tests whose scale and raw scores are not compatible (e.g., all scores are converted to z scores and then compared).

Raw Scores Compared with a Standard

A few measures (or scores), like age, body temperature, or wrist circumference in inches, have immediate intuitive meaning and therefore rarely need further attention unless they are to be compared with scores from other persons in a research study. Their scale is known and is the standard against which a score for an individual is compared. Most raw scores, however, are just about meaningless all by themselves, because their scale is not known, and when it is it still does not provide enough information, a standard, against which a raw score can be compared. For example, even if you know a score of 85 means 85 correct answers out of 100, you still do not know if 85 is average performance, above average, or below. Thus, we seek norms or standards.

Most standardized tests of intelligence, achievement, aptitude, interest, personality, and so forth yield a series of subscale scores that can be compared to norms presented in the test manual. If you read the manual for your particular test, interpretation is fairly straightforward. **Profile analysis,** analysis of a person's entire set of subscales relative to each other, usually via a visual depiction like the chart in Exhibit 12.1, can require special training beyond directions in the manual. Whenever you plan to use a standardized (i.e., normed) test, read the manual before you make your final decision to use the test.

Research scales and tests vary in the normative data that is available and therefore you sometimes must settle for comparisons between group means, which lead to such conclusions as that one group has less or more of the dependent variable than the other group. The value or meaning of scores in the sense of absolute values or even in comparison with norms may not be possible. Then again, some attitude scales, such as the Thurstone, place individuals along a unidimensional continuum on which one end is, say, negative and the other is positive. Thus, the midpoint of the **possible range of scores** (i.e., if the lowest possible score on a scale is 16 and the highest is 96, the possible range of scores is from 16 to 96 with a midpoint at 56) indicates neither negative nor positive. Intuitively, one can interpret individual scores as more negative or positive the closer they are to the respective ends of the continuum, while scores falling close to the midpoint of the possible (*not observed*) range are interpreted as undecided or a mixture of positive and negative. Thus, if you know the possible range of scores, you can find meaning in many attitude raw scores that were measured via such well researched techniques as the Thurstone method.

Derived Scores

There are a number of ways in which raw scores can be converted into scores that help us give them meaning. They can be converted into percentiles whereby an individual's relative standing within a group is evident (e.g., 86th percentile means 86 percent of the group had lower scores); a series of standard scores like the z score presented in Chapter 6; or developmental scores, such as age, which are used much less often in nursing research.

Percentiles

Percentile rank scores are expressed in terms of the percentage of persons in a sample who fall below a given raw score. The **50th percentile** corresponds to the median. In test manuals, percentile rank norms are sometimes reported in the form of a graph, called an *ogive,* which shows the cumulative percentage of

Exhibit 12-3. Conversion of raw scores to percentile rank scores.

X (1)	f (2)	CF (3)	$CF_{MP} = CF_{X-1} + 0.5f_X$ (4)	$P = 100(CF_{MP} \div n)$ (5)
84	0	180	$180 + 0 = 180.0$	100
83	5	180	$175 + 2.5 = 177.5$	98.6
82	11	175	$164 + 5.5 = 169.5$	94.2
81	14	164	$150 + 7 = 157$	87.2
80	11	150	$139 + 5.5 = 144.5$	80.3
79	9	139	$130 + 4.5 = 134.5$	74.7
78	10	130	$120 + 5 = 125$	69.4
77	10	120	$110 + 5 = 115$	63.9
76	11	110	$99 + 5.5 = 104.5$	58.1
75	13	99	$86 + 6.5 = 92.5$	51.4
74	15	86	$71 + 7.5 = 78.5$	43.6
73	18	71	$53 + 9 = 62.0$	34.4
72	20	53	$33 + 10 = 43.0$	23.9
71	15	33	$18 + 7.5 = 25.5$	14.2
70	9	18	$9 + 4.5 = 13.5$	7.5
69	6	9	$3 + 3 = 6.0$	3.3
68	3	3	$0 + 1.5 = 1.5$	0.8
67	0	0	$0 = 0$	0.0

$n = 180, \bar{X} = 75.44, SD = 4.08, \tilde{X} = 74.86$

cases falling below each score. Such a graph was presented in Chapter 6 as Exhibit 6.37. From it, you can determine the percentile of a raw score when precision to several decimal points is not required. Percentile can also be computed via the method presented in Exhibit 12.3.

To convert a raw score to a percentile score, the **cumulative frequency** (CF) as described in Chapter 6 is first computed (step 3 of Exhibit 12.3). Next, because a percentile rank is the proportion of people scoring below a given score and the raw scores are presented in Exhibit 12.3 as discrete although theoretically we have a continuous scale for them, we must find the **cumulative frequency to the midpoint** (CF_{MP}) or mark of the score interval by adding one-half the number of scores (frequencies) to the CF for the score interval just preceding it. (Remember, we start with the lowest score.) The formula is as follows:

$$CF_{MP} = CF_{X-1} + .5f_X \tag{12.3}$$

where CF_{MP} = cumulative frequency to the midpoint (of the data class interval) for score X

$$\text{CF}_{(X-1)} = \text{cumulative frequency for the class interval immediately preceding that for score } X$$
$$f_X = \text{frequency for } X$$

Formula 12.3 calculations are shown in column 4 of Exhibit 12.3. Last, the percentile rank is computed by dividing CF_{MP} by n and multiplying by 100 to yield percentages. This is shown in column 5 of Exhibit 12.3. The formula is as follows:

$$P_X = 100 \, (\text{CF}_{MP} \div n) \tag{12.4}$$

where P_X = percentile rank for score X
     CF_{MP} = cumulative frequency to the midpoint for score X
     n = total sample size

Percentiles have the advantage that they are easily understood. They are also used when a distribution of raw scores that is not normal is transformed so that it has a normal distribution—a process called, appropriately, normalizing. More will be said about this process in the following pages. There are also two major limitations to percentiles. First, they are ranks and constitute ordinal level data and as such do not guarantee equal intervals between points, as is readily apparent from Exhibit 12.4, where the z scores, the area under the normal curve, percentiles, and another derived score are compared. All have equal score intervals except percentiles (and the extremes of stanine scores, which are discussed later). As you can see, percentile ranks have the effect of spreading out scores disproportionately so that small raw score differences toward the center (or mean) produce relatively large percentile differences and, conversely, large raw score differences at the extremes or ends of the distribution produce only small percentile differences. This often leads to overinterpretation of seemingly large percentile differences in the center. The other limitation of percentiles is that none of the parametric statistical procedures, which are appropriate for interval level data, can be used with them. This limits further interpretation. Because percentiles are, in effect, the result of changing raw scores (presumably at the interval level) to ordinal level scores, their original raw score frequency distribution is lost. As percentiles, their distribution is flat or rectangular.

Standard Scores

Standard scores are considered interval level data and express a person's distance from the mean in terms of the standard deviation of the distribution. The **z score** presented in Chapter 6 is perhaps the most famous of these. Recall, it is computed by subtracting the mean from a score and dividing the difference by the standard deviation:

$$z = \frac{X - \bar{X}}{\text{SD}} \tag{12.5}$$

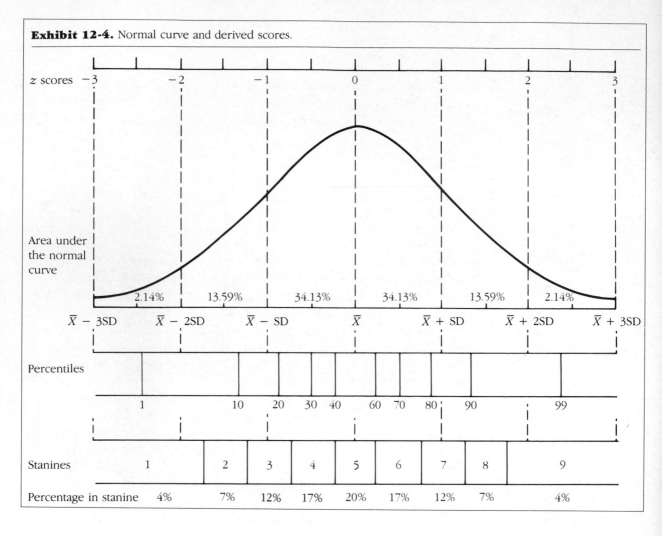

Exhibit 12-4. Normal curve and derived scores.

A group of raw scores that has been converted to z scores will have a mean of 0 and a standard deviation of 1. We can compute z scores for any distribution of scores without changing the *original* shape of the distribution of raw scores. When the distribution is normal or nearly normal, Table B of Appendix III can be used to calculate a percentile score equivalent to the z score. There are several other standard scores that have become very popular. They have the advantage of not having negative values as a z score does. The T score has a mean of 50 and a standard deviation of 10. The formula frequently used for the T score is

$$T = \frac{10}{SD} X + \left(50 - \frac{10\bar{X}}{SD}\right) \tag{12.6}$$

where X = raw score to be converted
$\bar{X}$ = mean of the group of raw scores
SD = standard deviation of the raw scores

Suppose you wished to convert a score of 80 to a T score from a group of raw scores were $\overline{X} = 75$ and SD $= 5$:

$$T = \frac{10}{5}(80) + \left(50 - \frac{10\,(75)}{5}\right) = 2\,(80) + (50 - 150) = 160 - 100 = 60$$

If you already knew the z score for 80 the computation is even easier. The z score is simply multiplied by 10 and then added to 50:

$$T = 10\,z + 50 \tag{12.7}$$

The z score of 80 can be easily computed:

$$Z = \frac{80 - 75}{5} = \frac{5}{5} = 1$$

As a check on our previous calculation, we will compute t via formula 12.7:

$$T = (10)(1) + 50 = 10 + 50 = 60$$

There are still other standard scores that are frequently used. Tests for admission to graduate and undergraduate schools (e.g., the Graduate Record Exam) typically use a type of standardized score that is based on a mean of 500 and a standard deviation of 100. Assuming prior calculation of a z score, the formula for the College Entrance Examination Board (CEEB) scores is

$$\text{CEEB} = 100\,z + 500 \tag{12.8}$$

Many intelligence tests (e.g., Stanford-Binet) use what is called a **deviation IQ score,** which is based on a mean of 100 and a standard deviation of 16. Assuming prior calculation of a z score, the formula for a deviation IQ score is as follows:

$$\text{IQ} = 16\,z + 100 \tag{12.9}$$

Finally, one other type of standard score should be mentioned. This well known transformation is known as the **stanine** (a contraction of *standard nine*) and was developed to provide single-digit numbers for handier use with calculators and computers. There are nine stanines and all but the first and ninth equal .5 standard deviation. The stanine scale is shown in comparison with percentile, z scores, and the normal curve in Exhibit 12.4. Note how the first and ninth stanines encompass a wider area on the horizontal axis than the other seven stanines. Raw scores can be readily converted to stanines by rank-ordering them and then assigning them to the percentages given in Exhibit 12.5.

Exhibit 12-5. Percentages and percentile equivalents for stanines.

Stanine	1	2	3	4	5	6	7	8	9
Percentile	2	7.5	17	31.5	50	68.5	83	92.5	98
Percentage in stanine	4	7	12	17	20	17	12	7	4

Normalized Standard Scores

So far we have talked about **linear standard scores.** That is, when the raw scores were transformed to standard scores via the various formulas, whatever was the shape of the raw score distribution was also the shape of the new standard score distribution. (This was not true for percentile scores, the distribution of which is rectangular; however, percentiles are not standard scores either.) As emphasized in Chapter 6, raw scores do not have to have a normal distribution to be converted to derived scores. If they do have a normal distribution, their interpretation is sometimes more straightforward via areas under the normal curve (using Table B, Appendix III). Conversion of scores that are not normally distributed to percentiles, as shown in Exhibit 12.3, fulfills this same purpose, however.

Sometimes we desire a normal distribution for our sample data because of the statistical advantage it allows or because we wish to compare (or correlate) with raw scores or another measure that is normally distributed. This is especially appropriate when the sample is large and representative of the population, and the reason for the nonnormal distribution is primarily attributed to measurement error rather than a nonnormal distribution of the variable in the population. Although nonlinear transformation could convert a distribution to many different kinds of distributions, the normal curve is usually used. This is because most raw score distributions approximate the normal curve more closely than other curves. The other advantage is that the normal curve has many useful mathematical qualities that permit more statistical analyses.

The transformation of raw scores to **normalized standard scores** (i.e., scores whose distribution is normal) is easily completed in two steps. The first involves converting a raw score to a percentile as explained in the discussion of percentiles. Next, the pecentiles are converted to z scores via Exhibit 12.6 or a table of the distribution for a normal curve, like Table B in Appendix III. The resulting z scores are now normally distributed. If further conversion to T or other scores is desired, use the formulas provided in this chapter. The distribution will remain normal.

When normalizing scores, remember that the frequency of a raw score is no longer relevant because only half of it was used to compute CF_{MP} for percentile rank. Therefore, to make a frequency graph of transformed scores, you cannot use the old raw score frequencies *as they were* in making the frequency distribution for the raw scores.

Exhibit 12-6. Normalized standard scores via conversion of percentile raw score equivalents to z scores.

Percentile	z	Percentile	z	Percentile	z	Percentile	z
99.9	3.09	74.5	0.66	49.5	-0.01	24.5	-0.69
99.5	2.58	74.0	0.64	49.0	-0.03	24.0	-0.71
99.0	2.33	73.5	0.63	48.5	-0.04	23.5	-0.72
98.5	2.17	73.0	0.61	48.0	-0.05	23.0	-0.74
98.0	2.05	72.5	0.60	47.5	-0.06	22.5	-0.76
97.5	1.96	72.0	0.58	47.0	-0.07	22.0	-0.77
97.0	1.88	71.5	0.57	46.5	-0.09	21.5	-0.79
96.5	1.81	71.0	0.55	46.0	-0.10	21.0	-0.80
96.0	1.75	70.5	0.54	45.5	-0.11	20.5	-0.82
95.5	1.70	70.0	0.52	45.0	-0.12	20.0	-0.84
95.0	1.64	69.5	0.51	44.5	-0.14	19.5	-0.86
94.5	1.60	69.0	0.49	44.0	-0.15	19.0	-0.88
94.0	1.55	68.5	0.48	43.5	-0.16	18.5	-0.90
93.5	1.51	68.0	0.47	43.0	-0.18	18.0	-0.91
93.0	1.40	67.5	0.45	42.5	-0.19	17.5	-0.93
92.5	1.44	67.0	0.44	42.0	-0.20	17.0	-0.95
92.0	1.41	66.5	0.43	41.5	-0.21	16.5	-0.97
91.5	1.37	66.0	0.41	41.0	-0.23	16.0	-0.99
91.0	1.34	65.5	0.40	40.5	-0.24	15.5	-1.01
90.5	1.31	65.0	0.39	40.0	-0.25	15.0	-1.03
90.0	1.28	64.5	0.37	39.5	-0.27	14.5	-1.06
89.5	1.25	64.0	0.36	39.0	-0.28	14.0	-1.08
89.0	1.22	63.5	0.35	38.5	-0.29	13.5	-1.10
88.5	1.20	63.0	0.33	38.0	-0.31	13.0	-1.13
88.0	1.18	62.5	0.32	37.5	-0.32	12.5	-1.15
87.5	1.15	62.0	0.31	37.0	-0.33	12.0	-1.18
87.0	1.13	61.5	0.29	36.5	-0.35	11.5	-1.20
86.5	1.10	61.0	0.28	36.0	-0.36	11.0	1.22
86.0	1.08	60.5	0.27	35.5	-0.37	10.5	-1.25
85.5	1.06	60.0	0.25	35.0	-0.39	10.0	-1.28
85.0	1.04	59.5	0.24	34.5	-0.40	9.5	-1.31
84.5	1.01	59.0	0.23	34.0	-0.41	9.0	-1.34
84.0	0.99	58.5	0.21	33.5	-0.43	8.5	-1.37
83.5	0.97	58.0	0.20	33.0	-0.44	8.0	-1.41
83.0	0.95	57.5	0.19	32.5	-0.45	7.5	-1.44
82.5	0.93	57.0	0.18	32.0	-0.47	7.0	-1.48
82.0	0.91	56.5	0.16	31.5	-0.48	6.5	-1.51
81.5	0.90	56.0	0.15	31.0	-0.49	6.0	-1.55
81.0	0.88	55.5	0.14	30.5	-0.51	5.5	-1.60
80.5	0.86	55.0	0.12	30.0	-0.52	5.0	-1.64
80.0	0.84	54.5	0.11	29.5	-0.54	4.5	-1.70
79.5	0.82	54.0	0.10	29.0	-0.55	4.0	-1.75
79.0	0.80	53.5	0.09	28.5	-0.57	3.5	-1.81
78.5	0.79	53.0	0.07	28.0	-0.58	3.0	-1.88
78.0	0.77	52.5	0.06	27.5	-0.60	2.5	-1.96
77.5	0.76	52.0	0.05	27.0	-0.61	2.0	-2.05
77.0	0.74	51.5	0.04	26.5	-0.63	1.5	-2.17
76.5	0.72	51.0	0.03	26.0	-0.64	1.0	-2.33
76.0	0.71	50.5	0.01	25.5	-0.66	0.5	-2.58
75.5	0.69	50.0	0.00	25.0	-0.67	0.1	-3.09
75.0	0.67						

O*ther Scoring Issues*

The decision about how raw scores will be computed and in what form they will be presented for interpretation (i.e., raw versus derived) is usually determined by the test developer after consideration of the theoretical underpinnings of the research (e.g., ipsativity as in the EPPS, Thurstone scaling to give meaning to points along the continuum for the possible range of scores) and common practice in the area under study or discipline (e.g., psychologists tend to use *T* scores; deviation IQ scores are used for major intelligence tests). Certainly, anything that facilitates easy comparisons within an area is of value as long as recent advances in instrument development are not ignored.

Missing Data

Quite often subjects skip answers or otherwise fail to respond. When these instances are infrequent, say, less than 5 percent to 10 percent of the items, it is possible to use the data anyway. In tests that have an ideal or correct answer (i.e., a standard), the subject is considered as having *not* responded to an item. Thus it would be considered *wrong* or as having deliberately *not been selected*. With attitude scales, the midpoint of the *possible range* is generally used when hand scoring is necessary. When computer scoring is used, it is often possible to substitute the mean of a subject's other answers, thereby having less effect on the total score. Some researchers substitute the mean response to the item (by all others in the group), although the rationale of such a practice seems dubious if the purpose is really to place subjects on a continuum.

There is no foolproof way of treating missing data. The more missing data with which you must contend, obviously, the greater are your risks for increasing measurement error. In our kind of research, where subjects are difficult to obtain, throwing out incomplete questionnaires may dangerously reduce sample size, thereby increasing the probability of error even further. It should go without saying that you should take precautions during data collection to minimize the probability of missing data.

Residualized Scores

Sometimes change scores are required. A group may be pre- and posttested with an intervention, instruction, or even therapy in between. A design of this sort for assessing change is weak and vulnerable to many rival hypotheses as presented in Chapters 3 and 4. However, that is not the concern of this chapter. It so happens, nevertheless, that pre- and posttests are often given to assess change. When change scores for individual subjects are desired, there is an alternate method of obtaining them than just subtracting one from the other and calling that difference change. It is the use of residualized scores.

Residualized scores are simply the difference between the expected score on the posttest as predicted by the pretest and the observed posttest score. Chapter 7 introduced **bivariate regression** and demonstrated how scores on one test could be predicted on another using the correlation between the two tests (r_{XY}). This is the procedure used with residualized scores. A formula for a predicted posttest score is as follows:

$$\hat{Y} = r_{XY}\left(\frac{SD_Y}{SD_X}\right) X + \left[\bar{Y} - r_{XY}\left(\frac{SD_Y}{SD_X}\right) \bar{X}\right] \tag{12.10}$$

where $\hat{Y}$ = predicted score on posttest Y
$\quad r_{XY}$ = correlation between the pretest X and posttest Y
$\quad SD_Y$ = standard deviation of the posttest Y
$\quad SD_X$ = standard deviation of the pretest X
$\quad\quad X$ = a person's pretest scores
$\quad\quad \bar{X}$ = mean of the pretest scores
$\quad\quad \bar{Y}$ = mean of the posttest scores

Once an individual's predicted posttest score ($\hat{Y}$) has been computed, it is subtracted from his or her observed score on Y:

$$R = Y - \hat{Y} \tag{12.11}$$

This is a person's "change" score. It reflects that portion that cannot be accounted for by the pretest. It controls for the correlation between the two measures. It also includes measurement error.

Suppose a group of 50 individuals was tested twice, before and after a programmed instruction program designed to change attitudes toward alcoholic patients. The pretest yielded $\bar{X}$ of 46 and $SD_X = 5$ and the posttest $\bar{Y} = 60$ and $SD = 4$. The pretest and posttest correlated .80. For subject A, his pretest score was 50 and posttest score was 62. Did he change or is the apparent difference of 12 points misleading? First, his predicted score ($\hat{Y}$) based upon his pretest score should be computed:

$$\hat{Y} = .80\left(\frac{4}{5}\right) 50 + \left[60 - .80\left(\frac{4}{5}\right) 46\right] = (.80)(.80)50 + [60 - (.80)(.80)46]$$

$$= 32 + (60 - 29.44) = 32 + 30.56 = 63$$

Next, his observed score and predicted score are compared in order to compute his residualized score:

$$R = Y - \hat{Y} = 62 - 63 = -1$$

What seemed to be a big difference is no longer such a difference when correlation to the pretest is removed from consideration. Of course, to the extent that all posttest scores for r_{XY} and $\bar{Y}$ reflect change due to the intervention, use of residualized scores can also be misleading.

Recap

Returning to the examples presented at the beginning of this chapter, you now understand more about what they mean and what you need to know in order to give them meaning. If you were a parent receiving the following scores for Johnny, how would you interpret them?

Stanford-Binet deviation IQ	125
Scholastic and aptitude test stanines	
Verbal	8
Quantitative	9
Nonverbal	8
Schoolwork	C
Recent achievement test percentile	80

We have enough information from this chapter to estimate the percentile rank for all scores. This will allow us to compare Johnny's performance on the various tests. First, we convert the deviation IQ score to a z score by using the inverse of formula 12.9.

$$z = \frac{IQ - 100}{16} = \frac{125 - 100}{16} = 1.56$$

We can then use Table B, Appendix III, to determine the area under the normal curve for $z = 1.56$. This corresponds to a percentile rank of 94. Next, the stanine scores are converted via Exhibit 12.5, where we see that 8 stanine = 92.5th percentile rank and 9 stanine = 98th percentile. We have no easy conversion for his C letter grade from school. However, we reason that since C work is considered "average," it should be at about the 50th percentile. Now, let us review the scores as percentile conversions to see if they make more sense:

Stanford-Binet	94
Scholastic and aptitude test	
Verbal	92.5
Quantitative	98
Nonverbal	92.5
Schoolwork	50
Recent achievement test	80

It does seem that Johnny should be doing better than he is in school. On the basis of his IQ and aptitude tests he should be able to perform better than over 90 percent of those in his age group. His recent national achievement tests shows his current performance as better than only 80 percent of his age or grade group. This would suggest that he is probably not learning as well as he could in school. Then again, measurement error could bias his scores—a question about the standard error of measurement (see Chapter 13) for the tests might be appropriate when you visit the school. Finally, although it is unlikely, Johnny could be attending a school where almost all students are ranking above the 90th percentile on national standardized tests. If school grades are based on comparison with other students, Johnny's C could be accurate—albeit unfair to him psychologically in terms of his self-concept.

One other example was presented at the beginning of this chapter. It involved scores for a subject in a stress reduction study:

Blood pressure	160/110
Checklist of agitated behaviors	40
Paired adjectives checklist	26
Self-report on a Likert scale of 1 to 5	3
Memory tests for digits	23

The question was whether or not the subject was stressed. Only measures 1 and 4 are decipherable without additional information. The blood pressure reading is high and could indicate stress. However, this subject could be an untreated hypertensive rather than stressed. The self-report measure indicates that this individual considers herself as only moderately stressed. Then again, some of us are sometimes unaware of being stressed—or so some personality theories suggest. The behavioral observation checklist, the paired adjectives checklist (a semantic differential scale whose purpose is less apparent than the Likert scale), and the memory test, a performance test on which highly stressed persons are unable to remember complex digits, require norms (and, of course, scoring instructions) before we can interpret them. If you, the researcher, do not have them, you should not use the measures. The measures are meaningless and thereby useless without this information.

Vocabulary

Absolute magnitude	Likert scales
Answer key	Linear standard scores
Attitude scores	Missing data
Card sort	Normalized standard scores
CEEB scores	Norm-referenced testing
Content scores	Norms
Criterion-referenced testing	Observed score
Cumulative frequency	Percentile rank scores
Cumulative frequency to midpoint	Possible range of scores
Derived score	Profile (of subscales)
Deviation IQ scores	Profile analysis
Error score	Q sort
Flipped (items)	Raw score
Guttman scales	Relative intensity
Ipsative testing	Residualized scores
Item	Response alternative

Scaling	Stem
Score	*T* scores
Scoring stencils	Test manual
Semantic differential scales	Thurstone scales
Standard scores	True score
Stanine scores	*z* scores

References

1. Anastasi, A. *Psychological Testing* (4th ed.). New York: Macmillan, 1976.
2. Brown, F. G. *Principles of Educational and Psychological Testing.* Hinsdale, Ill.: Dryden Press, 1970.
3. Burns, B. J., Lapine, L., and Andrews, P. M. Personality profile of pediatric nurse practitioners. *Nurs. Res.* 27:286, 1978.
4. Buros, O. K. (ed.). *The Eighth Mental Measurements Yearbook.* Highland Park, N.J.: Greyphon Press, 1978.
5. Edwards, A. L. *The Edwards Personal Preference Schedule.* New York: Psychological Corp., 1953.
6. Ghiselli, E. E., Campbell, J. P., and Zedeck, S. *Measurement Theory for the Behavioral Sciences.* San Francisco: W. H. Freeman, 1981.
7. Guttman, L. The Cornell technique for scale and intensity analysis. *Educ. Psychol. Meas.* 7:247, 1947.
8. Likert, R. A technique for the measurement of attitude scales. *Arch. Psychol.* No. 140, 1932.
9. Martuza, V. R. *Applying Norm-Referenced and Criterion-Referenced Measurement in Education.* Boston: Allyn and Bacon, 1977.
10. Navran, L. and Stauffacher, J. C. A comparative analysis of the personality structure of psychiatric and nonpsychiatric nurses. *Nurs. Res.* 7:64, 1958.
11. Nunally, J. *Popular Conceptions of Mental Health.* New York: Holt, Rinehart, 1961.
12. Nunally, J. C. *Psychometric Theory* (2nd ed.). New York: McGraw-Hill, 1978.
13. Osgood, C., Suci, G., and Tannenbaum, P. *The Measurement of Meaning.* Urbana, Ill: University of Illinois Press, 1957.
14. Thurstone, L. L. *The Measurement of Values.* Chicago: University of Chicago Press, 1959.
15. Thurstone, L. L. Theory of attitude measurement. *Psychol. Bull.* 36:222, 1929.
16. Thurstone, L. L., and Chave, E. J. *The Measurement of Attitude.* Chicago: University of Chicago Press, 1929.
17. Wiggins, J. S. *Personality and Prediction: Principles of Personality Assessment.* Reading, Mass.: Addison-Wesley, 1973.

Instrument credentialing refers to the process and procedures used to demonstrate that a measure or instrument is good for use under certain conditions and with subjects who have certain characteristics. In the self report and observation modes these procedures must include reliability coefficients and evidence from which validity can be inferred. They can include item analysis, norms for various groups, and even guidelines for interpretation of the subscale profiles of large standardized tests. For the standardized tests and scales, this material is presented in a test or observer manual. For research scales and tests there may be manuals, but generally there are none. More often, the instrument's credentials are either presented in an article published in a scholarly research journal or available from the test developer who may not yet be ready to publish results.

This chapter presents the more common reliability, item analysis, and validity procedures used with **norm-referenced tests** and scales. There are additional procedures available for use, particularly with **criterion-referenced scales;** however, they could fill an entire book and are used much less often in research. Once the basic approaches that are presented in this chapter are understood, many of the procedures that are found in the literature or test manuals should be easily understood and emulated when appropriate.

Reliability and validity are never so well established or proven that no more work in this area need be done. Each must be continuously assessed, especially when different samples are used. The concepts of reliability and validity apply to both the self-report (e.g., tests and scales) and behavioral observation modes of measurement as well as the subgroup of observation measures from the physical assessment mode. Although most of the discussion in this chapter focuses on tests and scales, it does not mean to suggest that reliability and validity are less important in the other modes of measurement.

Reliability

Whenever an instrument is used, a realiability coefficient should be computed based on the data from the research subjects—even if many coefficients are available for similar subjects. This calculation lets you know how well your measure performed in your research setting, because it can vary from setting to setting depending on a number of factors such as variability of scores and the presence or absence of measurement error.

Unlike most correlation coefficients based on the Pearson product moment correlation coefficient, **reliability coefficients** based upon the product moment coefficient are never squared for interpretation. If a reliability coefficient is .86, the shared variance is 86 percent. Sources of error account for 14 percent (100 − .86). The reliability coefficient represents a ratio of a person's **true score** variance to the person's **observed score** variance. The true score is the real amount of a variable possessed by a person. We never know this amount. Instead, we know a person's observed score, which we calculate via our measurement instrument. An observed score consists of a person's true score plus error. Error can either inflate or deflate the true score. The higher a reliability coefficient is, the less likely it is that error has greatly changed a true score. More will be said about this in the next few pages.

Error of Measurement

As stated in Chapter 11, sources of measurement error include reactivity; personal states like hunger, fatigue, and mood; ambiguous or poor questions; differences in how measures are scored; which questions out of all possible questions are included (content sampling); the number of items (a large number is usually better up to a ceiling amount, beyond which no additional information is yielded and subjects become tired and cranky); guessing; and even clerical error (a subject may mark one alternative *a* when intending to mark *b*, or halfway through a test a subject may discover he misinterpreted instructions, not have time to go back to redo his responses, and therefore respond appropriately to only the last half). When too much time is given to respond, subjects often go back over responses and change many. It is a known fact that on achievement tests, as on final examinations in college courses, these changes usually make correct responses wrong. Moreover, many personality tests depend on "gut reactions," which are considered more accurate than premeditated responses. Therefore, test directions often tell respondents not to go back over their responses. If the respondents do so, **measurement error** is often introduced.

Standard Error of Measurement

There is almost always significant error associated with the self-report and behavioral observation modes of measurement, particularly when compared with physical assessment measures. When scales and tests are used to make clinical judgments, give grades to students, and so forth, knowledge of just how much error might be associated with an individual's score is important. It can be easily computed if you know the standard deviation of the measure and its reliability coefficient, and is known as the **standard error of measurement**:

$$SEm = SD_X \sqrt{1 - r_{XX}}$$

(13.1)

where SEm = standard error of measurement
SD_X = the standard deviation of test X
r_{XX} = the reliability of test X

[handwritten: like sampling distribution]

The standard error of measurement is an estimated standard deviation of a hypothetical group of observed scores obtained by the same person on a large number of similar or alternate form measures. It can therefore be used to establish **confidence intervals** within which a person's true score can be expected to fall. Thus, the range of scores between points that are plus and minus the value of 1.96 standard errors from a person's score could represent, with 95 percent confidence of being correct, a range within which a person's true score would fall. If 99 percent confidence were required, the range of scores would be based on the value of 2.58 standard errors (of measurement). There is one further calculation required, however, in order to calculate the range of scores within which the true score falls. This is a modification of a person's observed score.

It is incorrect to establish confidence zones symmetrically around an observed score, because obtained scores tend to be biased. High scores tend to be biased upward and low scores tend to be biased downward. Therefore, an **unbiased observed score** must be calculated in order to have a value from which to add or subtract standard errors of measurement. It is a simple calculation:

$$\hat{X} = {}_{xx}(X - \bar{X}) + \bar{X} \tag{13.2}$$

where $\hat{X}$ = unbiased score
r_{xx} = reliability coefficient
X = observed score
$\bar{X}$ = mean of scores

If a person's observed score was 64 on an anxiety scale and the mean of the scale was 50, the standard deviation 10, and the reliability .90, the person's unbiased score would be

$$\hat{X} = r_{xx} (X - \bar{X}) + \bar{X} = .90 (64 - 50) + 50 = 62.6$$

The standard error of measurement is

$$SEm = SD_X \sqrt{1 - r_{xx}} = 10 \sqrt{1 - .90} = 10 (3.16) = 3.16$$

Thus, with 95 percent probability, the person's true score falls within $\pm$ 1.96 (3.16) (or 6.19) of 62.6 or within the range of scores from 56.4 to 68.79 (or, to round, 56 to 69 as compared with his observed score of 64).

In research settings, if the standard deviation of scores in a sample is not much larger than the SEm (which means reliability is extremely low), it is hopeless to continue investigation with that measure, because its correlations to other variables will be too low. In addition, the SEm may demonstrate that the same measure may be less useful in one group than it is in another, even though the reliability coefficients may be the same. For example, suppose one group of subjects had a standard deviation of 16 for obtained scores and another had a standard deviation of 8 for its obtained scores, although both measures yielded .78 reliability:

Group 1: $SEm = 16 \sqrt{1 - .78} = (16) (.469) = 7.5$

Group 2: $SEm = 8 \sqrt{1 - .78} = (8) (.469) = 3.7$

Obviously, you would place more confidence in a Group 2 individual's obtained score than in one from Group 1.

The unbiased score is generally used only for establishing confidence intervals. The observed score is used in calculation of statistical tests and interpretation of individual performance. In fact, in most research, particularly basic research, there is seldom any need to compute confidence intervals for a true score. In research the major concern is how much measurement error reduces correlations to other variables and the effects of experimental variables. There is one situation, however, in which unbiased scores might be used. Suppose extreme groups on a pretest measure (e.g., high anxiety, low IQ) were subjected to an experimental intervention (independent variable) and then given a posttest that was the same or an alternate form. The gain or loss scores for the experimental and control groups may be due to regression effects. Therefore, unbiased scores for both groups on both pretest and posttest could be computed and the differences between the unbiased scores compared for the two groups [12].

Alternate Forms Reliability

Exhibit 13.1 shows samples from **alternate forms** of two tests designed to assess research knowledge and attitudes toward research of nursing students. The particular items in Exhibit 13.1 were deleted from the final test forms during instrument development. The authors [15] plan to establish sufficient test credentials so that they will become standardized measures. These alternate forms are especially interesting because the parallel items are so similar. This is one approach to alternate forms. Other approaches vary in the degree to which they deviate from the strict parallelism shown in Exhibit 13.1. The degree of permissible deviation, of course, depends on the alternate forms reliability coefficient.

The traditional method (Nunnally [12]) for determining alternate forms reliability has been to administer the two forms 2 weeks apart in order to provide time for variations in ability and attitude to occur. Total scores on the two forms for each subject are correlated using a Pearson *r* coefficient. At least 30 people should participate, half receiving Form A first and the other half completing Form B first.

When this reliability coefficient is lower by 20 points than the internal consistency reliability coefficients for each form, the error can be attributed to errors in (1) scoring (e.g., subjectivity), (2) differences in the content of the two forms, or (3) large changes in people over a short period of time. To investigate the latter, the correlation between forms administered 2 weeks apart is compared to one between forms that were both administered the same day. If both are low, the problem is probably due to content (if scoring errors have been ruled out) and this can necessitate development of a new alternate form.

Internal Consistency Reliability

Internal consistency refers to the extent to which all items on a scale measure the same variable. This is a very old and traditional attribute of measures and

---

Exhibit 13-1. Alternate forms of the Thomas-Price [15] test.

Form *A*	Form *B*

Attitudes

1. Research is an important component of nursing today.	1. Research is an important part of contemporary nursing practice.
2. Nursing research has not advanced nursing practice.	2. Nursing research has not advanced nursing as far as I can determine.

Knowledge

1. Pulse rate is an example of measurement at the
  a. Nominal level
  b. Ordinal level
  c. Interval/ratio level
  d. None of the above
	1. Body temperature in degrees Celsius is an example of measurement at the
	  a. Nominal level
	  b. Ordinal level
	  c. Interval/ratio level
	  d. None of the above

2. A descriptive study is planned in which data are to be collected from 200 mothers of preschool children. Advantages of a questionnaire over an interview for this study are:
  a. Less expensive; data are more likely to be comparable
  b. Less expensive; less time-consuming
  c. Greater flexibility; easier coding
  d. Higher proportion of responses; no need for a pretest
	2. A descriptive study is planned in which data are to be collected from 200 mothers of preschool children. Advantages of an interview over a questionnaire for this study include:
	  a. Less expensive; easier coding
	  b. Easier coding; use of interviewer reduces bias
	  c. Questions can be clarified, more flexibility
	  d. Less time-consuming; no need for a pretest

---

comes from a basic philosophy and goal of **psychometricians** (i.e., test developers). The long-term goal of measurement science involves being able to measure all human attributes and behaviors perfectly. The thousands of existing measures would then be reduced by more than one-half, as measures were developed to measure well each single attribute or behavior known to man. Then, various combinations of these, which would correlate perfectly with various combinations of criterion or predicted behaviors, could be used as needed. In order to achieve this goal, of course, each measure must be homogeneous in regard to content or, in other words, possess internal consistency reliability.

Another way of explaining internal consistency reliability is to say that it is based on the average correlation among items within a test and the number of items. **Coefficient alpha (α),** developed by Cronbach, is the basic formula for determining internal consistency reliability. It should be used whenever possible. However, when the number of items and subjects each exceed 10 or 15, computation without the aid of a computer is tedious and, due to numerous calculations, very vulnerable to human error. In that case the **split-half method** is used. In addition, 2 other approaches to calculating internal consistency include (1) the **Kuder-Richardson 20** (KR-20), a special form of coefficient alpha for data having correct/incorrect responses and (2) the **Kuder-Richardson 21** (KR-21), a calculation for correct/incorrect data that yields lower estimates but does not require information about each subject's response to each item. Instead, the test mean, variance, and number of items are all that is needed to do the computation.

Coefficient Alpha

Exhibit 13.2 gives fictitious data for a 10-item scale administered to five subjects. As you will note, variances for each item and for the total scores on the scale are computed. Once these are calculated, the formula for α is easy to use. The formula is as follows:

$$\text{alpha } (\alpha) = \left(\frac{K}{K - 1} \right) \left[1 - \left(\frac{\Sigma V_{\text{items}}}{V_{\text{total}}} \right) \right] \tag{13.3}$$

where K = the number of items in the scale
ΣV_{items} = sum of all item variances
V_{total} = variance of the total scores on the scale

To use the data in Exhibit 13.2 to calculate alpha, the following simple steps are followed:

(1) $\left(\dfrac{10}{10 - 1} \right) \left[1 - \left(\dfrac{.24 + .16 + .24 + .16 + .24 + .16 + .24 + .16 + .24 + .16}{14} \right) \right] =$

(2) $\dfrac{10}{9} \left[1 - \left(\dfrac{2}{14} \right) \right] = 1.11(1 - .14) = 1.11(.86) = .95$

In step 1, all values are substituted into the formula; in step 2, the calculations are carried out in successive reductions.

Split-Half Reliability

Split-half reliability involves splitting a scale in half, usually grouping all even-numbered items and all odd-numbered items. Other methods such as random assignment can be used also. Once the two groups of items have been determined, a subject's total score on each split-half is computed. Then, a correlation coefficient between the two sets of scores is calculated. Because this correlation is based on total scores with only half as many items as the actual measure, it is likely to be smaller than one based upon the longer scale. Therefore, the **Spear-**

Exhibit 13-2. Fictitious data for calculation of coefficient alpha.

| | Scale Items | | | | | | | | | | |
	1	2	3	4	5	6	7	8	9	10	Total
Subject											
01	5	4	2	3	4	5	4	3	5	4	39
02	5	3	2	2	4	4	4	2	5	3	34
03	4	3	1	2	3	4	3	2	4	3	29
04	4	3	1	2	3	4	3	2	4	3	29
05	5	3	2	2	4	4	4	2	5	3	34
Total	23	16	8	11	18	21	18	11	23	16	165
$\overline{X}$	4.6	3.2	1.6	2.2	3.6	4.2	3.6	2.2	4.6	3.2	33
V	0.24	0.16	0.24	0.16	0.24	0.16	0.24	0.16	0.24	0.16	14

man-Brown formula can be used to correct the correlation upward in order to approximate what it would be for the longer scale. When two equal halves are made from a larger scale, the Spearman-Brown formula is as follows:

$$r_{tt} = \frac{2\, r_{XY}}{1 - r_{XY}}$$
(13.4)

where r_{tt} = corrected reliability coefficient
r_{XY} = correlation between the two halves

Other versions of the Spearman-Brown formula exist for other purposes. These are discussed later in this chapter.

If the data in Exhibit 13.2 were used to compute a Pearson correlation coefficient for split halves using the odd-even numbers method, the resulting coefficient would be .42. Using the Spearman-Brown formula, the corrected reliability coefficient is calculated as follows:

$$r_{tt} = \frac{2(.42)}{1 + .42} = \frac{.84}{1.42} = .59$$

The reliability is therefore increased substantially (from .42 to .59) but it is still much lower than the alpha coefficient of .96.

Using a random assignment (to one of the two halves) method we might have items 1, 2, 3, 7, and 8 in one half and items 4, 5, 6, 9, and 10 in the other half. The Pearson correlation coefficient between these halves is .97, substantially larger than the odd-even coefficient. Using the Spearman-Brown formula, the corrected coefficient is computed as follows:

$$r_{tt} = \frac{2(.97)}{1 + .97} = \frac{1.94}{1.97} = .98$$

Thus, the corrected coefficient is not much larger. This is because the correlation between the two halves was larger to begin with.

Why are these two correlation coefficients so different from each other and, of course, also different from coefficient alpha? Coefficient alpha can be considered the *average* of all possible split halves using the split-half method and Spearman-Brown formula. Therefore, it would follow that various split-half coefficients would be higher or lower than each other and alpha. This is why coefficient alpha is the preferred method for computing internal consistency reliability.

The Kuder-Richardson Formulas

Two other formulas, specialized versions of coefficient alpha, are available for computation of internal consistency reliability coefficients. They can be used only with items that have correct answers. Therefore they are inappropriate for attitude scales and such. They are somewhat easier to use than coefficient alpha, because they do not require computation of item variances according to our usual method via sum of squares.

The KR-20 can be used when you know the variance for the test, the number of items on the test, and the number of persons getting *each* item correct. The formula is as follows:

$$r_{tt} = \left(\frac{K}{K - 1}\right)\left(1 - \frac{\Sigma pq}{V_{total}}\right) \tag{13.5}$$

where K = number of items
   V_{total} = variance of the test
      p = proportion of persons answering an item correctly (i.e., those answering the item correctly divided by the number taking test)
      $q = 1 - p$
   $\Sigma\,pq$ = sum of p times q for each item

Exhibit 13.3 presents fictitious data for use in illustrating computation of the KR-20 reliability coefficient. KR-20 is a special version of coefficient α and therefore represents the average of all possible split halves. Using the data from Exhibit 13.3, computation is as follows:

$$r_{tt} = \left(\frac{10}{10 - 1}\right)\left(1 - \frac{1.20}{4.64}\right) = (1.11)(.741) = .82$$

The KR-21 formula can be used when data for individual items are missing. All that is needed are the test mean, variance, and number of items. This is especially helpful when you wish to compute reliability for, say, a test that was

Exhibit 13-3. Fictitious data for calculation of KR-20.

| | Scale Items | | | | | | | | | | |
	1	2	3	4	5	6	7	8	9	10	Total
Subject											
01	1	1	0	1	1	0	0	1	1	1	7
02	1	1	0	1	1	1	1	1	1	1	9
03	1	1	0	1	1	0	0	1	0	0	5
04	1	1	0	1	1	0	1	1	1	1	8
05	0	0	0	1	1	0	0	1	0	0	3
Total correct	4	4	0	5	5	1	2	5	3	3	32
p	0.80	0.80	0	1.00	1.00	0.20	0.40	1.00	0.60	0.60	
q	0.20	0.20	1.00	0	0	0.80	0.60	0	0.40	0.40	
pq	0.16	0.16	0	0	0	0.16	0.24	0	0.24	0.24	1.20

$\bar{X} = 6.4$; SD $= 2.15$; $V = 4.64$.

used in a journal article, but for which no reliability coefficient was reported. The major limitations of the KR-21 are that (1) the coefficient is conservative (i.e., can be lower than those computed by other methods) and (2) it is limited for use with tests where there are correct and incorrect answers. The formula is as follows:

$$r_{tt} = \left(\frac{K}{K-1} \right) \left[1 - \frac{\bar{X}\left(1 - \frac{\hat{X}}{K}\right)}{V_{total}} \right] \tag{13.6}$$

Using the data from Exhibit 13.3, internal consistency reliability calculated according to the KR-21 formula is as follows:

$$r_{tt} = \left(\frac{10}{10-1} \right) \left[1 - \frac{6.4\left(1 - \frac{6.4}{10}\right)}{4.64} \right] = (1.11)(5.043) = .559 = .56$$

In this example, the coefficients derived from the KR-20 and KR-21 formulas are different. The KR-21 is considerably lower, illustrating how much more conservative this formula is than the KR-20, which is the average of all possible split halves.

Test-Retest Reliability

Test-retest reliability involves correlating, usually with a Pearson r, scores from a single test that was administered on two separate occasions—anywhere from 2 weeks (short term) to 6 months (long term) apart and more. Test-retest reliability is dependent on the **stability** of the variable being measured. If change in the variable being measured occurs during the time interval, a low reliability coefficient will result. When stability over time is of interest, for example in pretest-posttest designs, and only one scale is available, split halves administered 2 weeks apart and corrected upward with the Spearman-Brown formula can give an indication of this type of reliability. If the resulting coefficient is considerably lower than coefficient alpha (say, 20 points) the measure may not be stable enough to incorporate into a pretest-posttest design.

Sometimes this type of reliability is the only kind it is possible to calculate. By all means do so if stability over time is appropriate for your research setting. However, alternative forms and internal consistency reliability are both considered better indices (Nunnally [12]). The final decision, of course, depends on the sources of measurement error anticipated in your research setting.

Speeded Tests

The foregoing procedures for internal consistency reliability cannot be used with speeded (i.e., timed) tests. There is a distinction, although not clear, between **power tests** and **speeded tests.** Power tests and scales are those in which at least 75 percent of the respondents are able to complete or at least attempt all items in the time allocated. The reason internal consistency methods are inappropriate for speeded tests is that the unanswered items can either inflate or deflate the coefficient, depending on how it is calculated. For example if an odd-even approach were used, the unanswered items would correlate and contribute to an inflated coefficient.

The best approach for computing reliability of speeded tests is alternate forms. If this is not possible, test-retest can be used in some circumstances. However, then you must beware of practice effect, which may contribute to measurement error.

Increasing Reliability

Low reliability can be attributed to the many sources of measurement error, not enough variability among scores as a result of using a homogeneous (on the variable being measured) sample rather than a heterogeneous one, and not including enough items on a scale. When the standard deviation of a scale is unusually small when compared with the mean, the sample may be too homogeneous to yield a strong correlation coefficient. This is due to the mathematical properties of the Pearson correlation coefficient in which greater variability among scores produces a higher coefficient. An "eyeball" estimate to determine whether this is the reason for a low coefficient involves using the KR-21 formula to calculate reliability based on sample data (mean, variance, and number of items) and then calculating it again with a variance figure that is doubled. If the new coefficient is significantly larger than the one that is based on the observed variance, you may wish to use a more heterogeneous sample.

By far the major source of low reliability rests with too few items. The number of items that must be added to increase reliability can be estimated by using another version of the Spearman-Brown formula. When using it, keep in mind the fact that it is assumed that the additional items will be similar in content and average correlation to the other items already included in the scales. This formula is surprisingly accurate when there are at least 20 items in the original scale. Before using it, however, you should investigate all other sources of measurement error as well as **sample homogeneity,** because generation of good additional items is no easy task.

The formula is as follows:

$$K = \frac{r_{KK}(1 - r_{tt})}{r_{tt}(1 - r_{KK})} \tag{13.7}$$

where K = number of *times* the test must be lengthened to obtain the desired reliability (r_{KK}) or number of items on proposed test divided by the number of items on the current test

r_{KK} = desired reliability

r_{tt} = observed reliability

In the case of a scale with a .55 reliability and 25 items, the calculation to determine how many items must be added to achieve .85 reliability is as follows:

$$K = \frac{.85(1 - .55)}{.55(1 - .85)} = \frac{.85(.45)}{.55(.15)} = \frac{.38}{.08} = 4.75$$

Thus, 4.75 *times* 25 or 119 items would be required to raise the reliability to .85. This involves writing 94 more items, which may or may not be prohibitive. Depending on the research setting, 119 items may make the scale too long for subjects, also. It is apparent, of course, that the items have low correlations among themselves. This may be due to measurement of more than a single variable or, simply, the need to sample more amply the content domain of the variable being measured. When it is necessary to generate a significant number of additional items, you are essentially developing a new measure. The principles presented in the section describing item analysis in the following pages should be used, then, to avoid repeating previous errors.

The Spearman-Brown formula can also be used to determine how much a reliability coefficient will be reduced if some items are deleted. Again, the assumption in using the formula is that all items correlate equally with each other and are similar in content. The formula is as follows:

$$r_{KK} = \frac{(K)(r_{tt})}{1 + (K - 1)r_{tt}} \tag{13.8}$$

where r_{KK} = new reliability of the shortened test

K = number of items in the proposed (shortened) test divided by the number of items on the current (longer) test

r_{tt} = reliability of the longer test

Suppose you have a 200 item true-false midterm course examination, with a .93 reliability, that you wish to shorten to 100 items because of time constraints:

$$r_{KK} = \frac{\frac{1}{2}(.93)}{1 + (\frac{1}{2} - 1).93} = \frac{.465}{1 + (-\frac{1}{2}).93} = \frac{.465}{1 - .465} = \frac{.465}{.535} = .869 = .87$$

Obviously, shortening the test will not appreciably affect reliability. Finally, this formula can also be used to correct a coefficient when the number of items is not simply doubled as is assumed in formula 13.4. In this case, K is calculated as the ratio of the number of items in the proposed larger scale to the number of items in the current smaller scale.

Observer Agreement

The measurement of **interrater reliability** (i.e., two or more raters observing the same thing) and **intrarater reliability** (i.e., the same rater observing the same thing on two or more occasions) is not nearly as well developed as reliability of tests and scales. In fact, there is considerable disagreement among experts about what is the best approach. Traditionally, researchers have used (1) percentage of agreement or (2) a correlation coefficient when time sampling, or many time intervals for observing a behavior were used for each observation period. As an example, suppose the frequency of coughing was observed via tape recording. A cough, moreover, was defined as lasting no longer than one exhalation. Therefore, a single coughing episode might be coded anywhere from 1 to 20 or so. Two observers record the occurrence of coughs continuously over a 1-hour period. Observer A records 100 coughs and Observer B records 85 coughs. To obtain the percentage of agreement, the smaller frequency is divided by the larger frequency (i.e., $85 \div 100 = .85$). Interrater reliability is 85 percent. Eighty-five percent agreement is perfectly acceptable. However, is it really 85 percent agreement? When frequently occurring behaviors are observed over a long period of time, the possibility exists that the two observers may not be recording the same behaviors at precisely the same time. One observer may record accurately for the first half hour and, because of fatigue, underrecord for the second half hour. The other observer may underrecord for the first half hour, due to lack of practice, and record accurately for the second half hour. Yet, the percentage of agreement score would be high. In addition, consider our example that used number of coughs. If the frequencies had been 35 and 50 instead of 85 and 100, the percentage would be 70 percent instead of 85 percent. The more often the target behavior occurs, the greater are the chances of obtaining a higher reliability coefficient.

A solution to these problems has been to use a correlation coefficient based on a number of smaller intervals via **time sampling.** For example, the number of coughs would be recorded for a 1-minute **time interval** followed by a 2-minute **time-out interval** followed by a 1-minute observation interval, 2-minute time-out interval, and so forth, until 20 1-minute intervals had been recorded during a 1-hour observation period. A Pearson correlation could then be computed between frequencies for each corresponding time interval. It would be the same as correlating the scores of 20 people. Exhibit 13.4 demonstrates the computational procedure. It also depicts a percentage of agreement for each interval, the mean of these and the standard deviation, and, finally, the overall percentage of agreement calculated by dividing the smaller total frequency by the larger one. Using time sampling, interrater reliability is .87 and .81. Using just total frequencies, agreement is .94. Obviously there is less agreement when smaller intervals are considered, which is masked when overall percent of agreement is used. If six kinds of behavior were being observed (e.g., crying, moaning, talking), this procedure would be followed for each category; or, using total frequencies for a series of variables, a correlation could be computed between raters. In this case, each variable would be like a "subject pair" in the calculation of r.

Using a correlation rather than percentage of agreement has the advantages of being able to use the standard error of measurement to generate confidence intervals and estimate the number of time intervals required to achieve better reliability (via the Spearman-Brown formula) or detect significant effects. However, correlation procedures have disadvantages, sometimes of limited variability in observations, hence lower values for coefficients, and, on the other hand, inflated correlations when one observer consistently overrecords or underrecords. It is possible to obtain a correlation over .90 when the interobserver agreement is really very poor (e.g., Observer A consistently records two coughs fewer than Observer B).

One solution is to compute both percentage of agreement and a correlation. When time intervals are used, a percentage of agreement for each time interval is computed and then the mean percentage, standard deviation and range, and number of calculations are reported. Agreement refers to nonoccurrence as well as occurrence of behaviors.

An issue that concerns experts is that agreement calculated by the previous methods is dependent on the frequency with which the observed behaviors occur. As mentioned previously, rates of behavior drastically affect agreement. The more often the behavior occurs, the greater is the probability that raters could reach a reasonably high level of agreement by chance alone. Therefore, many investigators believe that in computing the agreement coefficient, researchers should consider the level of agreement by chance alone. This has opened a "bucket of worms." Numerous methods are beginning to appear in the literature (e.g., Cohen's k or the *kappa* statistic [4, 8]), which are not really comparable with each other. Moreover, there is still controversy about the criterion for judging whether or not agreement coefficients are significantly beyond levels that would be expected to occur by chance. Therefore, until more agreement is reached, it seems inappropriate to present one of those procedures in a book about the basics, such as is this text.

Exhibit 13-4. Interrater reliability calculations.

One-Minute Intervals	X = Observer A	Y = Observer B	$x^2 = (X - \bar{X})^2$	$y^2 = (Y - \bar{Y})^2$	$xy = (X - \bar{X})(Y - \bar{Y})$	Percentage of Agreement
1	4	4	1.69	2.25	1.95	100
2	8	7	28.09	20.25	23.85	88
3	4	3	1.69	0.25	0.65	75
4	0	0	0	0	0	100
5	0	1	0	2.25	0	0
6	4	4	1.69	2.25	1.95	100
7	5	5	5.29	6.25	5.75	100
8	4	4	1.69	2.25	1.95	100
9	0	0	0	0	0	100
10	1	0	2.89	0	0	0
11	1	1	2.89	2.25	2.55	100
12	0	0	0	0	0	100
13	1	1	2.89	2.25	2.55	100
14	0	0	0	0	0	100
15	0	1	0	2.25	0	0
16	3	3	0.09	0.25	0.15	100
17	7	7	18.49	20.25	19.35	100
18	6	5	10.89	6.25	8.25	83
19	4	3	1.69	0.25	0.65	75
20	2	2	0.49	0.25	0.35	100
Σ	54	51	80.46	80.37	69.95	1,621
	$\bar{X}$ = 2.7	$\bar{Y}$ = 2.5				

$$SD_X = \sqrt{\frac{80.46}{20}} = \sqrt{4.02} = 2.00 \qquad SD_Y = \sqrt{\frac{80.37}{20}} = \sqrt{4.01} = 2.00$$

$$r_{XY} = \frac{69.95}{20(2)(2)} = \frac{69.95}{80} = 0.87$$

Percentage of agreement for intervals: $\bar{X}$ = 81%; SD = 15.52

Overall percentage of agreement: $\frac{51}{54}$ = 94%

Agreement for Ratings

Although most observations involve recording frequency of occurrence, there are times when observers rank-order individuals or behaviors. There is yet another approach that can be used in this situation. When two or more raters are involved and their ratings are rank orderings from highest to lowest for an interval or for individuals, the following method is appropriate. It was developed by Guilford [6] as a revision of the earlier work by Hollingsworth [7]. The formula is as follows:

$$\bar{r} = 1 - \left[\frac{K\,(4N + 2)}{(K - 1)\,(N - 1)} + \frac{12\Sigma S^2}{K\,(K - 1)\,N\,(N^2 - 1)} \right] \tag{13.9}$$

where $\bar{r}$ = the average intercorrelation among judges or the reliability for *one* judge
　　K = number of judges
　　N = number of observations or subjects
　　S = sum of the ranks for any observation or subject

This $\bar{r}$ is reliability for one rater. Therefore, the Spearman-Brown formula should be used to adjust it upward to determine reliability for K judges. For example, in an in-service evaluation of the efficacy of triage nursing, four emergency room nurses were asked to rank-order six patients according to the order in which they should receive care. Data for this example are presented as Exhibit 13.5. To compute:

$$\bar{r} = 1 - \frac{4\,(4 \times 6 + 2)}{(4 - 1)\,(6 - 1)} + \frac{12\,(1436)}{4\,(4 - 1)\,(6)\,(6 \times 6 - 1)}$$

$$= 1 - \frac{(4)\,(26)}{(3)\,(5)} + \frac{(12)\,(1436)}{(4)\,(3)\,(6)\,(35)} = 1 - 6.93 + 6.83 = .90$$

Exhibit 13-5. Reliability of four raters rank ordering six patients.

Patient	Rater 1	2	3	4	S = Sum of Ranks	S^2
01	4	4	5	4	17	289
02	1	1	1	1	4	16
03	3	2	3	3	11	121
04	2	3	2	2	9	81
05	5	5	4	6	20	400
06	6	6	6	5	23	529
						$\Sigma S^2 = 1,436$

Using the Spearman-Brown formula, 13.8, to increase the coefficient fourfold, where ($K = 4/1$):

$$\tilde{r} = \frac{(4)(.90)}{1 + (3)(.90)} = \frac{3.6}{3.7} = .97$$

Reliability is increased from .90 to .97 because four raters are used to obtain each subject's rank.

In conclusion, as already discussed in this section, the situation or state of the art with respect to computing reliability of raters is not as well defined as that for self-report measures. For a thorough and informative discussion of this area of concern, you are directed to a series of articles presented in 1977 in the *Journal of Applied Behavior Analysis,* Volume 10.

Although it is obvious why *inter*rater reliability is essential, the importance of *intra*rater reliability is equally so—even when there is only one rater. The primary reason for assessing intrarater reliability is to guard against **observer drift.** As discussed in Chapter 11, many experts believe that drift is a very serious problem, even over short periods of time. Some believe that almost continuous monitoring is necessary in order to maintain acceptable levels of reliability. Therefore, intrarater reliability, unlike its counterpart, test-retest reliability, is considered a very important and necessary form of reliability in settings that involve multiple observations extending over weeks and, sometimes, over a few days. The research literature related to your content area and the methodologic literature focusing on observation are good sources for determining when this reliability is essential. When in doubt, assess it.

Correction for Attenuation

As the discussion of reliability draws to an end, a somewhat controversial procedure known as the correction for attenuation deserves introduction. The **correction for attenuation** can revise upward the correlation between two variables that have been measured with scales that are not 100 percent reliable. What it does is estimate what the correlation would be if the reliability of both scales were perfect. The basic formula is as follows:

$$\tilde{r}_{XY} = \frac{r_{XY}}{\sqrt{r_{XX}\, r_{YY}}} \tag{13.10}$$

where $\tilde{r}_{XY}$ = expected correlation if both measures were perfectly reliable
$\quad r_{XY}$ = observed correlation between the two variables X and Y
$\quad r_{XX}$ = observed reliability of the scale measuring variable X
$\quad r_{YY}$ = observed reliability of the scale measuring variable Y

Thus, if scale X has a reliability of .50, scale Y has a reliability of .60, and the observed correlation between the two variables is .21, it would have been .38 had the two measures been perfectly reliable:

$$\bar{r}_{XY} = \frac{.21}{\sqrt{(.50)(.60)}} = \frac{.21}{.55} = .38$$

Because perfect reliability is fiction, the .38 correlation is equally fictional. The usefulness of the formula therefore rests with what a correlation would be if reliabilities were raised to some attainable figure. In that case, the formula is

$$\bar{r}_{XY} = r_{XY} \sqrt{\frac{\bar{r}_{XX}\, \bar{r}_{YY}}{r_{XX}\, r_{YY}}} \qquad (13.11)$$

where $\bar{r}_{XY}$ = expected correlation
$\quad\quad r_{XY}$ = observed correlation between X and Y
$\quad\quad r_{XX}$ = observed reliability of scale X
$\quad\quad r_{YY}$ = observed reliability of scale Y
$\quad\quad \bar{r}_{XX}$ = improved reliability of scale X
$\quad\quad \bar{r}_{YY}$ = improved reliability of scale Y

Using the previous example and assuming both scale reliabilities could be raised to .90, the correlation between the two variables could be .34:

$$\bar{r}_{XY} = .21 \sqrt{\frac{(.90)(.90)}{(.50)(.60)}} = .21 \sqrt{\frac{.81}{.30}} = .21 \sqrt{2.7} = .21(1.64) = .34$$

The researcher can then decide if the research is worth further pursuit. If reliability of only one variable is to be changed, the following formula is appropriate:

$$\bar{r}_{XY} = r_{XY} \sqrt{\frac{\bar{r}_{XX}}{r_{XX}}} \qquad (13.12)$$

The correction for attenuation can also be used when reliabilities are lowered. For example, it is often necessary to use shortened versions of scales. The lowered reliabilities can be calculated by pilot testing or estimated by the Spearman-Brown formula. Then, if the correlation between the two longer versions of the scales is known, the correction for attenuation can be used to estimate the value of the correlation between the two shortened scales. The reliabilities of the shortened versions are inserted into the formula as $\bar{r}_{XX}$ and $\bar{r}_{YY}$.

There is controversy about some applications of the correction for attenuation. Few experts support routine use of the correction in order to increase correlations obtained via poor measures (i.e., reliabilities below .50 or .60). Many agree that it is a very poor estimate of a real correlation when reliabilities are less than .50 or .60, because it can drastically underestimate. One of the major values of the correction, according to this author, is in letting researchers know just how much higher a correlation would be if reliabilities were higher. This is because researchers often expect considerably higher correlations than is realistic and often unjustifiably blame lower reliabilities for a lack of significant results when the real blame rests elsewhere, perhaps with the hypothesis itself.

As stated elsewhere in this book, reliabilities as high as .90 should be required when those measures are the bases for major clinical decisions. The standard error of measurement must also be considered when clinical decisions are made. However, reliabilities as low as .60, sometimes .50 when few items are available, are adequate when using scales or tests for research. Rater agreement should reach at least .80. Obviously, higher reliabilities are better. A goal in scale development might be .85. It should be accompanied by a willingness to compromise downward however far is appropriate for the research setting. Use of the formulas presented previously can provide a guide to how far downward is acceptable.

In basic research, experts agree that increasing reliabilities beyond .80 can sometimes be wasteful. At .80 or better, correlations are not raised substantially, as shown by application of the correction for attenuation. To obtain reliabilities of .90 would require excessive time and work to add many additional items and develop strict standards for administration. The resulting scale might then become too time consuming and complex to administer in a research setting.

As demonstrated in the discussion of reliability, the number of items greatly affects the reliability of a measure. The other factor related to reliability is the extent to which items correlate with each other and are measuring the same variable or trait. It follows, then, that scales must include an adequate number of items that all correlate well to the total score, because if they correlate well with each other, they would also correlate well to the total score. Norm-referenced scale construction, therefore, is focused on developing a sufficient number of items that correlate well with the total score. In so doing, it is anticipated that the resulting instrument will also provide for variability among scores.

Item Analysis

Item analysis is an integral part of test development. It is often needed when tests and scales are modified for use in new research settings or with a different population of subjects. That is why three kinds of item analysis are presented here. Although you are not encouraged to develop your own scales or tests when you are just beginning as a researcher, you may well have to modify some or develop a questionnaire (see Chapter 14).

Item analysis occurs after you have conducted a **pilot test** of the instrument. Typically, twice as many items are administered as are intended for the final instrument to at least five (and preferably ten) times as many persons as items. Persons participating in the pilot testing of an instrument should be selected to be similar to the target population for which the instrument is intended, and the conditions for the pilot test should be the conditions under which the instrument is administered. If measurement conditions in the actual research setting are to be highly controlled, so too should be the conditions under which pilot data are gathered.

Difficulty Index, p Value

The p value, or **difficulty index,** of an item is, simply, the proportion of persons who answered it correctly. It is the number of persons answering correctly divided by the total number of persons responding to the item. If a trait such as anxiety is measured dichotomously by "yes" or "no" or "high" or "low," it would be the proportion of persons responding "yes" or "high." The difficulty index is used only with dichotomous items.

The p values are important for two reasons. First, they relate to the mean of the total set of observed scores, because it is the sum of p values. More importantly, they reflect the distribution of scores. If the average p value is considerably higher or lower than .5, the distribution of scores is likely to be skewed, especially when the number of items is small (e.g., 20). The standard deviation of test scores is larger when all the p values are near .5 rather than widely scattered. Second, items with p values that are extreme in either direction tend to have low correlations with each other, and, therefore, coefficient alpha tends to be lower for scales with extreme (e.g., high or low) values as compared to those with p values that are near the middle of the range. Therefore, items with p values between .4 and .6 are desirable.

The p value is easy to compute. Therefore, there is a tendency for some to use it as the sole criterion in test development. This can sometimes lead to serious errors. For example, any item that is highly ambiguous will tend to have a p value near .5 because of guessing. Guessing also tends to raise p values on other types of items and introduce measurement error. This can lead to less measurement error on easy items and more measurement error with more difficult items. Consequently, the difficulty index, or p value, should not be used as the only criterion for retention of items. Moreover, p values refer only to dichotomously scored items. They cannot be used with multipoint items such as a Likert scale, and some believe they are inappropriate with multiple choice questions. One of the two following approaches to determining item to total score correlations is more appropriate for these.

Discrimination Index

One approach to describing item to total score relationships is the **discrimination index.**[*] It has the advantage of being manageable when a computer is not available. It is relatively straightforward to compute:

1. In terms of their total scores, group the highest and lowest 25 percent of scores together. Set aside the middle group. They are not used in this analysis.

[*]There are several versions of the discrimination index. This is only one. They all do the same thing—yield an index of the item to total score relationship.

2. For each item, count the number of persons from the high group getting the question correct (C_{high}) and the number of persons from the low group getting it correct (C_{low}).
3. Subtract the number of persons in the low group who got it correct (C_{low}) from the number of persons in the high group who got it correct (C_{high}).
4. Calculate D_{max}, the largest difference *possible*. This occurs when everyone in the high group answers correctly and no one in the lower group does.
5. Divide the observed difference between the high and low groups. (C_{high} − C_{low}) by D_{max}, the largest difference possible. This is the discrimination index.

The procedure can be summarized as follows:

$$\text{Discrim} = \frac{C_{high} - C_{low}}{D_{max}} \qquad (13.13)$$

where C_{high} = number of persons in the upper 25 percent (of total scores) group answering the item correctly

C_{low} = number of persons in the low 25 percent (of total scores) group answering the item correctly

D_{max} = maximum difference if everyone in the high group answered correctly and no one in the lower group did

Exhibit 13.6 gives fictitious data that can be used to demonstrate computation of the discrimination index. For Item 1, suppose that it is a multiple choice question where alternative 5 is the correct answer. The number correct in the high group is 6 and the number correct in the low group is 0. The maximum difference occurs when all 10 persons in the high group are correct and none in the low group are. Therefore, D_{max} is 10. Calculation of the index is as follows:

$$\text{Discrim} = \frac{6 - 0}{10} = \frac{6}{10} = .60$$

If alternative 4 were correct, on the other hand, the discrimination index would be .30. For item 2, the discrimination index when alternative 4 is correct is − .10, because more persons in the lower group were correct than in the higher group.

The discrimination index can range from − 1.00 to + 1.00. When the index is negative, more persons in the low group than in the high group got the item correct. As a rule, .40 or better indicates good discrimination. When items are below .20, they are usually discarded and when they range from .20 to .40 they are examined for rewording. For example, with multiple choice items this involves looking at *distractors* (incorrect response alternatives) to see if they have about the same number of persons in the low group selecting each alterna-

Exhibit 13-6. Fictitious data for computing the discrimination index.

	Item Response Alternative				
Group*	1	2	3	4	5
Item 1					
Upper 25 percent	0	0	1	3	6
Lower 25 percent	4	4	2	0	0
Item 2					
Upper 25 percent	0	0	0	2	8
Lower 25 percent	1	3	2	3	1

*Groups determined on the basis of total score. Numbers in the body of the table represent the number of persons in that group selecting that alternative.

tive. If none selects an alternative, it may be too obvious and need rewording. If a large number in the high group selects a distractor, it may be either correct or ambiguous. The .20 cutting point, although often used, is arbitrary when the distribution of total scores is skewed upward. For example, a pilot test group may be too homogeneous to use .20 as the point at which items are dropped. In this case, it may have to be lowered.

So far, the discrimination index has been illustrated with correct-incorrect items. Unlike the difficulty index, it can also be used with multipoint responses like semantic differential or Likert scales. Only slight modifications are required:

1. **Total points** instead of **number correct** are computed separately for each group. For example, in a high group of 15 persons, if 3 people select 1, they each contribute 1 point for a total of 3 points. If 3 people select 2, they each contribute 2 points for a total of 6 points. If 2 people select 3 and 5 people select 4, the items are given 6 and 20 points respectively. Two people select 5 (for a total of 10). The total points for each alternative are summed (e.g., 3 + 6 + 6 + 20 + 10 = 45) to yield the total points for the high group, which, in this case, are 45. The same procedure is followed for the low group.
2. The difference between points for the high and low groups is calculated by subtracting lower group points from higher group points.
3. D_{max} is calculated. The high group ($n = 15$) would be expected to all select the highest value, 5, yielding the maximum possible of $5 \times 15 = 75$. The low group ($n = 15$) would all select 1 if the lowest number of points were to be obtained, thus yielding a point score of $15 \times 1 = 15$. D_{max} is therefore calculated by subtracting 15 from 75. It is 60.
4. As usual, the observed difference in groups is divided by the maximum difference in groups to get the discrimination index.
5. Make sure you flip item responses where necessary, before beginning this analysis. Then use the flipped rather than the original response.

This procedure can be summarized as follows:

$$\text{Discrim} = \frac{P_{\text{high}} - P_{\text{low}}}{D_{\text{max}}} \tag{13.14}$$

where P_{high} = the number of points for the high group
P_{low} = the number of points for the low group
D_{max} = the maximum possible difference in points between the two groups

Referring to Exhibit 13.6 again, suppose Item 1 were a Likert type response scale where 1 indicated strong disagreement, 3 was undecided, and 5 was strongly agree. To compute the discrimination index, you would proceed as follows:

$$\text{Discrim} = \frac{(1 \times 3) + (3 \times 4) + (6 \times 5) - (4 \times 1) + (4 \times 2) + (2 \times 3)}{(10 \times 5) - (10 \times 1)}$$

$$= \frac{45 - 18}{40} = .68$$

Using the same procedure for Item 2, the discrimination index is .45. Can you compute it?

To summarize, the discrimination index can be used when a computer is not available and data are not overwhelmingly large in number. Of course, a random sample from a larger data base is always preferable to nothing. Some researchers, when using this index, point out that because only 25 percent from the upper and lower ends of the total score distributions are used, a situation similar to the split-half reliability procedure exists. They therefore argue that the Spearman-Brown formula should be used to correct upward any correlations based on only half the sample. The discrimination index does not usually seem to need this added boost, and there is some question about its qualification as a correlation coefficient. Therefore, this author does not recommend using the Spearman-Brown formula with it. However, sometimes other correlations are computed once data are summarized as shown in Exhibit 13.6. For some of these it may be perfectly appropriate to correct the correlation upward with the Spearman-Brown formula.

Item to Total Score Correlations*

This approach to **item to total score correlation** requires computer assistance. It is the preferred approach when it is at all possible, particularly when a major research instrument is being developed. It is presented in the following steps.

---

*This approach assumes that tests are power tests rather than speeded tests. It also assumes an equal "weight" for each item, because there is little evidence to suggest weights make significant contributions. In fact, in tests with at least 20 dichotomous items, tests scored both with and without weights correlate in the high .90s.

1. Devise a scoring system that allows all ideal item to total score correlations to be positive. This is really no problem in tests of achievement or ability. However, in some scales that word half the attitudes positively (to which a high score would agree) and the other half negatively (to which a high score would disagree), half of the responses must be converted via **flipping** to look like the other half before total scores can be computed or the item to total score correlations computed. For example, on a 7 point Likert scale in which 7 equals strongly agree and high scores indicate strong agreement, the numerical responses to negatively worded items (to which high scores would disagree) must be subtracted from 8 (one more than the highest number of points). The resulting (i.e., flipped) value would be the response recorded for that item and used in calculations using the item. The flipping option is available with some (not all) computer programs.

2. If the number of items is considerably less than 80 and the number of subjects small (less than 5 per item), remove the **spurious** (inflated) effects of including the item in the calculation of the total score by calculating the total score without the item before the item to total score correlation (known therefore as the **corrected correlation**) is computed.

3. Using the Pearson product moment correlation coefficient, calculate a correlation between each item and the "corrected" total score.

4. Retain items that correlate .20 or better. (Typically, two-thirds of items will correlate between .10 and .30 for dichotomous scales—somewhat higher for multipoint scales.) If not enough items are retained, additional items whose corrected correlations meet standards for statistical significance at the .05 level can be added. If the number of retained items is still too small to allow further screening, start over.

5. Rank items according to the value of their item to total score correlations. If an equal number of agree-disagree or true-false response items are desired, it may be appropriate to make two separate rank orderings, one for each.

6. Investigate (via computer) the reliability of successive sets of items using coefficient alpha or KR-20, beginning with the highest ranking 30 items for dichotomous data and for multipoint items the highest ranking 15. (Thirty and fifteen items, respectively, are generally the minimum required for .80 reliability.) If alternate forms are being developed via this method, assign every other item in the rank ordering to one form and the remaining to the other form. Sixty and/or thirty items are therefore used.* If reliability for this group of items is .85

---

*Sometimes assignment to alternate forms is made by first rank-ordering item means (after flipping, if appropriate) for two groups of items, those with high and those with adequate correlations to the total score. Then, every other item on the rank ordering of means is assigned to the alternate form. This method results in about equal total scores for an individual on both forms.

or higher, go to the next step. If not, begin adding the next-ranking items until the desired reliability is achieved. The exact number of items required depends upon their correlations to the total score and the reliability of the first set of items. Usually, items can be added in sets of five or ten, or an estimate of the number to be added can be calculated by using the Spearman-Brown formula. If the reliability does not increase, or even decreases when an additional set of items is added, stop and delete that set.

7. After an adequate reliability has been obtained, plot a frequency distribution of total scores. If the distribution is nearly normal or symmetrical, item selection is completed. If the distribution is badly skewed, examine items that correlated satisfactorily with the total score but that were not included in the final collection of items and substitute those representing content opposite to the skewed scores for some of the lower ranking items which have responses contributing to the skewedness (e.g., negative attitudes if total scores are too positive, easy items if total scores are too low). Be sure to calculate a new reliability coefficient (and then a frequency distribution) for this collection of items. You may find it necessary to add a few items. Generally, item substitution, if at all necessary, can be accomplished intuitively. However, for those wishing a more definitive approach, p values (difficulty index) can be used. (On multipoint items, e.g., Likert scale, the item mean can be used in determining items to add.) In exchanging items to improve a test distribution, exchange a value of .70 for a .30, a .60 for a .40, a .80 for a .20, and vice versa. However, please note that the shape of the test distribution is not particularly important in most research uses, so avoid spending too much time at this step, unnecessarily lowering reliability, or adding items just to get a perfect bell shape.

8. If the preceding approach fails, it may be owing to any of three reasons:
   a. Items may be from a domain where correlations among items and item to total score correlations are low. This would then require a very large number of items to reach high reliability.
   b. The items may cluster into many "factors" or groups, each of which correlates weakly among items in the group and does not correlate with items from other groups, thereby yielding low item to total score correlations. (A scale with only a few factors or groups of items usually yields a sufficiently high reliability. See Nunnally [12].)
   c. Some items correlate well with one another and others (poor items) do not correlate with any items. This is apparent when the value of ranked item correlations suddenly drops .10 from one item to the next. The remedy for this is to retain the good items, replace the poor ones with new ones, and start over. If either (A) or (B) is suspected, the remedies are obscure and partly art. Consult a good psychometrician. Factor analysis, the so-called cure-all advocated by many, will probably not work. The probability is great that a different approach to measuring the variable under study is needed unless all the items are just very poorly constructed.

9. Although experts disagree, factor analysis prior to this point will probably not be helpful except in using much of your time and money. It also requires a minimum of ten subjects per item. When you believe you have your instrument constructed (with an adequate reliability and frequency distribution), factor analysis may then be appropriate.

10. After the first computation of item to total score correlations, you may discover that 30 percent to 50 percent of the items have very low correlations and therefore may be "watering down" the other correlations since these weak ones are still contributing to the total score. **Successive approximations** might therefore be used. This simply involves eliminating all items which do not correlate at the .05 level of significance and then recomputing item to total score correlations using only the retained items in calculating total scores. Then begin at step 4. This can be done as many times as necessary, although it is not generally needed more than once unless there are many negative correlations among items. This can happen with personality tests.

Prior to undertaking the preceding steps, it is sometimes prudent to conduct a mini-pilot study or **feasibility study.** For this, 30 dichotomous or 15 multipoint items are administered to 100 persons and then item to total score corrected correlations are calculated. If half or more items are retained and yield an alpha reliability coefficient of .50 or better, generate more items and begin full-fledged test construction or item analysis. If, however, your results are discouraging, abandon the project to avoid further loss of time and effort.

Another kind of two-stage procedure may also be appropriate in some circumstances. It involves screening of subjects (stage 1) according to some variable prior to the actual pilot testing to gather data for item analysis. For example, suppose a researcher of patient compliance wished to develop a scale to measure ability to delay gratification or satisfaction. She also wished to use it with persons with limited verbal ability. The procedure, therefore, might involve a double item analysis to first reduce the effects of verbal ability. The first stage would use a verbal comprehension test as an external criterion. Those scale items with a low discrimination index (according to high and low verbal ability) would be retained. The second stage, then, would involve an item to total score correlation analysis for the delay of gratification scale (DGS). Those items with low discrimination on the verbal ability scale and good discrimination (or correlation to total score) on the DGS would therefore be included in the final collection of items.

In conclusion, the final decision to include items is yours. There are sometimes reasons other than adequate item to total score correlations for retaining items. For example, many achievement tests include a few easy questions at the beginning to prevent discouragement and give practice in answering that type of question. These items could easily appear worthless during item analysis. Moreover, with reference to behavioral observations, accuracy of observation is considered an index of content validity. This is inferred from observer agreement (i.e., the interrater reliability coefficient). Thus, just as the boundaries between the three kinds of validity are not distinct, not even the boundary between reliability and validity is sacred. It all depends on your purpose. You are therefore encouraged to concentrate on the concepts and logical inferences of the kinds of reliability and validity as they fulfill various purposes, instead of undue categorizing and labeling of examples according to type. If you have extra time, devote it to asking "why?" and "why not?"

A measure must have good reliability before validity can be inferred. Reliability is essential, a prerequisite. To repeat, a measure cannot be considered valid if it is not reliable. When a measure is inconsistent and unstable, it is useless to be concerned about what a score means. Instead, we ignore it or throw it away. It is meaningless.

V*alidity*

When you investigate the validity of a measure, you are asking what can be *inferred* from the total score. Validity is inferred, not measured, from evidence which is presented. Two major areas of concern are (1) the internal nature or properties of the measure itself and (2) how the total score relates to measures of other variables and criteria. There are many so-called kinds of validity. However, because most of these refer to a method for establishing *evidence* of validity, the principles of gathering this evidence, for the sake of discussion, can be conceptualized as three types: content, construct, and criterion-related. To define simply, content validity is concerned with the internal properties of a measure; the other two refer to the measure's correlation with other measures of either the same concept/behavior (i.e., criterion-related) or other variables as specified by theory (i.e., construct). These three categories, like many others, are not mutually exclusive. They are interdependent; evidence of only one is rarely sufficient to infer validity. Content validity is almost always a concern during test development. Then, if the purpose of the measure is, say, prediction, criterion-related validity becomes paramount. If, however, the characteristics of other variables in relationship to the variable being measured are of major interest, construct validity becomes important.

Content Validity

Content validity involves the systematic examination of test content to determine whether it adequately covers a representative sample from the domain of the variable being measured. It might appear that mere inspection of items to see if they measure the content would suffice. However, it is not so simple.

The content area to be tested must first be studied to make certain that all major aspects or subcategories are represented and in the correct proportion. Sometimes an additional dimension is added to specify at what level of cognitive functioning (e.g., knowledge, comprehension, application, synthesis according to Bloom [2]) the items within the subcategories should be constructed. Once the test specifications have been drawn up, items are generated for each cate-

Exhibit 13-7. Content analysis for SSM.

			Judge		
Item	A	B	C	D	E
1. A Friend					
a. Should make life worthwhile by offering help and guidance along the rocky road of life.	4	4	3	5	4
b. Will work through any disagreements until true understanding is reached.	6	6	7	6	6
c. Is one who has common interests with you and who enjoys friendly competition.	5	7	5	7	5
d. Has self-worth independent of your needs for him or her.	7	5	7	4	7
e. Will always agree with you and will do anything for you if she or he is a true friend.	3	3	4	3	3
2. Men and Women					
a. Are different and can learn from each other's ways of being.	7	6	7	7	7
b. Do not need formal roles or stuffy morals to get along with one another.	6	7	6	6	5
c. Are essentially equal and should treat one another as such.	5	5	5	5	6
d. Should respect one another's God-given role in life.	4	4	4	4	4
e. Get along best when each knows his or her proper place.	3	3	3	3	3

Note: Numbers in judge columns opposite alternatives indicate system that item represents, according to the judge.

gory and these items are then reviewed by experts to assess, on a three-point scale, for example, how well the item measures the domain category. From these are chosen the items that will compose the pilot test. Judges also point out errors and ambiguities in items and make recommendations for changes.

Content validity is sometimes assessed before pilot testing. For example, the author and colleagues developed a multidimensional scale, called the SSM, to assess biopsychosocial systems according to Graves' theory [5]. The test was designed to determine in which of the five possible systems, or combination of systems, an individual was operating. The final format of the instrument, after several attempts at others failed, was a forced-choice one in which respondents distributed 11 points between 5 alternatives, each of which represented one of the 5 systems. The content validity question for this measure, therefore, involved evidence that each of the five alternatives represented only one of the systems and that all five systems were represented in each question. Therefore, the judges who were expert in the theory were asked to determine which system each alternative represented. Exhibit 13.7 presents data for two of the questions.

Exhibit 13-8. Step I table of specifications—Knowledge of nursing research.

Category	Percentage Assigned Each Category by Panel Member								
	I	II	III	IV	V	VI	VII	VIII	Average
1. Development of nursing research	16.5	9	2.5	10	10	10	7	7	8
2. Types of nursing research	1.7	9	2.5	10	15	10	3	4	4
3. Formulating the problem	6.5	5	5	25	15	20	9	10	8
4. Review of literature	8.2	27	5	10	15	10	10	10	12
5. Delimiting the problem	9.0	9	10	10	15	20	20	16	14
6. Methodology	32.5	23	55	25	15	20	30	40	34
7. Findings, conclusions, and recommendations	23	18	20	10	15	10	18	13	17
8. Elements of a critique	3.3								3

Reprinted with permission [15].

It is apparent that question 1 was poor. The judges could not agree. It was therefore deleted before pilot testing. Question 2, on the other hand, was not as poor. Alternatives D and E had no disagreement and alternatives A and C had only slight disagreement—being confused for the system that alternative B was designed to represent. Alternative B was therefore rewritten and, along with all others, reevaluated by a panel of judges. Those receiving 100 percent agreement the second time around were used for pilot testing. Question 2 was used for pilot testing but was eliminated during item analysis of item to total score correlations.

Another example of content validity assessment involves a more elaborate multistage procedure which occurred even before items were written. Exhibit 13.1 presented examples of alternate form items developed by Thomas and Price [15] for their standardized tests of knowledge about research methodology for nursing students. Prior to developing these and other items, Thomas and Price presented to a panel of eight experts a list of subtopics and asked them to determine the percentage of items for each category. These results are shown in Exhibit 13.8. It is apparent that there was disagreement among panel members. Thomas and Price therefore used means for each category to determine the proportion of items to be devoted to each. The second stage of content validity then involved asking the same panel of judges to apportion the percentage of items for each category among three levels of cognitive functioning. The results of this are shown in Exhibit 13.9. At this point, an appropriate number of items was generated to measure functioning at these levels within each of the categories. Two alternative forms were developed and the panel of judges was asked to evaluate each item, including assessing appropriateness on a 1 to 3 scale. After poor items were deleted and others reworded, pilot testing on a national sample began. Item analysis was then used to develop the final form of the tests. National norms are now being developed as many schools of nursing use these tests to pretest and posttest undergraduate and graduate students.

After item analysis to determine inclusion of the final set of items, content validity may need to be assessed again to determine if the correct proportion of items for each subcategory has been maintained. If the proportion has not been maintained, exchanges of items and sometimes addition of items occurs until the content is sampled appropriately while retaining an acceptable level of reliability.

Construct Validity

Most variables that require development of a measure with properties of reliability and validity cannot be directly assessed as can variables like height and weight. They are variables like anxiety, creativity, locus of control, attitudes toward numerous phenomena, intelligence, dependency, power, self-concept, and so forth. All are **constructs.** These variables have been *constructed* from theory and **empirical data** (i.e., quantitative data from research). For measures of variables that are constructs, evidence must be presented that scores represent the degree to which an individual does indeed possess or exhibit the construct. This is known as **construct validity.** Constructs, because they are constructed variables, are related to other variables, many of which are also constructs. Sometimes, in addition, their description and definition may include variables to which they are *not* related. This is the theory relationship network, called a **nomological network,** to which construct validity is addressed. According to the American Psychological Association (APA) Standards for Educational and Psychological Tests [9], the test developer begins by generating hypotheses about the characteristics of those with high and low scores on the measure to be validated. They form a network of relationships which composes a theory about the construct that is being measured. Sometimes more than one theory (competing theories) emerges. At any rate, the construct being measured may be an independent variable in some hypotheses and a dependent variable in others. If the test developer's theory (i.e., the relationship or nomological network) about what the test measures is correct, most of these relationship hypotheses will be supported. If not, she must revise her definition of the construct, revise the test to measure the construct better as she conceived it, or question the theory from which the hypotheses were generated. Researchers in the behavioral sciences, unfortunately, have usually chosen the first two alternatives rather than questioned the theory. When it has been questioned, it has usually been because an alternative or competing theory was available. This may be too conservative an approach.

You may wonder why content validity is not also a way of establishing construct validity, because constructs are often comprised of factors or subconstructs. It is. Recall, in the introduction to this section of the chapter, the fact that the three types of validity are not really separate and mutually exclusive was

Exhibit 13-9. Step II table of specifications—Knowledge of nursing research.

| | Bloom's Taxonomy (%) | | | |
Category	Weighting	Knowledge and Comprehension	Application and Analysis	Synthesis and Evaluation
1. Development of nursing research (historical background and landmark studies)	8 (4)	4	2	2
2. Types of nursing research (categorization schemes such as exploratory, descriptive, experimental or clinical, administrative, historical, educational)	4 (2)	1	1	2
3. Formulating the problem (sources for ideas—clinical practice, literature, theory, need, significance)	8 (4)	2	2	4
4. Review of literature (establishing framework, previous relevant studies, tools)	12 (6)	6	3	3
5. Delimiting the problem [feasibility; identifying variables; formulation of statement(s), question(s), or hypotheses; assumptions and limitations]	14 (7)	3	4	7
6. Methodology (selecting approach; population and sampling tools; planning, collecting, and analyzing data)	34 (24)	7	7	20

7. Findings, conclusions, and recommendations (reporting findings, limitations, recommendations for practice and research)	17 (11)	4	4	9
8. Elements of a critique	3 (2)	1	1	1

Note: Numbers in parentheses following percentages in the weighting column indicate the number of items in each category.
Reprinted with permission [15].

stated. Trying to keep the boundaries sacred is a waste of time. Content validity can provide evidence for construct validity. So can criterion-related validity. Content validity refers to the internal properties of a test. This discussion of construct validity refers to the external situation—what the test relates to, except for the small portion reserved for criterion-related validity (relationships to other measures or criteria for the *same* construct).

Construct validity accumulates over time. Through the process of **successive verification,** modifications are made and hypotheses eliminated or retained. The test developer gradually increases her knowledge of what is measured by the test, and knowledge about the usefulness of the test as a measure of the construct improves. At some point the researcher decides the instrument can be used for research purposes—usually once content and a few construct or criterion-related validity studies have been successfully completed. Many correlational research studies that use research tests and scales are, in addition to their intended goals, actually contributing to the further construct validity of the scale. That is why a wise test developer requests copies of all research reports of studies using the scale when permission is granted for its use. Construct validity builds, as if part of a chain letter, as the scale is used in more and more research over many years. The instrument's other credentials also begin to accumulate via, for example, new reliability coefficients for different samples, norms for various groups, and so forth.

Chapter 4 introduced construct validity as it relates to the research design itself. It, of course, is different from the construct validity of a measure, because it considers how all aspects of a research design are operationalized. By **operationalized** we mean how all aspects of the design are converted from theoretical constructs to research manipulations (or operations) that yield quantitative data. As a beginning researcher, it is probably best that you consider these two uses of the term construct validity as two different research concepts—like random sampling versus random assignment or internal validity versus external validity. Another way of viewing these which is even more accurate (but more confusing, unfortunately) is that **construct validity of operational definitions** is a subset of **construct validity of research designs.** However you wish to view these two construct validities, keep in mind that this chapter presents construct validity only as it relates to a measurement instrument.

Experimental Manipulation

There are a number of special techniques that have been developed to establish evidence of construct validity. A few are presented here. Others can be found by reading test manuals and the research literature. One approach is by **experimental manipulation.** For example, Martuza [11] administered the Spielberger, Gorauch, and Lushene [14] trait and state anxiety scales to students in his class studying tests and measurements at 10 successive class meetings. According to the theory on which the two scales were based, trait anxiety is a relatively enduring quality over time. That is, it indicates a basic personality trait that describes how an individual perceives and reacts to the myriad of life events that constitute the business of living. A person scoring low would tend to remain calm in most routine situations, while a person scoring high would either become anxious whenever minor threatening events occurred, or, in extreme cases, remain anxious all the time because the whole business of living seemed threatening. Changes in an individual's trait anxiety score occur infrequently, if ever, because it represents a habitual way of life. State anxiety, on the other hand, refers to an individual's emotional response when an especially threatening event occurs, such as taking a final examination or even a quiz when the material being covered is not well understood. Therefore, Martuza used two course tests as the experimental intervention. Anxiety was measured at each of 10 class sessions. The first seven class sessions were routine. Course tests were administered at the eighth and ninth sessions. The tenth session was another routine class. Results demonstrated the same mean on trait anxiety across all 10 sessions, demonstrating the enduring quality or stability of the trait. State anxiety, on the other hand, remained the same for the first six sessions, began rising at the seventh (in anticipation of the tests), peaked very high on the eighth day (the first test), and was back at the baseline of the first six sessions at the tenth testing. Thus, potent evidence was produced for the state-trait anxiety scales.

The Multitrait-Multimethod Matrix

The **multitrait-multimethod matrix** approach is based on the principle that two different measures of the same construct should have high correlation coefficients while two kinds of measures of two different constructs should have low correlations. The former is called **convergent validity** and the later is called **divergent validity.** Convergent validity is conceived of as the correlation between the test and other constructs to which it was expected to correlate. On

Exhibit 13-10. Multitrait-multimethod matrix.

	Method A		Method B	
	Variable *X*	Variable *Y*	Variable *X*	Variable *Y*
Method A				
Variable *X*	I	IV	II	III
Variable *Y*	IV	I	III	II
Method B				
Variable *X*	II	III	I	IV
Variable *Y*	III	II	IV	I

I = Reliability of measure. When observers are used, it is usually interrater reliability; with self-report measures, it is generally alternate forms. However, depending on the research situation, other kinds of reliability (e.g., internal consistency) might be justified. These coefficients, of course, should be high—at least 0.80 and preferably higher.

II = Convergent validity form of construct validity. Indicated by high II correlation (same trait, two methods) and low III and IV correlations; II correlations below 0.70 are suspect because less than half the variance is shared by the trait.

III = Divergent validity. Indicated by low III correlations (as compared to II) but not as low as IV.

IV = Divergent validity. Indicated by the very lowest correlations of all.

the other hand, support for no correlation between constructs that are not suppose to correlate is called divergent validity.

In 1959 Campbell and Fiske [3] proposed an experimental design to assess convergent and discriminant validity, which they called the multitract-multimethod matrix. Essentially, the design called for the measurement of two or more traits (or variables), each by two or more methods (e.g., Likert scale versus behavioral observation versus semantic differential scale versus physical assessment measures of each variable). According to theory, the variables selected would not be related (or correlated). All measures would then be correlated and entered into a matrix like that shown in Exhibit 13.10. In addition, reliability coefficients are also entered. Reliability, in this context, represents agreement between two measures of the same trait obtained through maximally similar methods, such as parallel forms of the same test; validity represents agreement between two measures of the same trait obtained by maximally different methods, such as a Likert scale and behavioral observation.

The "coefficients" shown in Exhibit 13.10 are labeled from I to IV according to expected magnitude rather than actual correlations in order to better explain this procedure. Alternate forms reliability (I)* measurement of the same trait by the same method would obviously be high. Measurement of the same trait by

---

*Sometimes internal consistency reliability measures are substituted for alternate forms, because in most cases it is considered a good predictor of alternate forms. If you have any reason to believe it is not, then you should not use it.

two different methods (II) would also be high, and that is the convergent validity coefficient. However, it can be expected to be somewhat lower than I, because of the measurement error introduced as a result of using two different methods to measure the trait. This same reasoning applies to the III and IV correlations. While both are expected to be low, thereby providing evidence of divergent validity, IV correlations would be expected to be lower than III because of the error introduced by using two different methods. If III correlations were too high, an individual's scores may be unduly affected by some irrelevant common factor, such as ability to understand the directions or questions or the desire to make himself appear favorable on all traits.

This approach, in a more complex design with three variables, was used by Reisinger and Ora [13] in a (research) methodologic study comparing naturalistic and laboratory settings (the two methods). Parent–child interactions were observed in the laboratory for 20 minutes by two observers who were separated from each other by a wooden partition. They are also observed in the home by live observers and by radio transmitters worn by mothers for 2 hours and activated only for the last 30 minutes. Live observations and transmitted tapes were coded by the same observation code as the laboratory one. Support for construct validity was *inferred* when two of the three II coefficients were .80 and all of the III and IV coefficients were low.

Factor Analysis

Once a measure has achieved an adequate reliability coefficient, it may be appropriate to use factor analysis. Factor analysis is an advanced statistical procedure (beyond the scope of this book) in which, say, scores from 20 tests are correlated and clusters of highly correlated tests defined. These are called factors. Five or six factors might result from analysis of the 20 tests. Therefore an individual might be described in terms of these factors instead of all 20 tests. The major purposes of factor analysis, therefore, it to simplify descriptions of behavior by reducing the number of variables to a few common factors or traits. In essence, a few new constructs are constructed to account for the 20 constructs measured by the 20 tests. After factors have been identified and named, in view of the combination of tests (constructs) which are comprised by the factor, the measure being studied can be described in terms of its factorial composition.

The factorial composition of a single measure can also be examined by combining items that are closely correlated to each other. Each measure can be described in terms of the major factors determining the total score together with the factor weight or loading for each factor. The factor loading (weight) represents the correlation of the measure with the factor and is known as the **factorial validity** of the measure. Thus, if a dependency factor has a weight of .62 for a measure of the locus of control construct, the factorial validity of the locus of control measure is .62 as a measure of the trait of dependency. To summarize, factorial validity is, simply, the correlation of the test with whatever is common to a group of items included in the measure.

Other Construct Validity Techniques

The number of other approaches to establishing construct validation are limited only by the creativity of those conducting research studies of this type. Moreover, the following is an incomplete list of names that have been generated to describe the many approaches, usually according to their purposes. They are all construct validity:

Congruent validity	Population validity
Divergent validity	Structural validity
Ecologic validity	Substantive validity
External validity	Task validity
Factorial validity	Temporal validity
Nomological validity	Trait validity

You probably recognize some of these. Others you may wish to look up. If you come across any of these terms in your readings, remember they all mean the same thing—construct validity.

Criterion-Related Validity

Criterion-related validity is the empirical technique of studying the relationship between test scores and an independent, external criterion or measure of the same variable. In essence, you are asking whether or not the test score can be substituted for some less efficient way of gathering data about the variable that is being measured. Some measurement experts go so far as to say it compares test performance with an independent measure of what that test was designed to measure (e.g., Anastasi [1]). The APA Standards of Educational and Psychological Tests [9] broadens this somewhat to include investigations designed to enhance understanding of what the test measures, thereby introducing some ambiguity in terms of a clear distinction between criterion-related and construct validity. This need not concern us, however, since all forms of validity could be considered construct validity, depending on your point of view (purpose and interpretation of evidence). Thus, it is sufficient here to say that criterion-related validity concerns the relationship between test (or observed) performance and an independent, external criterion that the test or observational code is expected to substitute for or predict. Criterion-related validity may be characterized as presenting more applied research, as distinguished from construct validity which is more basic and theoretical, and as such its results pertain to specified situations and are sometimes less generalizable.

Two kinds of criterion-related validity are universally recognized—concurrent and predictive. The distinction between them pertains to the time period when data are gathered. In concurrent validity, both the test and criterion are measured about the same time. In predictive validity, there is a time lapse between the two measures.

In **predictive validity,** performance on the criterion is predicted based on test scores measuring the predictor variable. Later, the criterion is assessed and compared to the prediction. A **hit or miss table** is then sometimes developed. For example, suppose a 28-item scale was designed to measure student nurses' interpersonal communication skills with patients. The test developers hoped the test could replace observation of these skills in the clinical setting and thereby reduce the costs of nurse education. The test was administered at the end of a class unit focusing on the principles of interpersonal communication. On the basis of total scores, students' skill was predicted as (1) meets or exceeds standards or (2) is below standards. At a later date, the criterion measure, observation (according to a nine-category code) of student interactions with patients on five randomly selected separate occasions, was made. Exhibit 13.11 summarizes data from this hypothetical research study. From this Exhibit it is apparent that the scale predicts with about 85 percent accuracy, because only five persons who are predicted to be below standard actually performed according to standards and just 10 persons who were predicted as performing adequately failed to do so. This, then, is the validity evidence from which you, a potential user, must infer predictive validity. Surprises are always nice and therefore the 5 percent who performed better may not be a major concern. However, 10 percent of the students failed to perform as predicted. In a profession such as nursing in which safe patient care is a concern, you would have to decide if you could live with the 10 percent (or 15 percent) error rate in exchange for the cost savings of not needing to assess this skill in a clinical setting. Perhaps no more than 1 percent error rate is permissible, or perhaps 5 percent is permissible because interpersonal skill is less critical than, say, physical care, for which tolerating more than 1 percent is unacceptable. You must decide. One alternative might involve examination of the scores for the 15 percent in order to develop a range of scores where clinical supervision and observation was necessary and another "safe" range, from the 75 percent who performed satisfactorily as expected, where no clinical assessment would be necessary. This could reduce costs while still providing terminal assessment when needed.

Concurrent validity, on the other hand, involves concurrent (i.e., simultaneous) measurement of the scale or code being validated and the criterion. In the previous example, if the question or purpose was determining which students needed clinical supervision for interpersonal skills and which ones did not, the validity question would be one of concurrent validity to assess via the measure those whose skills were already developed at acceptable standards.

While prediction validity is sometimes inferred from concurrent validity data, it is usually very dangerous to do so. Some test developers, moreover, present only correlation coefficients to describe the relationship to the criterion. At times this may be acceptable, particularly if your major concern is with construct validity. However, the hit or miss table, perhaps accompanied by a correlation coefficient, provides practical data for decision making that cannot be inferred from just the coefficient.

Exhibit 13-11. Hit-or-miss criterion-related validity table.

Predicted Interpersonal Behavior	Criterion: Observed Behavior	
	Meets or Exceeds Standards	Below Standards
Meets or exceeds standards	75	10
Below standards	5	10

Note: In an actual research setting, more than 100 subjects would be used. Moreover, these data are fictitious.

There are, of course, as with all things, pitfalls to be aware of with criterion-related validity. These largely pertain to selection and measurement of the criterion. If this were easy to do, in most cases it would not be necessary to develop the new measure. Numerous methods have been tried by college admissions staff to predict success in school. Often the criterion has been student grade point average, which is, to be sure, an incomplete if not misleading criterion. Professional judgement after psychiatric interview has been used as criterion for personality tests and is very suspect if dependent upon one interview rather than a series of them over a period of time. One of the hardest aspects of criterion-related validity, therefore, is selection and measurement of the criterion. It must (1) be relevant, (2) possess reliability and validity, and (3) be free from **criterion contamination** (e.g., bias due to an observer knowing a subject's test score). Often, other variables as well as the one measured by the new scale relate to (i.e., compose) criterion characteristics. This is known as **criterion complexity,** and it is the reason extensive study of the criterion variable's known and theoretical properties must be undertaken prior to data gathering.

A popular method of establishing criterion-related validity is the **contrasted groups approach.** With this, a group known to possess the characteristic being measured and another assumed or known to not possess it (or possess it to a lesser degree) complete the scale. The group means are then compared. For example, suppose a researcher developed a humanistic caring scale and administered it to a group of nurses and a group of computer programmers, reasoning that nurses would be much higher. Results might very well turn out in the expected direction. Then again, they might not, owing to criterion complexity. When criterion complexity is a major concern, other approaches to defining a criterion must be found. Simulation in laboratory settings where more potential confounding variables can be controlled has been used. In other situations, a more complex and lengthy test measuring the same construct has been used. To summarize, when selecting a criterion, ask yourself, "What else is it measuring besides the variable I am testing? How much of the total score on the criterion is accounted for by these other variables?" Failure to investigate these questions can result in low correlations and poor hit or miss tables.

A *Case Study in Instrument Credentialing*

The following case study is presented in order to make the preceding principles of instrument credentialing more clear and show how they were used in an actual instrument development research setting.

As a class project in their graduate level nursing research course, four students and their instructor began development of an instrument to measure exercise of self-care agency (Kearney & Fleischer [10]). Conceptually based on the work of Orem and others, this construct was considered more appropriate in the self-report mode than the behavioral observation mode, because observation did not distinguish between a person using all of very limited self-care knowledge and a person using very little of much more knowledge. To begin, six open-ended questions were completed by four class members, all of whom were familiar with the self-care concept in nursing. First, each wrote what she believed it to be. Next, the salient characteristics of persons with low and high self-care agency and the factors affecting a person's exercise of it were described. Five questions you would use to assess exercise of self-care agency were then elicited and, finally, the conditions under which you would decide to use (or not use) it were listed. The responses were then discussed by the class and four **subconstructs** that contribute to the exercise of self-care agency and five related **indicants** of an individual's exercise of self-care agency were agreed on (i.e., each subconstruct had two indicants). Five-point Likert-type items ranging from characteristic to uncharacteristic for each indicant were then designed by the researchers (i.e., the same four students) resulting in 83 items, each rated as positive or negative toward exercise of self-care agency and rated as good or fair or poor in terms of appropriateness to the subconstruct. Forty-five items were ranked good and twenty-one were ranked with a mixture of good and fair. Of these 66, twenty-two were removed because they duplicated others. This resulted in 44 items for the initial instrument.

Content validity was assessed by asking five faculty members, all experts in the self-care concept of nursing, to rate each item's worth as an indicator of self-care agency. Twenty-nine of the forty-four items were rated as good with 80 percent rater agreement. These were left unchanged. The remaining 15 items had 60 percent agreement as good or fair. Based on rater feedback, one item was reworded and one was eliminated. The resulting scale now had 43 items.

The self-care literature was examined to find theoretical relationships between self care and other characteristics of the individual. These would be used to establish construct validity, the relationship between exercise of self-care agency as measured by the scale, and other variables as measured by already established instruments. If the scale correlated as hypothesized, then chances were high that it was indeed measuring what it purported to measure. Based on the literature review, it was hypothesized that the scale would correlate positively with internal locus of control (as measured by the Rotter scale), self-confidence, achievement, and intraception, and correlate negatively with abasement and lability (the foregoing five constructs all being measured by the Gough and Heilbrun adjective check list).

Next, a test "battery" consisting of the research scale, the Rotter scale, and the adjective check list was administered to volunteer nursing and psychology students in order to determine reliability (split-half and test-retest) and construct validity. In all, between 232 and 292 students participated in at least part of the research with 76 nursing students available for test-retest (5-week) reliability.

The results showed .77 test-retest reliability and split-half reliabilities of .80 (n = 79), .81 (n = 84) and .77 (n = 153), using an odd-even split and the Spearman-Brown formula. Significant positive correlations were found with self confidence ($r = .23, p < .05$), achievement ($r = .32, p < .01$), and intraception ($r = .26, p < .05$) and a negative correlation was found with abasement ($r = .35, p < .01$). No correlation was found with locus of control, as measured by the Rotter scale, and lability. **Serendipitous findings** (i.e., extra findings) included positive correlations with the number of favorable adjectives checked ($r = .27, p < .05$), defensiveness ($r = .41, p < .01$), endurance ($r = .32, p < .05$), self-control ($r = .29, p < .05$), dominance ($r = 26, p < .05$), nurturance ($r = .28, p < .05$), and affiliation ($r = .26, p < 05$) and negative correlations with the number of unfavorable adjectives checked ($r = -.30, p < .01$), succorance ($r = -.47, p < .01$) and aggression ($r = -.27, p < .05$).

Critique

Taken as a whole, this was a very successful project. A few things need further discussion, however. The scale should have been subjected to item analysis in order to reduce the number of items and increase the reliability coefficients, which are minimal and may not replicate. A "tighter" instrument might have led to stronger validity correlations. The correlation of item to total score approach should certainly be tried before settling for a more lengthy scale than is necessary.

The item analysis approach might have begun with either the first 20 items correlating best with the total score or the best correlating 20 items from among the 29 which received good ratings by 80 percent of the content validity raters. The author tends to favor the latter but would certainly try the former if the other approach failed.

Did the content validity experts judge appropriateness to each of the subconstructs or did they simply judge appropriateness to the global self-care construct? The results of content validity might easily have been presented in the article in a column next to the items, thereby aiding researchers who may wish to refine this instrument further.

The various testings and sample sizes and compositions of each were not clear in the article. Presumably, these are convenience samples. However, it appears there were pilot testings within larger testings or some such. It also seems a shame, given the frequent use of computers by all researchers, that coefficient alpha (the average of all split halves) could not be reported instead of an odd-even split. Finally, this research did *not* demonstrate a *lack* of relationship with locus of control or lability. The research quite simply failed to observe them.

Vocabulary

Alternate forms reliability	Item to total score correlation
Coefficient *alpha* (α)	Kuder-Richardson 20
Concurrent validity	Kuder-Richardson 21
Confidence intervals	Measurement error
Construct	Multitrait-multimethod matrix
Construct validity (of a measure)	Nomological network
Construct validity (of a research design)	Norm-referenced tests
Content validity	Observed score
Contrasted groups	Observer drift
Convergent validity	Operationalization
Corrected correlation	Pilot test
Correction for attenuation	Power test
Criterion complexity	Predictive validity
Criterion contamination	Psychometricians
Criterion-referenced tests	Reliability coefficient
Criterion-related validity	Sample homogeneity
Difficulty index (*p* value)	Serendipitous findings
Discrimination index	Spearman-Brown formula
Distractor	Speeded test
Divergent validity	Split-half reliability method
Empirical data	Spurious
Experimental manipulation	Standard error of measurement
Factorial validity	Sub-constructs
Feasibility study	Successive approximations
Flipping	Successive verification
Hit or miss tables	Test-retest reliability
Indicants	Time interval
Instrument credentialing	Time sampling
Internal consistency reliability	Time-out interval
Interrater reliability	True score
Intrarater reliability	Unbiased observed score
Item analysis	

References

1. Anastasi, A. *Psychological Testing* (4th ed.). London: Macmillan, Collier-Macmillan Ltd, 1976.

2. Bloom, B. S. (ed.). *Taxonomy of Educational Objectives: Handbook I: Cognitive Domain.* New York: David McKays, 1956.
3. Campbell, D. T., and Fiske, D. W. Convergent and discriminant validation by the multi-trait-multimethod matrix. *Psychol. Bull.* 56:81, 1959.
4. Cohen, J. A coefficient of agreement for nominal scales. *Educ. Psychol. Meas.* 20:27, 1960.
5. Graves, C. W. Levels of existence: An open system of values. *J. Hum. Psychol.* 10:131, 1970.
6. Guilford, J. P. *Psychometric Methods* (2nd ed.). New York: McGraw-Hill, 1954.
7. Hollingsworth, H. L. *Experimental Studies in Judgement.* New York: Science Press, 1913.
8. Hopkins, B. L., and Hermann, J. A. Evaluating interobserver reliability of interval data. *J. Appl. Behav. Anal.* 10:121, 1977.
9. Joint Committee of the American Psychological Association, American Educational Research Association, National Council on Measurement in Education; Davis, F. B., chair. *Standards for Educational and Psychological Tests.* Washington: American Psychological Association, 1974.
10. Kearney, B. Y., and Fleisher, B. J. Development of an instrument to measure exercise of self-care agency. *Res. Nurs. Health* 2:25, 1979.
11. Martuza, V. R. *Applying Norm-Referenced and Criterion-Referenced Measurement in Education.* Boston: Allyn and Bacon, 1977.
12. Nunnally, J. C. *Psychometric Theory* (2nd ed.). New York: McGraw-Hill, 1978.
13. Reisinger, J. J., and Ora, J. P. Parent-child clinic and home interaction during toddler management training. *Behav. Ther.* 8:771, 1977.
14. Spielberger, C. D., Gorsuck, R., and Luschene, R. E. *Manual for the State-Trait Anxiety Inventory.* Palo Alto: Consulting Psychologists Press, 1970.
15. Thomas, B., and Price, M. *Evaluating Research Preparation in Baccalaureate Nursing Programs.* Iowa City: University of Iowa College of Nursing, 1982.

After failing to reach agreement on whether it is a sin to smoke and pray at the same time, two nuns from different orders agreed to consult their respective Mother Superiors and meet in 2 days. When they met again, one nun asked, "Well, what did she say?"

The other responded, "She said there was no problem."

"My word," said the first nun, "my Mother Superior says it is a sin."

"Well, what did you ask?" said the second nun.

"I asked if it was all right to smoke while praying."

"Oh," said the second nun. "I asked if it was all right to pray while smoking."

This example has been used often in various forms to illustrate the relationship between the way questions are asked and the responses they receive. Researchers in questionnaire design know that small changes in the wording, method of asking questions, and setting in which questions are asked can cause large differences in responses. However, these findings are not always heeded by researchers who consider questionnaire design one of the easiest parts of research and therefore devote too little effort and time to it.

This book does not advocate (or teach) the development of tests and scales that yield interval level data on abstract variables (e.g., empathy, assertiveness, attitudes toward euthanasia), because it is an advanced skill requiring more knowledge than basic quantitative methods, and many tests and scales are already available for use either intact or with slight modification. However, it is important to know the basic elements of designing simple questionnaires, because many people are called upon to develop a questionnaire or two at some point, and nurses, in particular, can expect to do so even more often.

In general, a **questionnaire** involves written questions that a subject reads and responds to by writing in a space provided on the questionnaire. Often, to remove the suggestion of a test with *correct* answers, researchers will call the instrument an **opinionnaire** rather than a questionnaire. The researcher may or may not be present when a subject responds to a questionnaire/opinionnaire. An **interview schedule**, on the other hand, is an instrument that includes a series of questions to be asked by an interviewer and spaces for the interviewer to record a subject's responses to each question. Because most of the principles for questionnaire design pertain to interviews as well, these two methods of gathering self-report data are treated simultaneously throughout this chapter and their differences pointed out when appropriate.

Questionnaire development never begins with the generation of questions. Several steps in the process occur before this, including a search for questions that have been used successfully by others. Some researchers have ethical concerns about using the questions of others, but practice in the social and behavioral sciences not only permits but also encourages the use of such questions. It facilitates comparisons among different studies because the same questions are used. Normally, no permission from the originator of uncopyrighted questions is required or expected, although your source is cited in the report of your research. Often it is advisable to communicate with the originator to learn whether there were problems with the questions that were not discussed in the report. If you use items from a questionnaire that has been copyrighted, permission from the copyright holder is needed. Sometimes a small fee is charged. Questionnaires produced by the United States government, either directly or under contract, such as the National Institute of Mental Health (NIMH) Diagnostic Interview Schedule [4] and U.S. census forms, are in the public domain and may be used without permission. If a journal article does not include a copy of a questionnaire (and it usually does not), you must write to the author for a copy. Common courtesy dictates that you then request permission to use questions from it, and custom is that you will receive it, perhaps with a request for a copy of your results. Sometimes the search for existing questions becomes time consuming and tedious. It is time well spent, however. Your search usually helps to sharpen your research questions and improve the quality of any new questions that must be generated.

There are seven basic steps in questionnaire/interview schedule development. They are the following:

1. Determining what information is sought and why
2. Determining the appropriate type of questionnaire/schedule
3. Formulating the questions
4. Determining question sequence, format, and directions
5. Obtaining outside review
6. Revising and giving a pilot test
7. Making the final revision

Determining What Information Is Needed and Why

As stated previously, questionnaire development does not begin with formulating the questions. It does not even begin with finding those that have been used by others. It begins with *writing down* your answers to the following questions:

1. For what reasons am I proposing to conduct this research?
2. What hypotheses, research questions, and/or objectives am I using in this research?
3. What information is needed in order to complete this research? What *kind* of information is it? How many questions are needed for each kind of information?

The first question, which involves why you are conducting this research, usually evolves from your literature review, which has summarized existing knowledge about a topic and pointed out gaps—some of which you intend to fill. Of course, there are other research situations in which your motives are far less lofty. You may simply wish to elicit opinions about hospital food or rotation shifts for presentation to hospital administration in the hope that an existing policy will be modified. You may wish simply to assess health care practices and needs in a community or attitudes toward various aspects of care. Ask yourself how you intend to use your findings. Your hypotheses or research questions should be focused on the information you will need in order to use your findings as you have described. If they are not, they should be revised until they accurately reflect your overall purpose.

The third question requires a detailed listing of the information needed to address the hypotheses or research questions. The more detailed and precise you can be, the easier it will be to avoid ambiguity in writing or selecting the actual questions. At this point you may feel that this list is merely time consuming busywork. It is not. Writing down the information needed helps you to eliminate uncertainty about the direction your research should take and enables you to focus on only those areas in which information is needed. It helps prevent the "Wouldn't it be nice to know" trap, into which even experienced researchers have been known to fall. As you list the information needed, ask yourself, "Why do I want to know this?" Needing it to answer your research question is an appropriate response, but that it would just be interesting to know is not. After you have listed the information you need, it is helpful to determine what *kind* of information it is, because questions for the various kinds of information are often formulated differently. Generally, information needed can be categorized as requiring questions about the following:

1. *Behavior.* These questions describe all things a subject might do, from obtaining immunizations to wife beating. The behaviors should, in principle, be verifiable by an observer, although doing so may be extremely difficult.
2. *Knowledge.* These questions have *correct* answers. They generally focus on current issues and persons or attempt to measure educational achievement or intelligence. Knowledge questions are sometimes considered a form of behavior question.
3. *Attitudes, Beliefs, Opinions, and Values.* In contrast to knowledge questions, these questions have no correct answers. Often the response alternatives represent a continuum of possible views.
4. *Demographics.* These are the basic variables that classify or characterize individuals, such as sex, age, marital status, occupation, and income.

Finally, determine how many questions are needed for each piece of information required. The information needed, the kind of information it is, and the number of questions can be summarized in a **specification matrix**, which is similar to the content validity matrices presented in Chapter 13. Let us consider an example. Suppose your supervisor, the Director of Nursing at a large urban hospital, requests that you gather information to illuminate and suggest solutions for growing problems in the hospital—high R.N. turnover rate and frequent absenteeism. The director has already ascertained that these are significantly higher than the averages for prior years, and she suspects that they may be higher than citywide averages. She assumes that job satisfaction is low, and she wishes to find out whether any aspects of the work environment are correlated with it. Finally, she would like to know what job factors (e.g., salary, shift work, being appreciated) are most important to the nurses in order to begin devising strategies to alleviate the problems.

You begin to organize for this project by asking yourself the three questions posed at the beginning of this section:

1. *For what reasons am I proposing to conduct this research?* The Director of Nursing is concerned about high R.N. turnover rates and absenteeism. She would like to know what factors may be contributing to these (e.g., poor job satisfaction) and what might help alleviate them. You have been asked to gather relevant data and suggest solutions based on these data.

2. *What hypotheses, research questions, and/or objectives am I using in this research?* The goals of this research are to (1) describe the current situation and (2) suggest solutions. Based on your conversation with the director and a literature review of this topic area, however, you can devise a series of questions to guide your research and thereby make your task more specific:

A. What is the level of job satisfaction among R.N.s?
B. Is absenteeism related to job satisfaction?
C. How do various job-related factors (e.g., salary; fringe benefits like insurance; amount of paid vacation; shift work; beds per R.N.; being appreciated; security and safety; respect for R.N.s as equal members of the health care team; tension among coworkers; quality of care; opportunity for continued education; responsibility appropriate to education and experience) relate to job satisfaction?
D. How are these same factors perceived to occur in other area hospitals?
E. What job-related factors are most important to R.N.s?
F. Why do R.N.s resign?
G. What suggestions for improvement do R.N.s have?

3. *What information is needed in order to complete this research? What kind of information is it? How many questions are needed for each kind of information?* The research questions can now be used as guides for generating the information needed, classifying it as to kind, and determining the number of questions needed. Exhibit 14.1 displays a specification matrix for our example. It includes a fourth column heading called Comments, under which additional information or needs can be placed for use at future decision points. In the example, this space was used to suggest possible kinds of response alternatives. As shown, job satisfaction will be measured by one of the many scales already developed. You have selected a 20-item scale, whose questions seem most relevant for nurses and which has already been used in similar research. In this way, results from this study can be compared with other studies that used this

Exhibit 14-1. Specification matrix.

Information Needed	Kind of Information	Number of Questions	Comments
Level of job satisfaction	Attitudes, beliefs	20	Use an already developed Likert scale
Absenteeism	Behavior	1	
Evaluation of 12 job-related factors	Attitudes, beliefs	12	5-point Likert type: 1 = needs improvement; 5 = outstanding
Evaluation of 12 job-related factors in other hospitals	Attitudes, beliefs	12	3-point scale: 1 = below average; 2 = average; 3 = above average
Three most important job-related factors	Attitudes, beliefs	1	Fill in the blank
Reasons why colleagues have quit	Attitudes, beliefs	1	Open-ended
Suggestions for improvement	Attitudes, beliefs	1	Open-ended
Years worked as a nurse	Behavior/ demographic	1	
Time worked at this hospital	Behavior/ demographic	1	
Present assignment (i.e., unit)	Demographic	1	

same instrument. Absenteeism could be obtained from personnel files; however, this would require obtaining respondents' names (or a code). Because these questions are potentially threatening, a decision to give complete anonymity disallows this option. Therefore, subjects in the research (Ss) will be asked how often they were absent from work during a specified period (e.g., last year). This assessment will, of course, contain error, which can be estimated by comparing the sample mean with the observed figure from the personnel department. It could be an underestimate. Based on the literature search and a pilot test, 12 job-related factors have been generated. These will be used twice, first to obtain a five-point evaluation of each as it applies to this hospital and second to obtain a three-point evaluation of each as it is perceived to occur in area hospitals (i.e., the competition). From these 12, subjects in the research will then select the three that are most important to them. Two open-ended questions (i.e., reasons for resigning given by colleagues who have left and suggestions for improvement) will capture additional factors not anticipated and validate those being assessed. Only three demographic questions are needed beyond the staff characteristics already available from the personnel department. The number of years worked as a nurse and present assignment will allow comparisons among specialties and number of years in nursing. If not measured and incorporated into the design, both might become confounding variables.

Determining the Appropriate Type of Questionnaire/Schedule

To determine the type of interview or questionnaire to use, you must consider a number of things:

1. What are the special characteristics of your study population? How many subjects are needed?
2. What resources (e.g., time, money, person power, duplicating equipment, office space) are available? Do you have a deadline?
3. Which type of administration—interview or questionnaire; single or group; face-to-face, telephone, or mail—best suits your purposes, considering your resources and the characteristics of the study population? With which will refusals be minimized?
4. What type of response options are appropriate? Are open- or closed-ended responses most appropriate? What level of measurement is needed? Are questionnaires/interview schedules to be precoded for easy data entry into a computer?

The educational level and language/vocabulary of the study population is particularly important to assess so that errors in communication do not occur. There may be special needs if hearing- or vision-impaired persons are targeted. Interviews rather than questionnaires may be required. A translator may be necessary for non-English-speaking subjects. If your research questions involve sensitive topics for a particular group, anonymity rather than confidentiality may be required and this, of course, can be obtained only via questionnaire. If your sample is to be, say, burn patients, the time involved in answering questions must be kept short. They may not be able to cope with a self-administered questionnaire, either, thus mandating an interview. Are potential subjects in one location or must home visits be made? In general, relevant parameters to consider are age range, educational level, occupation, and even geographic location. Major differences in these variables produce very different capacities to respond to questions. By creating a profile of your study population, then, you will not only be better able to tailor the level of language (simple or complex) used in questions and directions but also be better able to select intelligently the best vehicle for obtaining *enough* accurate answers.

Another major consideration for deciding between the two kinds of interviews (i.e., face-to-face or telephone) and three kinds of questionnaires (i.e., mail, one-to-one, or group administered) involves the resources available to you and any deadlines you might have for obtaining and reporting the information. Obviously, interviews will cost more and take longer. They allow greater flexibility, however, for probing and obtaining observational data. Are trained interviewers available or must a training program be developed? Is there office or conference room space available to do this? Are funds available for postage, home visits, telephone interviews, travel expenses, salaries, or printing a questionnaire? How will data be coded and analyzed? Are computer time and programming available? If analysis "by hand" is necessary, fewer questions might be used, particularly if a short turnaround time is involved for reporting results.

Tempered by the characteristics of the study population and the resources available, you must select the best vehicle for meeting your purpose. If your purpose is to assess a level of knowledge, for example, you would not use a mailed questionnaire because subjects could look up answers. On the other hand, if records or other persons must be consulted before complete information can be given, a mailed questionnaire is the best choice. The pros and cons of questionnaires and interviews have already been presented in Chapter 11. The following points (and also many in the next section on formulating questions) should also be considered:

1. The number and complexity of **skip instructions** (i.e., directions indicating which question to answer next, usually skipping over some questions, based on a person's answer to the question just asked) is limited on questionnaires, particularly mailed questionnaires, on which confusing instructions generally lead to a lower participation rate.
2. The number and difficulty of open-ended questions is also limited on questionnaires. Never start a questionnaire with such a question. Instead, place them toward the end to give subjects a chance to make additional comments. Most open-ended responses are only a sentence or two. When longer responses are requested, refusals to answer the question or even the entire questionnaire occur. Many written answers need to be discarded anyway, because they are inappropriate or unable to be coded for analysis.
3. Because probing is impossible and long written answers should be avoided on questionnaires, it is unwise to ask subjects *why* they answered a question in a certain way. This type of question is much more successful in interviews.
4. The appearance of mailed questionnaires is very important to high response rates and few omissions. Questionnaires should also be short (i.e., four pages or less) unless the topic is highly salient.
5. With telephone interviews, cards with response alternatives obviously cannot be used with more complex questions. Therefore, because respondents can keep only a small number of alternatives in mind, questions should have no more than three or four alternatives. Sometimes a numerical display of sorts can be provided by using the telephone dial or a thermometer as a reference on which to base responses. If pictures, products, or response cards must be used, they can be mailed to subjects prior to a telephone interview.
6. Telephone questions about sensitive items like income are difficult because of subject suspicion. A longer introduction or other introductory questions sometimes help. Questions about race or the condition of the home, which

are ordinarily just observed and recorded by a face-to-face interviewer are also difficult.

7. Complex skip instructions are possible on telephone interviews as well as face-to-face interviews. Moreover, telephone interviews can be just as lengthy as face-to-face and considerably longer and more complex than questionnaires.

Having made the decisions between questionnaire or interview and face-to-face, telephone, or mail, you must make a few other decisions about response options in order to meet requirements for data analysis. First, the number and extent of open-ended responses should be determined. Some information can be captured only with this type of response; however, it generally requires content analysis of responses prior to any statistical analysis. Content analysis requires a lot of time, person power, and devotion. The first two are more possible when you have sufficient funding. With devotion and funding, almost anything is possible. However, open-ended and closed-ended responses to the same question might be different. For example, it is known that omitted non-threatening behavior alternatives and answers lumped into an "other" category will be substantially underreported as compared with items that are listed separately (Belson and Duncan, [3]). On the other hand, open-ended responses are better than closed-ended for obtaining information on *frequency* of socially undesirable behavior. This type of open-minded response does not carry with it the usual drawbacks, however, because the *frequency* is all that is desired, and it can be easily coded for data analysis.

A second consideration about response options must be the level of measurement desired. Sometimes this cannot be manipulated, but in other cases, as with knowledge and attitude questions, it can easily be designed for interval level measurement or lower. Age, income, and some other demographic variables can also be measured at either the interval or nominal level. Data analysis plans to test your hypotheses/research questions should be considered and these needs balanced with practicality (e.g., subjects generally prefer to report income in categories, like less than $10,000 or from $10,001 to $20,000, rather than as the exact amount). When undecided or in the absence of arguments either way, try for interval level measurement. You will have more options later on.

Third, questionnaires and interview schedules, whenever possible, should be designed with computer analysis coding, so that data can be entered onto cards or tape directly, thereby bypassing data coding onto 80-column sheets as described in Chapter 6. Instead, the column number of the coding sheet on which the response would have been coded is written next to the place where the response is recorded. Column numbers range consecutively from 1 to whatever is needed—where 1 through 80 indicate one "card," 81 through 160 the next, 161 through 250 the next, and so on. Thus, the questionnaire, or schedule, serves also as a coding sheet. This is illustrated in several of the Exhibits represented in this chapter.

Formulating Questions

We are all aware of how the wording of questions can affect responses. This chapter began with such an example. Consider the following questions as an additional example:

1. Do you feel there is too much power over our education concentrated in the hands of absent-minded professors?
2. Are you in favor of allowing department chairperson czars the power to cancel an entire course just because not enough students signed up, thereby forcing those who wanted the course to be deprived and suffer the consequences?
3. Should all students be forced into being dues-paying members of the Student Association, thus raising the cost of education for students?

Words like "absent-minded," "czars," "power," "deprived," "suffer," and "forced" are considered **loaded words**, words that can be expected to produce a specific response. **Loaded questions** are worded so that certain desired answers are more likely to be given by respondents. In the second question, chairpersons are labeled as "czars" in an effort to depict them as being dictators not considering input from students or the consequences of their actions. Furthermore, to bring the point home, the question loads for the desired response by also describing the students as "deprived" and "suffering." In the third question, the idea of "forced" membership combined with mentioning only the consequences rather than benefits also produces another loaded question. These questions are obviously inappropriate. No one would take responses to them very seriously. However, loading can become much more subtle. Consider the following two examples from two national surveys about United States involvement in the Korean war:

1. *Gallup, January 1951:* Do you think the U.S. made a mistake in deciding to defend Korea, or not?
Wrong	49%
Right	38%
Don't know	13%
2. *National Opinion Research Center, January 1951:* Do you think the U.S. was right or wrong in sending American troops to stop the Communist invasion of South Korea?
Wrong	36%
Right	55%
Don't know	6%

Use of the word "mistake" in the first question encouraged respondents toward the negative, while in the second question "stop the Communist invasion" encouraged positive responses toward the war. In fact, researchers have found that U.S. foreign policy decisions are more often approved when the decision is described as trying "to stop communism." Thus, avoiding loaded questions can sometimes be difficult. The solution, of course, is to use good questions developed and tried by others.

In addition to loaded questions that can bias responses, there are other sources of error in getting accurate data. These have to do with the subjects themselves and can be summarized into four sources:

1. *Knowledge*. Subjects may simply not know the answer or they may know only an incorrect one. Sometimes it is therefore wise to include a "don't know" response.
2. *Communication*. Subjects may not understand the question. This can be because of the use of vocabulary words or concepts that are too difficult for the population being sampled, ambiguous questions, or failure to give adequate directions. Pilot testing should bring communication problems to light.
3. *Motivation*. Subjects may want to look good in the eyes of the researcher and may therefore distort or not tell the truth. They may become bored and therefore given flippant answers or they could actually fear telling the truth because of possible consequences. Anonymity sometimes helps this with the use of questionnaires rather than interviewers. Careful phrasing, as in "Do you happen to . . . exercise, smoke marijuana, . . ." often reduces the tendency to give *socially desirable* answers. Explaining the purpose of the research and the good that will come from it often encourages subjects to take the research seriously by giving accurate answers.
4. *Memory*. When subjects are asked to report behavior that occurred in the past, they may make omissions because they have forgotten certain events. They may also telescope. **Telescoping** involves not remembering *when* behavior occurred. It usually involves remembering a behavior as having occurred during the time period of the question when, in reality, it occurred during an earlier time period. There are several **aided recall** procedures that can be used to help persons remember more accurately. These are discussed in the next section, involving questions about behavior.

Questions About Behavior

The most common questions asked relate to a subject's behavior, such as "How often do you take your baby to the clinic for a checkup?" or "Have you been immunized against polio?" This kind of question is sometimes not as easy and straightforward as you might expect. Such questions are subject to all the errors that have just been mentioned, although the major problem is likely to be memory. Therefore there are a number of pointers that should be kept in mind when you are formulating questions about behavior.

For nonthreatening behavior, subjects usually give more accurate information about themselves than about family members, friends, and coworkers. There are situations, however, especially when cost is a factor, in which **informants** can provide reasonably accurate information about others (e.g., spouses about each other, parents about children). Research has shown that, in general, reports about others are 10 percent to 20 percent less accurate than reports about self, unless the behavior is threatening [8]. Informants may not know about the behavior or may have forgotten about it because it was not considered salient. If an informant does know about the behavior and it is salient (e.g., hospitalization), it is an especially good way to screen a population to find those with certain characteristics.

Second, use words that everyone understands *and* defines in the same way. Slang and colloquialisms should be avoided unless all respondents would understand them. Our language has words that have multiple meanings (e.g., "fair" can mean "average," "pretty good," "not bad," "favorable," "barely acceptable," "just") and these should be avoided. In order to have single words that everyone understands and that have only one meaning, researchers often give explanations of a word first and then use the word itself. For example, consider the question "Do you tithe?" It could confuse subjects who do not know what the word *tithe* means. Some researchers therefore ask "Do you tithe—that is, give 10 percent of your income to your church and charity?" This, however, could be considered talking down. It is as if the researcher did not expect the subject to know what the word means. A better approach, therefore, is "Do you give 10 percent of your income to your church and charity—that is, tithe?" A careful pilot test conducted by an experienced researcher who is sensitive to respondents is the best way of discovering problem words. It is often helpful to ask subjects at the end of the pilot test, "What did you think we meant when we asked . . . ?"

Third, practice has been to make questions as short as possible. This is known to be most effective with attitude questions. However, with questions about behavior, longer questions can help to reduce the number of omitted events and thus improve memory cues of the events. A longer question also takes more time for an interviewer to read and provides more time for subjects to think and recall. Of course, longer questions do have the disadvantage of increasing the chance of telescoping, remembering an event from a prior time period as belonging to the one in question. Sudman and Bradburn [11] give an example of short and long questions about wine drinking, in which the possible uses of wine in the long question help subjects to remember occasions when they might have had wine:

Short: Did you ever drink, even once, wine or champagne?
(If yes) Have you drunk any wine or champagne in the past year?

Long: Wines have been increasingly popular in this country over the last few years; by wines, we mean liqueurs, cordials, sherries, and similar drinks, as well as table wines, sparkling wines, and champagne. Did you ever drink, even once, wine or champagne?
(If yes) You might have drunk wine to build your appetite before dinner, to accompany dinner to celebrate some occasion, to enjoy a party, or for some other reason. Have you drunk any wine or champagne in the last year?

The longer question would be appropriate with subjects who had drunk little wine during the time period. It would be a waste of time with more frequent drinkers. It is also more appropriate with interviews than with questionnaires in which subjects must read all the additional material and could well quit. Longer questions are especially appropriate with behavior that might be socially undesirable.

Fourth, selecting the time period within which the behaviors being asked about would have occurred must be done carefully. As a rule, forgetting is related to the importance attached to a behavior and the length of time since it occurred. Major events that do not occur often, such as marriage, the birth of a child, the purchase of a home, graduation, and the death of a parent are generally remembered indefinitely. Ordinary, habitual events like brushing teeth or taking pills can become difficult to remember for even a day or two. Holding unusualness constant, the greater the cost or benefit of a behavior, the more likely we are to remember it. Thus, for highly salient events (e.g., major accidents or illness), periods of a year or even more may be possible. For low salience behaviors (e.g., foods eaten) periods of 2 weeks to a month are more appropriate. For intermediate saliency (e.g., clinic visits) 1 to 3 months may be all that is appropriate. Of course, saliency of events will vary from population to population and this must be ascertained prior to formulating questions. For example, among a reasonably healthy population the number of physician visits might be remembered for a year or more, while among the chronically ill for whom these visits have become habitual, a month may yield the most accurate data. In addition, if summary information is available for a longer period (e.g., clinic visits from medical charts or insurance reimbursement forms), it is best to use the information for this longer period rather than ask respondents about a shorter period and then extrapolating it to, say, a year. Diaries are another useful technique, especially for habitual behaviors like food intake. For food diaries, for instance, researchers have found that a minimum of 4 days over a weekend (Friday through Monday) are necessary, with a 7-day record yielding even better, more accurate data. Trained coders will then extract from the diaries the amount of carbohydrate intake, deficiencies (from RDA standards), or whatever are the dependent variables. Diaries, of course, should be kept relatively short (i.e., 10 to 20 pages) to avoid underreporting. It is also important to ask for reports of several items rather than just the target behavior to prevent too much focus on a single behavior and the risk of changing it as a result of the diary, as discussed in Chapter 11.

Fifth, make questions as specific as possible. Instead of asking about *usual* behavior, ask about behavior during a specific time period. It should always be clear whether subjects are responding for only themselves or for others also. Therefore, because "you" is both singular and plural, it is best to use "you, yourself," "you or any member of the household," or "you and all other members of this household." "Household" can be replaced by "organization," "team," and the like. Where the behavior occurred should also be specified. Does it include job-related behavior, activity while on vacation, or behavior not related to the job that occurs on weekdays only? For example, consider the following wording for questions about jogging [11].

1. During the past month, aside from any work you do home or at work, did you do anything regularly—that is, on a daily basis—that helped you keep physically fit?

    _____ Yes

    _____ No

2. A. Do you happen to jog, or not?

    _____ Yes

    _____ No

    B. On the average, how far do you usually jog in terms of miles or fractions of miles? _____

Exercise is clearly limited to that which is not work at home or at a job and also to that which occurs on a daily basis. Notice how the vague term "regularly" is defined as on a "daily basis." Words like "regularly," "usually," "weekday," "children," "young people," "generally," and "proportion" are often misunderstood. (Subjects interpret broad terms less broadly than intended and often distort questions to fit their own situations.) Also note the use of "Do you happen to" and "or not." These are intended to give the appearance of equal importance to a negative answer and minimize a tendency to say "yes" when, in fact, it is not on or nearly on a daily basis. Finally, the time period, the past month, is specified. Few persons could answer "yes" to daily exercise without some time period being specified. By using the last month, those *currently* getting some form of exercise can be determined. In fact, whenever possible the best wording is "In the past two weeks, that is, since October 10, . . ."

Last, behavior questions are helped by aided-recall procedures, particularly when **underreporting** of behavior is of concern. **Aided-recall procedures** provide memory cues for behavior and knowledge questions. These can include the use of lists, inventories, pictures, and detailed questions. Rather than ask if subjects have strong fears of things that they therefore try to avoid—phobias, the NIMH Diagnostic Interview Schedule [4] used the following approach:

68. Some people have phobias, that is, such a strong fear of something or some situation that they try to avoid, even though they know there is no real danger. Have you ever had such an *unreasonable* fear of_____(phobia)_____ that you tried to avoid it? (Repeat for each phobia listed. If the answer is "yes" or "it doesn't interfere with my life a lot, because I avoid it," record an example).

    A. Heights

    B. Tunnels or bridges

    C. Being in a crowd

    D. Being on any kind of public transportation like airplanes, buses, or elevators

    E. Going out of the house alone

    F. Being in a closed place

    G. Being alone

    H. Eating in front of other people (either people you know or in public)

I. Speaking in front of a small group of people you know
J. Speaking to strangers or meeting new people
K. Storms
L. Being in water, for instance in a swimming pool or lake
M. Spiders, bugs, mice, snakes, or bats
N. Being near any harmless animal or a dangerous animal that couldn't get to you
O. Is there anything else you were unreasonably terrified to do or be near?

By actually listing each phobia, you provide memory cues. In this particular case, in addition, it may be much easier to say "yes" than to name the actual fear. Another form of aided recall is to put some examples into questions, like "How many kinds of exercise do you participate in at least once a month—baseball, jogging, bowling, golf, hiking, or tennis for example?" Similarly, subjects can be shown a card with all possible responses listed. A final form of aided recall is the joint inventory, conducted by both the respondent and interviewer. Home visits conducted as part of compliance research often use this approach. Subjects are asked to bring all their medicine to the interviewer, who then tests their knowledge about the instructions for use and often counts the number of pills taken (or remaining) as one measure of compliance. Researchers have found that use of aided-recall procedures produces higher levels of reported behavior. Certain precautions are necessary with these procedures, however:

1. Lists should be as exhaustive as possible. Behaviors not listed or included only in "other" will be underreported as compared with those that are listed.
2. When the number of alternatives is great, you will have to limit the number of listed items to the *most likely*.
3. Always include an "other" category. It is useful in building rapport and allows subjects to have their say. However, data from "other" cannot be combined with listed data.
4. Sometimes you can proceed in stages. Instead of listing all journals, they could be listed by major categories (e.g., nursing journals) with a few examples of each. Next the actual journals could be listed for only those categories that were selected.
5. The order of long lists can be important, especially those that subjects read. Items given first receive more attention and more positive responses. Thus, researchers often have several alternate forms of a list in which items have been reordered randomly.
6. Long lists (e.g., 50 behaviors) suggest to subjects that some behaviors should have "yes" responses. This results in deliberate fibbing or unconscious misremembering. Having lists on which everyone could answer "yes" to a few items or **screening questions**, like "Do you happen to have read any research journals in the past 2 months?" before using the list can counteract this.
7. In situations in which omissions are not frequent because behaviors are very salient or recent, aided recall can lead to overreporting.

8. Screening questions, when used frequently, teach respondents that saying "no" saves them the trouble of dealing with a long list. Therefore, vary the format to avoid deliberate fibbing and make the process more interesting for subjects.

Exhibit 14.2 illustrates a series of questions about smoking from the NIMH Diagnostic Interview Schedule [4]. They serve to summarize via illustrations this discussion of questions about behavior. On the extreme right are the column numbers for data coding and computer entry. Because this is an interview, notice the many **skip instructions**. "Have you ever . . ." makes the question less threatening and more casual. Smoking "daily" and "for a month or so" makes the question more specific and ties down the time period of interest. The list of problems in D is aided recall. Note how F very carefully determines when the subject quit smoking "half a pack or more in one day." Are there any words that may be ambiguous or unknown to some respondents (e.g., serious illness, nervous, drowsy)? How might these be improved?

Threatening Questions About Behavior

If you believe a question may be threatening, there are some additional considerations to keep in mind. A rule of thumb for determining whether a question is threatening is that a subject may think there is a right or wrong answer. If certain behaviors are seen as socially desirable or undesirable, these questions may also be threatening and therefore result in overreporting or underreporting, respectively. Barton [2] presented an amusing primer of traditional techniques a number of years ago:

The pollster's greatest ingenuity has been devoted to finding ways to ask embarrassing questions in nonembarrassing ways. We give here examples of a number of these techniques, as applied to the question "Did you kill your wife?"

The Casual Approach:

"Do you happen to have murdered your wife?"

The Numbered Card:

"Would you please read off the number on this card which corresponds to what became of your wife?" (Hand card to respondent.)

1. Natural death
2. I killed her
3. Other (What)?

(Get the card back from respondent before proceeding!)

The Everybody Approach:

"As you know, many people have been killing their wives these days. Do you happened to have killed yours?"

Exhibit 14-2. Smoking behavior questions.

15. Have you ever smoked cigarettes daily for a month or more?

38/

No   (SKIP TO Q. 16)   ①
Yes   (ASK A-C)   ⑤

a. How old were you when you first smoked daily?

Enter age: ⓪ ① ② ③ ④ ⑤ ⑥ ⑦ ⑧ ⑨
             ⓪ ① ② ③ ④ ⑤ ⑥ ⑦ ⑧ ⑨   39/

b. Have you ever continued to smoke when you had a serious illness that you knew made it unwise for you to smoke?
   No   ①   41/
   Yes   ⑤

c. Have you ever tried to quit or reduce your smoking?
   No   (Answer C1)   ①   42/
   Yes   (Ask D)   ⑤
   C1: IF Q. 15B is coded 1, skip to Q. 16.
       If Q. 15B is coded 5, skip to E.

d. I'm going to ask about some problems you might have had in the first day or so after you quit or cut down. READ ITEMS 1-8 AND CODE FOR EACH.

	No	Yes	
1) For instance, did you crave a cigarette?	①	⑤	43/
2) Were you irritable?	①	⑤	44/
3) Were you nervous?	①	⑤	45/
4) Were you restless?	①	⑤	46/
5) Did you have trouble concentrating?	①	⑤	47/
6) Did you have headaches?	①	⑤	48/
7) Were you drowsy?	①	⑤	49/
8) Did you have an upset stomach?	①	⑤	50/

e. Did you ever talk to a doctor about problems with smoking?
   No   ①   51/
   Yes   ⑤

f. How long ago did you last smoke half a pack or more in one day or do you still?

	Never smoked 1/2 pack per day	(SKIP TO Q. 16)	⑦
CODE MOST	Within last 2 weeks	(SKIP TO Q. 16)	①
RECENT TIME	Within last month	(SKIP TO Q. 16)	②
POSSIBLE	Within last 6 months	(SKIP TO Q. 16)	③
	Within last year	(SKIP TO Q. 16)	④
	More than 1 year ago	(ASK G)	⑤

g. IF MORE THAN ONE YEAR: How old were you then?

Enter age: ⓪ ① ② ③ ④ ⑤ ⑥ ⑦ ⑧ ⑨
             ⓪ ① ② ③ ④ ⑤ ⑥ ⑦ ⑧ ⑨   53/

Reprinted from the NIMH Diagnostic Interview Schedule [4].

The "Other People" Approach:

(a) "Do you know any people who have murdered their wives?"
(b) "How about yourself?"

The Sealed Ballot Technique:

In this version you explain that the survey respects people's right to anonymity in respect to their marital relations, and that they themselves are to fill out the answer to the question, seal it in an envelope, and drop it in a box conspicuously labeled "Sealed Ballot Box" carried by the interviewer.

The Kinsey Technique:

Stare firmly into respondent's eyes and ask in simple, clear-cut language such as that to which the respondent is accustomed, and with an air of assuming that everyone has done everything, "Did you ever kill your wife?"

Putting the question at the end of the interview.

Recent research results give us more guidance when the data we need are sensitive. First, when a question involves the occurrence of socially undesirable behavior, longer questions that are open-ended (although perhaps only coded as yes/no) are better. For example, the NIMH Diagnostic Interview Schedule [4] used the following long questions:

176. Some people have problems with feelings that they have to do something over and over again even though they know it is really foolish—but they can't resist doing it—things like washing their hands again and again or going back several times to be sure they've locked a door or turned off the stove. Have you ever had to do something like that over and over?
    A. Was there a time when you always had to do something—like getting dressed perhaps—in a certain order, and had to start all over if you got the order wrong? _____ No _____ Yes
177. Did you have to do this for a short time, or do you feel you had to do this over a period of several weeks?
    _____ Short time _____ Several weeks
179. How old were you when you first had to (do something over and over/check on things/ . . .)?
    A. If "can't remember," do you think it was before you were 40 or later than that? _____ Before _____ After _____ DK

These questions allow subjects to answer in their own fashion, volunteering as much as is comfortable. The interviewer, meanwhile, codes the answers in a predetermined way, as shown. Longer questions that are also open-ended have been found to yield the most accurate information about the *frequency* of the behavior, particularly since extreme scores are not omitted.

With socially undesirable behavior, the use of informants (e.g., family members) increases accuracy, although it is reduced with nonthreatening behavior.

An exception to the use of informants is asking parents about the behavior of their children. Parents are generally more threatened and will underreport or do not know.

For undesirable behavior, there are several **loading techniques** that have been used successfully. One is the use of the everybody-does-it approach. The question indicates that the behavior is common, thereby reducing the threat of reporting it. Another involves assuming the behavior exists and asking about frequency or other details. When this approach is used (e.g., how many alcoholic drinks do you have each week?), one response must be "none." A disadvantage of this approach is that some subjects may be uncomfortable with your assumption and therefore be less cooperative with the rest of the interview. A third loading technique involves the use of authority to justify behavior. The authorities are groups of persons, like lawyers, doctors, or scientists. An example might be "Scientists have found that sweets can be good now and then. How often during the past week did you have candy, cake, pie, and other sweets?" Fourth, the question can be embedded in a series of behavior questions of more and less threat in order to reduce the perceived importance of the topics. Finally, the "Did you happen to . . ." phrase, which is intended to reduce the importance of a topic, has been found *not to increase* reporting of socially *undesirable* behavior and possibly even to increase the threat.

There are also loading techniques used for reducing **overreporting** of socially desirable responses. First, use of words like "for certain" or "for sure" indicate that not remembering is a possible answer. Second, you can indicate that there are good reasons for not always engaging in the behavior. For example, you might ask "Did things come up that kept you from keeping your appointment, or did you keep it?" Third, the use of aided recall helps reduce telescoping and prevent confusion with similar behaviors. Another technique is to ask about the behavior in a series of questions about many behaviors in order to reduce its importance. The question might also be embedded among a series of attitude questions thereby placing the focus on the attitudes rather than behavior. Last, use of an informant or a single respondent for an entire household can also reduce overreporting.

Alternatives to the standard one-to-one interview can be used to reduce the threat of questions. The rationale here is that the more anonymous a respondent feels, the more truthful (assuming memory is accurate) will be the responses. Self-administered questionnaires, particularly group administered, provide the most anonymity. Although mail surveys without coding for follow-up are also completely anonymous, subjects often think the researcher knows who they are, anyway. Anonymity may work better for desirable behaviors because the need to impress an interviewer is removed. There is no research as yet that demonstrates the effectiveness of anonymity in reducing underreporting of socially undesirable behaviors. Researchers continue to use anonymity however, in the absence of anything else. It does seem reasonable to assume that subjects might be hesitant to express, say, their beliefs about abortion to an interviewer without knowing the interviewer's beliefs, while in an anonymous situation there would be no hesitation at all. Diaries have also been used successfully in dealing with threatening behaviors. Reporting these behaviors over time provides an **adaption period** whereby subjects become less inhibited.

Finally, try to check the accuracy of responses. Asking the same question more than once on a questionnaire is not recommended, because subjects either consider the researcher disorganized (or worse) or suspect the researcher of trickery. Either way, the result is usually a less cooperative subject. Researchers therefore ask questions at the end like, "Do you think these questions would make *most* people very uneasy, moderately uneasy, slightly uneasy, or not at all?" Use of a projective question about "most people" is less threatening than a direct one. This question not only helps determine the level of threat but also gives an indication of response accuracy, because those who report that the questions would make most people very uneasy are more likely than others to underreport [11]. A last way of assessing accuracy is to compare responses with aggregate data for that geographic region. What were donations per capita to charity and how does this figure compare to your sample statistic? How does your sample statistic on abortions received compare with local figures? None of these, of course is perfect. However, some indication of accuracy is better than none.

Questions About Knowledge

As stated before, the intent of this book is not the *development* of tests and scales. This is an advanced and specialized area, psychometrics, which is well beyond the scope of an introductory or intermediate level text. However, many of the commonly used methods of development were presented in Chapters 12 and 13 in order to give you the necessary background not only to select existing tests and scales but also to modify them for your purposes and then develop the necessary instrument credentials for your modified instruments. With this stated, some points are presented should you need to measure knowledge with a few questions on a questionnaire or interview schedule.

1. Ask knowledge questions to screen out subjects who lack sufficient knowledge to respond to attitude questions.
2. Reduce the threat of knowledge questions by asking them as opinions or using "Do you happen to know . . ." or "Can you recall, offhand . . ."
3. When testing ability to identify persons or organizations, ask for additional information or include fictitious names on your list. Some subjects will say they know so-and-so when they really do not.
4. Reduce the likelihood of successful guessing when using yes-no or true-false questions by asking several on the same topic.
5. For questions with numerical answers, use open-ended responses to avoid giving away the answer.

6. Ask only one question at a time. Beware of **double-barreled questions** (e.g., In your opinion, is the ocean purple because it reflects atmospheric conditions?), which are really two separate questions.
7. Administrations like mail surveys are inappropriate, because subjects can look up answers or consult with others.
8. If at all possible, use questions already developed by others.

All the other pointers about clarity and unambiguous language apply to questions about knowledge also. Finally, make sure the *correct* answer is also not ambiguous.

Questions About Attitudes

The best way to measure attitudes is with preexisting questions—as long as they measure the same attitude as the one you had in mind. Even if you use an entire scale developed by someone else, it can be embedded into your questionnaire in order to have a smooth "flow." More will be said about this later. Attitudes, opinions, beliefs, perceptions, intentions, and the like are used interchangeably here. Depending on which discipline (e.g., social psychology, political science, sociology) provides your theoretical framework, each may have subtle distinctions. As they are conceived of here, they all share the fact that they are psychological states that are unverifiable except by self-report. They have no "correct" or "accurate" answer in the sense that these terms are used with questions about knowledge or behavior. Attitudes and beliefs do not exist in the abstract altogether, however. They are always about or toward something. This something is called the **referent** or attitude object. It can be anything from health care to freedom to life force to Nurse Jones. The first step in measuring this group we shall call attitudes, then, is to know precisely what is your referent. All the principles of clarity and definition described in the section about behavior questions apply. Next, you must be clear about what aspects of an attitude toward a referent you wish to assess. These include (1) evaluative aspects (e.g., like/dislike, favor/disfavor, pro/con; (2) cognitive aspects (e.g., what a subject thinks, knows, believes, or perceives about the referent); and (3) action aspects (e.g., a subject's willingness or intention to do something toward or with the referent). In addition to these three aspects you may wish to assess the strength (e.g., extremely, somewhat, slightly, none) of any of these three aspects of attitudes toward the referent. In the case of the evaluative aspect, Likert scaling can combine the strength and evaluation itself with alternatives like "strongly agree, slightly agree, uncertain, slightly disagree, and strongly disagree." With the other two aspects it is less easy to combine them with strength in a *single* question. Another strategy for measuring the strength of an attitude in combination with one or more of the three aspects is to use one of the several attitude scale techniques (e.g., Likert, Thurstone, semantic differential) presented in Chapter 12. Development of scales like that (i.e., scales with two or more items) are beyond the scope of this discussion, however. Should you wish to develop several single attitude questions for a questionnaire, in addition to the suggestions made earlier in this chapter, keep the following pointers in mind:

1. Clearly define the referent and aspects to be assessed. Then, make sure the strength is also assessed, if appropriate.
2. Avoid double-barreled questions, which introduce multiple concepts and have no single answer.
3. The presence or absence of an explicitly stated alternative can greatly affect responses. Specification of alternative responses standardizes the question for respondents. Open-ended responses are often hard to compare and should be used sparingly.
4. Always **pilot test** new attitude items.
5. Because of **order effects**, ask general questions before specific ones. Respondents tend to subtract the referent of the preceding specific question from the referent of a general question when it is asked last. Results are therefore distorted.
6. When asking a series of questions about the same referent that are of varying popularity (or social desirability), ask the least popular first. In terms of alternative responses this is especially important. Otherwise, subjects tend to select a more popular or desirable alternative and never read or hear the others.
7. Do not have more than four or five response alternatives unless they are on a numerical scale. With telephone interviews, try to use only three nonnumerical alternatives. When lists or many alternatives must be used, have subjects rank the three most desirable and three least desirable. More complex rankings can be obtained via a series of paired comparisons, or yes-no type responses to each item on the list. However, respondent fatigue and boredom must be considered.
8. Complex ratings on several dimensions can sometimes be accomplished via card-sorting procedures.

When subjects are asked to rank-order a list of things during a telephone interview, a special memory problem emerges—unless written material has been mailed in advance. The first and last items on the list, no matter what they are, are selected more often. Therefore, the alternatives are sometimes broken up into a series of simpler questions:

1. What do you think is most important—friendly nurses or good physical care?
2. What do you think is most important—private rooms or longer visiting hours?
3. What do you think is most important—being taught all about your illness and how to care for it or having your doctor visit twice a day?
4. What is most important—good hospital food or separate television sets for each bed?
5. Which do you think is most important—Answer 1 or Answer 2?
6. And which do you think is most important—Answer 3 or Answer 4?
7. Between Answer 5 and Answer 6, which is most important?

As a final check, you might ask "I guess that you think Answer 7 is the most important. Is that right?" Another way to handle the question would be by asking the entire question first and then repeating each item for a Likert-type response:

I'm going to read you a list of things that hospitalized patients are concerned about. These include good physical care, friendly nurses, doctor visits twice a day, being taught all about your illness and how to care for it, private rooms, television sets for every bed not just each room, good food, and longer visiting hours. Assuming that not everything is equally important, please tell me, for each, whether it is (1) very important, (2) somewhat important, or (3) not so important.

		VI	*SI*	*NI*
A.	Good physical care	1	2	3
B.	Friendly nurses	1	2	3

The use of the phrase "Assuming that not everything is equally important" is intended to discourage the same response to each item. If the single most important issue is needed or if many ties result, an additional question can be asked:

(If more than one item is coded "Very Important") A, B, . . . were all considered "very important." Of these, which one would you say is the *most* important?

On the telephone, three possible responses are no problem, four are borderline, and five alternatives are too many. When five alternatives are needed, the following approach should be considered:

Do you favor, oppose or not care? (If favor) Are you strongly in favor or moderately in favor? (If oppose) Are you strongly opposed or moderately opposed?

Exhibit 14.3 presents a questionnaire used in a study conducted by the author in which health care providers' attitudes and beliefs about conducting a sex interview with five patients, each with a different diagnosis, were measured. Notice that a definition of a sex interview was given at the beginning of the questionnaire. Look at the first group of questions about R. Jones, a myocardial infarction patient. Item A measures the strength of and evaluative aspect of the referent, sex interview, which has already been clearly defined. The use of the visual "ruler" for these responses helps to give the respondent a better understanding of available choices and also helps to justify the scale of measurement as interval. Item B addresses action toward the referent and its strength. Item C gave some respondents trouble because no category was labeled "after hospitalization." Although the alternatives were intended to refer only to interviews during hospitalization, the fact that "after hospitalization" responses may have confounded the first two alternatives restricts any conclusion that may be drawn from this question. How would you reword it? Item D is straightforward. Notice how the directions are spelled out in detail.

Questions for Demographic Data

Demographic data are measures of variables like age, marital status, sex, occupation, income, race, ethnic origin, education, religion, and residence location. These basic classification variables characterize an individual or household. **Demographic questions** elicit these data from subjects. Although these variables are fairly straightforward (i.e., concrete variables) and their method of assessment rarely requires reliability and validity in the same sense that they are required for interval level tests and scales measuring abstract variables (e.g., anxiety, knowledge about research, or attitudes toward alcoholics), there are nevertheless several ways of "measuring" them. Some are better than others in terms of accuracy. Research studies investigating the accuracy of different ways of asking these questions have resulted in the questions shown in Exhibit 14.4.

The Social Science Research Council (SSRC [10]) has attempted to foster standardization of demographic questions and answers in order to make data from different researchers comparable and more useful for secondary and trend analysis. They have developed model items that are, for the most part, suggested in the following discussion. The SSRC recognizes also that certain research situations may require alternative or more elaborate questions, and, when this is true, researchers must of course use only items that meet their needs. In most research situations, however, the items that follow should be more than adequate.

Exhibit 14.4 presents a series of questions from which can be selected appropriate questions for an interview schedule assessing information about an entire household. The first and second questions are modified somewhat from the SSRC items, which ask first for the name of the *head of household* and then the names of others and their relationships to the *head of household*. The household *head* is used generally only as an anchor for relationship information about other household members rather than as an important variable. Therefore, more recently researchers have found it more convenient and appropriate to use the approach presented in Exhibit 14.4. Designating one member of a household as "head" implies authority structures that are not relevant in most households today and can offend potential respondents.

The age variable is very important because it is used so often in research. Therefore the exact age in years should be measured. The United States Census Bureau has found that a way to get a more accurate report is by asking two questions—age at last birthday and date of birth. These can be checked against each other during the interview and any discrepancy can be resolved at that time. If the date of birth is not known, the age at the last birthday can be accepted. Either way, the age variable should be coded in single-year rather than several-year intervals (e.g., wrong: age under 20, 20 to 30, 40 to 50). In studies in which many questions must be asked, two questions about age, as well as asking

Exhibit 14-3. Sex interview opinionnaire.

To fulfill a course requirement in our program of study for a degree in nursing, we are conducting a survey of nurses and physicians to determine their opinions about conducting a sex interview with various types of patients. We believe this survey will yield important information about which additions to curricula can be based.

We would appreciate your participation in this research. If you are willing, please answer the following questions. Your responses, of course, are completely anonymous. If you do not wish to participate, just return the opinionnaire unanswered.

Note: As used in this study, *sex interview* means obtaining information about a patient's sexual habits and values, perception of the illness or disability and its effect on sexual activity, and need for counseling or education in this regard.

1. R. Jones was admitted to the intensive coronary care unit for a myocardial infarction (MI). She remained in the ICU for 5 days before being transferred to the step-down special care unit. She was discharged 3 weeks after her MI and was seen by her physician in his private office 2 weeks later.

   a. How important is it for this patient to have a sex interview? Circle the number which reflects your belief.

1	2	3	4	5
Not important		Undecided		Very important

   b. How comfortable would you be in conducting a sex interview with this patient at an appropriate time? Circle the number which reflects your feelings.

1	2	3	4
Very uncomfortable	Somewhat uncomfort- able	Somewhat comfort- able	Very comfortable

   c. When should the sex interview be initiated? Please check only *one* response.

   _____ Only on orders of the patient's physician
   _____ Only when the patient asks
   _____ Soon after hospitalization
   _____ Shortly before discharge
   _____ Never

   d. Who should conduct the sex interview? If you select more than one response, please rank-order them. Put a 1 next to your first choice, a 2 next to your second choice, and, if you have one, a 3 next to your third choice.

   _____ Patient's physician
   _____ Any available physician
   _____ A nurse
   _____ A rehabilitation specialist
   _____ Someone from psychiatry

   · · ·

5. K. Mason, 34 years old, has had hypertension for the past 5 years. Shortly after hospitalization, Kim noticed that the medications administered in the hospital were different from those used before.

a. How important is it for this patient to have a sex interview? Circle the number which reflects your belief.

1	2	3	4	5
Not important		Undecided		Very important

b. How comfortable would you be in conducting a sex interview with this patient at an appropriate time? Circle the number which reflects your feelings.

1	2	3	4
Very uncomfortable	Somewhat uncomfortable	Somewhat comfortable	Very comfortable

c. When should the sex interview be initiated? Please check only *one* response.

_____ Only on orders of the patient's physician

_____ Only when the patient asks

_____ Soon after hospitalization

_____ Shortly before discharge

_____ Never

d. Who should conduct the sex interview? If you select more than one response, please rank-order them. Put a 1 next to your first choice, a 2 next to your second choice, and, if you have one, a 3 next to your third choice.

_____ Patient's physician

_____ Any available physician

_____ A nurse

_____ A rehabilitation specialist

_____ Someone from psychiatry

Directions: We would appreciate having some information about the participants in our study. Please complete the following:

6. What year were you born? _____   7. Sex: _____ Male _____ Female

8. Have you had a course in human sexuality or sex counseling? _____ Yes _____ No

9. What do you expect will be your specialty area?

Directions: We would like to know your opinions about other sexual matters also. Therefore, please indicate the extent to which you agree or disagree with the following statements by putting the appropriate number in the blank provided.

1. Strong agree
2. Moderately agree
3. Slightly agree
4. Slightly disagree
5. Moderately disagree
6. Strongly disagree

_____ 10. Premarital sexual relations often equip persons for more stable and happier marriages.

. . .

_____ 26. Homosexuals should be considered as no better than criminals.

Thank you very much for participating in our survey.

Exhibit 14-4. Sample interview schedule questions for demographic data.

1. Including yourself, how many people are living in this household? _____

	(1)	(2)
2. Including yourself, would you tell me the (first) name of each of these people and their relationship to you?	Name _____ Relationship _____	Name _____ Relationship _____
3. *If not obvious:* Is (name) male or female?	☐ 1. Male ☐ 2. Female	☐ 1. Male ☐ 2. Female
4. a. *For each person in the household, ask:* How old were you (name) on your birthday?	_____ years old	_____ years old
4. b. What is the month, day, and year of your (name's) birth?	Mo. Day Yr.	Mo. Day Yr.
5. a. Are you (Is name) now married (1) (to whom?); widowed (2); divorced (3); separated (4); or have you (has name) never been married (5)? Do you (does name) live with someone as husband and wife (6)?	Marital status ☐ 1. Married to _____ ☐ 2. Widowed ☐ 3. Divorced ☐ 4. Separated ☐ 5. Never Married ☐ 6. Cohabitating with _____	Marital status ☐ 1. Married to _____ ☐ 2. Widowed ☐ 3. Divorced ☐ 4. Separated ☐ 5. Never Married ☐ 6. Cohabitating with _____
5. b. *If married:* Is this your (name's) first marriage?	☐ 1. Yes ☐ 2. No	☐ 1. Yes ☐ 2. No
6. a. *Code by observation, or* what race do you consider yourself (name)?	☐ 1. White ☐ 2. Black ☐ 3. Asian ☐ 4. Other: _____	☐ 1. White ☐ 2. Black ☐ 3. Asian ☐ 4. Other: _____
	(1)	(2)
6. b. What is your (name's) origin or descent? (*Show flashcard or read list*).	☐ 1. German ☐ 2. Italian ☐ 3. Irish ☐ 4. French ☐ 5. Polish ☐ 6. Russian ☐ 7. English, Scottish, Welsh ☐ 11. Mexican-American ☐ 12. Chicano	☐ 1. German ☐ 2. Italian ☐ 3. Irish ☐ 4. French ☐ 5. Polish ☐ 6. Russian ☐ 7. English, Scottish, Welsh ☐ 11. Mexican-American ☐ 12. Chicano

	(1)	(2)
	☐ 13. Mexican (Mexicano)	☐ 13. Mexican (Mexicano)
	☐ 14. Puerto Rican	☐ 14. Puerto Rican
	☐ 15. Cuban	☐ 15. Cuban
	☐ 16. Central or South American	☐ 16. Central or South American
	☐ 17. Other Spanish	☐ 17. Other Spanish
	☐ 21. Negro or black	☐ 21. Negro or black
	☐ 31. Other (specify below)	☐ 31. Other (specify below)
	☐ 99. Don't know	☐ 99. Don't know
	Other: _____	Other: _____
	_____	_____

6. c. *If more than one origin is named,* which are you (would name be) more likely to identify with?

First choice: _____　　First choice: _____
Second choice: _____　　Second choice _____

7. What is your (name's) religion, if any? *If Protestant, specify denomination.*

☐ 1. Protestant	☐ 1. Protestant
☐ 2. Catholic	☐ 2. Catholic
☐ 3. Jewish	☐ 3. Jewish
☐ 4. None	☐ 4. None
☐ 7. Other: _____	☐ 7. Other: _____
_____	_____

8. a. Are you (Is name) now attending or enrolled in school? If yes, is that full-time or part-time?

☐ 1. Yes, full-time	☐ 1. Yes, full-time
☐ 2. Yes, part-time	☐ 2. Yes, part-time
☐ 3. No.	☐ 3. No

8. b. What is the highest grade or year you (name) finished and got credit for in regular school or college?

Education: _____　　Education: _____
(*Code highest grade completed in number of years*) (two digits; use 00 for none)　　(*Code highest grade completed in number of years*) (two digits; use 00 for none)

8. c. *If 8b is less than 12,* did you (name) receive a high school diploma or pass a high school equivalency test?

☐ 1. Yes	☐ 1. Yes
☐ 2. No	☐ 2. No

8. d. *If 8c was yes,* what school or schools did you (name) attend after you (name) completed high school? (If vocational school, ask 8g; or if college, ask 8e.)

Names of schools:　　Names of schools:
_____　　_____
_____　　_____
_____　　_____

Exhibit 14-4. (Continued)

	(1)	(2)
8. e. What degree(s) did you (name) receive?	☐ 1. Less than high school ☐ 2. High school ☐ 3. Associate degree ☐ 4. Bachelor's degree ☐ 5. Master's degree ☐ 6. Doctorate ☐ 7. Professional (M.D., J.D., D.D.S.) ☐ 8. Other: _____	☐ 1. Less than high school ☐ 2. High school ☐ 3. Associate degree ☐ 4. Bachelor's degree ☐ 5. Master's degree ☐ 6. Doctorate ☐ 7. Professional (M.D., J.D., D.D.S.) ☐ 8. Other: _____
8. f. Besides what you've already told me about your (name's) schooling, did you (name) ever attend any other kind of school, such as vocational or trade school?	☐ 1. Yes ☐ 2. No	☐ 1. Yes ☐ 2. No
8. g. *If yes to 8d or 8f,* what was your (name's) main field of vocational training?	☐ 1. Business, office work ☐ 2. Practical nurse, other health paraprofessionals ☐ 3. Trades and crafts (mechanic, electrician, beautician) ☐ 4. Engineering or science technician, drafter, computer technician ☐ 5. Agriculture, home economics ☐ 6. Other: _____	☐ 1. Business, office work ☐ 2. Practical nurse, other health paraprofessionals ☐ 3. Trades and crafts (mechanic, electrician, beautician) ☐ 4. Engineering or science technician, drafter, computer technician ☐ 5. Agriculture, home economics ☐ 6. Other: _____
9. a. Are you (name) presently employed or unemployed, retired, a student, homemaker, or what?	☐ 1. Working now Full-time Part-time (*go to 10a*) ☐ 2. Has job, but not at work due to temporary illness, vacation, labor dispute, bad weather, etc. (*go to 10a*) ☐ 3. Unemployed (*ask 9c*) ☐ 4. Retired (*ask 9b*)	☐ 1. Working now Full-time Part-time (*go to 10a*) ☐ 2. Has job, but not at work due to temporary illness, vacation, labor dispute, bad weather, etc. (*go to 10a*) ☐ 3. Unemployed (*ask 9c*) ☐ 4. Retired (*ask 9b*)

	(1)	(2)
	☐ 5. In school (*ask 9b*)	☐ 5. In school (*ask 9b*)
	☐ 6. Keeping house (*ask 9b*)	☐ 6. Keeping house (*ask 9b*)
	☐ 7. Disabled (*ask 9b*), too ill to work (*ask 9c*)	☐ 7. Disabled (*ask 9b*), too ill to work (*ask 9c*)
	☐ 8. Armed services (*ask 9c*)	☐ 8. Armed services (*ask 9c*)
	☐ 9. Other (specify): _____	☐ 9. Other (specify): _____

9. b. Are you (name) looking for work?

(*ask 9b*)

(1)	(2)
☐ 1. Yes, working full-time now (*go to 10a*)	☐ 1. Yes, working full-time now (*go to 10a*)
☐ 2. Yes, working part-time now (*go to 10a*)	☐ 2. Yes, working part-time now (*go to 10a*)
☐ 3. Yes, looking for work (*go to 9c*)	☐ 3. Yes, looking for work (*go to 9c*)
☐ 4. No (*go to 9c*)	☐ 4. No (*go to 9c*)

9. c. When did you (name) last work for pay at a regular job or business, either full-time or part-time? (code 1 for within the past 12 months, 2 for 1 to 2 years, 3 for 2 to 3 years, 4 for 3 to 4 years, 5 for 4 to 5 years, 6 for 5 or more years ago, 7 for never worked)

Last worked:	Last worked:
Mo. _____ Yr. _____ Code: _____	Mo. _____ Yr. _____ Code: _____

10. a. What kind of work do you (does name) do (or did you do on your last job)? What is your (name's) main occupation called?

Occupation	Occupation
_____	_____
_____	_____
_____	_____

10. b. Tell me a little about what you (name) do in the job. What are some of your (name's) main duties?

Duties	Duties
_____	_____
_____	_____
_____	_____

10. c. What kind of a business is that in? What do they do or make at the place where you (name) work?

(1)	(2)
Business/Industry	Business/Industry
_____	_____
_____	_____

Exhibit 14-4. (Continued)

10. d. *If subject worked at two or more kinds of work,* what kind of work have you (has name) done longer than any other? What is your (name's) usual occupation called?	Usual occupation _____ _____ _____	Usual occupation _____ _____ _____
10. e. *If 10d is asked,* tell a little more about what you (name) actually do in that job. What are some of your (name's) main duties?	Duties _____ _____ _____	Duties _____ _____ _____
If an additional probe is needed, What kind of business or industry is that in? What do they do or make at the place where you work?	Industry _____ _____	Industry _____ _____
10. f. Are you (Is name) an hourly wage worker, salaried, on commission, self-employed, or what?	☐ 1. Hourly wage ☐ 2. Salaried ☐ 3. Commission, tips ☐ 4. Self-employed in own business, professional practice, or farm ☐ 5. Works without pay in family business or farm	☐ 1. Hourly wage ☐ 2. Salaried ☐ 3. Commission, tips ☐ 4. Self-employed in own business, professional practice, or farm ☐ 5. Works without pay in family business or farm
10. g. Are you a member of a labor union?	☐ 1. Yes ☐ 2. No	☐ 1. Yes ☐ 2. No
11. a. *Hand flashcard and ask:* Would you please tell me the letter on the card which best represents your total family income in *19■■ before taxes?* This should include wages and salaries, net income from business or farm, pensions, dividends, interest, rent, and any other money income	Income Code: _____	

received by all those people in the household who are related to you.

11. b. *If probes are needed:* What would be your best guess?

Income Code: _____

11. c. *After initial response,* does that include everyone in your family who lives here? Is that before taxes or any deductions?

_____

_____

12. a. Do you (Does your family) own this house (apartment), are you buying it, do you pay rent, or what?

- ☐ 1. Living quarters other than a cooperative or condominium owned or being bought
- ☐ 2. Cooperative or condominium
- ☐ 3. Rented for cash rent
- ☐ 4. Occupied without payment of cash rent (living with relatives or living rent-free in exchange for work)
- ☐ 5. Other (specify): _____

12. b. *Code by observation:* Which best describes the building containing this housing unit (including all apartments, flats, etc., even if vacant)?

- ☐ 1. One-family detached
- ☐ 2. One-family attached to one or more houses
- ☐ 3. A building for 2 families or duplex
- ☐ 4. A building for 3 or 4 families
- ☐ 5. A building for 5 to 9 families
- ☐ 6. A building for 10 to 19 families
- ☐ 7. A building for 20 or more families
- ☐ 8. A mobile home or trailer
- ☐ 9. Other (specify): _____

12. c. How many years have you personally lived at this address? (*Enter actual number of years, rounded to the nearest year.*)

_____ years
- ☐ 00. Less than 6 months
- ☐ 90. All my life
- ☐ 98. Don't know
- ☐ 99. No answer

12. d. How many years have you personally lived here in (name of city, town, or county)? (*Enter actual number of years.*)

_____ years
- ☐ 00. Less than 6 months
- ☐ 90. All my life
- ☐ 98. Don't know
- ☐ 99. No answer

for the month and day of birth, may be too much. Researchers have found that when a single question is used, the best question is, "In what year were you (was name) born?"

Marital status is not as easily assessed as you might expect. A person can be married, divorced, and widowed. The SSRC questions entirely miss *cohabitation*. The term "single" is especially misleading and should never be used because it can mean divorced, separated, not married, or even widowed—although few people in the widowed category label themselves as "single." "Separated" should mean living apart from a spouse because of marital discord and not living apart because one spouse is in the armed forces, away on business, or some other reason. For this reason, some researchers ask, "What is your current marital status? Are you married, living with your husband/wife; married but not living with your husband/wife; widowed"; and so on. In addition to the basic questions on marital status shown in Exhibit 14.4, several follow-up questions are available depending on the purpose of the research:

5C. *If not a first marriage:* How many times have you (has name) been married, including your (name) present marriage? When did your (name's) first, second . . . marriage begin? How did this marriage end? *If death*, when did your husband/wife die? *If divorce or annulment*, what was the date of your divorce/annulment? *Data are coded as follows:*

Number of marriages: _____

Year began	Year ended	Cause of termination
_____	_____	_____
_____	_____	_____

The SSRC has resolved some of the problems with **ethnic identification** by separating it into race and ethnicity. They also believe a question on religion is a necessary part of ethnic identification. Exhibit 14.5 presents an alternative, longer list of countries of origin and their code numbers if you prefer to use those for question 6B. There is some ambiguity with national origin questions in a country like the United States, where mixtures are highly likely. Some surveys therefore focus only on descent through either the mother or the father. In the census of Canada, ethnic origin is defined as the birthplace of the paternal grandfather. Others believe the customs of the mother are more salient in the language of early childhood, food preferences, and so forth. Accordingly, complex questions have been developed to probe this area. For most purposes, however, the questions presented in Exhibit 14.4 are adequate. Certain follow-up questions on religion may involve, "In what religion were you (name) raised?" and, if more than one is given, "which one are you more likely to identify with?" In addition, with the growing tendency to name no religious preference or one of the nontraditional ones, it may be important to add a question identifying the religion of a subject's family of origin. Researchers have

Exhibit 14-5. National codes.

Africa	01	Korea	22
American Indian (Native American)	02	Lithuania	23
Austria	03	Mexico	24
Belgium	04	Netherlands (Dutch/Holland)	25
Canada (French)	05	Norway	26
Canada (Other)	06	Pakistan	27
Central or South America	07	Philippines	28
China	08	Poland	29
Cuba	09	Portugal	30
Czechoslovakia	10	Puerto Rico	31
Denmark	11	Russia (USSR)	32
England and Wales	12	Scotland (or Scottish Irish)	33
Finland	13	Spain	34
France	14	Sweden	35
Germany	15	Switzerland	36
Greece	16	West Indies	37
Hungary	17	Yugoslavia	38
India	18	Other (specify)	39
Ireland	19	More than one country;	
Italy	20	cannot choose one	88
Japan	21	Don't know	99

found that asking about religious *preference* rather than a subject's religion results in less accurate data (e.g., a Protestant who prefers, say, Catholicism).

Because the basic questions on education (8A and 8B) do not always identify people who have had special training, like vocational and on-the-job training, several additional questions (8C through 8G) may be necessary if this precision is advisable. For persons who have skipped or repeated grades, record the highest grade (e.g., 08 for eighth grade) regardless of the number of years involved. Needless to say, if you can get by with fewer questions, especially if your interview schedule is long, do so.

The employment and occupation questions must be sufficiently detailed to yield a true picture of a subject's status in order to classify him or her as unskilled, semiskilled, or skilled and the occupation into one of a series of occupational groups. The SSRC recommends against a respondent's trying to classify himself into one of a limited number of categories, because this is usually inaccurate. Instead, a series of probes is recommended to help elicit adequate job descriptions so that the researcher can code the data according to categories appropriate to the research, such as Hollingshead's Two Factor Socio-economic Status (SES [7]) or Green's SES for health research [6]. First, researchers have found it best to let respondents decide if they are working full-time or part-time. However, sometimes an additional question is asked about the number of hours worked in an average week. Some respondents will be in more than one category (e.g., working housewife) and all categories should be checked, although the "working now" sequence of questions is then followed. Current occupational information is recorded even though a subject may be looking for another job. In addition, persons who work 15 hours or more a week as unpaid workers on a farm or in a family business are considered as "working now" for the sequence of questions. Individuals whose only work is around their own home or volunteer work for religions, charitable, and other organizations are not considered as "working now" for the SSRC sequence of questions. A "job" is defined as working for pay; running a business, professional practice, or farm; or working without pay in a family business or farm. Farmers who cannot be considered hourly wage earners are considered self-employed. The name of the place where a person works is not a sufficient response to the occupation questions. For example, if an individual works at Mercy Hospital, he could be a nurse, physician, aide, janitor, or one of many other occupations. Thus, it is important to get an adequate job *description*. Job *titles* are often vague. For example, an engineer might design automobiles, operate a subway train, tend an engine, collect garbage, or shovel coal into a furnace. A nurse can be an aide, a practical nurse, a registered nurse, a nurse practitioner, or a paid companion. A teacher might teach in an elementary school or a large university. The first sequence of occupation questions in Exhibit 14.4 (10A to 10C) concern present occupation. However, because many persons change occupations when they change jobs, the present occupation may not reflect an individual's usual occupation. Questions 10D to 10G are designed for this and persons with more than one job.

Questions about income generally do not produce accurate information. Family income is often underreported both because it is a sensitive topic and because persons often do not know how much each member earns. Often take-home pay is reported instead of gross. Between 5 percent and 10 percent of respondents do not even answer. Therefore, some researchers begin the question by saying, "This information is being collected purely for statistical purposes." Although some researchers prefer to ask for income "during the last 12 months," the SSRC prefers using a calendar year, especially if it is in the spring when income tax returns are being prepared. Some researchers believe that chief wage earner information is more important, especially if the income is to be used to determine socioeconomic status. Others, and the SSRC, believe family income reflects the pool of resources upon which a family can draw. If this is what income data is used for, you may wish to know how many persons contribute to the family income and how many depend on it. People are often more willing to report income when it is represented by income ranges, as

---

Exhibit 14-6. Family-income flashcard.

Total Family Income in 1985—Before Taxes, All Members of Family Living in Your Household

A.	Under $3,000 a year	(or under $57.99 a week)
B.	$3,000 to $3,999 a year	(or $58 to $76.99 a week)
C.	$4,000 to $4,999 a year	(or $77 to $95.99 a week)
D.	$5,000 to $5,999 a year	(or $96 to $114.99 a week)
E.	$6,000 to $7,999 a year	(or $115 to $153.99 a week)
F.	$8,000 to $9,999 a year	(or $154 to $191.99 a week)
G.	$10,000 to $11,999 a year	(or $192 to $230.99 a week)
H.	$12,000 to $14,999 a year	(or $231 to $287.99 a week)
I.	$15,000 to $19,999 a year	(or $288 to $384.99 a week)
J.	$20,000 to $24,999 a year	(or $385 to $480.99 a week)
K.	$25,000 to $29,999 a year	(or $481 to $576.99 a week)
L.	$30,000 to $34,999 a year	(or $577 to $672.99 a week)
M.	$35,000 and over a year	(or $673 or more a week)

shown on the **flashcard** in Exhibit 14.6. Although some information is lost via this method, it seems to be the best approach. Weekly as well as yearly income is provided on the card. In some cases, monthly income might be provided. The intervals used on the flashcard, moreover, should be revised periodically to correspond with current U.S. Census Bureau intervals. On mailed or self-administered questionnaires, the intervals for income are reduced and broadened to increase cooperation. In telephone surveys, a series of dichotomous questions is asked until the income is bracketed. For example, you can start with the highest income and work down, start with the lowest and work up, or start in the middle and move either way. Usually starting at the top and working down is best with the general population or upper incomes because income is usually underreported. For low income or poverty groups, it is best to start low and move up. Starting in the middle usually involves fewer questions but also more underreporting.

For example, if you wished to start low:

Was it less than $5,000?
If no, was it less than $10,000?
If no, was it less than $15,000?
If no, was it less than $20,000?

On the other hand, if you wish to start high, you might begin:

Was it more than $50,000?
If no, was it more than $45,000?
If no, was it more than $40,000?

Starting in the middle you might begin:

Was it $15,000 or more, or less than that?

If 15,000 or more was it under $20,000 or over $20,000?	If less than $15,000, was it over $10,000 or under $10,000?
If over $20,000, was it under $25,000 or over $25,000?	If under $10,000, was it over $7,000 or under $7,000?
If over $25,000 was it under $30,000 or over $30,000?	If under $7,000, was it over $5,000 or under $5,000?

Although this is a time-consuming procedure, it is worth the effort when income is a key variable. It does not, however, alleviate the problem of underreporting. The Census Bureau has a lengthy format, used to overcome the tendency of persons to forget some sources of income when income is a key variable. In most cases, however, the sequence of 11A to 11C must be sufficient.

When housing questions (e.g., 12A to 12B) are used as measures of socioeconomic status, they are often followed by a question about the number of rooms or some index of crowding. No questions are needed to assess the region or size of place in which respondents reside. This is done by observation or coding zip codes, telephone exchanges, or other geographic identifiers. The Census Bureau divides the United States into four regions and nine divisions by states as follows:

Northeast
> *New England:* Maine, New Hampshire, Vermont, Massachusetts, Rhode Island, Connecticut
> *Middle Atlantic:* New York, New Jersey, Pennsylvania,

North Central
> *East North Central:* Ohio, Indiana, Illinois, Michigan, Wisconsin
> *West North Central:* Minnesota, Iowa, Missouri, North Dakota, South Dakota, Nebraska, Kansas

South
> *South Atlantic:* Delaware, Maryland, District of Columbia, Virginia, West Virginia, North Carolina, South Carolina, Georgia, Florida
> *East South Central:* Kentucky, Tennessee, Alabama, Mississippi
> *West South Central:* Arkansas, Louisiana, Oklahoma, Texas

West
> *Mountain:* Montana, Idaho, Wyoming, Colorado, Utah, New Mexico, Arizona, Nevada
> *Pacific:* Washington, Oregon, California, Alaska, Hawaii

Three categories are used to group places according to sizes:

Central Cities of Standard Metropolitan Statistical Areas (SMSAs)
Outside central cities of SMSAs
Nonmetropolitan areas

SMSAs are sometimes further broken down according to their total population:

3,000,000 or more
1,000,000 to 2,999,999
500,000 to 999,999
250,000 to 499,999
100,000 to 249,999
Less than 100,000

Similarly, nonmetropolitan areas are sometimes subdivided as follows:

25,000 or more
10,000 to 24,999
2,500 to 9,999
Under 2,500
Rural

There are rural or smaller places within many SMSAs. For most research, these are simply considered part of the SMSA because these residents usually behave more like people in the SMSA than like rural persons.

Determining Sequencing, Format, and Directions

Once questions have been formulated, your creativity has begun to flow and you are ready to continue with the *art* of developing an instrument. There are no clear-cut rules and operations to follow as there are, say, in computing a Pearson *r*. This section presents a series of flexible suggestions that seem to have worked for others. However, there are exceptions to most of these that have also been successful. You must use the skills of psychologist, novelist, detective, and politician. If you try to make the data collection experience as fun and interesting as possible for your particular target population, you will most likely be successful.

Sequencing Questions

There is, of course, no single best order for questions. There is, however, a number of rules of thumb that are helpful. Just as a great deal of thought must go into the formulation of questions, the same amount can go into the sequencing. To begin, it is wise to put each question on a separate card. If an already developed scale is to be used to measure a variable (e.g., 20-item Likert scale measuring patient satisfaction), make a single card for that scale because all the items must be presented as a group in the order of the original scale. Once questions are on cards, you can arrange and rearrange them until the best sequence has been found. Begin by sorting the cards into piles according to either the subtopics being covered or your specification matrix.

Keep your questionnaire as short as possible. Remove questions that are not likely to be used in data analysis or are redundant (particularly if you generated more than your specification matrix called for). If there are questions to which everyone will respond in the same way, that is, if some questions do not discriminate, remove them also. To make your final decision regarding the length of your questionnaire, consider the salience of the questions. If the questions are highly salient to subjects, personal interviews can last one and a half hours and mailed questionnaires can be up to 16 pages. For nonsalient topics, mailed questionnaires should be limited to two to four pages and interviews reduced similarly, probably to between 10 and 30 minutes.

Start with your most salient, easy, and nonthreatening questions. More difficult or threatening questions should be put toward the end. Never put an open-ended question requiring writing at the beginning of a mailed questionnaire. It will make the questionnaire seem too hard. Respondents like just to check answers. Give them this opportunity at the beginning in order to gain their commitment to the project. Because some demographic questions, such as those on income and age, can be threatening, researchers usually put them toward the end unless they are needed earlier for screening purposes. **Screening questions** determine whether respondents have certain characteristics (e.g., age, income, ethnic group, large medical expenses, recent death in the family) that make them eligible for a full-scale interview or questionnaire. At any rate, if at all possible, do not ask demographic questions first. When screening questions must be asked, other demographic questions can usually be deferred.

If questions deal with more than one topic, ask all the questions on a single topic before moving on to the next one. Check each of your card piles to make sure only one topic is included. Then you can either sequence the questions within each pile first or sequence your piles, keeping in mind the suggestions that follow. When collecting job or other histories, follow chronological order, either backward or forward in time. When you switch topics, use a transitional sentence or so to help subjects switch their thoughts to the new topic. In general, respondents resent answering the same question more than once and their resentment increases when they must constantly change their trains of thought. When the topic is changed without cues, you run the risk of having respondents become distracted from questions because they are trying to figure out why a question is being asked and in what logical order. Switching back and forth among topics is not the way to introduce variety and reduce boredom and response set, which are better handled with variety and change of pace in *how* questions are asked or responded to (e.g., closed-ended mixed with open-ended).

Questions within a topic, therefore, should follow a logical sequence. In interviews, funneling is often used. A **funnel sequence** begins with the most general question and goes on to progressively more restricted questions. Its purpose is to prevent early questions from influencing later questions. It is especially useful when you want first to learn about the frame of reference a subject uses to answer questions. On the other hand, if it is likely that a subject has not thought much about a topic, using an **inverted funnel sequence,** going from specific to general, may aid in his exploring various aspects of a topic before being asked to give a more general point of view. For example, a patient might be asked about several aspects of health care before being asked, "Now, taking all these into consideration, how satisfied are you with the care you have received?" Funneling is more appropriate for interviews than questionnaires, since respondents have the opportunity to look over the entire questionnaire before starting to answer. Inverted funneling, however can be used effectively with questionnaires.

Filter questions, those that determine which additional questions will be asked, allow more possibilities, encourage complete responses, and *usually* reduce error when used appropriately. A simple example of a filter question is "Do you have any children?" If the answer is "no," a **skip instruction** (e.g., "Go to question 6") is given. If the response is "yes," additional questions about the ages, sex, and so forth of offspring can be asked. Filter questions and skip instructions are more appropriate for interviews than for self-administered questionnaires. When they are used with questionnaires, they should be simple and used sparingly or else additional error will be introduced. The most complex filter question/skip instruction designs require computer administration, because even trained interviewers are known to make serious errors. Subjects who are not well motivated can find a polite way of reducing their involvement by answering filter questions so that no additional questions are asked. If you use the same format for filter questions, it is not long before they figure out that, say, a "no" answer saves answering five more questions. Therefore, researchers may ask a string of 10 or so filter questions and then return to get additional information. Because subjects at this point do not know how many additional questions accompany each affirmative response, they are more likely to answer honestly. For example, suppose you were interested in the effects on the family of several medical problems like myocardial infarction, hysterectomy, and so forth. First you would ask the respondent if he or she had had any of these problems. Then, for those with "yes" responses, you would follow with questions like these:

1. How many days were you hospitalized?
2. How many days were you unable to work?
3. Who took over your household chores? What did he/she do?
4. Were any of your usual household activities left undone?
5. Who cared for you?
6. All things considered, how did your illness affect each family member? The family as a group?

These questions, of course, could have open- or closed-ended responses, depending on the data needs of your research. If you use this approach more than once, some respondents may have become "test wise" the next time and may therefore give false-negative responses. Therefore, put your most important set of questions first.

Consider Exhibit 14.3, a questionnaire with three parts. The first part deals with four attitude/belief questions that refer to sex interviews with five specific patients. Question A is more global because it asks about importance. Question B becomes more personal and specific, because it asks about the comfort level of the respondent in terms of his or her conducting the interview. Having reflected on importance and personal comfort, the respondent is then ready to answer the questions about when and by whom the interview is to be conducted. These questions are repeated for each of the five patient vignettes. Note that the questionnaire is called an opinionnaire in order to underscore the fact that there are no correct answers. The second part includes a few demographic questions. This particular version was given to senior medical and nursing students, and therefore it asked about their *expected* specialty areas. The versions given to physicians and staff nurses, all of whom had worked a minimum of 5 years, simply asked what their specialty areas were. Each type of health care provider received opinionnaires printed on different colored paper, so it was unnecessary to ask occupation. Although these demographic questions seem innocuous, many physicians were upset about having to give their age, and some did not give it. Others accused the researchers of using the opinionnaire as a ruse to find out their age. Had the demographic questions been asked first, it is likely that many would have declined participation. Part III is the Athanasiou and Shaver [1] sexual liberalism-conservatism scale. Because it asks very personal and possibly threatening questions, it was placed last. Having "warmed up" with Part I, respondents were more ready for Part III.

Formatting the Questionnaire

A principle to follow in formatting a questionnaire is that the needs and convenience of your subjects come first, the needs of an interviewer or experimenter come second, and the needs of coders and data processing staff come last. If you can meet everyone's needs, you are that much further ahead. Furthermore, some researchers argue against changing improperly formatted questions from other researchers, because they believe that, for comparability to previous research, the original format should be retained. In the author's opinion, this reasoning is ridiculous. Poor formats lead to errors and lower participation, thereby reducing accuracy over time. Although you should avoid unnecessary changes, improving an undesirable format is almost always preferable.

If at all possible, use a booklet format for ease in turning pages and to reduce the likelihood of lost pages. For self-administered and mailed questionnaires, appearance impacts response rate. They should look easy and professionally designed. The front and back covers of self-administered questionnaires are especially important. Dillman [5] says the front cover should contain the study title, needed directions, the study sponsor and address, and an illustration (if the general population is involved). For short questionnaires, the illustration is often omitted. The back cover is usually blank and can be used for additional comments by a subject. In some studies the back cover has a mailing label, which can then be used with a window envelope. The mailing label can include a code number for the respondent to allow follow-up. Otherwise, if it is appropriate to use one, the code number goes on the first page. For interviews, allow space on the front page of the schedule to record the time the interview started and ended, the date, and any special problems that were encountered.

Leave enough space. Do not crowd questions (or reduce them) in order to limit the number of pages. The result will not look good and your response rate will be reduced. A less crowded questionnaire with a fair amount of clear space looks easier, and it results in higher cooperation and fewer errors. Be sure sufficient space is allowed for open-ended questions. Use lines for responses only if short answers are expected. Remember, as a rule, responses will be only as long as the space provided. Few respondents will continue their responses on the blank last page, even if you request them to do so. Also, use a sufficiently large and clear type so that it is easy to read. This is especially important with older (and very young) respondents.

Number all questions and use letters, indented, for subparts. With interview schedules, as shown in Exhibit 14.4, interviewers might skip to the next number as soon as a certain (usually negative) response is received. The use of numbers and letters facilitates the use of skip instructions, which should be placed immediately following an answer.

Exhibit 14.7 demonstrates a poor format for self-administered questionnaires. Not only are subjects asked to respond to a vertical (versus horizontal) format of answers, but they are expected to answer two questions at once. A better format for this same scale is shown in Exhibit 14.8. Here all responses are vertical, so that respondents do not have to turn their questionnaires sideways to figure out what to respond. Furthermore, it does not have the grid work, which many consider ominous. The second question, which consists of three additional questions, is separated out from the original first question. Even this requires fairly sophisticated respondents for self-administered formats or else an interviewer type format. You can, of course, use boxes instead of blanks. This depends on your printing options. Whether subjects put a check on a line or put an X in a box is irrelevant to accuracy or completeness of response.

Do not split questions between two pages. Interviewers or respondents may think all options are on one page and therefore miss some. When asking identical questions about the members of a household, use parallel columns as shown in Exhibit 14.4, or even spread them across facing pages if necessary. Similarly, if you are using a Likert-type scale formatted as shown in Exhibit 14.8 and the items run to the next page, repeat the response alternative numbers and their meanings (e.g., 1 = strongly agree) at the top of each page. An alternative format for a Likert-type scale is shown in Exhibit 14.9.

Position on the page is also important. Respondents must know *in which blank* to place their answers and they need enough room for their answers. Exhibit 14.10 presents a questionnaire in which spacing and the places for

Exhibit 14-7. Unacceptable vertical answers.

Directions: Please disagree/agree with the following statements by putting an X in the space provided. In addition, rank-order the three questions with which you agree most by putting a 1 for the most agreement and a 3 for the least agreement in the space provided.	Strongly Agree	Agree	Uncertain	Disagree	Strongly Disagree	Rank
1. The fantasy of wanting to grow up to be Santa's dry cleaner—what with all the chimneys to come down—is perfectly healthy for a child.						
2. Who knows, in a figurative sense, maybe the Easter Bunny does scatter colored eggs and candies.						
3. The idea of a tooth fairy giving money for a lost body part teaches a value decent human beings should abhor.						
4. Witches flying on brooms and ghosts and skeletons behind bushes is a novel way to teach bravery.						
5. Halloween candy and goodies are a child's just reward for bravery in the face of witches, ghosts, skeletons, and the like.						
6. No one, even children, should be allowed to believe reindeer can fly through the sky.						
7. The tooth fairy idea is great at easing the pain and loss of a body part.						
8. Dressing up in costumes of favorite characters at Halloween is really no different than adult costume balls and the theater itself.						
9. Trick-or-treating does not teach the appropriate values for living in peace and harmony with your neighbors.						

nominal

Exhibit 14-8. Fantasies-of-childhood opinionnaire.

Directions: For each of the following statements about childhood fantasies, please indicate the extent to which you agree or disagree by putting the appropriate number in the blank provided.

> 1 = Strongly agree
> 2 = Agree
> 3 = Uncertain
> 4 = Disagree
> 5 = Strongly disagree

_____ 1. The fantasy of growing up to be Santa's dry cleaner—what with all the chimneys to come down—is perfectly healthy for a child.

. . .

_____ 9. Trick-or-treating does not teach the appropriate values for living in peace and harmony with your neighbors.

Directions: From the preceding nine statements, select the three with which you agree most. Put the number of the statement in the blank provided.

_____ 1. First choice
_____ 2. Second choice
_____ 3. Third choice

Directions: From the preceding nine statements select the three with which you agree least. Put the number of the statement in the blank provided.

_____ 1. Least favorite
_____ 2. Second least favorite
_____ 3. Third least favorite

Directions: From your previous selections for most and least favored responses, select the two with which you have the strongest feelings.

_____ 1. Most important:
   I favor _____; disfavor _____ this question
_____ 2. Second most important:
   I favor _____; disfavor _____ this question

---

responses are not adequate. This questionnaire was designed to ascertain reasons why nurses who had been out of nursing for a number of years were returning to work as nurses. Although the format as presented might yield the needed data, a more engaging format is presented in Exhibit 14.11. Here, easy questions begin the series, leading directly to the major question, item 5, of why nurses return to nursing. The introductory paragraph references agency nurse shortages and the list of reasons effectively disguise the hypotheses of economic need as the major reason. The use of an "other" alternative is good public relations. It allows for all possible responses even though additional reasons presented in this section will probably not be analyzed with the others. Demographic questions are placed last, with the less threatening questions about education preceding age and marital status. A thank-you ends the questionnaire. Notice how alternatives are lined up underneath each other with the blanks

---

Exhibit 14-9. Alternative formats for Likert scale.

Directions: For each of the following statements about childhood fantasies, please indicate the extent to which you agree or disagree by *circling the most appropriate response.*

Strongly agree	Agree	Uncertain	Disagree	Strongly disagree	
SA	A	U	D	SD	1. The fantasy of growing up to be Santa's dry cleaner—what with all the chimneys to come down—is perfectly healthy for a child.
					. . .
SA	A	U	D	SD	9. Trick-or-treating does not teach the appropriate values for living in peace and harmony with your neighbors.

Directions: For each of the following statements about childhood fantasies, please indicate the extent to which you agree or disagree by *circling the most appropriate response.* Use the following code for your responses:

SA = Strongly agree
A = Agree
U = Uncertain
D = Disagree
SP = Strongly disagree

SA A U D SD 1. The fantasy of growing up to be Santa's dry cleaner—what with all the chimneys to come down—is perfectly healthy for a child.

. . .

SA A U D SD 9. Trick-or-treating does not teach the appropriate values for living in peace and harmony with your neighbors.

---

immediately *preceding* each alternative. This gives a much more professional appearance and prevents confusion about where to put an answer. Numbering of questions provides a guide for the respondent and also assists data coders. The questionnaire is **precolumned** for computer coding at the extreme right. The numbers indicate in which column of a computer card (or tape) the response to that question is to be coded. This allows data entry directly from the questionnaire, assuming response codes are clear, thereby skipping the tiresome task of data encoding onto 80 column sheets which was presented in Chapter 6. Finally, note the additional questions for married nurses with children (11 and 12). Even with their improved format, a few respondents will not

Exhibit 14-10. Poor spacing and unclear response blanks.

General Information:

Age _____ Date of birth _____

Sex _____

Marital status:

Married _____ Husband   Working _____

                             Unemployed _____

                             Retired _____

Divorced _____ Separated _____

Widowed _____

Single _____

Children: No _____ Yes _____ How many: 0–6 _____

                                          7–12 _____

                                          12–18 _____

                                          over 18 _____

Number of dependents _____

When did you graduate? _____ (Year)

Education:

LPN _____ 2-year AA _____ 3-year diploma _____ BSN _____

Other: _____

Clinical specialty: _____

How long have you been out of nursing? _____

Reasons for leaving nursing? _____

Did you work outside of nursing during your leave? _____

Are you going to work full-time? _____ Part-time? _____

Why are you reentering nursing? _____

complete them. The chances for completion are improved over the original, however. Pilot testing with the target group might yield suggestions for improving the questionnaire even more.

Cover Letters and Directions

The introduction of a questionnaire often must allay fear that you are conducting bogus research and that your real purpose is, for example, to sell magazine subscriptions. Introductions do not necessarily need to be long. However, they should clearly identify the researchers and their purpose. An example is shown in Exhibit 14.3. It quickly identifies the researchers and their purpose as well as guarantees anonymity and shows how refusal to participate can be handled unobtrusively. The potential benefits of the research are also given. Because administration of the sex interview opinionnaire was handled in person, experimenters solicited participation by repeating this material and adding that it would take between 10 and 15 minutes to participate. The time involvement could have also been included on the opinionnaire. As long as subjects are told, where they are told is a matter of researcher preference.

Consider the following *draft* of an introduction to a questionnaire designed to

Exhibit 14-11. Improved questionnaire.

We are a group of graduate students in nursing interested in why nurses return to nursing after a prolonged absence of 5 years or more. We believe this information may have implications for agencies with nursing shortages.

We would appreciate your participation in this research. If you are willing, please answer the following questions. Your responses, of course, will be completely anonymous. If you do not wish to participate, just return the questionnaire unanswered.

Card 1

1. How many years has it been since you stopped working in nursing?   5–6
   —— years

2. Why did you leave nursing? In the blanks provided, please put a 1 for the most important, a 2 for the second most important, and a 3 for the third most important.

   ———— a. Marriage   8
   ———— b. Pregnancy/motherhood   9
   ———— c. Couldn't take the stress   10
   ———— d. Poor hours and shift work   11
   ———— e. Moved to another area   12

   · · ·

   ———— i. Lack of appreciation for what I was doing   16
   ———— j. Other (specify): ————————————————————   17

3. Did you work at another kind of job since you left nursing?   19
   ———— Yes ———— No
   If yes, what kind of job? ————————————————————————   20–21

4. Do you plan to work ———— full-time? ———— part-time?   22

5. The following statements are reasons given by many who are returning to nursing. In the blanks provided, please indicate how important each reason is to you in terms of why you are reentering nursing. Use the following responses:

   $$1 = \text{Very important}$$
   $$2 = \text{Important}$$
   $$3 = \text{Not important}$$

   ———— a. I miss nursing.   24
   ———— b. I'm bored at home.   25
   ———— c. Prefer nursing to my current job.   26
   ———— d. Need the money.   27

   · · ·

   ———— g. I want to help reduce the nursing shortage.   30
   ———— h. Other (Please specify): ————————————————   31

Directions: We would also like to know something about the characteristics of the participants in our survey. Please answer the following questions in the blanks provided.

6. What year did you graduate from nursing school? ————   34–35

7. Education:

    _____ LPN

    _____ 2-year AA

    _____ 3-year diploma

    _____ BSN

8. Clinical specialty: 36–37

    _____

9. Year of birth _____

10. Sex _____ Female   39–40,41

    _____ Male

11. Marital status: 43–44

    _____ Married ⟶ If married, is your husband

    _____ Separated   _____ Working

    _____ Divorced   _____ Retired

    _____ Widowed   _____ Unemployed

    _____ Single

12. Do you have any children?   45,46–47

    _____ Yes ⟶ If yes, how many? _____

    _____ No   What are their ages? _____

Thank you for participating in our survey.

measure variables for a correlational research design. There are several ways in which it can be improved.

You are invited to participate in a graduate level nursing study designed to look at the "buffering effects" of exercise and hardiness on levels of stress on nursing.

You are asked to complete the following questions related to this study, being assured of anonymity. This should take about 10 minutes of your time.

The results of the study will be available upon request at a later date through the graduate nursing student helping to conduct the study in your hospital. Thus far nursing research has not looked at these variables together. The results should show an interesting correlation among the three.

First, the identity of the researchers remains uncertain and the purpose of this correlational research study misleading because no "buffering effects" were being assessed. Had they been, labeling the variables as buffers in this way could easily "lead the subjects" because they would immediately infer the hypothesis being tested. Stress among nurses rather than *on* nursing was the third variable being assessed. How not to participate was not even mentioned. A better wording for the introduction is as follows.

We are a group of nurses conducting research as part of the requirements in our research methodology course at the University of *XXXX*. You are invited to participate in our study, which is designed to examine the relationships among daily activities like exercise, stress, and a personality trait known as hardiness. We believe it may have implications for reducing any stressful effects of nursing practice that might exist.

Please complete the following questions, which should take about 10 minutes. Your responses are completely anonymous. If you do not wish to participate, simply return the questionnaire unanswered.

A summary of results from the research will be available through your Director in about 3 months. Thank you for your cooperation.

The second (but not necessarily perfect) version begins by identifying the researchers and then inviting participation. The study purpose and benefits are then explained. Introduction of benefits at the beginning should give added inducement to reluctant subjects, especially when the benefits fall close to home. Next, the mechanics of participation/nonparticipation are explained— including time involvements. Finally, another benefit, study results, is offered as a final inducement to participate. The thank-you could be here or at the end of the questionnaire as it is in Exhibit 14.3.

Some researchers believe that the first page should not include any actual questions. This is really a matter of personal taste and the specific target population being solicited. In studies that are not anonymous, the method of coding or recording names is usually explained, also. In another of the author's research studies, volunteers from among the sample were solicited for future studies on the first page. Because volunteering involved completing identifying information, the following was used:

This opinionnaire is one part of a several part research study. If you would be willing to participate in future studies, please fill in the following information:
Name: _____
Address: _____
_____
Telephone: (   ) _____
The above information will be kept confidential, and your answers to this opinionnaire will be filed apart from any identifying information on this cover page.

Verbal *and* written introductions are appropriate with interviews and questionnaires administered by the researchers [5]. Sometimes a written introduction is given even to interview subjects. However, when mailed questionnaires are used, a cover letter becomes necessary.

Cover Letters

A well written **cover letter** is a persuasive and motivating device. It presents the reasons for the study and why it is important for the respondent to complete the instrument personally. It should never be more than one page long. You should do the following in the cover letter:

1. Present the purpose and value of the study.
2. Identify the researcher(s) and sponsoring agency (or even faculty supervisor) if appropriate.

3. Do not forget to actually invite participation. If possible, tell why the respondent is important to the research.
4. Explain how data will be used (e.g., grouped data, anonymity). Promise confidentiality if anonymity is not assured and explain how code numbers or identifiers will be used.
5. Estimate the time involved in participating in the study.
6. Give explicit directions for completing the questionnaire.
7. Provide a reasonable deadline for returning the questionnaire.
8. If possible, offer rewards for participation or state how results of the research may be obtained. If you cannot, stress the social importance of the research.
9. Provide a stamped self-addressed envelope.
10. Date your letter.
11. Sign the letter personally.
12. Use an original or an extremely high-quality copy.

Exhibit 14.12 and 13 present two versions of cover letters. Exhibit 14.12 begins with an invitation to participate, and then goes on to explain the purpose of the research and identity of the researchers. Note how it is made more "official" by giving the name of the faculty sponsor and university as well as the foundation that is providing funds. Of course, you need permission to use these names. It is also helpful to use university letterhead if you can get permission to do so. Directions for participation are clear. Asking nonparticipants to return unanswered questionnaires not only helps you account for all subjects but may actually increase participation, because even nonparticipation requires some effort. Be careful in your use of this technique, however, because it may anger some recipients who wish to be left alone to do nothing. The letter ends with one last encouragement to participate, which brings the reader back from thinking about the mechanics of participation to actual participation. Exhibit 14.13 is a follow-up solicitation. It gives some results of the previous research and then requests additional participation. In the research in which it was used, only one subject did not respond. However, the sample had become one of self-selected volunteers, because these subjects had already expressed a willingness to continue participation during the earlier stage of the research.

If more than a 50 percent response rate is needed, it is likely that follow-up procedures within a week of the deadline date will be necessary. There are several such approaches. One is to send a second letter that gently asks for return of the questionnaire. Postcards can also be used, although they may be slightly less effective. Some researchers telephone delinquent subjects. Of course, if you have granted anonymity, you have no way of knowing who did not respond. In this case a letter is sent to everyone with "disregard" instructions for those who have already returned their questionnaires. Another method is to send a second questionnaire and return envelope with the second letter. This is

---

Exhibit 14-12. Cover letter I.

Dear XXXX,

You are invited to participate in a national survey to determine the level of activity and interest in research by staff nurses. Problems that you encounter in your daily practice and believe need further research are also of interest. As a result of this survey, we hope to establish priorities and guidelines for nursing research in clinical settings.

We are a group of nursing students under the supervision of Dr. XXXX XXXXXX-XXX, University of XXXX School of Nursing. This study is part of the requirements for completion of our program; and, because of its potential usefulness to nursing, it has been funded by the XXXX Foundation. Your participation is very important to the success of our project. Won't you do so today?

To participate, simply fill out the enclosed questionnaire and return it in the stamped, addressed envelope, which is also enclosed. It should take about 20 minutes. If you do not wish to participate, just return the unanswered questionnaire in the envelope provided. Then you will not receive any follow-up notices. The return mailing label is coded to identify participants. It will be destroyed after we receive it and note that you have responded. The questionnaire itself will be immediately separated from the return envelope, and then your response will be completely anonymous.

Please return the questionnaire by October 10. If you have any questions, feel free to contact us through Dr. XXXX XXXXXX-XXX. We expect to publish the results of this study in the *Journal of Nursing* in about one year. We hope you'll take advantage of this opportunity to have your opinions included.

Thank you for giving this matter your attention.

Sincerely yours,

Lucile J. Smith, RN

also for   Mary L. Quiote, RN

           Linda Carethers, RN

           Sally J. Jenkins, RN

Enclosures

---

certainly necessary for later follow-ups. Exhibit 14.14 presents Orlich's [9] system for achieving almost 100 percent returns.

Directions

As stated previously, transitions from one topic to another are important. These are often made via a new set of directions as shown in Exhibit 14.3. Just prior to the demographic questions, subjects are told that the researchers would appreciate having some information about the participants in the study. Then, prior to the final, most threatening set of questions, their opinions about other sexual matters are requested.

It is often helpful to point out that there are no right or wrong answers (assuming there are none). Exhibit 14.15 uses this approach in a study that

---

Exhibit 14-13. Cover letter II.

Dear XXXX,

    A year ago you helped us in our research by completing an opinionnaire to assist health care providers and others in knowing how best to help people. In all, 230 persons responded, and we were therefore able to test the questions and delete or change poor ones. Thank you!

    We are now ready to do part II of our study which involves looking at changes, if any, in your opinions after a year's time.

    Since you indicated a willingness to participate in additional research, we are asking you to complete the enclosed Opinionnaire-II and return it to us in the stamped, addressed envelope (also enclosed). You will find that this one is much shorter than the first opinionnaire, and that almost half the questions have been removed. A few have changed. In all, it should take you about an hour to complete. Won't you do so today? We would appreciate your returning it to us within a week or two.

    Thank you for helping us.

Sincerely,

Sonya I. Shelley, Ph.D.
Professor
Center for Research

Enclosures

---

involved a more complex response mode than usual. To ensure that instructions are not mistaken as part of a question, be sure to label them clearly or set them apart with different type faces. It is often helpful to put "please go to the next page" at the bottom of each page. This is especially important when the back of pages are used, in order to avoid having respondents miss the back. In that case directions would state "please go to the back of this page."

Exhibit 14-14. Orlich's system for almost 100 percent returns.

---

1. Mail the questionnaire—first mailing.
2. Within 1 week, mail a first follow-up postcard to all nonrespondents. (Some surveyors automatically mail a postcard to every sample member 1 week after the first mailing.)
3. Within 3 weeks of the first mailing, send a second questionnaire—with a second cover letter stressing the importance of the instrument being returned.
4. Within 1 week of the mailing of the second instrument, mail a second follow-up postcard.
5. Within 2 weeks of the second instrument, mail a third instrument.
6. Within 1 week of the third instrument, follow up with a letter.
7. Last effort—telephone the nonrespondents.

Reprinted from Orlich [9].

> **Exhibit 14-15.** Directions for using the SSM.
>
> ---
>
> *Directions:* Each of the following 28 questions has five possible responses. Indicate to what extent you agree with some or all of the five responses by giving them a numerical value, the total of which will add up to 11 points for each question. The more you agree with any particular response, the higher the number you should assign to it. For example,
>
> > If you agree with several responses in differing degrees, you should assign a proportionate amount of points to each response with which you agree, for a total of 11 for the whole question.
>
> > If you agree with only one response, you should assign all 11 points for that question to that response.
>
> This is not a test—there are no "right" or "wrong" answers. People have different beliefs and values about life. Please distribute the 11 points for each question in such a way as to reflect your particular beliefs and values.
>
> Please go on to the next page.

Obtaining Outside Review

At this point you should have a draft of your instrument from beginning to end. Put it aside for a day or two and then go over it carefully and critically, putting yourself in the place of one of your subjects. Make any revisions you think appropriate and type your final rough draft. Obviously, it is going to be very difficult for you to be completely objective as you critique your questionnaire. If you have worked with it for an extended period of time, you won't even see some mistakes if they "jump off the page and hit you in the eye." Therefore, when you have given it your "best shot," seek outside help in reviewing the items.

For outside review, select one person with expertise in questionnaire design and one with expertise in the subject matter. An optional third person for proofreading is sometimes helpful also. The reviewer with questionnaire design expertise can help with the wording of questions as well as sequencing, format, and directions. The subject matter specialist can give feedback about the technical and factual accuracy of items as well as less obvious errors in design, such as experimenter bias or omission of an important subtopic. Beware of only positive critiques. They are not what you need at this point. Select reviewers who are not afraid to give negative feedback. Assure them that you need help, not praise. Avoid someone who works for you or is in a more subtle but nevertheless subservient position.

When your outside reviewers have completed their work, revise the questionnaire, incorporating the suggestions that make sense and contribute to your objectives. You will no doubt receive some suggestions that are beyond your specification matrix or just plain inappropriate. You are, as usual, the final judge.

You should not fear ignoring a reviewer's comments any more than a reviewer should fear giving negative feedback. If this seems impossible, have a friend seek the reviews and keep all identities, including yours, anonymous.

Finally, develop your code book (see Chapter 6) and precolumn responses. This often points out errors that might otherwise go undetected. You are now ready to pilot test your questionnaire.

P*ilot Testing*

The pilot test is a trial run of your interview/questionnaire. It will reveal whether and how the instrument will work under administration conditions with "real" subjects. Pilot test subjects should be selected from your target population if not your study population. If this group is so small that you cannot reduce your study sample for pilot test purposes, your only alternative is to find another group with as many of the same characteristics as possible.

You will obtain the most feedback if you can conduct an individual session with each subject. Administer your questionnaire just as you have planned during your research. However, remain present to note each subject's responses to the various parts. When finished, interview each subject briefly to get overall reactions, comments about trouble spots, and suggestions. Some researchers prefer to read questionnaires to *some* (not all) subjects in order to catch ambiguities and misunderstandings as they occur rather than rely on memory.

If you use a one-to-one situation that includes an "exit" interview, you may need only about five subjects. If you use a group administration without individual interviews, you need at least twice as many subjects. In addition, provide the subjects with an evaluation form or reaction sheet on which to write their comments, suggestions, and criticisms. Also encourage them to write on the questionnaire. Be sure to stress that the questionnaire, and not the participant, is under scrutiny.

F*inal Revision*

Having pilot tested your questionnaire, you make final revisions and are ready to go. If you have carefully followed the steps presented in this chapter, you will probably not have major changes. If you do, consider a second pilot test. Code data according to your code book. Do as many data analyses as possible given the small sample size. Does your code book yield the data you need for your planned contingency tables and other analyses? If not, revise it or even the questions being coded.

As you analyze pilot test data, pay special attention to open-ended questions. If responses to these seem to fall into distinct categories, you may want to convert the question to closed-ended. This will certainly expedite data analysis. Also, check to see that question responses are spread across several alternatives. If all subjects select the same response, consider the question. If an alternative is never selected, consider deleting it. However, keep in mind the number of subjects included in your pilot test. It might not have been large enough to represent typical responses. Again, you must be the judge—a fact that should not come as any great surprise.

Vocabulary

Adaption period	Loaded questions
Aided recall	Loaded words
Cover letter	Loading techniques
Demographic data	Opinionnaire
Demographic questions	Order effects
Double-barreled question	Pilot test
Ethnic identification	Precolumned questionnaire
Filter questions	Questionnaire
Flashcard	Referent
Funnel sequence	Screening question
Informants	Skip instructions
Interview schedule	Specification matrix
Inverted funnel sequence	Telescoping

References

1. Athanasiou, R., and Shaver, P. A research questionnaire on sex. *Psychol. Today*, July 1969. Pp. 64–69.
2. Barton, A. J. Asking the embarrassing question. *Public Opin. Q.* 22:67, 1958.
3. Belson, W. A., and Duncan, J. A. A comparison of the checklist and open response questioning systems. *Appl. Stat.* 11:120, 1962.
4. Department of Health and Human Services, Public Health Service, Division of Alcohol, Drug Abuse, and Mental Health Administration, National Institute of Mental Health. *NIMH Diagnostic Interview Schedule: Version III*, 1981.
5. Dillman, D. *Mail and Telephone Surveys: The Total Design Method*. New York: Wiley, 1978.
6. Green, L. W. Manual for scoring socioeconomic status for research on health behavior. *Public Health Rep*. 85:815, 1970.
7. Hollingshead, A. B. *Two Factor Index of Social Position*. New Haven: Hollingshead, 1957.
8. Marquis, K. H., and Cannell, C. F. Effects of Some Experimental Interviewing Techniques on Reporting in the Health Interview Survey. In *Vital and Health Statistics*, Series 2, No. 41. Rockville, Md.: U.S. National Center for Health Statistics, 1971.
9. Orlich, D. C. *Designing Sensible Surveys*. Pleasantville, N.Y.: Redgrave, 1978.
10. Social Science Research Council. *Basic Background Items for U.S. Household Surveys*. Washington: Center for Coordination of Research on Social Indicators, 1975.
11. Sudman, S., and Bradburn, N. M. *Asking Questions: A Practical Guide to Questionnaire Design*. San Francisco: Jossey-Bass, 1982.

VI: *Inferential Statistics*

The chapters in this Unit describe common tests for statistical significance. They are organized according to whether they are

1. Parametric or nonparametric
2. Bivariate or multivariate
3. Designed for independent variables that are dichotomous (two groups) or multivalued (three or more groups).

Chapter 15 introduces the notion of inference testing, sampling distributions and standard errors, degrees of freedom, power, and the probabilities of Type I and II errors. The Z test is used to explain the statistical test. The Pearson r is used to illustrate power analysis for sample size and the probability of Type II error when a null hypothesis is retained. Finally, threats to statistical conclusion validity are presented and "when a null is a null is a null" is explored. This chapter provides basic material that should be part of the repertoire of all those who seek to use statistical tests. Without it, and with only the recipe for computing a specific test, the probability for abuse and statistical hocus pocus remains high.

Chapter 16 focuses on the *t* test and related *parametric* procedures for one or two groups. It is best studied immediately following Chapter 15, although some parts of it may be skipped by introductory level students. Chapter 17 presents one-way ANOVA and other parametric multivalue group procedures, and Chapters 18 and 19 present nonparametric procedures. Chapter 20 introduces multivariate techniques with presentation of computer analysis for multiple regression, factorial ANOVA, and ANCOVA and simple descriptions of yet other techniques. Once Chapters 15 and 16 have been read, Chapters 17, 18, and 19 can follow in any order. Chapter 17 is required before Chapter 20.

Use of the vocabulary words and short data analysis problems from your instructor will help you understand the material in this unit. However, do not stop there. Generate three or four hypotheses appropriate for each test you study. If the analyses of these hypotheses are statistically significant, or *not* significant, what can you conclude? Are rival hypotheses present? How might they be controlled? Next, review the statistical analyses presented in the articles of a recent nursing research journal. If the null hypothesis is accepted, do power analysis for Type II error. If the null is rejected, calculate magnitude estimates or confidence intervals. Now, what is the *practical significance* of this research? How might it be improved?

Statistical analysis serves two functions. First, it allows you to organize, describe, and summarize a series or group of data points. For this you use measures of central tendency—the mean, median, and mode—and dispersion—the range, variance, and standard deviation. Often, frequency distributions, percentages, scatter diagrams, rates, proportions, and correlation coefficients are used. The first function, called descriptive statistics, was presented in Chapters 6 through 8.

The second function, inferential statistics, allows you to determine, for example, if an experimental and control group are significantly different or if a correlation coefficient is significantly different from zero. Inferential statistics is presented in Chapters 15 through 20.

Statistical Hypotheses

As discussed in Chapter 2, the focus of research can be stated as a research hypothesis, research question, or objective. They are all comparable and selection of one or another depends largely on the nature of your research. However, when you use inferential statistics, you translate, conceptually at least, your question into statistical hypotheses as the first part of your number manipulations. The statistical hypothesis usually takes the form of a **null hypothesis** (H_0) and an **alternate hypothesis** (H_a). For example, if you wish to determine whether males are different from females on a criterion (i.e., dependent) variable that is measured at the interval level, such as response to touch, the null hypothesis would be

$$H_0: \mu_M = \mu_F$$

where H_0 = null hypothesis

μ_M = mean of male population on the dependent variable

μ_F = mean of female population on the dependent variable.

The equal sign indicates that, under the null hypothesis, you expect male and female responses to be equal. You are, of course, hoping to reject your null hypothesis. Therefore, you propose an alternate hypothesis (H_a), which corresponds to a research hypothesis and describes what you expect to find. It could be $H_a: \mu_M \neq \mu_F$ if you do not have a basis for knowing how males and females will differ. This would be called **nondirectional,** because you have not specified in which direction (or how) the two means are expected to differ. However, if you have a theoretical basis for predicting the direction in which they will differ, your alternate hypothesis could be $H_a: \mu_M > \mu_F$ or $Ha: \mu_M < \mu_F$ and would therefore be considered **directional.** Note that the Greek letter μ (*mu,* pronounced *mew*) rather than $\overline{X}$ is used to symbolize the means. This is because statistical hypotheses are written in terms of population **parameters** rather than sample descriptive statistics. According to custom, the values of variables in a population are called parameters and are symbolized by Greek letters while values of variables describing samples are called statistics and are symbolized by English letters.

Statistical hypotheses are rarely included in journal reports of research. It is simply assumed that researchers have conceptualized their research in these terms when they use inferential procedures. In theses and other student reports, however, they are sometimes required as proof of a student's understanding of these concepts.

Power Analysis

Suppose an experimental group was taught a special relaxation technique for use during proctoscopic examinations, while the control group received no special instruction. A stress index, consisting of the physiological measures for blood pressure and pulse, a checklist of observed stress response behaviors, and a self-report anxiety scale is used as a measure of the dependent variable. Means for each group are computed. Because group means tend to vary somewhat owing to chance or factors unrelated to an independent variable, it is essential that the researcher determine if the observed difference between the two groups is due to chance variation alone or due to the effect of the relaxation technique. To do this, first a level of significance is selected.

Level of Significance

In order to decide objectively which differences are so unusual that we will not consider them chance occurrences, we agree on a conventional statistical definition of *unusual* by establishing a level of significance *before* data analysis begins. In effect, we are setting odds on how often we would be incorrect in concluding that the independent variable caused change in the dependent variable. This level of significance is often called **alpha,** or the *alpha* level, and in statistical shorthand is signified by α, the Greek letter for alpha.

One thing we could do is set the chance of error so low that it would be almost impossible to make a mistake. In so doing, however, it would also be almost impossible for observed differences to be attributed to experimental effects. We would seldom obtain a **significant difference.** We would, in essence, be agreeing to attribute no causality to an experimental variable. In addition, we would be running a high risk of actually obtaining a significant difference and yet not declaring it as such. Our conclusions, then, would be wrong. The more sensible combination of reality with research precision is, therefore, to choose a low but realistic level at which to draw the line, or establish a cutting point, between chance and experimental effects. In the behavioral sciences two such levels of significance are commonly used, one at 1 percent and the other at 5 percent. In statistical shorthand, these are written as $\alpha = .01$ or $\alpha = .05$, respectively. *After* statistical analysis, moreover, these are written as $p < .01$ or $p < .05$, respectively, or even $p < .03$ or $p < .04$. The *less than* sign ($<$) indicates that probabilities of error lower but not higher than the indicated value are possible. The p stands for the **observed probability of**

error in declaring that a difference is due to an independent variable when, in fact, it is due to chance fluctuation. In the past, when most statistical tests were calculated without the aid of computers, researchers labeled results as either $p < .05$, $p < .01$, or $p < .001$, selecting the most stringent p level applicable to each test statistic. These three p levels were all the information statistical tables could easily yield. Thus, while a result might actually be $p < .03$, a researcher would label it with the less stringent $p < .05$. With the widespread use of computers that calculate exact observed probability levels, this practice is now changing. More often, researchers report exact observed probability levels, so that readers have this additional piece of information to use in evaluating a given research project.

Nursing research typically uses the 5 percent level of significance. Again, this means that you are willing to run a 5 percent chance of making an error when you declare a significant difference. Five percent may not seem large. However, it means that if a study in which there were no real differences was conducted twenty times, one of those times, or 5 percent, you would conclude that there was an experimental effect when, in reality, there was none. By the standards of fields such as medical engineering, the 1 percent and 5 percent error rates are grotesquely large. Thus, in setting the level of significance, a researcher must be guided by the nature of the research. A study involving a radical surgical procedure would set the risk of error low because of hazards involved in erroneously advocating a radical technique. A study correlating clinic appointment keeping with greater geographic distance traveled might set the risk of error low if a false negative correlation might result in reduced funding for neighborhood clinics. However, in most nursing research, because of measurement error, threats to validity, and various confounding variables, we must often run a 5 percent risk if we want ever to obtain statistically significant results.

Type I and Type II Errors

When a researcher sets out to test a research hypothesis and establishes a 5 percent level of significance before analyzing the data, this particular error, labeling a difference real or significant when it is not, is called a **type I error.** Thus, the odds of incorrectly concluding significant results can be called the level of significance, α level, p level, p value, and probability of type I error. Moreover, via the exact observed probabilities associated with findings, the p value, a research report reader decides whether or not the null hypothesis should have been rejected. While the researcher may believe $p < .05$ is adequate, a reader may not accept findings unless they are significant at .01 or .001. Other readers may be content with .08 or .10 if the sample size is small. Standards for this can be inferred from related research.

There is another possible error—incorrectly labeling a difference as due to chance, or not significant, when it is actually a real difference. It is called **type II error.** This is an equally important problem and involves a risk rate that is relatively easy to estimate by use of tables. In reports of research, however, you will seldom see any reference to the probability of type II error when researchers have failed to obtain significant results. Ignoring this leaves us at an imprecise level of research, which is inexcusable. Part of the blame for this rests with professional journals whose practice is to publish only studies that report significant results. Publication of results that failed to reject the null hypothesis while maintaining a relatively low rate of type II error (20 percent or less) would also enhance building a body of knowledge as well as preventing future researchers from needlessly repeating the fruitless efforts of others.

Determination of the type II error rate, sometimes called the ***beta*** (β) **level,** involves power analysis. **Power** is defined as the probability that the inferential procedure (i.e., statistical test) will reject a null hypothesis *when it should be rejected.* In other words, it is the probability that an inferential procedure will support a research or alternate hypothesis when it should be supported. Both power and the probability of type II error can vary from zero to 100 percent, as can the probability of type I error. Furthermore, power and the probability of type II error always sum to 100 percent or unity (i.e., 1). This is not so for type I error in combination with either power or type II error. Exhibit 15.1 illustrates the four possible outcomes of statistical analysis and should clarify the distinctions between Type I and Type II error and between power and Type II error. To summarize Exhibit 15.1, in any research situation in which inferential statistics are used, there are four possible outcomes. You can declare significant results when, in real life, there indeed are significant results. This is power. (In Exhibit 15.1, this is outcome 1.) Second, you can make another correct conclusion when you fail to reject your null hypothesis and, indeed, in real life your null hypothesis was correct. (This is outcome 4 in Exhibit 15.1.) Third, you can make a type I error by declaring that you have significant results when in real life there is no significant difference or effect. (Outcome 3 in Exhibit 15.1.) The chances of your having done this are described by your α level. Fourth, you can make a type II error by failing to reject your null hypothesis when, in real life, there is a significant difference. (This is outcome 2 in Exhibit 15.1)

Power

Power analysis is useful in determining sample size before research is implemented and the type II error rate after failure to reject the null hypothesis. Power is a function of (1) the level of significance, (2) sample size, and (3) effect size. **Effect size** (ES) is the *amount* of differences or the *strength* of relationships found in the sample. The ES must be calculated after a statistical test, usually using the test statistic or sample statistics in a simple formula. Only with a Pearson r is this not necessary. Thus, for illustrative purposes, we will use the Pearson r in this chapter. As each statistical test is presented in subsequent chapters, so too is the simple formula for calculating ES. You can use these formulas to calculate ES from information given in journal articles so that you can use power analysis in planning your own research or critiquing the research of others.

Exhibit 15.2 illustrates the relationship among power, α level, sample size,

Exhibit 15-1. Four possible outcomes of research.

Results of data analysis	What Really Exists in the Population	
	In real life, the null hypothesis is false (or the research hypothesis is true)	In real life, the null hypothesis is true (or the research hypothesis is false)
Inferential data analysis yields significant results (or the null hypothesis is rejected)	(1) Correct conclusion (power)	(3) Type I error (described by alpha level)
Inferential data analysis yields no significant results (or the null hypothesis is accepted)	(2) Type II error (described by beta level; β = 1 − power)	(4) Correct conclusion

and effect size for the Pearson r. Note that power increases as the type I error rate, or α level, becomes larger. For example, for r = .30 and n = 50, power is 33 percent at α = .01, 57 percent at α = .05, and 69 percent at α = .10. Recalling that type II error equals one (or 100 percent) minus power, this can be stated another way. For r = .30 and n = 50, type II error is 67 percent (100 − 33) when type I error is set at 1 percent, type II error is 43 percent (100 − 57) when type I error is 5 percent, and type II error is 31 percent (100 − 69) when type I error is 10 percent. Thus, type II error decreases as the α level, type I error rate, increases. Power also increases (thereby reducing the chance of type II error) as sample size increases. For r = .30, power is 9 percent when n = 20, while it is 25 percent for n = 40 and 41 percent for n = 60. Finally, power increases as the effect size increases. For n = 50 at α = .05, power is 11 percent for r = .10, 29 percent for r = .20, and 57 percent for r = .30.

The computational procedures for power analysis are beyond the scope of this textbook. However, tables that use power analysis to estimate the probability of Type II error in research utilizing α = .05 are provided in Appendix IV for many commonly used statistical procedures. The chapters discussing each procedure demonstrate how ES is calculated for that particular statistical test. Furthermore, the tables in Appendix IV can also be used to estimate needed sample size before you begin your research. Using an effect size based on results reported by studies included in your literature review (or the minimum ES you can accept as practically significant), enter the table and move down the ES column until you find a type II probability of 20 (or power of 80) opposite a row

Exhibit 15-2. Percentage of power of nondirectional r as a function of effect size (ES), sample size (n), and alpha level (α).

		ES = r				
		Small		Medium		Large
n	α	.10	.20	.30	.40	.50
20	.01	02	04	09	20	38
	.05	07	14	25	43	64
	.10	13	22	37	56	75
30	.01	02	06	17	36	62
	.05	08	19	37	61	83
	.10	15	29	50	72	90
40	.01	02	09	25	50	78
	.05	09	24	48	74	92
	.10	16	35	60	83	96
50	.01	03	12	33	63	89
	.05	11	29	57	83	97
	.10	18	41	69	90	98
60	.01	03	15	41	74	94
	.05	12	34	65	90	99
	.10	20	46	76	94	99
80	.01	04	21	56	87	99
	.05	14	43	78	96	>99
	.10	23	56	86	98	
100	.01	06	29	69	95	>99
	.05	17	52	86	99	>99
	.10	27	64	92	99	
120	.01	06	29	69	95	>99
	.05	19	59	92	>99	>99
	.10	29	71	96		
140	.01	08	42	85	99	>99
	.05	22	66	95	>99	>99
	.10	32	82	99		
160	.01	09	49	90	99	>99
	.05	24	72	97		
	.10	35	82	99		
180	.01	11	55	94	>99	>99
	.05	27	77	98		
	.10	38	86	99		
200	.01	12	61	96	>99	>99
	.05	29	81	99		
	.10	41	89			
250	.01	16	73	99	>99	>99
	.05	35	89			
	.10	47	94			

Note: Type II error rate is 1 − power.

that has $\alpha = .05$. Then, move across the row to the value of n that corresponds to that value. For example, using Exhibit 15.2, if your literature review suggests an ideal (or realistic) ES of .30, start at the top of the .30 column and move down until you reach the first power = 80 for a row with $\alpha = .05$ and left across the row to n. You find $n = 80$ for a power of 78 percent and $n = 100$ for power = 86 percent. Sample size should be between 80 and 100. To be more exact, $n = 85$ will yield power = .80 or beta, β, type II error rate = .20. Using $n = 85$, if you still fail to reject your null hypothesis, you might consider other avenues of research. Refer to Cohen's *Statistical Power Analysis for the Behavioral Sciences* [1] for additional tables using other values of α that are not included in the tables in this book. For values of n or ES not given in the tables, linear interpolation between the two nearest values will give an adequate estimate.

Just how much should power be? How large can the type II error rate be? There are no right or wrong answers to these questions, just as there is no right or wrong α level, although by custom most behavioral scientists use $\alpha = .05$. Cohen [1] suggests a type II error rate of .20 (and thus ideal power set at .80) and type I error rate of .05, based upon the rationale that it is four times worse to make a type I error—declare significant results when there are none—than it is to make a type II error—fail to declare significant results when they exist. If you have a good reason for using different values of α and power, you should do so. As nursing research incorporates more physiological measures with their decreased measurement error, it is quite possible that power will be increased and the risk for error reduced.

If you fail to reject a null hypothesis and you find that your type II error rate is 20 percent or less, you probably have good reason to abandon that line of inquiry. If, on the other hand, your type II error rate is higher, you would do well to redesign your research. Moreover, after doing power analysis before a study begins, you may find that some research is simply not worth doing. For example, you know ahead of time that your sample size is small—say 20, the practical significance test demands at least a medium effect size of $r = .30$ (or $r^2 = .09$), and you have no legitimate reason for increasing the α level beyond .05. Using Exhibit 15.2 for $r = .30$ and $n = 20$, you find that your chance of type II error is 63 percent at $\alpha = .10$, 75 percent at $\alpha = .05$, and 91 percent at .01. (An r of .44 is needed to reach statistical significance at $\alpha = .05$ when $n = 20$.) Clearly, a well designed study should not set up the researcher for the failure that this analysis forecasts. The most obvious solutions are to increase the sample size or abandon the project. Proponents of small sample size, however, argue that only large effects ($r = .50$ or $r^2 = .25$) are practically significant and at these levels power increases dramatically. This is a valid argument. However, base your decision to proceed on your literature review, which should have revealed the magnitude of effect sizes found in related research studies. If these are large, then you can feel reasonably confident in proceeding with a small sample size. In most cases, however, effect sizes are small.

The Statistical Test

Before we discuss specific statistical tests, we will discuss what all statistical tests have in common and what these tests are, in fact, doing. This involves four concepts: the sampling distribution, the standard error, degrees of freedom, and directionality or tailedness.

Sampling Distribution

You can think of one type of **sampling distribution** as similar to the normal curve distribution with one difference. Instead of describing individual scores dispersed around the group mean of a *sample,* like the normal curve distribution studied in Chapter 6, the sampling distribution describes a distribution of values (e.g., standard deviations or means) that have been calculated for many separate samples drawn from the *same* population. Each sampling distribution has a mean (e.g., mean of all the sample standard deviations, mean for all the sample means) and standard deviation, which is called its standard error. For purposes of this discussion, consider as an example a sampling distribution of means of samples, each with $n = 100$, drawn from the same population. The mean of the sampling distribution would be the **mean of means,** the mean of all the $n = 100$ sample means. The values on which each sample mean is based can be scores on a specific measure, differences observed between two groups, or correlations between variables. *The sampling distribution describes all the different values that can be expected to occur.* To make a sampling distribution, you would randomly select (and measure) from the population all possible samples of a given size. Each sample mean would be one data point in the sampling distribution. By computing the mean of all those means, you obtain a value, equal to the value of the population mean, called the mean of means. In reality, of course, we do not develop sampling distributions. This has already been done mathematically, and we simply make use of this previous work.

Standard Error

You have already seen how the standard error is used to establish confidence intervals. More will be said about this later in the chapter. Now we wish to examine the standard error as it is used in a statistical test. The **standard error** is simply the standard deviation of the sampling distribution. Because the sampling distribution includes many more individual subjects than the frequency distribution of just one sample, it stands to reason that there will be less error in estimating the true mean of the population. Therefore, the standard error of a sampling distribution is smaller than the standard deviation of a corresponding frequency distribution for a single sample. Thus, when you are using the standard deviation of a sample to *estimate** the standard error of the sampling distribution (which you must do in some of the statistical tests), you must, so to speak, use a "correction factor." If you used $(n - 1)$ to compute your standard

---

*The actual standard error is the *population* standard deviation, σ, divided by the square root of the size of the samples, $\sqrt{n}$. Since we rarely know σ, we substitute SD, which introduces little error when sample sizes are large enough.

deviation, you divide the standard deviation of your sample by the square root of n, ($\sqrt{n}$), the number of subjects in each of the samples which compose the sampling distribution.* Notice that as the sample size increases, the standard error decreases. This seems logical because there would be less error in estimating the population values, **parameters,** from sample values, **statistics,** if you had more members of the population included in each sample. Just as with the sampling distribution, you rarely compute the actual standard error ($SE_{\bar{x}}$). You simply estimate it by using the standard deviation of a sample and dividing it by the square root of the number of subjects in the sample.

In reality, the sampling distribution and standard error are theoretical notions that we use to evaluate our results. We compare sample values with them when using a statistical test to *infer* significant differences or significant relationships. If a sample value is more than 1.96 or 2.56 standard errors from the mean of means, we conclude that the observed value or test statistic is not likely to be due to chance variation. Therefore it is statistically significant. Our conclusion is based upon a 95 percent (1.96 $SE_{\bar{x}}$) or 99 percent (2.56 $SE_{\bar{x}}$) probability of being correct (i.e., an α level of .05 or .01). This should be clearer when these principles are illustrated using the Z test. First, a few other concepts must be introduced.

Degrees of Freedom

The concept of degrees of freedom (df) is used in most of the statistical tests. There is an appropriate method of computing df associated with each statistical test. It will be presented with each test.

To illustrate the general concept of degrees of freedom, suppose you asked a subject to name any five numbers. We could say that she had five df. Now, suppose that you asked her to name eight numbers but to make sure that the mean of these numbers equaled 40. She is now free to name any numbers she chooses for the first seven, but for the last number she must name the number that will make a total of 320 for the eight numbers, in order to arrive at a mean of 40. If she names as her first seven numbers 16, 0.5, .75, 100, − 4, 45, and − 65, then her eighth number must be 226.75. She has eight numbers to name and one restriction, so her df equals eight minus one, or seven. Suppose you asked another subject to name seven numbers in such a way that the first three had a mean of 19 and all seven had a mean of 10. Here, there are seven numbers and two restrictions, so the df equals seven minus two, or five.

Directionality or Tailedness

At the beginning of this chapter, directionality was mentioned. When the alternate hypothesis specified only that a difference would be present but not which group would have higher means, it was called *nondirectional*. When one group was specified as having a higher mean than the other, the hypothesis was consid-

---

*If, for some reason, the sum of squares was divided by n rather than $n − 1$ when the SD was computed, the standard error is computed by dividing the sample SD by $\sqrt{n − 1}$. See Spence, Cotton, Underwood, and Duncan [3] for details.

ered *directional.* This is what is known as *directionality.* It is also referred to as *tailedness.* A **two-tailed** hypothesis is the same as a nondirectional hypothesis, implying that the difference can be in either of two directions. A **one-tailed** test is directional; the hypothesis specifies which way the groups will differ or whether a correlation is positive or negative.

How a Statistical Test Works

You now have the basic essentials of statistical tests. Statistical tests enable you to attach a probability estimate to an inference you draw from your data. A statistical test says, in effect, "The inference you have drawn is correct at the specified level of significance. You may act as though your research hypothesis were true, remembering that the probability that it is in error or untrue is equal to your level of significance." It can also say, "Your failure to reject the null hypothesis is the result of a statistical test with power equal to one minus the Type II error rate. Therefore, this line of research should be abandoned or pursued, depending on the error rate acceptable to you."

Just how do you draw an inference? Based on your level of measurement and the type of statement you wish to make, causal-comparative or correlational, you select a statistical test whose assumptions or rules can be met by your research situation. The statistical test is a mathematical procedure or formula that converts the raw data or the descriptive statistics for your sample into a numerical value, a **test statistic,** which is then compared with the sampling distribution for that statistical test. Each statistical test has a unique sampling distribution (or series of sampling distributions for each degree of freedom) that is summarized in the form of a table and included in the appendices of most statistics books. Appendix III in this book includes statistical tables. Entering the table developed for the specific statistical test you are employing and using (1) the df you calculated according to the rules for that statistical test and (2) the level of significance you have established before beginning your research, you extract a **critical value.** You then compare the value of the test statistic you have computed with the critical value you extracted from the table. In most cases, when the value of your test statistic is equal to or larger than the critical value in the table, your results are statistically significant. In some tests, it must be less than the critical value. The directions for each statistical test tell you which. This is all there is to significance testing.

Sometimes, you can calculate "by hand" this numerical value or test statistic. Most of the time, especially with large sample sizes or the more sophisticated statistical tests, the calculation is complicated and you therefore use a computer. Most of the computer routines, in addition, print out the level of significance for your value or test statistic, so you do not have to consult a statistical table. You just look to see if the p value is equal to or less than your α level. If it is, your results are *significant.* Beware of computer errors. In addition to being subject to human error, machines can malfunction while still printing out what appear to be valid results. You should periodically test the accuracy of a computer by submitting problems for which you already have an answer—such as examples from your textbook.

The One-Sample Z Test

The one-sample Z test, which is not often used in research because it requires samples larger than 30 and knowledge of both the mean and standard deviation of the population from which a sample is drawn, illustrates how a statistical test works more clearly than most. Since you have already studied the normal curve, as well as the transformation of a raw score into a z score and its resultant position on the normal curve distribution, the process of statistical testing should be easier to understand within the context of the Z test.

Suppose you are working at a community health agency that serves a special neighborhood area. It seems to you that venereal disease is first occurring at younger ages at your clinic as compared with the city at large. You decide to see if your clinic is significantly different. If it is, you believe more funds should be allocated to your clinic to provide additional services for youth. Because you know the population (city) mean (14.2 years) and standard deviation (7.34), and you have a sample size of 40, you can use the one-sample Z statistic. You set .05 as your α level.

Computing a one-sample Z statistic is similar to computing a z score. In effect, you are computing a z score for one sample mean in the sampling distribution. The formula is

$$Z = \frac{\bar{X} - \bar{\bar{X}}}{SE_{\bar{X}}} \tag{15.1}$$

where $\bar{\bar{X}}$ = the population mean, or mean of means

$\bar{X}$ = the sample mean

$SE_{\bar{X}}$ = the standard error of the sampling distribution

The standard error, recall, can be estimated by dividing the standard deviation of the city population by the square root of n ($7.34/\sqrt{40} = 1.16$).* Because the mean age in your clinic sample is 12.1, the mean age citywide is 14.2, and the standard error is 1.16, the Z statistic is computed as follows:

$$Z = \frac{12.1 - 14.2}{1.16} = \frac{-2.1}{1.16} = -1.81$$

The Z test does not have df.

You are now ready to compare the test statistic (-1.81) with the critical value from the distribution for Z, which is the normal curve distribution. Recall, on the

---

*The sampling distribution is made up of samples of equal sizes (n), which are the same as the sample n. Therefore, when estimating the SE from the σ, the n that is used is the sample size.

normal curve, 95 percent of all z scores will fall between ± 1.96 standard deviations and 99 percent will fall between ± 2.58 standard deviations. Therefore, if your Z test statistic is greater than ± 1.96, the chances are 95 percent that your value did not occur by chance alone. It is not just a chance fluctuation within the population. Conversely, the chances are 5 percent that you will be in error if you declare a value greater than ± 1.96 as significant. Because your level of significance was set at .05, the critical value is ± 1.96. (If the level of significance had been set at .01, the critical value would have been ± 2.58, the points within which 99 percent of the z scores on a normal curve fall.) The Z statistic for our example is -1.81. Because it is not equal to or greater than the critical value of ± 1.96, it appears that it is *not significant*.

This brings up an important point. The preceding example was treated as nondirectional or two-tailed. That is, the sample difference could be either greater or less than the population mean. The "tailed" term refers to the tails or extremes of the sampling distribution, in this case the normal distribution curve. If a direction is not specified, then you must select a critical value of Z *in each tail* of the curve so that you will be able to determine the significance of either of two possible differences (or changes)—higher or lower than the population mean. To use the 5 percent level of significance we divided the 5 percent so that some of it was in each of the two tails of the Z distribution. The typical procedure is to do this symmetrically—identifying the extreme 2.5 percent of the curve at either end. This is what was done for the nondirectional test and therefore the critical value of ± 1.96 was used.

If we hypothesize that the mean is significantly *less than* the population mean, we can use a directional or one-tailed test. At $\alpha < .05$, this means that only *negative Z* values of -1.643 or greater indicate a significant difference. (At $\alpha < .01$, only negative Z values of -2.33 or greater indicate a significant difference.) When the research hypothesis specifies the nature of change or difference that is expected, a one-tailed test is sufficient to test that hypothesis. When the research hypothesis does not specify the direction of the difference or change to be expected, then a two-tailed test is required to test the hypothesis fully. There is a practical issue involved here: it is always easier to achieve statistically significant results using the one-tailed rather than the two-tailed test *when the results come out in the direction expected.* Exhibit 15.3 illustrates this point. The two points representing 1.96 in each tail are the critical values for a two-tailed test of significance at $\alpha = .05$. The grey area represents the basis of some controversy. All the research results that fall into the grey area would be statistically significant by the one-tailed test but would not be statistically significant by the two-tailed test. This difference has led to some criticism of the one-tailed procedure. Critics state that in almost every research situation one direction is more logical than the other. Therefore, almost any researcher can state a directional hypothesis and justify use of the one-tailed test, with its greater ease of obtaining a statistically significant result. Critics of the one-tailed test also state if the researcher was wrong in selecting the direction and statistical significance

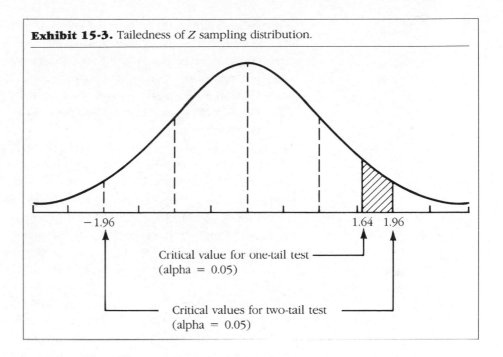

Exhibit 15-3. Tailedness of Z sampling distribution.

occurs in the opposite direction, a type II error would occur. Thus, the one-tailed alternate hypothesis may be rejected when, in fact, a two tailed alternate hypothesis might have been supported.

Returning to our example, because a negative one-tailed test was specified, the Z value of -1.81 is greater than the critical value of -1.64. Thus, the H_0 is rejected and the H_a supported. The age at first onset of venereal disease in the neighborhood clinic is significantly lower than that in the citywide population. Of course, directionality, like level of significance, must be determined *before* data analysis. We cannot change our minds and add directionality after we see the results of data analysis. It would be akin to placing a bet on a horse after the race was finished.

Parametric and Nonparametric Tests

There are two major categories of inferential statistics, parametric and non-parametric. **Parametric** statistical tests make assumptions about the population from which the sample was drawn and demand interval level measurement. **Nonparametric** statistical tests, on the other hand, are not restricted by assumptions about the population and can be used with nominal and ordinal data as well. The advantages of nonparametric tests are that (1) they do not assume the sample represents some specific type of population, (2) they are applicable to small samples of less than 8 when their parallel parametric tests might require, as a minimum, 12 or 15 and, (3) they require no more than ordinal level measurement and some, such as chi square, require only nominal level data.

Since nonparametric statistical tests have fewer restrictions, you may wonder why every researcher does not use them to avoid the assumptions of parametric statistical tests. One reason is power, the probability that an inferential procedure will reject H_0 when it should be rejected. For comparable situations, any one nonparametric procedure is less powerful than the parallel parametric procedure, and therefore you pay a price in loss of power if you routinely use a nonparametric procedure. However, parametric tests are more powerful only when the assumptions underlying their use are met. Otherwise, a nonparametric test may be as powerful as the parallel parametric test. Why are nonparametric procedures less powerful? It is because nonparametric procedures use less information about the data than parametric procedures. Data are treated as ordinal or nominal. The information gained by the interval quality (equal distances between points) is ignored. With less precise measurement, greater differences must occur before significant results can be obtained. Of course, there are times when both procedures would lead to the same conclusion. However, there are other times when a parametric procedure would yield significant results while the comparable nonparametric procedure would not. In addition, some parametric tests are much more complex than any existing nonparametric tests. These allow more sophisticated analysis, such as simultaneous consideration of many independent and/or dependent variables. This can be an important advantage to research that studies holistic man. Therefore, when you have interval level data and can meet the assumptions, use parametric tests. Some of the widely used nonparametric statistical tests are discussed in Chapters 18 and 19. Chapters 16, 17, and 20 describe parametric tests.

Assumptions of Parametric Statistical Tests

Although parametric statistical tests have more power and sophistication, they also have certain requirements or basic assumptions that must be met before they can be used. The rationale behind these asumptions requires extensive mathematical theory that is beyond the scope of this book. We will simply describe the assumptions.

The first requirement is that data are measured at the interval level. The second requirement is called the **assumption of normality.** Your data are assumed to have been drawn from a population that has a nearly normal distribution of values for the dependent or criterion variable being researched. If you could measure the entire population on the variable, the resultant frequency distribution would look similar to the normal curve. The third, and last, assumption is known as the **homogeneity of variance** assumption. Variances in each of your sample groups are assumed to be homogeneous or about equal, within the bounds of chance variation. In rare cases when variances or groups are not homogeneous, especially in complex parametric tests, even large differences between means can result in type II errors.

The first assumption, interval data, is the most important. The second and third assumptions have been examined extensively by researchers in mathematical statistical theory who have found that many parametric tests are relatively insensitive to violation of these two assumptions, especially when only one occurs at a given time and groups are nearly equal in size. Therefore, unless there is good evidence to believe that populations are rather seriously nonnormal or that variances are extremely *heterogeneous,* it is usually unwise to use a nonparametric statistical test in place of a parametric one.

Many of the parametric procedures have additional assumptions or rules that are unique to a specific statistical test. These, of course, are presented in this book when that test is described. If a researcher cannot meet the assumptions, a parallel nonparametric procedure is generally used. This usually involves converting interval data to ordinal data.

Selecting the Appropriate Inferential Test

Each parametric or nonparametric statistical test is designed to test a specific type of research statement. For example, there is a specific test to use when you wish to compare the pretest mean of a single group of subjects with its posttest mean or when you wish to compare means of two groups in which the subjects have been matched. These tests are called **dependent groups** or **correlated means,** because there exist, in addition to any differences due to an independent or other variable, similarities due to matching or the same person's being measured more than once. There are tests for only two related measures and others for more than two related measures. Other tests compare two, or more than two, groups that have been randomly assigned or are otherwise independent of each other. These tests are called **independent groups** or **independent means.** There are also parametric and nonparametric correlational procedures. Some use only two variables while others use three or more. As you progress through this Unit you will become familiar with many of the tests available to you.

Statistical Conclusion Validity

As stated in Chapter 4, the many rival explanations to support a research hypothesis can be, for the sake of expediency, grouped into four categories: threats to (1) internal validity, (2) construct validity, (3) external validity, and (4) statistical conclusion validity. The first two groups were discussed in Chapter 4 and the third, threats to external validity, was discussed in Chapter 10. The last group of threats, threats to statistical conclusion validity, is discussed in this chapter.

Statistical conclusion validity is concerned with whether or not statistical analysis has been correctly applied to data and the interpretation of either rejection or acceptance of a null hypothesis. Power analysis is essential for statistical conclusion validity. If sample size is not large enough, even true effects may not be observed. Therefore, when a null hypothesis is not rejected, power analysis to detect the probability of type II error is appropriate. On the other hand, even small effects (i.e., small ES) can be declared statistically significant when sample size is excessively large.

Magnitude Estimates

Because an ES can sometimes be statistically but not practically significant, it is important to examine the magnitude of, say, differences between two groups— just how large is this difference? Because a correlation coefficient provides a measure of magnitude that is independent of the scale of the raw scores involved, it can help to assess the practical significance of differences between means. Therefore, the statistical tests presented in the succeeding chapters include procedures, whenever possible, for estimating both the ES and the **magnitude of effect** via a correlation coefficient as an alternative to using differences between raw score means. The correlations allow examination of the shared variance and amount of unexplained variance. Thus, if a *t* test between two groups was statistically significant and an *r* of .26 was calculated as an estimate of the magnitude of the observed differences, the researcher can readily see that only 7 percent (r^2) of the variance in the dependent variable is accounted for by the independent variable—not such a very big deal after all. You would do well to look for *additional* variables with which to explain changes in the dependent variables, rather than considering that line of research complete because the groups were significantly different.

Confidence Intervals

Cook and Campbell [2], two of the leading authors on the topic of research design, moreover, urge researchers to consider not only tests of statistical significance (including the probability of Type II error if the null hypothesis is accepted) *and* magnitude estimates, but also **confidence intervals** when appropriate. The concept of confidence intervals has been presented previously in this book. In Chapter 6, the standard error was used to place confidence intervals around a sample mean in order to estimate with a given probability the value of the population mean. In Chapter 7, the standard error of estimate was used to place confidence intervals around a predicted score in order to describe, with a given probability, the range within which a true score could be expected to fall. Finally, the standard error of measurement was presented in Chapter 13 for the purpose of placing confidence intervals around corrected observed scores.

Although confidence intervals and even magnitude estimates are rarely reported in research articles at the present time, you can easily compute them from the information presented in the article and this book and thereby have much more information on which to base your evaluation of the efficacy of research you are critiquing. For example, in a survey of weight reduction techniques, suppose a given intervention with 100 subjects yielded a mean weight loss of 32 pounds in 2 months with a SD = 20. The SE = $20/\sqrt{100}$ or 2. By adding and subtracting 2.56 SEs (i.e., 2.56 × 2 = 5.12) from the sample mean of 32, we have confidence limits at 99 percent of 26.88 and 37.12. Within that interval, 99 percent of all future replications with that same population can be expected to fall. Knowing that a range from 27 to 37 pounds lost can be expected 99 percent of the time tells more than that 32 pounds were lost in only one sample.

Threats to Statistical Conclusion Validity

The following threats to statistical conclusion validity are not equally damaging or equal in the probability that they might occur. Although the list includes many of those that occur fairly often, there may be others, peculiar to your research situation, that have been omitted. The threats as listed are not mutually exclusive, either. They are simply meant to provide a core you can modify to suit the unique purposes of your research situation.

Low Statistical Power

The probability of type II error, as you know, increases when n is low. Moreover, certain statistical tests have inherently lower power (e.g., test of the difference between independent correlation coefficients and most nonparametric tests) than others.

Violated Assumptions of Statistical Tests

Although some assumptions like normality can be violated with little problem in some tests, other violations render the results suspect. With the widespread use of computers, it is particularly important to *look* at the data that is input. Computers will always grind out numbers, however irrelevant. Do not forget the saying, "garbage in–garbage out." Look at your data and how they are distributed.

Family Type I Error

The widespread use of computers has also enabled data snooping and fishing. Often, many tests are run on the *same* data. This increases the risk of type I error, called **family type I error,** which is discussed further in Chapter 17, where the *post hoc* tests to be used after successful analysis of variance are introduced.

Low Reliability of Measures

As discussed in Chapters 11 and 13, poor reliability of measures places severe restrictions upon the upper limits of effect sizes ($\sqrt{r_{tt}}$). Low reliability inflates standard errors, which, as you know, play important roles in calculating inferential statistics and confidence intervals. There is a statistical correction for poor reliability (i.e., correction for attenuation), but its use is rarely justified.

Low Reliability of Independent Variables

When an experimental variable is administered differently to some subjects, it is unstable. That difference may account for observed differences instead of the independent variable per se. Therefore, when there is a risk of instability for the independent variable, your research design should include gathering data to assess its stability. Furthermore, if there are planned systematic changes in the independent variable per se. Therefore, when there is a risk of instability for the clude those changes in the statistical analysis itself, thereby increasing power and reducing error.

Random Variables from the Experimental Setting

Some other aspects of the experimental setting may account for some variance in the dependent variable. When these can be anticipated, they should be either eliminated or measured and included in the statistical analysis via use of multivariate techniques. When these variables remain unmeasured, they become part of error, which, in turn, both decreases the chance of achieving statistical significance and increases confidence intervals.

Random Differences Among Subjects

When subject heterogeneity is related to the dependent variable (e.g., intelligence and success in a patient education program), that variable becomes part of error unless it is measured and included in the analysis, the same way as do random variables from the experimental setting. Matching subjects on a key variable often ameliorates this threat.

Accepting the Null Hypothesis

Although a null hypothesis cannot, technically, be "proven," there are many times in research, especially applied research, when we must make decisions based on accepting the null. Thus, at issue is under what conditions can we feel confident in accepting the null hypothesis.

The first condition, of course, is that statistically significant results are opposite to expected results. Even when not significant, if the results are like those of many other replications, one can have some confidence in accepting the null. However, you should always look to see if the absence of effects is due to a **suppressor variable,** a (third) variable not included in the analysis that might account for the absence of effects. For example, most weight reduction intervention studies report only a 10 percent success rate over time. This has led the public and many scientists to conclude that maintenance of weight loss is unlikely. This statistic and conclusion are very misleading, however, because they are based on a population of persons who seek or need help with weight loss. In reality, around 60 percent of the general population has achieved and maintained major weight loss. The suppressor variable here is whether or not persons must seek help to lose weight.

A second condition under which acting as though the null were true may be justified is when a desired effect size is specified *in advance* and power analysis is used to determine an appropriate sample size. Failure to reject the null cannot then be attributed to an excessively large type II error probability. Certainly analysis for type II error should always accompany a report in which a null is accepted.

Third, it is often possible to calculate the ES required in order to achieve statistical significance after a test is run, given the *n* and *α* used in the original analysis. Sometimes, it turns out to be unreasonably large. In this case, you would have little confidence in accepting the null at the level of significance originally specified. Instead, you should raise the level of significance.

Fourth, when results are not statistically significant but are in the expected direction and the analysis includes few variables, the error term (i.e., the denominator of the test statistic in most cases) may be unduly inflated owing to random variables from the experimental setting or random differences among subjects. If these have been reliably measured and can then be incorporated into the analysis via multivariate methods (e.g., analysis of covariance), they will then be removed from error. This is called **reducing error variance.** If all attempts fail, and all rival hypotheses and threats that can reasonably be expected to be present are accounted for, then you can probably act as though the null is true.

V*ocabulary*

Alpha (*α*) level	Normality assumption
Beta (*β*) level	Observed probability of error
Bivariate	One-tailed test
Confidence interval	*p* value
Correlated means	Parameter
Critical value	Parameters and statistics
Degrees of freedom (df)	Parametric test
Dependent groups	Power
Directional test	Reducing error variance
Directionality	Sampling distribution
Effect size	Significant difference
Family type I error	Standard error of the sampling distribution
H_a (alternate hypothesis)	Statistical conclusion validity
H_0 (null hypothesis)	Statistical hypothesis
Heterogeneous groups	Suppressor variable
Homogeneity of variance	Tailedness
Independent groups	Test statistic
Level of significance	Two-tailed test
Magnitude estimate	Type I error
Mean of means	Type II error
Nondirectional test	Univariate
Nonparametric test	

References

1. Cohen, J. *Statistical Power Analysis for the Behavioral Sciences* (rev. ed.). New York: Academic Press, 1977.
2. Cook, T. D., and Campbell, D. T. *Quasi-experimentation Design and Analysis Issues for Field Settings.* Chicago: Rand McNally, 1979.
3. Spense, J. T., Cotton, J. W., Underwood, B. J., and Duncan, C. P. *Elementary Statistics* (3rd ed.). Englewood Cliffs, N.J.: Prentice-Hall, 1976.

16: *Parametric Tests for One or Two Groups*

In Chapter 15, the one-sample Z test was used to illustrate how a statistical test works. The Z test is a parametric test that requires a sample size larger than 30 and knowledge of the values of the population mean (μ) and standard deviation (σ).* The Z test can be used to compare a sample mean with the population mean or to compare two sample means. The difficulty with the Z test comes from the need to know the population parameters. Because these are rarely known, such forms of the Z test are of little practical use in studying most research topics.

The t *Statistic*

Fortunately, a comparable test, the *t* test, exists.† The *t* test allows you to estimate the standard error of the sampling distribution by using the standard deviation of the sample. It is also useful when *n* is less than 30, although it can be used for larger samples as well. When *n* is 30, in fact, the sampling distribution for *t* looks very similar to the (normal curve) sampling distribution for Z. When *n* is less than 30, the *t* sampling distributions flatten out somewhat and have more area in the two tails. The *t* test has been one of the most widely used parametric tests because of its easy computation and wide applicability. Like the Z test, it can be used to test the difference between two independent group means or between a sample and population mean. It can also test the difference between two correlated or related means that result from (1) pre- and posttest measures from the same persons in a single group or (2) measures from two groups of subjects who have been matched on some variable that is correlated with the dependent or criterion variable.

The *t* test requires the three assumptions of parametric tests about the causal comparative hypotheses it tests. The first is that the dependent variable is measured at the interval level; the second is that the scores in the population under study are about normally distributed; and the third is that the score variances (σ^2) are about equal. Generally, we do not know the population distribution of scores or variances. Instead, our information about the population is based on inferences from our sample statistics. If the sample distribution is drastically skewed or the sample variances are very different, a nonparametric statistic is more appropriate. However, it has been found that even when one of these assumptions is seriously violated, the *t* test provides an accurate estimate of the significance level for differences between sample means. If both assumptions appear violated as a result of inspecting sample data and group sizes are unequal as well, a parallel nonparametric procedure, presented in Chapter 19, will most likely yield more accurate results.

Unlike the Z test, the *t* test requires calculation of **degrees of freedom** (*df*). A

---

*When population values rather than sample values are referred to, the Greek letters μ and σ are used to designate the mean and standard deviation. $\bar{X}$ and SD (or S) are used for sample values.
†The *t* test is sometimes called Student's *t*. This is because the originator, William Gosset, first published his description of the procedure under the pseudonym Student.

different sampling distribution is used for different degrees of freedom. The *t* test, furthermore, can be one-tailed or two-tailed, because only two groups of scores are being compared.

The t *Test for Two Independent Groups*

Suppose you are interested in testing the effects on postoperative adjustment of a special educational program in the use of prostheses. Adjustment is measured by a personality test with .91 reliability and good criterion validity as indicated by a .89 correlation with another well-established, but much longer, test measuring psychological adjustment. Other physical and observational measures compose the multimodal approach to measuring adjustment. However, for the sake of the discussion, only the self-report personality test will be used. A sample of 26 patients is randomly assigned to experimental and control groups of 13 patients each. You hypothesize that the experimental group will be significantly more adjusted as a result of your training program, and you select a .05 level of significance.

The data for this example are given in Exhibit 16.1. The appropriate statistical test for these data is the *t* test for independent groups, because the data are interval level and a causal comparative statement involving two *independent* groups is being tested. Note that one control group subject was lost. This does not affect use of this *t* test, because groups do not have to be equal in size.

The Conceptual Formula

Computation of the *t* statistic is similar to that of the *Z* statistic. The numerator is the difference between the two independent means and the denominator is the standard error of the *t* sampling distribution for a specific number of degrees of freedom. The standard error, moreover, is estimated by using the **pooled standard deviations** of the two groups in the sample. The **conceptual formula** for the *t* test for independent groups is

$$t = \frac{\bar{X}_A - \bar{X}_B}{\sqrt{\dfrac{\Sigma X_A^2 + \Sigma X_B^2}{n_A + n_B - 2}\left(\dfrac{1}{n_A} + \dfrac{1}{n_B}\right)}}$$

(16.1)

where $df = n_A + n_B - 2$

This impressive formula for the *t* statistic, particularly the denominator, which estimates the **standard error,** is fairly easy to compute by using the same type of computations involved in calculating the standard deviation.

In theory, the numerator of the *t* statistic involves subtracting from the observed difference between means of the two groups $(\bar{X}_A - \bar{X}_B)$ the difference between the means for the two populations from which the groups are sampled $(\mu_A - \mu_B)$. Strictly speaking, therefore, the numerator is $(\bar{X}_A - \bar{X}_B) - (\mu_A - \mu_B)$. However, under the null hypothesis, there is no difference between the population means and therefore $\mu_A - \mu_B = 0$. Thus, this part of the numerator is left out of the conceptual formula, because it equals zero anyway and would just add needless complexity to the formula. The *df* for this *t* test equal

Exhibit 16-1. Experimental and control group adjustment scores.

Experimental (*A*)			Control (*B*)	
12	16		10	11
17	16		13	11
16	14		11	12
15	16		12	15
15	14		12	10
13	15		14	—*
16			13	

*One control Ss lost.

Exhibit 16-2. Data organization for computation of t according to the conceptual formula.

X_A (1)	f (2)	fX_A (3)	$X_A - \bar{X}_A = x$ (6)	x_A^2 (7)	fx_A^2 (8)
17	1	17	$17 - 15 = 2$	4	$(1)(4) = 4$
16	5	80	$16 - 15 = 1$	1	$(5)(1) = 5$
15	3	45	$15 - 15 = 0$	0	$(3)(0) = 0$
14	2	28	$14 - 15 = -1$	1	$(2)(1) = 2$
13	1	13	$13 - 15 = -2$	4	$(1)(4) = 4$
12	1	$\underline{12}$	$12 - 15 = -3$	9	$(1)(9) = \underline{9}$

$(4)\ \Sigma fX_A = 195$

$(9)\ \Sigma fx^2 = 24$

$(5)\quad \bar{X}_A = 15$

$(10)\quad V = \dfrac{24}{12} = 2$

$\qquad\qquad SD = \sqrt{2} = 1.44$

$n_A = 13$

X_B (11)	f (12)	fX_B (13)	$X_B - \bar{X}_B = x_B$ (16)	x_B^2 (17)	fx_B^2 (18)
15	1	15	$15 - 12 = 3$	9	$(1)(9) = 9$
14	1	14	$14 - 12 = 2$	4	$(1)(4) = 4$
13	2	26	$13 - 12 = 1$	1	$(2)(1) = 2$
12	3	36	$12 - 12 = 0$	0	$(3)(0) = 0$
11	3	33	$11 - 12 = -1$	1	$(3)(1) = 3$
10	2	$\underline{20}$	$10 - 12 = -2$	4	$(2)(4) = \underline{8}$

$(14)\ \Sigma fx_B = 144$

$(19)\ \Sigma fx_B^2 = 26$

$(15)\quad \bar{X}_B = 12$

$(20)\quad V = \dfrac{26}{11} = 2.364$

$\qquad\qquad SD = \sqrt{2.364} = 1.537$

$n_B = 12$

the number of observations in the total sample ($n_A + n_B$) minus two restrictions that relate to computation of the two group means. Therefore, $df = n_A + n_B - 2$.

Exhibit 16.2 uses the data from Exhibit 16.1 to compute the t statistic for independent groups. Once a sum of squares, $\Sigma (X - \bar{X})^2$ or Σx^2, for each group is calculated, numbers can be easily substituted in the t statistic formula. First, data for the first group (A) are rank ordered in magnitude from largest to smallest (step 1). The frequency of occurrence is then given opposite each score (step 2). In step 3, each raw score is multiplied by its **frequency of occurrence.** The sum of raw scores is then computed (ΣX) (step 4) and divided by the n in Group A to yield the mean of Group A (step 5). You could list all scores separately rather than use frequency of occurrence to compute the sum of raw scores; however, this method is shorter. Next, the deviation of each score from the mean of its group is computed ($X_A - \bar{X}_A$) = x_A (step 7) and squared (step 8). The deviation scores are then multiplied by their frequency of occurrence (step 9) and summed (step 10) to yield the sum of squared deviation scores (or **sum of squares**) for group A. As an extra step not needed to compute t, the variance (V) is computed by dividing the sum of squares (in step 10) by $n - 1$. The standard deviation is then computed by simply taking the square root of the variance. This is called the unbiased SD because $n - 1$, instead of n, was used to calculate the variance. This whole process is then repeated for Group B and is shown in Exhibit 16.2 as steps 11 through 20. The t statistic can then be computed by substituting the values of the means, sums of squares, and n into the t test formula. (For an explanation of how the denominator of the t test statistic relates to the standard error presented in Chapter 15, please see Reference Note 1 of this chapter.)

$$t = \frac{15 - 12}{\sqrt{[(24 + 26)/(13 + 12 - 2)]\,(\frac{1}{13} + \frac{1}{12})}} = \frac{3}{\sqrt{\frac{50}{23}\,(.16)}}$$

$$= \frac{3}{\sqrt{(2.174)\,(.16)}} = \frac{3}{\sqrt{.348}} = \frac{3}{.59} = 5.08$$

$df = 13 + 12 - 2 = 23$

Using the **degrees of freedom** ($df = 23$) and the level of significance ($\alpha = .05$), enter Table D, Appendix III, to extract the **critical value** of t. If the computed **t test statistic** is *equal to or greater than* the critical value, the two groups are significantly different. From Table D, the critical value is 2.069, well below 5.08. It is apparent from the table that not only is t significant at $p<.05$, it is significant at $p<.001$. The .001 level is therefore reported. We reject the null hypothesis and conclude that the experimental educational program *caused* greater adjustment—if the threats to internal validity and any probable confounding variables have been controlled. Statistical significance does not *prove* causality. It merely allows you to draw a causal conclusion if, and only if, the research design and methodology produce no rival hypotheses.

The Computational Formula

Just as there is a computational formula for the SD there is also one for t. The same formula used for computing the sum of squares, $\Sigma X^2 - (\Sigma X)^2/n$, can be extended for use with the t statistic for independent groups. The computational formula for t, to be used when a computer is not available, is as follows:

$$t = \frac{\overline{X}_A - \overline{X}_B}{\sqrt{\dfrac{\Sigma X_A^2 - \dfrac{(\Sigma X_A)^2}{n_A} + \Sigma X_B^2 - \dfrac{(\Sigma X_B)^2}{n_B}}{(n_A + n_B - 2)}\left(\dfrac{1}{n_A} + \dfrac{1}{n_B}\right)}} \tag{16.2}$$

Using data organized in Exhibit 16.3, this rather menancing formula is easily solved as follows:

$$t = \frac{15 - 12}{\sqrt{\dfrac{2949 - \dfrac{38025}{13} + 1754 - \dfrac{20736}{12}}{13 + 12 - 2}\left(\dfrac{1}{13} + \dfrac{1}{12}\right)}}$$

$$= \frac{3}{\sqrt{\dfrac{24 + 26}{23}(.16)}} = \frac{3}{.59} = 5.08$$

Once the test statistic is calculated, the decision about significance is the same as previously presented. This formula is superior to the conceptual formula when large data sets are used and a computer is not available. There is less danger of error due to rounding.

Computing t from $\overline{X}$, SD, and n

If you are given the $\overline{X}$, SD, and n of each group, you can compute a t statistic from these data. All you need to do is calculate for each group the sum of squares (i.e., the sum of squared deviation scores for X, Σx^2), which is used in the denominator for the t statistic. Recall that when the sum of squares is divided by $n - 1$, the variance results. Therefore, when the variance is multiplied by $n - 1$, the sum of squares results (and, of course, the variance is the standard deviation squared, SD^2). Thus, you have all the information you need.

For example, suppose you have the following information: Group A: $\overline{X} = 14$, $SD = 3, n = 15$; Group B: $\overline{X} = 81$, $SD = 4, n = 17$. The sum of squares for each group is calculated as follows: Group A: $\Sigma x_A^2 = (n-1)(SD_A)^2 = (14)(3)^2 = 126$; Group B: $\Sigma x_B^2 = (n-1)(SD_B)^2 = (16)(4)^2 = 256$.

Exhibit 16-3. Data organization for computation of t according to the computational formula.

X_A (1)	f (2)	fX_A (3)	X_A^2 (7)	fX_A^2 (8)
17	1	17	289	289
16	5	80	256	1280
15	3	45	225	675
14	2	28	196	392
13	1	13	169	169
12	1	12	144	144

(4) $\quad \Sigma fX_A = 195$ $\qquad$ (9) $\Sigma fx_A^2 = 2{,}949$

(5) $\quad \bar{X}_A = 15$
$\qquad n_A = 13$

(6) $(\Sigma X_A)^2 = 38{,}025$ $\qquad$ (10) $\quad SD_A = \sqrt{\dfrac{\Sigma X^2 - \dfrac{(\Sigma X)^2}{n}}{n-1}} =$

$$\sqrt{\dfrac{2{,}949 - \dfrac{38{,}025}{13}}{12}} = \sqrt{\dfrac{24}{12}} = 1.44$$

X_B (1)	f (2)	fX_B (3)	X_B^2 (7)	fX_B^2 (8)
15	1	15	225	225
14	1	14	196	196
13	2	26	169	338
12	3	36	144	432
11	3	33	121	363
10	2	20	100	200

(4) $\quad \Sigma fX_B = 144$ $\qquad$ (9) $\Sigma fx_B^2 = 1{,}754$

(5) $\quad \bar{X}_B = 12$
$\qquad n_B = 12$

(6) $(\Sigma X_B)^2 = 20{,}736$ $\qquad$ (10) $\quad SD_B = \sqrt{\dfrac{1{,}754 - \dfrac{20{,}736}{12}}{11}} = \sqrt{\dfrac{26}{11}} = 1.537$

Using the *conceptual* formula for t, the values are inserted and t is computed as follows:

$$t = \frac{\bar{X}_A - \bar{X}_B}{\sqrt{[(\Sigma x_A^2 + \Sigma x_B^2)/(n_A + n_B - 2)]\,(1/n_A + 1/n_B)}}$$

$$= \frac{14 - 8}{\sqrt{[(126 + 256)/(15 + 17 - 2)]\,(1/15 + 1/17)}} = \frac{6}{\sqrt{382/30\,(17/255 + 15/255)}}$$

$$= \frac{6}{\sqrt{(382/30)(32/255)}} = \frac{6}{\sqrt{(12.73)(.125)}} = \frac{6}{\sqrt{1.59}} = \frac{6}{1.26} = 4.76$$

$$df = n_A + n_B - 2 = 15 + 17 - 2 = 30$$

The t *Test for Two Dependent Groups*

Sometimes you may wish to match subjects (Ss) according to some qualities that are important to the purpose of the research or compare means obtained by the same subjects in a group under two different conditions. In this case, the two groups of observations are no longer independent, because the composition of one group is related to the composition of the second group. Scores on the dependent variable during the first observation are most likely correlated to scores during the second observation. Therefore, the *t* test for dependent groups (or correlated means) is used. Instead of comparing means to get an observed difference, the computational formula is based on the **sum of squared differences** between each of the **paired scores.**

Suppose that data in the example in Exhibit 16.1 were believed to be confounded by severity of disability. Therefore, the subjects' nurses were asked to rank-order them according to severity of impairment. The two highest ranking were then paired and one was randomly assigned to the experimental group and the other to the control group. The third and fourth highest ranks were next paired and randomly assigned, the fifth and sixth paired and randomly assigned, and so on until twelve pairs had been assigned to an experimental or control condition. For the sake of simplicity, (and also to make a later point), we will use

Exhibit 16-4. Data organization for computation of *t* test for dependent groups.

Pair	X_A (1)	X_B	$D = X_A - X_B$ (2)	$(D - \bar{D})^2 = d^2$ (5)
01	12	10	2	$(2 - 3)^2 = 1$
02	17	13	4	$(4 - 3)^2 = 1$
03	16	11	5	$(5 - 3)^2 = 4$
04	15	12	3	$(3 - 3)^2 = 0$
05	15	12	3	$(3 - 3)^2 = 0$
06	13	14	-1	$(-1 - 3)^2 = 16$
07	16	13	3	$(3 - 3)^2 = 0$
08	16	11	5	$(5 - 3)^2 = 4$
09	16	11	5	$(5 - 3)^2 = 4$
10	14	12	2	$(2 - 3)^2 = 1$
11	16	15	1	$(1 - 3)^2 = 4$
12	14	10	4	$(4 - 3)^2 = 1$

$(3) \Sigma D = 36$

$(4)\ \bar{D} = 3$

$n = 12$

$(6) \Sigma d^2 = 36$

the same data as used for the t test for independent groups. Exhibit 16.4 illustrates the data organization for computation of t for dependent groups. First, for each pair, the scores on measure A and measure B are listed. This is step 1. Next the difference, D, between each pair is computed, (step 2). Sometimes this is negative. If so, the pair is added as negative numbers which means that, in effect, the two are subtracted from the sum of all D, ΣD (step 3). The mean difference score, $\bar{D}$, is then computed by dividing ΣD by n; this is step 4. Deviation scores based on the deviation of each difference score, D, from the difference score mean, $\bar{D}$, are computed for each pair and then squared (step 5). These are slightly different deviation scores from those used for the SD, because each individual "score" is based on a *difference* between two other scores rather than the set of scores themselves. However, the principle of a score's deviation from its mean remains the same. As step 6, these squared deviation scores are then summed to yield the **sum of squares for difference deviation scores** Σd^2. Again, this sum of squares is slightly different because it is based on the score calculations of step 5. However, the principle of adding all the squared deviation scores to get the sum of squares remains the same. With the information computed in Exhibit 16.4, the t statistic for correlated means can be computed:

$$t = \frac{\bar{D}}{\sqrt{\dfrac{\Sigma d^2}{n(n-1)}}} \tag{16.3}$$

where $df = n - 1$

$\qquad \bar{D}$ = mean difference between paired scores

$\qquad \Sigma d^2$ = sum of squared deviation difference scores

$\qquad n$ = number of pairs

For a more detailed explanation of the denominator of formula 16.3, see Reference Note 2. Substituting the data summarized in Exhibit 16.4, we get

$$t = \frac{3}{\sqrt{36/[12\,(12-1)]}} = \frac{3}{\sqrt{36/132}} = \frac{3}{\sqrt{.272}} = \frac{3}{.52} = 5.76$$

$df = 12 - 1 = 11$

Using Table D, Appendix III, the critical value of t at $\alpha = .05$ is 2.201. Further inspection reveals that this t statistic is significant at $p < .001$.

　　Let us compare the two t tests using the same data. In the first, Ss were randomly assigned to either experimental or control groups. The t statistic which resulted was 5.08. In the second example, we wished to control for severity of disability and therefore matched Ss on this variable. We controlled a potential confounding variable. The t statistic which resulted was 5.76, 13 percent larger than the first t test.* This is because the severity of disability con-

---

*Recall that one of the simple versions of the formula for the t test for independent groups (see

founded the first analysis and it was controlled in the second. In controlling it, we did reduce the *df* from 23 to 11 and thereby increased the critical value from 2.069 to 2.201. This increase of the critical value might make a difference in rejection of a null hypothesis in cases in which the confounding variable turned out not to be present or to be present to only a small extent. However, controlling confounding variables that are indeed present by incorporating them into the design, as we did, usually more than makes up for this slight handicap because it increases the *t* test statistic more than it increases the critical value (in our example, 13% versus 6%). Of course, sometimes the attempt to control one confounding variable introduces others, such as making the staff more aware of the research and thereby changing their behavior toward patients. Your research setting and your interactions with it largely determine the presence and extent of rival hypotheses and the conclusions you may draw from data analysis. Sometimes, as in this case, statistical analysis can help you add more control. The challenge to be creative and thoughtful is ever present. Once a study is completed, otherwise obscure confounding variables usually become apparent. Better ways of doing the research appear. In your follow-up study you incorporate them, increasing precision and the body of knowledge in your topic area.

The One-Sample t *Test*

The one-sample *t* test does just what the one-sample *Z* test does, except that it is more widely applicable because you do not need to know the population SD (i.e., σ) and it can be used with samples of less than 30. The SE of the *t* sampling distribution for $df = n - 1$ is estimated by using the unbiased sample SD and dividing it by $\sqrt{n}$. Thus the formula for the one-sample *t* is

$$t = \frac{\bar{X} - \mu}{\sqrt{\dfrac{\Sigma x^2}{n(n-1)}}} \qquad (16.4)$$

where $df = n - 1$

$\bar{X}$ = sample mean

μ = population mean

Σx^2 = sum of squared deviations from the sample mean (i.e., sum of squares for X)

n = sample size

Reference Note 1) was:

$$t = \frac{\bar{X}_A - \bar{X}_B}{\sqrt{V_A/n_A + V_B/n_B}}$$

A similar version can be written for the *t* test for dependent groups (which would not be used in actual practice because of all the added calculations involved):

$$t = \frac{\bar{X}_A - \bar{X}_B}{\sqrt{V_A/n_A + V_B/n_B - 2(r_{AB})(SD_A/\sqrt{n_A})(SD_B/\sqrt{n_B})}}$$

This second formula when compared with the first illustrates the added *reduction* to the denominator or error term that can be achieved when a research design allows matching.

Exhibit 16-5. Data organization for computation of one-sample t test.

X (1)	f (2)	fX (3)	$X - \overline{X} = x$ (6)	x^2 (7)	fx^2 (8)
17	1	17	$(17 - 15) = 2$	4	$(1)(4) = 4$
16	5	80	$(16 - 15) = 1$	1	$(5)(1) = 5$
15	3	45	$(15 - 15) = 0$	0	$(3)(0) = 0$
14	2	28	$(14 - 15) = -1$	1	$(2)(1) = 2$
13	1	13	$(13 - 15) = -2$	4	$(1)(4) = 4$
12	1	12	$(12 - 15) = -3$	9	$(1)(9) = 9$

$(4)\ \Sigma X = 195$

$(5)\ \overline{X} = 15$

$n = 13$

$(9)\ \Sigma fx^2 = 24$

$(10)\quad V = \dfrac{24}{12} = 2$

$SD = \sqrt{2} = 1.44$

Given that $\mu = 13$:

$$t = \frac{15 - 13}{\sqrt{24/[13(13 - 1)]}} = \frac{2}{\sqrt{24/156}} = \frac{2}{0.392} = 5.102$$

$df = 13 - 1 = 12$

From Table D, Appendix III, critical values (CV) (two-tailed) are 2.179 ($\alpha = .05$), 3.055 ($\alpha = .01$), and 4.318 ($\alpha = .001$). Therefore H_0 is rejected at $p < .001$.

Exhibit 16.5 illustrates computation of the one-sample t test using Group A data from Exhibit 16.1 and a population mean (μ) of 13. By now, the steps should not require additional discussion.

The t *Test for the Significance of* r

Another use for the t statistic, a special case of the one-sample t, is testing the significance of the Pearson Product Moment Correlation Coefficient, r. The computational formula is

$$t = r\frac{\sqrt{n - 2}}{\sqrt{1 - r^2}} \tag{16.5}$$

$df = n - 2$

where n = number of pairs

r = the correlation coefficient being tested

It is also used to test the significance of other correlation coefficients, such as the Spearman *rho*. Table C, Appendix III, gives critical values for r so that you do not need to compute t. If your r is significant, you can conclude with 5 percent (or 1 percent) probability of error that the r is not zero. This may not be your most relevant or meaningful conclusion. Remember that with r you can square the correlation coefficient and know just how much variability is shared by the two variables which were correlated.

Power Analysis for t

As stated in Chapter 15, when the null hypothesis is not rejected it is important to estimate the probability of **type II error,** the probability of having *incorrectly* accepted the null hypothesis. Table A in Appendix IV yields the probability of such errors after failing to reject the null hypothesis when using the *t* statistic at the .05 level of significance. Before using the table, however, it is necessary to compute *effect size* (ES).

If we were simply to use $\bar{X}_A - \bar{X}_B$ as the ES (i.e., the magnitude of difference between means), it would be very misleading, because the difference would depend on the range of the metric scale used to measure the dependent variable. For example, one operational definition of a dependent variable might be a metric scale, AA, that ranged from zero to twenty. Here, $\bar{X}_A - \bar{X}_B$ might be $14.85 - 12.17 = 2.68$. If you used a different measure, BB, which could range from zero to sixty and was perfectly correlated with the AA, the means would be 44.55 and 36.51. Using measure BB, $\bar{X}_A - \bar{X}_B$ would be 8.04 for the very same difference that was 2.68 using measure AA. Difference BB would appear larger than difference AA, although in reality they were the same. Clearly, this cannot be tolerated. An ES that is independent of the scale must be used so that an ES of, say, 1.3 means the same thing no matter what type of metric scale was used to operationally define the dependent variable. For most statistical tests, therefore, there are simple procedures to follow to calculate ES. The major exception to this is with the Pearson *r*, because it is already independent of the metric range used to operationally define the two variables being correlated. It does not require calculation of a special ES. Instead, ES is the value of *r*.

ES for the *t* Test for Independent Groups

The ES for the *t* statistic for independent groups is computed by using the following formula:

$$ES = \frac{|\bar{X}_A - \bar{X}_B|}{SD} \tag{16.6}$$

where $n_A = n_B$ and the SD is from either group A or group B because they are assumed to be about equal

Suppose that a comparison of two independent groups of equal size ($n = 10$) yielded a *t* of 1.09, the group means were 20 and 22, and the standard deviations were 4 and 4.2, respectively. The critical value of *t* at $\alpha = .05$ is 2.101 (see Table D, Appendix III). The *t* statistic of 1.09 is certainly not equal to or greater than 2.101, and H_0 is therefore not rejected. You therefore wish to assess the probability of type II error. ES is computed by

$$ES = \frac{|\bar{X}_A - \bar{X}_B|}{SD} = \frac{|20 - 22|}{4} = \frac{2}{4} = .50$$

Entering Table A, Appendix IV, for $n = 10$, a two-tailed test, and ES = .50, the probability of type II error is found to be 82 percent. You therefore have little faith in your results and decide to repeat your study using a larger sample. Note that had you performed a one-tailed test, the probability of type II error would have been somewhat less, 71 percent.

Unequal *n*. When the two groups being compared do not have the same *n* in each group, it is necessary to do an extra computation. The *n* with which the table is entered is computed by averaging the *n* in each group via the **harmonic mean:**

$$\bar{n}_{\text{H}} = \frac{2(n_{\text{A}})(n_{\text{B}})}{n_{\text{A}} + n_{\text{B}}} \tag{16.7}$$

For example, suppose $n_{\text{A}} = 20$ and $n_{\text{B}} = 36$:

$$\bar{n}_{\text{H}} = \frac{2(20)(36)}{20 + 36} = \frac{1440}{56} = 25.71$$

This is slightly smaller than the **arithmetic mean** of 28. In order to use the tables, the $\bar{n}_{\text{H}}$ is rounded to a whole number, 26. From Table A, Appendix IV, we see that for ES = .50, two-tailed, the probability of type II error is 58 percent using the harmonic mean and 55 percent using the arithmetic mean. This slight loss of power (3 percent) is the price that is paid for the extremely unequal *n*s of 20 and 36.

Unequal Variances. Although one of the assumptions of parametric tests is equal variances, it is often violated without serious consequences. If group variances are *significantly different,* the **root mean square,** or square root of the mean of the two variances, is used as the denominator in the ES formula:

$$\widehat{\text{SD}} = \sqrt{\frac{V_{\text{A}} + V_{\text{B}}}{2}} \tag{16.8}$$

The root mean square is not much different than the arithmetic $\bar{X}$ of the two SDs unless they are extremely different. For example, suppose $\text{SD}_{\text{A}} = 4$ and $\text{SD}_{\text{B}} = 8$.

$$\widehat{\text{SD}} = \sqrt{\frac{16 + 64}{2}} = \sqrt{40} = 6.32$$

The arithmetic mean of 8 and 4 is 6, slightly less than 6.32. If $\bar{X}_{\text{A}} - \bar{X}_{\text{B}}$ were 45.2 − 41.4 = 3.8, ES using 6.32 would be .60 and ES using 6 would be .63. Thus, the ES is slightly smaller to compensate for unequal variances. Referring to Table A, Appendix IV, for $n = 16$, probability of type II error is 63 percent (two-tailed) and 49 percent (one-tailed) for ES = .60, while it decreases to 59 percent (two-tailed) and 45 percent (one-tailed) for ES = .63. (See Reference Note 3 for a description of **linear interpolation,** which was used to calculate probability of type II error for ES = .63, which is not tabulated.) The slight difference demonstrates the small effect on power associated with violating the equivariance assumption.

Unequal *n* and Variances. If group *n*'s are unequal and group variances are significantly different (statistically), the probability of type II error cannot be estimated by using Appendix IV's Table A. The values in the table would contain too much error.

Interpreting ES as *r*

The ES, recall, describes the magnitude of the difference between means, independent of the metric scale used to operationally define the dependent variable. It is an **absolute value.** ES of .60 is half the magnitude of ES = 1.20. This we can tell intuitively. However, we do not attach meaning to ES = .60 as we would, for example, to weight in pounds. A difference of 60 pounds would have meaning. As ES of .60 does not. Therefore, it is often more meaningful to convert ES to a correlation coefficient (r), which does have meaning intuitively, especially in terms of r^2 and unexplained variance ($1 - r^2$). The ES for *t* can be converted to a **point biserial correlation,** r_{PB}, a special version of Pearson *r* in which the variables correlated are group membership, a dichotomous discrete variable, and whatever the interval level dependent variable may be. Exhibit 16.6 presents r_{PB} equivalents for various ESs associated with the *t* statistic. Note that it is based on the assumption that the subjects in population A are as numerous as the subjects in population B. We usually make that assumption, although in the case of males and females in the general population, we might be stretching the point. If this assumption cannot be met, use the formula for r_{PB} presented at the bottom of Exhibit 16.6.

As the discussion of statistical conclusion validity in Chapter 15 pointed out, just knowing that there is a significant difference between two groups is really not enough information. We need to know if this difference is practically significant, also. To do this we examine the means of the two groups, because a *large n* can produce statistical significance for *small* differences between two means. Because it is sometimes hard to decide how large a difference between means is *large enough* to, say, make changes in clinical practice or implement new costly programs, another way of examining effects is to look at the *magnitude* of difference in terms of explained variance. To do this, convert *t* to an *r* by means of Exhibit 16.6. Then the amount of unexplained variance is calculated:

$$V_u = 1 - r^2 \tag{16.10}$$

For the data presented in Exhibits 16.1 and 16.2 the r_{PB} of the *t* statistic is

Exhibit 16-6. Point biserial equivalents[a] for ES of the *t* statistic[b].

ES	r	r^2	ES	r	r^2
.10	.05	.00	1.60	.63	.39
.20	.10	.01	1.70	.65	.42
.30	.15	.02	1.80	.67	.45
.40	.20	.04	1.90	.69	.47
.50	.24	.06	2.00	.71	.50
.60	.29	.08	2.20	.74	.55
.70	.33	.11	2.40	.77	.59
.80	.37	.14	2.60	.79	.63
.90	.41	.17	2.80	.81	.66
1.00	.45	.20	3.00	.83	.69
1.10	.48	.23	3.20	.85	.72
1.20	.51	.27	3.40	.86	.74
1.30	.55	.30	3.60	.87	.76
1.40	.57	.33	3.80	.88	.78
1.50	.60	.36	4.00	.89	.80

Note: The *r* values are based on the assumption of two equally numerous populations. If samples cannot be assumed to come from equally large populations, use

$$r_{PB} = \frac{ES}{\sqrt{ES^2 - (1/pq)}} \tag{16.9}$$

where p = the proportion of *A*'s in the combined *A* and *B* populations
$q = 1 - p$

[a]Based upon $r = \dfrac{ES}{\sqrt{ES^2 + 4}}$.
[b]Abridged from table 2.21 of Cohen [2].

computed by first calculating ES_t from formula 16.6:

$$ES_t = \frac{|\bar{X}_A - \bar{X}_B|}{SD} = \frac{|115 - 121|}{1.5} = \frac{3}{1.5} = 2$$

The value 1.5 is used for the SD to simplify calculation and approximate the midpoint of the two SD values, 1.44 and 1.537, as shown in Exhibit 16.2. Next, using the ES of 2, Exhibit 16.6 is consulted and an *r* of .71 and r^2 of .50 results. The unexplained variance, $1 - r^2$, is only .50. This is a very strong intervention and is worthy of implementation, as you will see in the following discussion of ES for planning sample size. It is clear that the conversion of ES to r_{PB} helps in attaching meaning to ES and a significant *t* statistic.

Planning Sample Size

The calculation of ES from related literature during the literature review can help determine sample size before research begins. In the behavioral sciences,

small effect size for t is usually defined as .2 (or $r = .10, r^2 = .01$); **medium effect size** as ES $= .5$ (or $r = .24, r^2 = .06$); and **large effect size** as ES $= .8$ (or $r = .37, r^2 = .14$). These effects are really quite small when r^2 is considered. However, they represent the magnitude of differences for t currently reported in the literature.

When planning a research study, you should be guided in determining sample size via an ES by those found by other researchers in research areas closely related to yours. You can easily calculate ES from the value of sample statistics, which are almost always given in a report of research, by using the formulas presented in this book. On the other hand, if there is no related research or other rational means of selecting an ES before you do your own research, the small, medium, and large ES values generally found in behavioral research are helpful. The tables in Appendix IV, which present probability levels for type II error, can also be used to determine sample size before research begins. First, find your permissible probability of type II error (usually 20 percent) in the body of the table in the column for your ES. Then read across the row to extract n. These tables are all based upon $\alpha = .05$. If you are using .01 or .10, consult Cohen [2].

ES for *t* Test for Dependent Groups

The calculation of ES_t for correlated means begins by proceeding in the same way as we would if the groups were independent (formula 16.6):

$$ES_t = \frac{|\overline{X}_A - \overline{X}_B|}{SD}$$

where SD = either SD_A or SD_B because they are assumed about equal

The value of ES_t that is calculated in this manner can be used to determine r and r^2 from Exhibit 16.6 for interpretive purposes. However, it will not be as accurate for power analysis using Table A, Appendix IV. The values yielded in Exhibit 16.6 are based on independence of groups. Although this can be ignored when interpreting the ES of correlated means, ES must be more accurate in determining probability of type II error. The correlation between the two groups of observations, used in the t test for dependent groups, makes ES_t more precise and thereby *increases* power. The ES_t for correlated means with which you enter Table A, Appendix IV, is calculated by

$$\widehat{ES}_t = \frac{ES_t}{\sqrt{1 - r_{AB}}} \tag{16.11}$$

where $\widehat{ES}_t$ = the ES for correlated means

ES_t = the ES computed from formula 16.6

r_{AB} = the correlation between paired scores

Note that as r increases, the denominator will decrease, thereby increasing the size of $\widehat{ES}_t$. Because $1 - r$ will always be less than one (unless no correlation exists), $\widehat{ES}_t$ is always *increased* by this additional step. Moreover, because correlations between dependent groups are usually .30 or greater, power estimates are considerably improved by using this operation. The difference between the power associated with ES_t and that associated with $\widehat{ES}_t$ is the increase in power due to matching.

For example, using the data from power analysis for the t test for independent groups where $ES_t = .50, n = 10$, and probability of type II error was 82 percent (two-tailed), we add an r of .45 between scores for each pair and calculate $\widehat{ES}_t$:

$$\widehat{ES}_t = \frac{ES_t}{\sqrt{1 - r}} = \frac{.50}{\sqrt{1 - .45}} = \frac{.50}{.74} = .68$$

$\widehat{ES}_t$ has increased from .50 to .68. Using Table A, Appendix IV, the probability of type II error is calculated by linear interpolation to be 71 percent, as compared with 82 percent for independent groups. Power has increased 11 percent by matching. (Remember that the probability of type II error is one minus power.) The statistical advantages of matching are apparent.

$\widehat{ES}_t$ leads to a slight overestimate of power (and therefore an underestimate of type II error probability) in samples of less than 30, because Table A assumes $2n - 2$ degrees of freedom when there are actually only $n - 1$. If an r between two dependent observations in the t test for two dependent groups is not available, $\widehat{ES}_t$ can be modified by using the procedure for the ES in the one-sample t test, which is presented in the following section. However, power may be slightly underestimated with this procedure.

ES for the One-Sample *t* Test

The one-sample t test has many of the same problems as the t test for dependent groups in calculating ES. In fact, the procedure also involves calculating ES_t and then modifying it as follows:

$$\widehat{ES}_t = ES_t\sqrt{2} \tag{16.12}$$

The modification is needed because Table A, Appendix IV, assumes two sample means, each of which contributes sampling error and thereby reduces power. Although the table assumes $df = 2n - 2$ and the one-sample t has only $df = n - 1$, the slight overestimate due to this does not offset the underestimate due to twice as much sampling error. $\widehat{ES}_t$ must also be used for the estimates of r and r^2 from Exhibit 16.6.

ES of *r*

Exhibit 15.2 in Chapter 15 provides probability values of *power* for the Pearson r. The probability of type II error is then determined by subtracting the value of power from one. No calculation of ES is required because r is already free from the influence of the metric scales used to measure the variables.

Difference Between Two Correlation Coefficients

Difference Between Two Independent Correlation Coefficients

Interest in relationships in nursing research often goes beyond the simple question of whether or not a relationship exists. Whether a relationship is stronger in one group than another is often of more interest.

Suppose a nurse researcher were interested in the relationship between state (i.e., short duration) anxiety, as measured by the Spielberger, Gorsuch, and Lushene scale [3], and systolic blood pressure. (Researchers have long used both or either as an operational definition for anxiety of patients.) The nurse further hypothesizes that the conflicting results that occur in the literature (i.e., sometimes the two are correlated and sometimes they are not) may be due to the patient's locus of control.* Externals, that is, might experience physiological reactions to cognitively experienced anxiety, while internals would not. Two groups, one consisting of 30 externals and another consisting of 30 internals, are measured on the two indices of anxiety. Correlations of .31 (internals) and .49 (externals) result. To test the hypothesis of a difference between them, a special Z statistic must be computed. The difference between the two correlations cannot be observed by simple subtraction, because differences between rs at various points between 0 and 1 are not comparable. For example, although the difference between .55 and .30 and the difference between .80 and .55 may both appear to be .25, they do not represent the same difference in terms of magnitude or shared variance. Recall, the amount of shared variance is r^2. Thus, $(.55)^2 - (.30)^2 = .30 - .09 = 21$ percent shared variance. On the other hand, $(.80)^2 - (.55)^2 = .64 - .30 = 34$ percent shared variance. The difference between .80 and .55 is clearly greater than the difference between .55 and .30. Therefore, when computing the difference between two independent r's, the Fisher's Z transformation is used to convert each r to a z score. These conversions are easily made by using Table N, Appendix III.

Exhibit 16.7 summarizes the computation of $Z_{r_A} - Z_{r_B}$. Note from the formula for Z in Exhibit 16.7 that, for the same difference between rs, Z becomes larger (thereby approaching significance) as sample size increases. In our example, the difference between .49 and .31, although amounting to shared variance of 15 percent, is not significant, because the Z of .73 is less than the critical value of 1.643 at $\alpha = .05$, one-tailed. No support for locus of control as a mediating or intervening variable in the correlation between self-report and physiological measures of anxiety has been found. The researcher cannot conclude, however,

---

*Locus of control involves the source of control over life as perceived by the individual. *Internals* perceive themselves as controlling most life events and *externals* perceive events as coming from the outside via fate or powerful others.

Exhibit 16-7. Calculation of the Z test for difference between two independent correlations.

The following formula is used to compute Z:

$$Z_{r_A - r_B} = \frac{Z_{r_A} - Z_{r_B}}{\sqrt{\dfrac{1}{(n_A - 3)} + \dfrac{1}{(n_B - 3)}}} \tag{16.13}$$

1. Let r_A be the larger of the two coefficients.
2. Convert r_A and r_B to z scores, using Table N, Appendix IV.
3. Divide 1 by $(n_A - 3)$, carrying out four places, and divide 1 by $(n_B - 3)$, carrying out four places.
4. Substitute the values derived in steps 2 and 3 into the formula, and solve for Z. If Z equals or is greater than 1.96 (two-tailed) or 1.643 (one-tailed), it is significant at .05. If Z equals or is greater than 2.58 (two-tailed) or 2.33 (one-tailed), it is significant at .01.

Example: Given $r_A = .49$, $n_A = 30$; $r_B = .31$, $n_B = 30$.

1. Z_{r_A} for .49 is .536, and Z_{r_B} for .31 is .321.
2. $1 \div (30 - 3) = .0370$
3. $Z = \dfrac{.536 - .321}{\sqrt{.0370 + .0370}} = \dfrac{.215}{\sqrt{.0740}} = \dfrac{.215}{.272} = .79$
4. Z is *not* significant.

---

that it is *not* an intervening variable. (If no difference is the research hypothesis, an α of .20 or .25 must be used.) Moreover, it would be *very, very incorrect* to conclude that "while no significance was found there was a trend toward stronger correlation among externals, thus *partially* supporting the research hypothesis." This interpretation is wrong, wrong, wrong.

Difference Between a Sample r *and a Known* r

Occasionally, researchers wish to see if an observed r is significantly different from a known r. For example, it might be considerably more relevant to know if a correlation is significantly greater than a given amount, determined by theory or previous research, than just zero. Before implementation of a screening test in clinical practice, administrators might require a research correlation to be significantly greater than, say, .50, which has a shared variance of 25 percent. The computation of the difference between a sample r and an existing population r essentially follows the procedure for a difference between two rs except that the denominator reflects only one sample and the Z transformation of the population r is substituted for the second r in the numerator:

$$Z = \frac{Z_r - Z_c}{\sqrt{\dfrac{1}{n-3}}} \qquad\qquad (16.14)$$

where Z_r = Fisher transformation of r

Z_c = Fisher transformation of the constant or population value

n = number of pairs in r

Power Analysis for Differences Between rs

In Exhibit 16.7 the difference between the two coefficients of .49 and .31 was not significant at $\alpha = .05$. Therefore it is appropriate to estimate the probability of a type II error. Effect size is computed as follows:

$$ES_{r_A - r_B} = |Z_{r_A} - Z_{r_B}| = .536 - .321 = .215 \qquad\qquad (16.15)$$

Using Table B in Appendix IV, the one-tailed probability of type II error for $n = 30$ is 80 percent. A larger sample might better test H_0.

Interpreting $ES_{r_A - r_B}$

The magnitude of $ES_{r_A - r_B}$ can be interpreted by using the index $r_A^2 - r_B^2$. For example, $(.49)^2 - (.31)^2 = .24 - .09 = .15$ or 15 percent more variance explained by r_A than by r_B. In terms of estimating $ES_{r_A - r_B}$ for planning sample size when no other research results are appropriate, small ES is .10 (or ranging from 4 percent to 8 percent variance for $r_A^2 - r_B^2$), medium is .30 (or ranging 15 percent to 23 percent for $r_A^2 - r_B^2$), and large is .50 (or ranging from 32 percent to 38 percent for $r_A^2 - r_B^2$).

Unequal n

When the two correlations being compared result from samples of different sizes, the n with which Table B, Appendix IV, is entered is calculated as follows:

$$\hat{n} = \frac{2(n_A - 3)(n_B - 3)}{n_A + n_B - 6} + 3 \qquad\qquad (16.16)$$

If n_A were 30 and n_B were 60, $\hat{n}$ would equal 40 while the arithmetic mean would be 45. Using Table B, Appendix IV, for ES = .50, the probability of type II error is 31 percent using an n of 40 and 25 percent if both samples were equal at n of 45. Again, unequal n results in a slight loss of power.

ES for the Difference Between a Sample r and a Known r

Just as with the one-sample t test, a one-sample r has sampling error from only one set of observations rather than two. Therefore, the ES must be modified in order to account for this. This modification simply involves multiplying the ES as computed in the regular manner by $\sqrt{2}$.

$$\widehat{ES} = ES \sqrt{2} \tag{16.17}$$

This has the effect of enlarging the ES, thereby increasing the power of the test.

Equivariance Tests

One of the basic assumptions of parametric tests is that the variances of groups are equal. Not wishing to leave any stones unturned, therefore, statisticians have developed statistical tests of this assumption. In addition, there occasionally exists a research situation in which differences in the variability or dispersion of two groups might be of more interest than the difference between means. For example, perhaps an experimental intervention reduced the variability in patient compliance, operationally defined as a ratio of appointments kept to appointments made, although the mean rates did not change. In this case, the reduction in variability might help administrators to staff the clinic more economically and therefore the intervention would be worth implementing, even if no difference in group means is found. If "no shows" *consistently* amount to 10 percent of daily appointments, this could be used in staffing. Also, suppose a nursing intervention were aimed at improving patient performance in a self-care activity (e.g., developing the capabilities of partially paralyzed stroke victims to dress themselves). From the theory and literature it is known that competition has different effects on different individuals. Among fairly bright, outgoing persons, competition might stimulate even better performance. Among more introverted individuals, competition might cause poor performance. A researcher therefore hypothesizes that the *variability* of effects due to a routinely administered intervention that uses small group interactions and competition between teams might be *significantly reduced* by careful screening to include only bright, outgoing patients. Support of this hypothesis might then lead to more individually tailored interventions for these two types of patients, so that the introverted as well as extroverted develop capabilities for self-care.

Exhibit 16.8 displays frequency distributions for four experimental groups and also illustrates the various differences possible between two groups. There is no difference in means between Groups A and B, but there is a difference in means between Groups B and D. The two sample Z and t tests apply to these comparisons. They might also be used to test the difference between the means of Groups A and C (no difference) or Groups C and D (a difference). However, in the later two comparisons, it appears that the variances may be unequal also. Thus, the F test for variances is appropriate.

Exhibit 16-8. Frequency distributions for illustrating dispersion and central tendency of four groups.

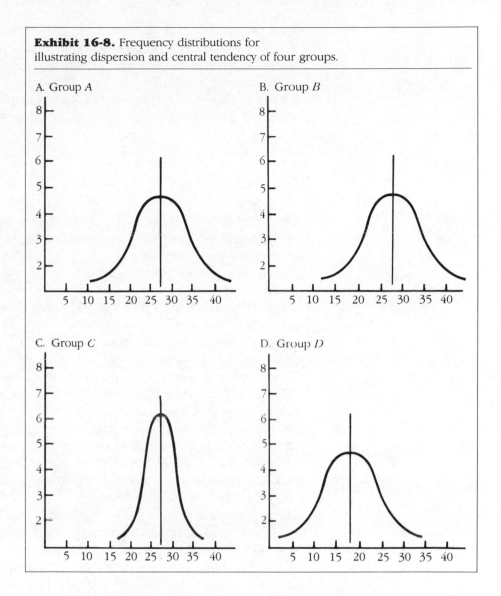

A. Group *A*

B. Group *B*

C. Group *C*

D. Group *D*

F Test for Homogeneity of Two Independent Variances

This *F* test, as it is often referred to, is just about the easiest statistical test there is. It involves dividing the largest variance (not standard deviation) by the smallest variance.*

$$F = \frac{V \text{ (largest)}}{V \text{ (smallest)}} \qquad (16.16)$$

*Recall that the SD is the square root of the variance. The variance is the sum of squares divided by $n-1$.

It has two values, rather than one, associated with *df*. For the numerator *df* = *n* − 1 for the group with the largest variance; for the denominator, *df* = *n* − 1 for the group with the smallest variance. Group sizes do not have to be equal.

For example, if Group A had a SD of 3.6 and *n* = 26, and Group B had a SD of 5.3 and *n* = 13, the SDs would first be squared to yield the variances. Next, the *F* would be computed using Group B for the numerator, because its variance is larger.

$$F = \frac{28.09}{12.96} = 2.167$$

Degrees of freedom are 13 − 1 = 12 for the numerator and 26 − 1 = 25 for the denominator. Note that the *n* associated with the variance in the numerator is used (not the *n* that is larger).

Two special rules are associated with this *F* test. First, if you test the homogeneity of variance assumption of parametric tests, you are really testing a research hypothesis that calls for *no difference*. Therefore, an α level of .20 (or .25) is used instead of .05. Second, when using *a two-tailed test,* you need a correction before finding the critical value from Table E, Appendix III, in order to account for having selected only the largest variance as the numerator. This correction involves multiplying the probability value in the table by 2. Thus, for α = .05, the critical value associated with α = .025 is used. For α = .01, the critical value associated with .005 is used. For α = .20 (as when the homogeneity of variance assumption is tested), you use the critical value associated with α = .10. *If a one-tailed test is desired, the* p *value is not multiplied by 2.* A one-tailed test is not usually used to test the equivariance (or homogeneity of variance) assumption of parametric tests because variances are assumed equal, and thus you could not hypothesize directionality beforehand. However, for testing a research hypothesis involving differences between variances, a one-tailed test could be of interest. In that case, the probability values in Table E, Appendix III, would remain as they are given.

The critical value (CV) at α = .20, two-tailed, for *df* = 12, 25 is found opposite α = .10 in Table E, Appendix III. This CV is 1.82. Because our *F* statistic is 2.167, greater than 1.82, we conclude that the variances are not homogeneous. A *t* test to compare means of Groups A and B would be violating the parametric assumptions of this test and thus would be reducing its power. Because the groups are also not equal in size, one of the nonparametric procedures presented in Chapter 19 should be considered.

If our *F* statistic of 2.167 had represented a one-tailed research hypothesis, the critical value at α = .05 would be 2.16 and we would reject H_0, concluding that the variance of Group B is significantly larger than that of Group A. If the research setting were experimental and well controlled, we might even conclude causality. As you are aware, the exact interpretation of significant results depends on the research itself rather than the statistical test.

Exhibit 16-9. t Test for homogeneity of two related variances.

---

1. Let the largest variance be V_1 and the smallest be V_2.
2. Compute the correlation r between the two sets of related observations.

$$t = \frac{(V_1 - V_2)\sqrt{n - 2}}{4(V_1)(V_2)(1 - r)} \qquad (16.19)$$

where $df = n - 2$ and $n = $ the number of observations in one group.

Example: Given: a pretest score variance of 7.78, posttest score variance of 3.17 for a group of 25 Ss, an r of .45 between pretest and posttest scores.

1. $t = \dfrac{(7.78 - 3.17)\sqrt{25 - 2}}{\sqrt{4(7.78)(3.17)(1 - .45)}} = \dfrac{(4.61)(4.795)}{54.258} = \dfrac{22.10}{54.258}$

   $= .41$

2. $df = n - 2 = 25 - 2 = 23$
3. From Table D, Appendix III, the CV at $\alpha = .20$ (two-tailed) for $df = 23$ is 1.319. Therefore, since the test statistic of .41 is less than 1.319, the variances are considered homogeneous.

---

t Test for Homogeneity of Two Related Variances

Occasionally a research hypothesis involves variances in matched groups, such as parent and child, or perhaps two measures on the same group of persons over a period of time. More often, a question emerges about the equivariance assumption underlying the t test for dependent groups. Bruning and Kintz [1] present a procedure for testing homogeneity of related variances, summarized in Exhibit 16.9, that uses the t distributions for $n - 2$ degrees of freedom. The computational procedure as illustrated is straightforward, given your experience with the earlier sections of this chapter.

Reference Notes

---

1. It is beyond the scope of this book to dwell on the derivations of formulas. However, the rationale for the standard error of the sampling distribution of differences between means bears some mention as a reference note, because you were asked to accept on faith that

$$SE_{\bar{x}} = \sqrt{\frac{\sum x_A^2 + \sum x_B^2}{n_A + n_B - 2}\left(\frac{1}{n_A} + \frac{1}{n_B}\right)}$$

Mathematical manipulation of the laws of probability as applied to random variables reveals a basic rule in dealing with differences between independent variables: the standard error of the sampling distribution of differences between independent means is the square root of the sum of each variable's squared standard error. Recall that in the one sample Z test, the standard error was estimated by the $\sigma/\sqrt{n}$. In the t test for two independent groups then, each sample $SE_{\bar{x}}$ would be its $SD/\sqrt{n}$. The square of this standard error is V/n. Using the basic rule, the SE of differences (or pooled standard errors) is therefore

$$\sqrt{\frac{V_A}{n_A} + \frac{V_B}{n_B}}$$

From the example in Exhibit 16.2, we can substitute the V and n values and get

$$\sqrt{\frac{2}{13} + \frac{2.364}{12}} = \sqrt{1.53 + .197} = \sqrt{.35} = .59$$

which is the same value as computed using the denominator of the formula for the t statistic. Thus, the formula for t could also be written

$$t = \frac{\bar{X}_A - \bar{X}_B}{\sqrt{V_A/n_A + V_B/n_B}}$$

2. The SE of the t sampling distribution for dependent groups is calculated by dividing the SD of the sample differences, $\sqrt{\Sigma d^2/n - 1}$, by the square root of n. Using the example, $SD = \sqrt{3.6/11} = \sqrt{3.273} = 1.80$. $SD \div \sqrt{12} = 1.80 \div \sqrt{12} = 1.80 \div 3.46 = .52$, which is the denominator of the t statistic.

3. Nontabulated values can often be adequately estimated from tables by a simple procedure known as *linear interpolation*. It assumes that the true curve which the tabular values represent does not differ appreciably from a straight line over the range that includes the sought-after value. Consider a table that gives values of some quantity, say Y, for a number of values of another variable, say X; (i.e., we have a table of Y versus X). Suppose the table gives values of $Y(1)$ for $X(1)$ and $Y(3)$ for $X(3)$ and you seek the value of $Y(2)$ for $X(2)$, where $X(2)$ falls between $X(1)$ and $X(3)$. The procedure of *linear interpolation* is based on a principle taught in high school math, which is that the sides of similar triangles are in the same proportion to each other. Algebraically, this is expressed as

$$\frac{X(2) - X(1)}{X(3) - X(1)} = \frac{Y(2) - Y(1)}{Y(3) - Y(1)}$$

We can solve this for $Y(2)$, the desired nontabulated value, and obtain

$$Y(2) = Y(1) + \left[\frac{X(2) - X(1)}{X(3) - X(1)} \right] [Y(3) - Y(1)]$$

In words, this expression says that the desired value, $Y(2)$ is equal to the tabulated value $Y(1)$ plus the percentage of the distance between $X(1)$ and $X(3)$ that $X(2)$ represents multiplied by the distance between $Y(1)$ and $Y(3)$. For the example, in the text, Table A of Appendix IV lists a probability value of 49 percent for ES = 0.60 and of 43 percent for ES = 0.65 for n = 16 and one tail. To find the probability value for ES = 0.63 we calculate

$$49 + \left(\frac{0.63 - 0.60}{0.65 - 0.60} \right)(43 - 49) = 49 + \frac{3}{5}(-6) = 45.4$$

What we have really done is to calculate the percent of the distance between ES = 0.60 and ES = 0.65 that ES = 0.63 represents, ⅗ or 60 percent, and multiplied it by the distance between the corresponding probability values, 6 in this case—with the minus sign accounting for the fact that the probability values are decreasing as ES increases (mathematically speaking, our line has a negative slope). When the result (-3.6) is arithmetically combined with the probability value of 49 (corresponding to ES = 0.60, the value from which we formed the distance ratio), we obtain (49 − 3.6) = 45.4 which, when rounded, is 45 percent.

Vocabulary

Absolute value	Medium effect size
Arithmetic mean	Point biserial correlation
Critical value	Power
Degrees of freedom	Root mean square
Effect size	Small effect size
Harmonic mean	Standard error of the sampling distribution
Homogeneity of variance	Sum of squares for difference deviation scores
Large effect size	Test statistic
Linear interpolation	Type II error

References

1. Bruning, J. L. and Kintz, B. L. *Computational Handbook of Statistics.* Glenview, Ill: Scott, Foresman & Co., 1977.
2. Cohen, J. *Statistical Power Analysis for the Behavioral Sciences* (Rev. ed.). New York: Academic Press, 1977.
3. Spielberger, C. D., Gorsuch, R. L., and Lushene, R. E. *The State-Trait Inventory.* Palo Alto, Calif.: Consulting Psychologists Press, 1970.

17: *One-Way Analysis of Variance (ANOVA) and Related Tests*

This chapter focuses on analysis of variance (ANOVA), another of the important concepts in statistics, like means, standard deviations, sums of squares, and *r*. Included, of course, are related statistical procedures such as whether or not three or more group variances are homogeneous. It is important to remember that these statistical tests are still bivariate: they have two variables, one of which is group membership (i.e., the nominal level independent variable) where the number of groups can be three or more. The *t* test and other procedures presented in Chapter 16 were limited to two groups or catagories of the independent variable.

One-Way Analysis of Variance (ANOVA)

Analysis of variance is a more versatile technique than the *t* test. A *t* test can be used only to test a difference between two sample means at one time. ANOVA can test the difference between two *or more* means at one time. Moreover, ANOVA and the *t* test are related. When two groups are compared using both methods, the *t* statistic equals the square root of the test statistic from ANOVA (i.e., the *F* ratio). Some statisticians never use the *t* test, because ANOVA can be used in almost any situation in which a *t* test can and, moreover, can do things the *t* test cannot do. However, others prefer the *t* test whenever possible because of its ease in computation and tailedness option. ANOVA is always two-tailed.

In ANOVA, just as in the *t* test, a ratio of the observed differences (the numerator) to an error term (the denominator) is used to test hypotheses. This ratio, called the **F ratio,** uses as a measure of observed differences among groups the variance (or distance) of group means from a grand mean. The **grand mean** is a mean calculated using observations from all subjects and ignoring to which group subjects belong.

Be particularly alert to the difference between the analysis of variance procedure itself and the use of the *F* test for homogeneity of variances.* These are two *different* inferential procedures, each of which leads to a different conclusion. ANOVA uses two estimates of the population variance as the basis for deciding whether or not the groups in the study differ significantly in *central tendency*. The *F* test is the procedure for testing the significance of the difference in two estimates of *variability*. The commonality of the two procedures is that both have two values for degrees of freedom and use of the *F* distribution table to get critical values for determining statistically significant differences. This is done because, in both, a ratio of two variances is computed; in other words, two variances are compared. If one variance is sufficiently larger than the other, you

---

*To avoid confusion in this book, the *F* test for homogeneity of variance is called the *F test* while the test statistic yielded from ANOVA is called the *F ratio*. Other books do not make such a clear distinction, however.

have significant results. Recall, in the *F* test, the larger variance is simply divided by the smaller variance. In ANOVA, computation of the two variances comprised by the *F* ratio is more complex.

Data to Illustrate ANOVA

Suppose a group of students wished to assess nurses' attitudes about the appropriateness or need for sexual counseling of three different types of patients—those with hypertension, diabetes, and amputation of a limb. They hypothesize that need would be perceived differently depending on diagnosis. The researchers decide on a simulation study approach in which a paragraph describing a patient is presented and followed by a 10-adjective-pair semantic differential type scale (i.e., adjective pairs like good–bad and happy–sad with five to seven continuum points between them) with which respondents assess the appropriateness of sexual counseling for that patient. The paragraphs are identical except for the diagnosis of the patient. Permission to conduct the study in a large teaching hospital is granted only on the condition that one vignette (i.e., paragraph) and scale per subject is completed and that the investigaters wait to collect responses while subjects complete their questionnaires. In this way a minimum of agency time is used by each subject, and the agency does not need to be bothered with collecting responses.

Therefore, the researchers decide to randomly assign one of the three vignettes to each subject, thereby considering them as three categories of the independent variable. Prior to full-scale data gathering, the researchers conduct a pilot study with 15 nurses from a medical-surgical unit. The data from this pilot study are presented in Exhibit 17.1. For purposes of demonstrating how

---

Exhibit 17-1. Summary data for attitudes toward sexual counseling needs of three patient groups: (A) Hypertensives, (B) diabetics, and (C) amputees.

Group A	Group B	Group C
20	34	29
22	39	34
31	47	41
33	48	41
34	47	40

$$\Sigma X_A = 140 \qquad \Sigma X_B = 215 \qquad \Sigma X_C = 185$$

$$\overline{X}_A = 28 \qquad \overline{X}_B = 43 \qquad \overline{X}_C = 37$$

$$SD_A = \sqrt{\frac{170}{4}} = 6.52 \qquad SD_B = \sqrt{\frac{154}{4}} = 6.20 \qquad SD_C = \sqrt{\frac{114}{4}} = 5.34$$

$$X = \frac{140 + 215 + 185}{5 + 5 + 5} = 36$$

Note: $\overline{X}$ denotes the grand mean, a mean based on all scores and ignoring group membership.

ANOVA and related procedures are computed, these few data are easier to use. However, in a real research setting, several hundred nurses stratified according to specialty or type of education would be solicited as well as physicians and/or other health care professionals. Differences in perceptions as well as patient diagnosis could then be examined for various specialties in order to assess needs for continuing education programs.

Conceptual Formula for ANOVA

In order to tell whether there are differences among the three diagnoses, ANOVA is the appropriate inferential statistic to use. To compute an ANOVA, we first compute a grand mean, $\overline{\overline{X}}$, which is the sum of all 15 scores (540) divided by N (15), the total number of subjects or observations in the study. Then, using the grand mean, a "variance" of the 15 scores is computed which is called the **total.** Two other "variances" are also computed, one that describes differences due to the independent variable, called the **between** or **among,** and one due to **error,** sometimes called **within.** These two "variances," between and error, add up to the total "variance." To look at it another way, the *total* "variance" of the 15 scores is divided into two separate "variances"—one representing the effects due to the independent variable called *between,* and one representing *error* (i.e., confounding variables, measurement error, and so forth). The *F* ratio is then just the ratio of the between to the error.

Computation of these three "variances" is done according to certain prescribed steps. First, three different **sums of squares** are calculated. These are then divided by special **degrees of freedom** *(df)* for each kind of sum of squares. These *df correspond* to the *n* or *n* − 1 by which the sum of squares for a variance/standard deviation of a sample is divided. The result of dividing each sum of squares by its degrees of freedom is called a **mean square** for total, between, and error instead of *variance* for total, between, and error. These mean squares are really just three kinds of variances. Last, the mean square for between is divided by the mean square for error to yield the *F* ratio test statistic.

To make this process clearer, we will use our example from Exhibit 17.1 to compute, via conceptual formulas, the three sums of squares. These are shown in Exhibit 17.2. The first of the three sums of squares to compute is the **total sum of squares,** denoted SS_{total}. Deviation scores are computed between each score and the grand mean, $\overline{\overline{X}}$, and then squared. These are summed for each group as shown and then the group sums are added, $\Sigma \Sigma (X - \overline{\overline{X}})^2$, to yield the SS_{total}: 490 + 399 + 119 = 1008.

The second kind of sum of squares is SS_{error}. This simply is the **sum of squares within** each group. That is, within each group, the group mean is subtracted from each score to yield a deviation score, this deviation score is squared, and then these squared scores are summed. Then, the sums for each group are added, $\Sigma \Sigma (X - \overline{X})^2$, to yield the SS_{error}: 170 + 154 + 114 = 438. It represents individual differences within the groups that go beyond those attributable to the group mean.

The last sum of squares, the **sum of squares for between** (or among), is for

Exhibit 17-2. ANOVA computations for use with the conceptual formulas.

Group A		Group B		Group C	

Total sum of squares:

$X_A - \bar{\bar{X}}$	$(X_A - \bar{\bar{X}})^2$	$X_B - \bar{\bar{X}}$	$(X_B - \bar{\bar{X}})^2$	$X_C - \bar{\bar{X}}$	$(X_C - \bar{\bar{X}})^2$
$20 - 36 = -16$	256	$34 - 36 = -2$	4	$29 - 36 = -7$	49
$22 - 36 = -14$	196	$39 - 36 = 3$	9	$34 - 36 = -2$	4
$31 - 36 = -5$	25	$47 - 36 = 11$	121	$41 - 36 = 5$	25
$33 - 36 = -3$	9	$48 - 36 = 12$	144	$41 - 36 = 5$	25
$34 - 36 = -2$	4	$47 - 36 = 11$	121	$40 - 36 = 4$	16

$\Sigma(X_A - \bar{\bar{X}})^2 = 490$ $\quad\quad\quad \Sigma(X_B - \bar{\bar{X}})^2 = 399$ $\quad\quad\quad \Sigma(X_C - \bar{\bar{X}})^2 = 119$

$\Sigma\Sigma(X - \bar{\bar{X}})^2 = 490 + 399 + 119 = 1008$

Error (or within) sum of squares:

$X_A - \bar{X}_A$	$(X_A - \bar{X}_A)^2$	$X_B - \bar{X}_B$	$(X_B - \bar{X}_B)^2$	$X_C - \bar{X}_C$	$(X_C - \bar{X}_C)^2$
$20 - 28 = -8$	64	$34 - 43 = -9$	81	$29 - 37 = -8$	64
$22 - 28 = -6$	36	$39 - 43 = -4$	16	$34 - 37 = -3$	9
$31 - 28 = -3$	9	$47 - 43 = 4$	16	$41 - 37 = 4$	16
$33 - 28 = 5$	25	$48 - 43 = 5$	25	$41 - 37 = 4$	16
$34 - 28 = 6$	36	$47 - 43 = 4$	16	$40 - 37 = 3$	9

$\Sigma(X_A - \bar{X}_A)^2 = 170$ $\quad\quad\quad \Sigma(X_B - \bar{X}_B)^2 = 154$ $\quad\quad\quad \Sigma(X_C - \bar{X}_C)^2 = 114$

$\Sigma\Sigma(X - \bar{X})^2 = 170 + 154 + 114 = 438$

Between or among sum of squares (experimental effects):

$\bar{X}_A - \bar{\bar{X}}$	$(\bar{X}_A - \bar{\bar{X}})^2$	$\bar{X}_B - \bar{\bar{X}}$	$(\bar{X}_B - \bar{\bar{X}})^2$	$\bar{X}_C - \bar{\bar{X}}$	$(\bar{X}_C - \bar{\bar{X}})^2$
$28 - 36 = -8$	64	$43 - 36 = 7$	49	$37 - 36 = 1$	1
	$\times 5$		$\times 5$		$\times 5$

$n_A(\bar{X}_A - \bar{\bar{X}})^2 = 320$ $\quad\quad\quad n_B(\bar{X}_B - \bar{\bar{X}})^2 = 399$ $\quad\quad\quad n_C(\bar{X}_C - \bar{\bar{X}})^2 = 5$

$\Sigma n(\bar{X} - \bar{\bar{X}})^2 = 320 + 245 + 5 = 570$

effects (of differences) due to the independent variable. Therefore, each group mean is compared to the grand mean in order to observe deviations. The greater the deviations, the greater the effects due to the independent variable. Therefore, deviation scores are computed for each mean from the grand mean and then squared. Because there is only one deviation score for each group and all other sums of squares are based on the number of individual scores in that group, 5, each squared deviation score for between is multiplied by n, the number of subjects in its group. (Please note that n is used when referring to the number of subjects in one group and N is used for the total number of subjects from all groups in the study.) For each group this is denoted, $n(\bar{X} = \bar{\bar{X}})^2$. The

Exhibit 17-3. One-way ANOVA tables.

(*a*)

Source	df	SS	MS	F
Between	$k - 1$	$\Sigma n(\bar{X} - \bar{\bar{X}})^2$	$\dfrac{SS_{between}}{k - 1}$	$\dfrac{MS_{between}}{MS_{error}}$
Error	$N - k$	$\Sigma\Sigma(X - \bar{X})^2$	$\dfrac{SS_{error}}{N - k}$	
Total	$N - 1$	$\Sigma\Sigma(X - \bar{\bar{X}})^2$		

where k = number of groups

N = total number of subjects

(*b*)

Source	df	SS	MS	F
Between	2	570	285	7.8
Error	12	438	36.5	
Total	14	1,008		

group sums are then added, $\Sigma\, n(\bar{X} - \bar{\bar{X}})^2$, to yield the $SS_{between}$: $320 + 245 + 5 = 570$.

After the sums of squares are computed they are inserted into an ANOVA table as shown in Exhibit 17.3. Table A shows how a one-way ANOVA table is structured. This ANOVA is called one-way because it involves only one independent variable. When it involves two independent variables, it is called two-way, and so on. Once the three sums of squares have been computed, all other calculations can be done easily as Table B is filled:

1. The sums of squares are inserted in Table B.
2. The df are computed (according to the formulas in Table A) and inserted in the table. Note that the $df_{total} = df_{between} + df_{error}$, just like with the sum of squares.
3. Mean squares for between and error are computed by dividing the SS by the df for each source. These are then inserted.
4. The F ratio is calculated by dividing the $MS_{between}$ by the MS_{error}.

The remaining task is to test the significance of the *F* ratio. The *F* Distribution Table, Table E of Appendix III, is used. This is the same table as the one used for the *F* test described in Chapter 16. Recall, this table requires two different kinds of *df*—one for the numerator, the $MS_{between}$, and one for the denominator, the MS_{error}. Thus, the table is entered at 2 *df* and 12 *df*. At α level of .05, the critical value is 3.88 and at the α level of .01, it is 6.93. Therefore, the *F* ratio is significant at $p < .01$.

Differences Among Levels of the Independent Variable

The assumption underlying the analysis of variance procedure is that if the groups to be compared are truly random samples from the *same* population, then the between mean square should not differ from the error mean square by more than the amount we would expect from chance alone. As the difference between these mean squares increase, the F ratio increases and the probability of obtaining that F if the null hypothesis is true decreases.

When the null hypothesis is rejected as a result of this analysis of variance procedure, we cannot say more than that the measures obtained from the groups involved differ and the differences are greater than one would expect to exist by chance alone. A significant F ratio does not necessarily mean that *all* groups differ significantly from *all* other groups. A significant F may be a result of a difference existing between one group and the rest of the groups. For instance, it might be that Group A is significantly different from Group B and Group C, but Groups B and C do not differ significantly from each other. There are simple statistical tests that must be applied *after* you get a significant F to find or verify the location of specific significant differences between levels of the independent variable. They are known as **post hoc group comparisons** and are discussed later in this chapter. Mere inspection of the means is not enough.

In our example, we selected our three groups randomly from the same population (i.e., nurses) and thus we can assume that they did not differ beyond the chance expectation prior to the independent variable (i.e., patient diagnoses). The significance of the F ratio indicates that differences among these groups after introduction of the independent variable are beyond chance expectation. We therefore attribute this to our independent variable and conclude that diagnosis affects how nurses perceive the appropriateness or need for sexual counseling. This is as far as we can go in our interpretation of the F ratio. If we need further statistical analysis, we can use the Newman-Keuls test, the Tukey test, the Scheffé test, or one of many others. These techniques can tell us how specific diagnoses differ in terms of nurses' perceptions of the need for sex counseling while keeping the risk of type I error at a minimum. If we were to simply compute three t tests (or ANOVAs) between each pair of means, we would have increased the probability of type I error from 5 to 14 percent. More will be said about this in the section on *post hoc* group comparisons.

Computing ANOVA From Group Descriptive Statistics

Suppose we had been given the mean, standard deviation, and n for each of the three groups in our Exhibit 17.1:

Group A: $\overline{X} = 28$; SD $= 6.52$; $n = 5$
Group B: $\overline{X} = 43$; SD $= 6.20$, $n = 5$
Group C: $\overline{X} = 37$; SD $= 5.34$, $n = 5$

Just as we could with the t test, we can compute ANOVA with these data instead of the original raw scores because the combined sums of squares for the three groups is the ANOVA sum of squares for within or error, and a sum of squares for between is easy to compute using the sample means. Notice how similar this approach is to the conceptual method of computing ANOVA. First, we compute the sum of squares for between:

1. The grand mean is calculated by summing the product of each group mean and n and then dividing this product by the total N.

$$\overline{\overline{X}} = \frac{(28 \times 5) + (43 \times 5) + (37 \times 5)}{5 + 5 + 5} = \frac{140 + 215 + 185}{15} = 36$$

2. The sum of squares for between is the sum of $n(\overline{X} - \overline{\overline{X}})^2$ for each group, just as in the conceptual formula procedure.

$$SS_{between} = 5(28 - 36)^2 + 5(43 - 36)^2 + 5(37 - 36)^2$$
$$= 5(64) + 5(49) + 5(1) = 320 + 399 + 5 = 570$$

Next, we compute the sum of squares for error:

1. Just as with the t test, we must first calculate the sum of squares (for deviation scores) for each group based on each group SD and n. Recall that when the sum of squares is divided by $n - 1$, the variance results. Therefore, when the variance is multiplied by $n - 1$, the sum of squares results (and, of course, the variance is the standard deviation squared, SD^2). Thus you have all the information you need. The sum of squares for each group is calculated as follows:

Group A: $SS_A = (n - 1)(SD_A)^2 = (4)(6.52)(6.52) = 170$
Group B: $SS_B = (n - 1)(SD_B)^2 = (4)(6.20)(6.20) = 154$
Group C: $SS_C = (n - 1)(SD_C)^2 = (4)(5.34)(5.34) = 114$

2. The sums of squares for each group are added to yield the sum of squares for error.

$170 + 154 + 114 = 438$

The last thing we do is complete the ANOVA table using these data. The sum of squares for total is obtained by adding those for between and error. The table would be the same as that presented in Exhibit 17.3.

Computational Formula for ANOVA

If you do not have a computer available and your sample size is large, you will find it easier to use the computational formulas for ANOVA than the conceptual formulas. The basic elements of each are presented and contrasted with the conceptual formula in Exhibit 17.4. Further, Exhibit 17.5 presents the methods for organizing the data prior to computing $SS_{between}$ and SS_{within}. They include

---

Exhibit 17-4. Comparison of conceptual and computational formulas for ANOVA sum of squares.

Source	Conceptual	Computational
$SS_{between}$	$(17.1)\ \Sigma n(\bar{X} - \bar{\bar{X}})^2$ (17.4)	$\left[\dfrac{(\Sigma X_A)^2}{n_A} + \dfrac{(\Sigma X_B)^2}{n_B} + \cdots + \dfrac{(\Sigma X_k)^2}{n_k} \right] - \dfrac{(\Sigma\Sigma X)^2}{N}$
SS_{within}	$(17.2)\ \Sigma\Sigma(X - \bar{X})^2$ (17.5)	$\left[\Sigma X_A^2 - \dfrac{(\Sigma X_A)^2}{n_A} \right] + \left[\Sigma X_B^2 - \dfrac{(\Sigma X_B)^2}{n_B} \right] + \cdots + \left[\Sigma X_k^2 - \dfrac{(\Sigma X_k)^2}{n_k} \right]$
SS_{total}	$(17.3)\ \Sigma\Sigma(X - \bar{\bar{X}})^2$ (17.6)	$SS_{between} + SS_{within}$

A. As indicated by step 1 in Exhibit 17.5, list all scores in each group (i.e., X_A, X_B, X_C) and sum them for each group (i.e., ΣX_A, ΣX_B, ΣX_C).

B. Square each score and sum the squared scores for each group (i.e., ΣX_A^2, ΣX_B^2, ΣX_C^2), step 2.

C. Square each group's sum of scores (i.e., $(\Sigma X_A)^2$, $(\Sigma X_B)^2$, $(\Sigma X_C)^2$ as step 3.

D. Sum all scores from all groups $\Sigma\Sigma X$, step 4.

E. Sum all squared scores from all groups, $\Sigma\Sigma X^2$, step 5.

F. Square the sum of all scores from all groups, $(\Sigma\Sigma X)^2$, step 6.

Using the formulas from Exhibit 17.4 and calculations from Exhibit 17.5, the ANOVA sums of squares can be computed as follows:

$$SS_{between} = \frac{19600}{5} + \frac{46225}{5} + \frac{34255}{5} - \frac{291600}{15}$$

$$= 3920 + 9245 + 6845 - 19440 = 20010 - 19440 = 570$$

$$SS_{within} = \left(4090 - \frac{19600}{5} \right) + \left(9299 - \frac{46225}{5} \right) + \left(6959 - \frac{34225}{5} \right)$$

Exhibit 17-5. ANOVA data organization for use with computational formulas.

Group A		Group B		Group C	
X_A	X_A^2	X_B	X_B^2	X_C	X_C^2
20	400	34	1,156	29	841
22	484	39	1,521	34	1,156
31	961	47	2,209	41	1,681
33	1,089	48	2,304	41	1,681
34	1,156	47	2,209	40	1,600

(1) $\Sigma X_A = 140$ (2) $\Sigma X_A^2 = 4,090$ (1) $\Sigma X_B = 215$ (2) $\Sigma X_B^2 = 9,399$ (1) $\Sigma X_C = 185$ (2) $\Sigma X_C^2 = 6,959$

(3) $(\Sigma X_A)^2 = 19,600$ (3) $(\Sigma X_B)^2 = 46,225$ (3) $(\Sigma X_C)^2 = 34,225$

(4) Sum of all scores = $\Sigma\Sigma X = 140 + 215 + 185 = 540$

(5) Sum of all squared scores = $\Sigma\Sigma X^2 = 4,090 + 9,399 + 6,959 = 20,448$

(6) Sum of all scores squared = $(\Sigma\Sigma X)^2 = (140 + 215 + 185)^2 = 540^2 = 291,600$

$$= (4090 - 3920) + (9399 - 9245) + (6959 - 6845)$$

$$= 170 + 154 + 114 = 438$$

$$SS_{total} = 570 + 438 = 1008$$

As you can observe, the results are the same as those computed with the conceptual formulas.

Unequal N One-way ANOVA, unlike certain of the more complex ANOVAs, can be computed as described previously even when the groups are not equal in size. Be sure not to confuse n, which refers to group size, and N, which refers to the size of the total sample. On the other hand, researchers have found that when groups are equal in size, the assumptions of parametric tests like homogeneity of variance can be violated without adversely affecting the results.

Comparisons Among Levels of the Independent Variable

Once a significant F is achieved for between, or the experimental variable, you cannot just look at means and say Group B is significantly different from, say, Group D. You must run special statistical tests in order to say that. When this is done after a significant ANOVA or after the researcher has seen the data, you select from the family of tests known as **post hoc group comparisons.** If you can hypothesize differences among various groups or levels of the independent variable ahead of time, you can use a priori tests, which use contrasts. Contrasts have an advantage over the post hoc tests in that it is easier to reach statistical significance. They use the α originally specified, while the post hoc tests reduce it in order to conform to the laws of probability and make up for the fact that the researcher has already seen the data. This section deals with the group of tests that usually accompanies statistically significant ANOVA when three or more groups, or levels, of an independent variable are involved.

Post Hoc Group Comparisons When the α level for an ANOVA is set, usually at 5 percent, you are saying that, on the average, one time in 20 you will make a type I error when an F ratio is declared statistically significant. If you have already computed an F for the between sum of squares and then compute a t test, say, between two of five means, you have now run two out of twenty tests, one of 20 which, by the laws of probability, will be wrong. Therefore, if you continued to make more comparisons, you would be running greater risk than five percent of making an error. This phenomenon is known as **family type I error.** Exhibit 17.6 gives the increased α level for the number of statistical tests performed on the same data set (i.e., subsets of the same dependent variable). As you can observe, it does not take many comparisons before the chance of error becomes intolerable. Therefore, after a significant F, the family of post hoc group comparisons is used.

Exhibit 17-6. Probability of family Type I error.

Number of Tests, Each at $\alpha = .05$	α Level, Compounded
2	.10
3	.14
4	.19
5	.23
6	.26
10	.40

Note: Compounded level based on the formula $1 - (1 - \alpha)^N$, where N = number of tests run and α is the alpha level of a single test.

Each, in its own *unique* way, minimizes the risk, usually by reducing the α level proportionate to the number of additional statistical tests performed.*

Concept of Ranges

Before discussing each of the more common post hoc procedures, it is necessary to understand the concept of ranges. Suppose a significant F ratio was found for the following group means:

$$\bar{X}_A = 36, \bar{X}_B = 47, \bar{X}_C = 29, \text{ and } \bar{X}_D = 53$$

Prior to conducting a post hoc group comparison test, you would first rank order the means from lowest to highest. (This is absolutely required for the Duncan Multiple Range and Neuman-Keuls tests.) It is then possible to define the various ranges:

$$
3 \begin{cases} \begin{aligned} \bar{X}_C &= 29 \\ \bar{X}_A &= 36 \\ \bar{X}_B &= 47 \\ \end{aligned} \end{cases} \begin{matrix} 2 \\ 2 \\ 2 \end{matrix} \quad 4
$$

3 $\bar{X}_D = 53$

The comparisons labeled *2* are of the two-**mean range** in which, obviously, two means are comprised by each range. This is one parameter, the number of means in the range, that must be used for the procedures. The comparisons labeled *3* are the three-mean range of comparisons, because the comparison required passing by one mean and therefore included three means. Last, the comparison labeled *4* is a four-mean range because two means are bypassed in order to make the comparison between the two others.

---

*Purists say that there are two additional sources of family type I error due to (1) replications of the same study and (2) the simultaneous F tests conducted when there is more than one independent variable. However, these are ignored by researchers except in complex ANOVA where interactions of four or more factors are not interpreted.

Harmonic Mean

Most of the post hoc tests are designed for use with equal n. However, when the largest group is not more than twice the size of the smallest group, the harmonic mean can be used to determine an n for use in the formulas. Suppose four groups had the following n: $n_A = 15$, $n_B = 25$, $n_C = 30$, and $n_D = 30$. The harmonic mean, n_H, also explained in Chapter 16, is calculated as follows:

$$n_H = \frac{k}{\Sigma \, (1/n)} \tag{17.7}$$

where k = the number of groups
$\Sigma \, (1/n)$ = sum of $1/n$ for all groups, where n in the number in each group

Using the hypothetical data, n is computed as follows:

$$n = \frac{4}{(\frac{1}{15} + \frac{1}{25} + \frac{1}{30} + \frac{1}{30})} = \frac{4}{(\frac{30}{450} + \frac{18}{450} + \frac{15}{450} + \frac{15}{450})} = \frac{4}{(\frac{78}{450})}$$

$$= \frac{4}{.1733} = 23.08$$

The harmonic mean of 23.08 is slightly smaller, in this case, than the arithmetic mean of 25.

Multiple *t* Test

The multiple t test does not control the level of α and therefore there is a high risk of type I error when more than a few comparisons are made. Because it is the least conservative (i.e., easiest to achieve statistical significance), it is the most powerful of the post hoc tests. Because the ANOVA table is already available, the following formula eases computation:

$$t = \frac{\overline{X}_A - \overline{X}_B}{\sqrt{MS_{error} \, (1/n_A + 1/n_B)}} \tag{17.8}$$

where $df = n_A + n_B - 2$

Recalling data from Exhibits 17.1 through 17.3, the $MS_{error} = 36.5$, $\overline{X}_A = 28$, $\overline{X}_B = 43$, $\overline{X}_C = 37$, and $n = 5$. All comparisons for t have $df = 8$; therefore a critical value of 2.306 at $\alpha = .05$. Each of the comparisons is as follows:

(1) $t_{\overline{X}_B - \overline{X}_C} = \dfrac{43 - 37}{\sqrt{36.5 \, (\frac{1}{5} + \frac{1}{5})}} = \dfrac{6}{\sqrt{(36.5)(.4)}} = \dfrac{6}{\sqrt{14.6}} = \dfrac{6}{3.82}$

$\qquad\qquad\qquad = 1.57$ (not significant)

(2) $t_{\overline{X}_B - \overline{X}_A} = \dfrac{43 - 28}{3.82} = \dfrac{15}{3.82} = 3.92$ (significant)

(3) $t_{\overline{X}_C - \overline{X}_A} = \dfrac{37 - 28}{3.82} = \dfrac{9}{3.82} = 2.35$ (significant)

We conclude that group A is significantly different from both group B and group C. However, groups B and C are not significantly different from one another. There is one major drawback to this analysis that must be considered. Using all pairwise comparisons as illustrated, the α level is .14.

Newman-Keuls Test

The Newman-Keuls test is used only for testing *all* possible pairs of means according to a specified order. It provides for computation of a different **critical mean difference** (CMD) for each **mean range.** As the mean range gets larger so does the CMD. That is, the farther apart two means are in a rank ordering of means, the larger the differences between them must be before this difference exceeds the CMD and is declared statistically significant. This test uses the studentized range distribution, Table O of Appendix III, in the computation of the CMDs. There is a prescribed sequence in which comparisons between means are made. Refer to Exhibit 17.7, where this sequencing is described along with the steps in data organization that lead to defining this required sequence.

The formula for determining a CMD via the Newman-Keuls Test is as follows:

$$NK_{CMD} = q \sqrt{\frac{MS_{error}}{n}} \tag{17.9}$$

where q = the studentized range statistic (Table O of Appendix III) for the number of means in the range, the *df* for the MS_{error}, and the .05 or .01 α level
n = number of subjects in one group

A CMD for *each* mean range is computed when using the Neuman-Keuls procedure. This is a decided advantage as you will see later in this section. Therefore, using the data shown in Exhibit 17.7 and formula 17.9, a CMD for each range at α = .05 is computed. From Table O, Appendix III, the q for two means is 2.95; for three is 3.58; for four is 3.96; and for five is 4.23. To deduce n from the information given in Exhibit 17.7, there are five means that, when added to the error *df* equal a total N of 25. Then, n is calculated by dividing the total N by the number of means or groups, n = (25 ÷ 5) = 5 in each group (assuming equal n). The calculations are as follows:

1. Two-mean range:

$$NK_{CMD} = 2.95 \sqrt{\frac{20}{5}} = (2.95)\,(2) = 5.9$$

2. Three-mean range:

$$NK_{CMD} = 3.58 \sqrt{\frac{20}{5}} = (3.58)\,(2) = 7.16$$

Exhibit 17-7. Data organization for computation of Neuman-Keuls test.

Example: A significant F was found among five means: $\bar{X}_A = 36, \bar{X}_B = 47, \bar{X}_C = 29, \bar{X}_D = 53, \bar{X}_E = 38$. From the ANOVA table, $MS_{error} = 20$ and df error $= 20$.

1. The means must be rank-ordered and the mean ranges labeled:

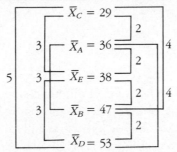

2. The differences between each pair of means are computed and tabled in a *Table of Differences*, which follows this pattern:

	Smallest Mean				Largest Mean
	C	A	E	B	D
C	—	$\bar{X}_A - \bar{X}_C$	$\bar{X}_E - \bar{X}_C$	$\bar{X}_B - \bar{X}_C$	$\bar{X}_D - \bar{X}_C$
A		—	$\bar{X}_E - \bar{X}_A$	$\bar{X}_B - \bar{X}_A$	$\bar{X}_D - \bar{X}_A$
E			—	$\bar{X}_B - \bar{X}_E$	$\bar{X}_D - \bar{X}_E$
B				—	$\bar{X}_D - \bar{X}_B$
D					

The value differences between means for this example are as follows:

	A	E	B	D
C	7	9	18	24
A		2	11	17
E			9	15
B				6

Note that column C and row D were not necessary since no differences can belong in these columns.

3. The order in which pairwise comparisons *must* be made is as follows:

   a. Begin with the comparison at the far right of the first row. If it is significant, move to the comparison in the same row that is just left of the one you have finished. Continue moving from right to left on the first row until you encounter a nonsignificant comparison D. Then stop. Comparisons can never come to this *column* again. Next, begin tests of comparisons in the second row, moving from right to left, until you reach a nonsignificant difference or the column where you stopped in row 1.

   b. Go to row 3, and move from right to left, stopping just before the column of row 2 that yielded a nonsignificant comparison.

   c. Continue until all rows have been examined or a nonsignificant comparison is encountered in the far right column of a row.

3. Four-mean range:

$$NK_{CMD} = 3.96 \sqrt{\frac{20}{5}} = (3.96)(2) = 7.92$$

4. Five-mean range:

$$NK_{CMD} = 4.23 \sqrt{\frac{20}{5}} = (4.23)(2) = 8.46$$

The actual post hoc tests of differences between means are now ready to be made. Using the table of differences from Exhibit 17.7, we start at the extreme right of the first row. $(\overline{X}_D - \overline{X}_C)$, 24, is a five-mean range comparison. Therefore 24 is compared to 8.46 and is significant. $(\overline{X}_B - \overline{X}_C)$, 18, is a four-mean range comparison so it is compared to 7.92 and found significant. $(\overline{X}_E - \overline{X}_C)$, 9, a three-mean range comparison, has a CMD of 7.16 and is therefore significant. $(\overline{X}_A - \overline{X}_C)$, 7, a two-mean comparison with CMD = 5.9, is also significant.

Next, the second row is tested. Because no nonsignificant comparisons were found in row 1, we do not have to stop comparisons in row 2 unless we reach a nonsignificant one. $(\overline{X}_D - \overline{X}_A)$, 17, a four-mean range comparison with a CMD of 7.92, is significant. Next, $(\overline{X}_B - \overline{X}_A)$, 11, a three-mean range comparison with a CMD of 7.16, is significant. Last, $(\overline{X}_E - \overline{X}_A)$, 2, a two-mean range comparison with a CMD of 5.9, is nonsignificant. We must therefore stop. And, *all subsequent comparisons must stop before the column headed E.* Of course, in this example, we could not go farther anyway. However, there may be times when you could but cannot.

Analysis continues by going to the next or third row. $(\overline{X}_D - \overline{X}_E)$, 15, a three-mean range comparison with CMD of 7.16, is significant. Next, $(\overline{X}_B - \overline{X}_E)$, 9, a two-mean range comparison with a CMD of 5.9, is significant. Finally, we come to the last row. $(\overline{X}_D - \overline{X}_B)$, 6, a two-mean range comparison, is significant.

As you can observe, computation of the NK procedure is not difficult. It just requires that you follow exactly the rules of order in testing the comparisons. To make sure this is clear and also to provide for comparison of the various procedures, we will do one more example, using our familiar data from Exhibits 17.1 through 17.3. First, the means must be rank-ordered, the mean ranges determined, and a *table of differences* constructed:

(1) *Mean Ranges*

$$3 \begin{bmatrix} \overline{X}_A = 28 \\ \overline{X}_C = 37 \\ \overline{X}_B = 43 \end{bmatrix} \begin{matrix} 2 \\ 2 \end{matrix}$$

(2) *Table of Differences*

	C	B
A	9	15
C		6

Next, the value of q is obtained from Table O in Appendix III. Entering the table at *df* for error = 12 and α = .05, q for a two-mean range = 2.08 and for a three-mean range is 3.77. Using formula 17.9, the CMD for the two ranges can now be computed:

1. Two-mean range:

$$ND_{r=2} = 3.08 \sqrt{\frac{36.5}{5}} = (3.08)\,(2.70) = 8.32$$

2. Three-mean range:

$$ND_{r=3} = 3.77 \sqrt{\frac{36.5}{5}} = (3.77)\,(2.70) = 10.18$$

Comparisons are tested in the order dictated by the table of differences beginning with the far right difference and working left across the row. $(\overline{X}_B - \overline{X}_A)$, 15, a three-mean range comparison with a CMD of 10.18, is significant. $(\overline{X}_C - \overline{X}_A)$, 9, is a two-mean range comparison with a CMD of 8.32, and also significant. Row 2, $(\overline{X}_B - \overline{X}_C)$, 6, has only a two-mean range comparison, which is not significant.

In the NK procedure the α level of *all* possible pairwise comparisons was kept at .05. However, had few comparisons been permitted owing to the rules of ordering, the overall α level for the few permitted tests could have been considerably lower than .05. To remedy this situation, a more lenient procedure called Duncan's multiple range is available. In it, α remains at .05 for the two- and three-mean ranges, but then rises for larger mean tests. Because of space limitations and the reluctance of some journals to accept this as a valid *post hoc* comparison owing to its leniency, its computation is not described in this book. It uses a special table developed by Duncan to obtain a k value that is similar to q in the Newman-Keuls procedure.

The Tukey HSD Test

Tukey's Honestly Significant Difference (HSD) test uses the same table of studentized ranges and formula as the Newman-Keuls. The Tukey procedure, however, computes only one CMD for the total number of means being compared, and therefore it is more stringent or conservative. It is easier to use and compute, because only one CMD must be determined and no special order of comparisons is required. While the Newman-Keuls procedure is limited to all pairwise comparisons, the Tukey procedure can be used for other kinds of comparisons, such as groups 1 and 2 with groups 3 and 4 or group 1 versus groups 2, 3, and 4 combined.* The formula for the Tukey test is as follows:

---

*For more complex designs, means can be formed by averaging across other factors. In computing T, use whatever MS, *df*, and *n* are appropriate for the effect being tested.

$$T_{CMD} = q\sqrt{\frac{MS_{error}}{n}} \tag{17.10}$$

where q = the studentized range statistic (Table O of Appendix III) for the number of means to be compared, df for error, and .05 or .01 level of significance

n = number is *one* group

To compute the CMD using our usual data, we enter the table for a three-mean range, $df = 12$, and $\alpha = .05$, and we find $q = 3.77$. We then compute the CMD:

$$T_{CMD} = 3.77 \sqrt{\frac{36.5}{5}} = (3.77)\,(2.70) = 10.18$$

It is the same value as the three-mean range CMD for the Newman-Keuls Test. Applying this to the three observed differences between means, 15, 9, and 8, we find that only one is significant: $\overline{X}_B - \overline{X}_A$.

The Tukey test is more conservative than the Newman-Keuls. Tukey has therefore proposed a second procedure, called the Tukey B procedure (versus the Tukey A procedure, which has just been presented.) In the Tukey B procedure, a compromise is struck by using as the CMD the mean of the Tukey A and Newman-Keuls CMDs for the particular comparison. Some statisticians believe that Tukey was less than serious when he proposed the Tukey B test.

The Scheffé Test

The Scheffé Test, sometimes called the S method, also computes only one CMD and is used with much more complex designs as well as all pairs. It has the advantage of using the same F table as ANOVA rather than the special table required by the preceding two tests. However, it is even more conservative than the Tukey test. The formula is as follows:

$$S_{CMD} = \sqrt{(k-1)F} \sqrt{\frac{2MS_{error}}{n}} \tag{17.11}$$

where k = number of means

F = the critical value for F using the between and error df from the ANOVA table and the desired α level

MS_{error} = mean square for error from the ANOVA table

n = number of observations in one group

To illustrate computation, we will again use the data from Exhibits 17.1 through 17.3. Therefore we enter the F table (Table E, Appendix III) to extract the critical value of F for 2, 12 df at $\alpha = .05$. It is 3.89.

$$S_{CMD} = \sqrt{(3-1)\,(3.89)} \sqrt{\frac{2(36.5)}{5}} = \sqrt{7.78}\,\sqrt{14.6}$$

$$= (2.78) (3.82) = 10.64$$

The CMD for this particular test is only larger by .46 than the Tukey test. The results are the same—only one comparison is significant. Both tests enjoy a good reputation among knowledgeable researchers because they are conservative and versatile. It is important to remember, however, that conservative tests have higher probabilities of type II error.

Dunnett's Test

Dunnett's test is a specialized test for comparing all means with a control group but not with each other. It uses a special table called Dunnett's t distribution, Table P, Appendix III. The error rate effectwise is α. The CMD is computed as follows:

$$D_{CMD} = \hat{t}\sqrt{\frac{2\ MS_{error}}{n}} \tag{17.12}$$

where t = the value found in the table of Dunnett's t distribution (Table P, Appendix III) for α, df for error, and whether the test is one-tailed or two-tailed
     n = number in one group

Under the assumption that our example data from Exhibits 17.1 through 17.3 could be converted for this use, D is computed as follows:

$$D = 2.11 \sqrt{\frac{2(36.5)}{5}} = (2.11) (3.82) = 8.06$$

As you can observe, it pays to use Dunnett's test whenever possible, because its CMD is smaller than that in the preceding tests.

Choosing a *Post Hoc* Test

There is no hard and fast rule for selecting one of the *post hoc* procedures. Certainly, if *only* comparisons with a control group are made, Dunnett's test is advantageous. From among the other three, if only pairwise comparisons are being made, the Newman-Keuls procedure seems appropriate. If other kinds of comparisons are wanted, the Tukey A or Scheffé test is a candidate. Instructors, thesis committees, and journal editors have their favorites. Therefore, your decision may be made for you. When writing for publication in a journal, it is certainly appropriate to study several issues of the journal to discover what *post hoc* procedures are popular among researchers who publish in that journal.

Sometimes it is possible to hypothesize which groups will be statistically different from each other *before* a study begins. In this case, instead of analyzing your data to see whether an overall main effect exists, you have a number of separate comparisons (of means) among the levels of the main effect you wish to make. This can be done by using planned comparisons or contrasts. This technique of **planned comparisons** is used *instead of* ordinary ANOVA and the *F* ratio. Discussion of this technique is beyond the scope of this book, however. The reader is referred to Hays [2] or Dayton [1].

Repeated-Measures ANOVA

In nursing research, subjects are usually people. Because people vary owing to experience and genetic makeup, those within a single group often show relatively large variability. This preexisting variation, as you have seen, is part of error and therefore reduces the likelihood of observing differences between groups. One way to reduce error due to uncontrolled sources of variation among subjects within a group is to use the **subjects as their own controls,** or otherwise **match** subjects as already demonstrated with the *t* test for dependent groups. Of course, many designs do not permit this.

When there are three or more matched groups, or observations on the same subjects, in a design, repeated-measures ANOVA is the appropriate statistical test. In this type of analysis, effects due to the independent variable are calculated the usual way. The variability due to differences in the average responsiveness of *each* subject, however, is eliminated from SS_{error}. The following is the computational formula for $SS_{subjects}$:

$$(17.13)$$

$$SS_{subjects} = \frac{[(A_1+B_1+ \cdots + K_1)^2 + (A_2+B_2+ \cdots +K_2)^2 + (A_n+B_n+ \cdots +K_n)^2]}{k}$$

$$- \left(\frac{\Sigma X^2}{N} \right)$$

where k = number of repeated measures per subject
n = number of subjects
N = total number of observations ($k \times n$)
$(A_1+B_1+ \cdots +K_1)^2$ = squared sum of all subject 1's scores
$(A_2+B_2+ \cdots +K_2)^2$ = squared sum of all subject 2's scores
$(A_n+B_n+ \cdots +K_n)^2$ = squared sum of all the last subject's scores
$(\Sigma\Sigma X)^2$ = sum of all scores ($k \times n$) across both subjects and repeated measures, which is then squared

$$df = n-1$$

If we were to change the focus of the data in Exhibit 17.1, which was used to illustrate calculation of one-way ANOVA, it could become an example for repeated-measures ANOVA. Suppose that, instead of randomly assigning one of the three vignettes to Ss, each Ss received and responded to all three. This design would then be appropriate for repeated-measures analysis, because each subject was exposed, in differing order, to each level of the independent variable. Using the data presented in Exhibits 17.1 through 17.5, we could calculate the $SS_{subjects}$ as follows:

$$SS_{subjects} = \frac{\begin{array}{c}(20+34+29)^2 + (22+39+34)^2 + (31+47+41)^2 \\ + (33+48+41)^2 + (34+47+40)^2\end{array}}{3} - \frac{(291600)}{15}$$

$$= \frac{(6889 + 9025 + 14161 + 14884 + 14641)}{3} - 19440$$

$$= \frac{59600}{3} - 19440 = 19866.66 - 19440 = 426.65$$

$$df_{subjects} = 5 - 1 = 4$$

$SS_{subjects}$ is subtracted from the original SS_{error} (see Exhibit 17.3). Similarly, the *df* for subjects is subtracted from the *df* for *error*. Therefore, the ANOVA table becomes:

Source	df	SS	MS	F
Subjects	4	426.65	—	—
Between	2	570	285	200.7
Error	8	11.35	1.42	
Total	14	1008		

The *F* is even more significant than before, because we have reduced the denominator of the *F* ratio from 26.5 to 1.42. The major impact of using repeated measures in this instance, however, is on the results of post hoc group comparisons and the conclusions drawn from the research. All post hoc comparisons of means become significantly different.

Power Analysis for ANOVA

As stated in Chapters 15 and 16, power analysis to determine the probability of type II error after failure of an *F* ratio to reach significance requires computation of an effect size (ES) and use of the power tables in Appendix IV. For one-way ANOVA, there are several methods for computing ES. A relatively easy and straightforward approach is with the following formula:

$$ES = \sqrt{\frac{SS_{between}}{SS_{error}}} \tag{17.14}$$

The *n* with which the table is entered is the size of *one* group, not the total sample. If groups have unequal *n*, the arithmetic mean of the *n* for the groups is used. The number of groups or levels of the independent variable must also be used when entering the table.

Table C in Appendix IV is the appropriate power table for ANOVA. Suppose a researcher completed a three-level experiment in which three equally sized groups had $n_A = 19, n_B = 20$, and $n_C = 21$ due to mortality. $F_{(2,57)}$ equalled 1.5

and was not significant. Therefore the probability of type II error is of interest. First the researcher computes ES and n as follows:

$$ES = \sqrt{\frac{96}{1728}} = \sqrt{.05} = .22$$

$$n = \frac{19 + 20 + 21}{3} = 20$$

Entering Table C, Appendix IV, with $n = 20$, ES $= .22$ and $df = 2$, we find that the probabilities of type II error are .74 for ES $= .20$ and .62 for ES $= .25$. Using linear interpolation, the probability for ES $= .22$ is .69 or 69 percent, considerably higher than our desired level, which is 20 percent. Thus, the researcher would do well to repeat the experiment with larger groups before concluding that the research is fruitless.

Correlation Ratio (Eta)

Eta (η) is a correlation coefficient that is used when (1) relationships are not linear or (2) after an ANOVA when you wish to know the **magnitude of effect** or extent of a relationship between an independent variable (usually group membership) and the dependent variable. The formula is as follows:

$$\eta = \sqrt{\frac{SS_{between}}{SS_{total}}} \tag{17.15}$$

By far the most common usage of *eta* is after an ANOVA table has been computed. Computation from raw data is considerably more complex and beyond the scope of this book. Therefore, when a computer is available and a relationship is curvilinear, the calculation is simplified by computing an ANOVA table in which the nonlinear variable is treated as the independent variable.

Eta squared can range from 0 to 1 and is interpreted just as is r^2, the proportion of variance shared by the two variables. If we return to the example used throughout most of this chapter, Exhibits 17.1 through 17.3, the relationship between patient diagnosis and nurse perception of the need for sexual counseling is as follows:

$$\eta = \sqrt{\frac{570}{1008}} = \sqrt{.565} = .75$$

To interpret, η is squared:

$$\eta^2 = (.75)^2 = .56$$

The relationship is strong. Over half of the variance is shared by the two variables. Since a much smaller F ratio (e.g., CV (.05) = 3.88) could also result in a significant F ratio, η^2 is useful additional information regarding the actual magnitude of the experimental effect. Moreover, the unexplained variance (using formula 16.10) is .44, very small indeed for behavioral research. Program changes are probably needed and justified. When this information about magnitude of effect is not presented in journal articles reporting the results of research, you can easily compute it yourself. In this way, you can judge the practical significance of experimental effects—particularly when large samples or other factors like repeated measures may have been used to achieve statistical significance for small effects.

$\mathbf{T}$*he* F_{max} *Test for Homogeneity of Variance*

The F test, described in Chapter 16, tests the equivariance assumption of parametric tests in which only two groups are used. When three or more groups are used, the F_{max} test can be employed. In this procedure, the largest group variance is divided by the smallest variance. The df are always $n - 1$, the number of subjects in one group minus one. A special table (Table Q, Appendix III) rather than the usual F table, is used for the F_{max} test. This simple test has one restriction. It *requires* equal n in all groups. When n is slightly unequal, some researchers randomly delete data points from some groups in order to achieve equal n.

Using data from the example used in this chapter (see Exhibits 17.1 through 17.3), the variances were $V_A = 42.5$, $V_B = 38.5$, and $V_C = 28.5$. The 3 groups had an equal n of 5. To test the equivariance assumption, the largest variance is divided by the smallest:

$$F_{max} = \frac{42.5}{28.5} = 1.9 \qquad df = n - 1 = 5 - 1 = 4$$

Entering Table Q, Appendix III, at $df = 4$, $\alpha = .05$ and $k = 3$, we find that the critical value is 15.5. The F_{max} test statistic must be equal to or larger than 15.5 if the variances are to be declared heterogeneous. Thus, the variances are not statistically different and this assumption of ANOVA is met.

Sometimes the n of groups is very unequal. There are other procedures that can then be used (i.e., Bartlett's, Cochran's, or Levine's tests). Discussion of these is beyond the scope of this book.

$\mathbf{V}$*ocabulary*

Among mean square	Error sum of squares
Between sum of squares	*Eta* squared
Degrees of freedom	F test versus F ratio

Family type I error

Grand mean

Harmonic mean

Magnitude of effect

Mean range

One-way ANOVA

Planned comparisons

Post hoc group comparisons

Subjects as their own controls

Table of differences

Total sum of squares

Within mean square

References

1. Dayton, C. M. *Design of Educational Experiments.* New York: McGraw-Hill, 1970.
2. Hays, W. L. *Statistics* (3rd ed.). New York: Holt, Reinhart & Winston, 1981.

Suppose a nurse practitioner who works in a primary care clinic conducted an experimental program to determine the effects on the stabilization of hypertensive patients of three experimental conditions. All patients had been in treatment for at least 6 months and had not stabilized. The first group of patients was given booklets describing their conditions, their specific medications and treatment regimens, and potential side effects and outcomes if they remained hypertensive. They were instructed in how to monitor their blood pressure and asked to do so weekly. A hotline was established to answer questions and provide additional information or support as needed. The second group received everything the first group did and, in addition, received weekly home visits for the first six weeks and monthly home visits for the next 3 months. A third group acted as controls and received the usual clinic care. A .05 level of significance was chosen. At the end of six months, patients were classified as having either stabilized or not stabilized.

Seventy-three systematically sampled patients were approached for inclusion in the study and four declined, stating they were too busy to be bothered by a research study. They were not interested in being "guinea pigs." Of the 69 patients who were included in the study, 8 were lost owing to death or relocation to another city. Group 2 lost five patients and Group 3 lost three. The dependent variable was whether or not a patient stabilized—reached his or her goal for blood pressure. The level of measurement for the dependent variable is nominal, therefore, because each subject was *classified* into one of two *categories*. The number of subjects in each category, a frequency count, is to be compared for each of the three experimental conditions. The null hypothesis states that there is no difference among the groups, or, in other words, the experimental variable is not related to stabilization. The alternate hypothesis states that the three groups are not only not equal, but that the experimental variable *caused* changes in stabilization.

The Chi Square Test of Independence

When you have **frequency counts** for **categories of variables,** and you want to know if these observed frequencies are significantly different (statistically) from each other for two or more groups, you can find out by calculating a chi square (χ^2) statistic. It is called the chi square test of independence. In the preceding example, we wish to find out if two variables, experimental condition (three categories) and stabilization (two categories), are independent (or not related). If they are independent, we accept the null hypothesis. If they are not, we reject the null hypothesis because we will have found that they are dependent (or related). We will have found that the experimental condition affects stabilization, a causal relationship between the variables. Essentially, chi square analysis compares what we observe in our research with what we would expect to observe if the two variables were independent. If the difference is large

Exhibit 18-1. Contingency table for experimental condition and stabilization.

		Stabilization	
		No	Yes
	Group 1: Booklet and self-monitoring	10	13
Experimental condition	Group 2: Booklet, self-monitoring, and home visits	3	15
	Group 3: Control	18	2

enough, we conclude that it is statistically significant. The chi square statistic is the most commonly used statistic with nominal data and, in addition, one of the most well known of all the inferential procedures. It ranks with the *t* test and ANOVA in terms of frequency of use, and it is the most popular of all the nonparametric statistical procedures.

The k × m *Table*

The first thing we must do is summarize the data for the 61 patients by making a contingency table. As you recall from Chapter 6, a contingency table has two variables. The categories (or levels) of one, group membership or the experimental condition, are represented as *k* rows in the table and the categories of the second, stabilization, are represented by the *m* columns in the table, as shown in Exhibit 18.1. It is a 2 × 3 contingency table and has 6 cells.

Computing Chi Squares

By inspecting the obsesrved frequencies, those we found as a result of the experimental program, we note that there appear to be differences in the percentages of patients who stabilized in each group. However, as usual, we want to be more objective in determining differences than mere inspection or "eyeballing" will allow. Because data are nominal, we compute chi square and use this statistic to test for independence. We begin by adding the cell frequencies (see Exhibit 18.2) to obtain totals for each row and column. There are 10 patients in cell U and 13 in cell V for a total of 23 in the first row. Similarly, the total in the second row is 18 (3 + 15) and in the third row, 20 (18 + 2). The total number of patients who did not stabilize is the sum of the cells U, W, and Y in column 1, 10 + 3 + 18 = 31. Similarly, the total for column 2, those patients who did stabilize, is 13 + 15 + 2 = 30. The grand total, or number of patients in the program, is 61 and is equal to the sum of all the rows or all the columns. Usually you sum each as a check on your arithmetic. You also calculate each sum on a percentage basis by dividing it by *N*, finding the percentage of column 1 to be

Exhibit 18-2. Row and column totals.

	Stabilization		
	No	Yes	
Group 1	Cell U	Cell V	23 (37.7%)
Group 2	Cell W	Cell X	18 (29.5%)
Group 3	Cell Y	Cell Z	20 (32.8%)
	31 (51%)	30 (49%)	$N = 61$

31/61 = 51 percent, of row 1 to be 23/61 = 37.7 percent, and so on. You can further double-check your calculations by noting that the column and row percentages each total 100 percent.

Next we calculate the **expected** (as opposed to **observed**) **frequencies** for each cell of the table. An expected frequency is the number of patients you would expect to find in a given cell if there were no group differences. Thus, you would expect to find 51 percent of the total of each row in the cells of column 1 and 49 percent of the total of each row in the cells of column 2. The formula for the expected frequency of a cell is as follows:

$$E = \frac{(Tr)(Tc)}{N} \tag{18.1}$$

where E = expected frequency of a cell
 Tr = cell's row total or number of Ss in that row
 Tc = cell's column total or number of Ss in that column
 N = total number of Ss in the study

Using formula 18.1, the expected frequency for cell Z is calculated as follows:

$$E_Z = \frac{(20)(30)}{61} = \frac{600}{61} = 9.8$$

You expect that of the 20 patients in row 3, 49 percent, or 9.8, stabilize, and thus this is the expected frequency for cell Z. Another way you can look at this is to consider the distribution of patients you would expect to find if you were given *only* the row and column totals as information on which to base an estimate of cell frequencies. As the formula shows, the expected frequency of a cell is calculated by multiplying its *row total* by its *column total* and dividing this product by N. The calculations of the expected frequencies are indicated in Exhibit 18.3. Note that the expected frequencies must add up to the grand total, or number of subjects (N) in the research study. The information now available

Exhibit 18-3. Computation of expected frequencies.

Cell	Row Total	Column Total	Product	Product ÷ Grand Total n	Expected Frequency
U	23	31	713	$713/61$	11.688
V	23	30	690	$690/61$	11.311
W	18	31	558	$558/61$	9.147
X	18	30	540	$540/61$	8.852
Y	20	31	620	$620/61$	10.166
Z	20	30	600	$600/61$	9.836
				Total	61.000

for this contingency table analysis is summarized in Exhibit 18.4, where O and E are used to indicate the observed and expected frequencies, respectively.

Once the expected frequencies of each cell are calculated, you are ready to see if the frequencies observed in the experiment are significantly different from the frequencies that would be expected if there were no group differences. The chi square statistic is calculated by summing the square of the difference between the observed and expected frequencies divided by the expected frequency for each cell. This calculation is depicted in Exhibit 18.5. The formula for calculation of the chi square statistic is as follows:

$$\chi^2 = \Sigma \frac{(O - E)^2}{E} \tag{18.2}$$

where O = the observed frequency
E = the expected frequency for each cell

In Exhibit 18.5, the first and second columns give the observed and expected frequencies. The third column gives the difference between the observed and

Exhibit 18-4. Contingency table with observed and expected frequencies and row and column totals.

		Stabilization		
		No	Yes	
	Group 1	$O = 10$ $E = 11.688$	$O = 13$ $E = 11.311$	23
Experimental Condition	Group 2	$O = 3$ $E = 9.147$	$O = 15$ $E = 8.852$	18
	Group 3	$O = 18$ $E = 10.166$	$O = 2$ $E = 9.836$	20
		31	30	61

Exhibit 18-5. Computation of chi-square statistic.

Cell	Observed Frequency O (1)	Expected Frequency E (2)	Difference, $(O - E)$ (3)	Difference Squared, $(O - E)^2$ (4)	$\dfrac{(O - E)^2}{E}$ (5)
U	10	11.688	-1.688	2.849	0.243
V	13	11.311	1.689	2.859	0.252
W	3	9.147	-6.147	37.785	4.130
X	15	8.852	6.148	37.797	4.269
Y	18	10.166	7.834	61.371	6.036
Z	2	9.836	-7.836	61.402	6.242
Sum	61	61.000	0		$\chi^2 = 21.172$

Note: χ^2 may be distorted by less than 1 due to rounding errors.

expected frequencies. Its total must be zero, or there has been an arithmetic error. The squared differences are shown in the fourth column. We cannot simply add these squared differences, however, because they do not take into account the degree of discrepancies or differences in the data. That is, the difference of 2 between 12 and 10, which would be 20 percent of the expected frequency, is not the same as a difference of 2 between 52 and 50, which is only 4 percent of the expected frequency. Therefore, to relate the difference to the data, or make it proportional, the squared differences are divided by their expected frequencies. These are given in the last column. They are then added and this sum is the chi square statistic. In statistical shorthand, the chi square statistic is symbolized by the Greek capital letter chi (χ) with a superscript of 2, representing squaring. The χ^2 value for this example is 21.172.

Computing the Degrees of Freedom

There is only one other value needed in order to be able to use the chi square table. The degrees of freedom (df) must be calculated. The df for chi square equal the product of the number of rows minus one and the number of columns minus one. The formula is as follows:

$$df = (R - 1)(C - 1)$$

where R = number of rows in the contingency table
C = number of columns

In our example, 3 rows minus 1 times 2 columns minus 1 produces 2 degrees of freedom:

$$df = (R - 1)(C - 1) = (3 - 1)(2 - 1) = 2$$

Using the Chi Square Table

We are now ready to use the chi square table, Table F, Appendix III, to get the critical value of chi square for $df = 2$ at $\alpha = .05$. If the chi square statistic is equal to or greater than the critical value, we will have found statistical significance. Most chi square tables are straightforward, but some are not. Exhibit 18.6 is part of a table that might be encountered. It is somewhat different in how the α level is located. Across the top, or the column headings, are the significance levels. They are written in a somewhat misleading version of statistical shorthand. With a .05 level of significance, you would use the column labeled $\chi^2_{.95}$. This is because you are seeking the smallest value needed to reject the null hypothesis with *95 percent confidence* that you are correct in rejecting it. It is important to note how a table is formatted when selecting a correct significance level. Selecting the critical value for $\chi^2_{.05}$ would be wrong. The consequence of this mistake would be declaring statistical significance when you did not have it, because the critical value for rejecting a null hypothesis with only 5 percent confidence of being correct (and a 95 percent probability of type I error) is, of course, much smaller. When in doubt about how a table is formatted, select as your critical value the *larger* of those given for $\chi^2_{.05}$ and $\chi^2_{.95}$.

As in the *t* and *F* tables, each row of the table represents a sampling distribution for a certain number of degrees of freedom. Because in our example there are 2 degrees of freedom and the level of significance is .05, or $\chi^2_{.95}$, the critical value is 6. Clearly, the test statistic, 21.172, is greater than 6; therefore, the result is statistically significant. In fact, it is significant at $p < .01$, and therefore this is the *p* level that is reported. In written reports of research, quite often contingency tables for only significant chi square analyses are given. This is due to the expense involved in printing additional tables and the fact that nonsignificant tables often do not reflect enough discrepancies or differences to merit such detailed reporting. Our table, for purposes of reporting, is shown in Exhibit 18.7. Note that neither the row and column totals nor the sample size is included. These can be calculated by the reader from the information given. Below the table are given the values of the chi square statistic, degrees of freedom (in parentheses), and probability level. Calculations for the chi square statistics are not included. There are variations of the table that are just as correct (e.g., sometimes the percentage is reported with the frequency in parentheses). In all, the same amount of information is presented. To get an idea of other ways tables are presented, consult journal articles reporting the results of research.

Interpreting Results

What have we proven? We have found a relationship between the experimental condition and stabilization. Because we were able to control or manipulate the independent variable, we can call this relationship *causal*. Had we just compared three intact groups of patients receiving different treatments, we could not conclude causality. Instead, we would have found that group membership

Exhibit 18-6. Abstract of chi-square table of critical values.

df	$\chi^2_{.01}$	$\chi^2_{.05}$	$\cdots\cdots$	$\chi^2_{.75}$	$\chi^2_{.90}$	$\chi^2_{.95}$	$\chi^2_{.975}$	$\chi^2_{.99}$
1	—	—		1.3	2.7	3.8	5.0	6.6
2	.02	.10		2.8	4.6	6.0	7.4	9.2
3	.11	.35		4.1	6.3	7.8	9.4	11.3

Exhibit 18-7. Specimen table for reporting chi-square results.

Experimental Condition	Stabilization	
	No	Yes
Group 1: Booklet and self-monitoring	10 (43%)	13 (57%)
Group 2: Booklet, self-monitoring, and home visits	3 (17%)	15 (83%)
Group 3: Control	18 (90%)	2 (20%)

$\chi^2(2) = 21.172, p < .01$

was related to stabilization. In either case, just as with three levels of ANOVA, we cannot say which group is significantly different from the others.

It is important to remember that chi square does not tell you which of the observed differences is statistically significant from the others, unless there are only two categories of a variable being compared. Chi square is a test of the significance of the differences in the overall pattern of data and that is all. This is often ignored in research. Researchers do a chi square analysis and, if it is significant, decide by observation which specific differences are worth singling out for conclusions. When you test an overall pattern of data and the test of the pattern is significant, further statistical analysis is required to single out specific differences. These post hoc comparisons are presented later in this chapter. Without such a test, we must technically restrict our discussion of differences to a global level. We cannot say that Group 2 was significantly different from group 3, or that group 1 was significantly different from the control group, group 3.

In practice, researchers often report the significant χ^2 and then simply describe the differences without declaring them significant. For example, we could state that, while only 20 percent of the control group stabilized, 57 percent (or over half) of those receiving the booklet and participating in the self-monitoring did so, and 83 percent of those who also received home visits stabilized. This is often enough. If, however, you suspect that, say, group 1 and group 3 may not really be significantly different, you can compute a post hoc test to make sure. Be alert to the need for further analysis because it is widely omitted. Specific differences noted in some research reports may be based on mere inspection of the data and may therefore be in error. Because the table is normally given, you can usually calculate a post hoc chi square statistic for differences that are doubtful.

In concluding that the experimental condition affected stabilization, we must also be mindful of possible rival hypotheses. Could differential mortality account for differences? None of the group 1 subjects was lost, but five (22 percent) were lost from group 2 and three (13 percent) were lost from the control group. If a sufficient number of stabilizers had been lost from the control group, this loss might account for observed differences. Therefore, we must check the records on the lost subjects. Perhaps we find that two were lost owing to death and six owing to relocation to another city. Because there is no reason to believe these individuals would all be stabilizers, we conclude that mortality is not a serious rival hypothesis. Could the nurses administering the experimental variable to group 1 and group 2 subjects have gone beyond expected procedures because they knew this was an experiment and wanted the patients to do better? You must decide. If you discover the presence of rival hypotheses, they should be reported. If you disprove one that might occur to the reader, you would do well to include that "disproof" in your report. However, do not present a listing of all possible threats to validity and rival hypotheses and then describe how they are controlled. This is very naive reporting. Simply discuss those few that may be relevant to your specific research study.

Requirements for $k \times m$ ($df > 1$) Chi Square Analysis

In order to use chi square analysis, you must be sure that the data in your contingency table meet several requirements. First, the *expected* frequency in any cell can never be zero. Second, *expected* frequencies of less than one can never occur in more than 20 percent of the cells. An old requirement used to be that expected frequencies could not be less than five in more than 20 percent of the cells. However, methodologic research [1] found this requirement to be too stringent, as would be using an $\alpha = .001$ level. These expected frequency requirements exist because such small expected frequencies could result in **spuriously** high chi square statistics. Recall that, in an effort to bring the squared differences into proportion with the data that produced them, you divided each squared difference by its corresponding expected value. This division contains the possibility of serious upward distortion when the expected value is zero or close to zero. The result of this division will be, as stated, spuriously high. You would make a type I error.

The old requirement that no more than 20 percent of cells have an expected frequency of less than 5 led to collapsing or combining categories in order to do the analysis. Because this was done *after* the first analysis (i.e., post hoc) when the violations were discovered, mathematical statisticians argued that the laws of probability were violated. In addition, **collapsing cells** often obscured the intent of the research hypothesis. Thus, tests of the requirement began, and it was found that lowering the expected values requirement (for no more than 20 percent of the cells) from 5 to 1 did not seriously distort results.

Nevertheless, change occurs slowly. Many still use the magic number of 5 for $k \times m$ tables and therefore collapse cells to meet it. This has led to, in reporting results, the practice of printing only the original table and not the collapsed table. When cells are combined, then, the reader of the research is informed about the extent to which the categories were collapsed by the number of degrees of freedom given at the bottom of the table. This means that you may be presented with the original data and not the data on which the statistical analysis was done. The text of an article should indicate the way in which the categories were combined for the purposes of the chi square analysis. Only with this information can you judge whether the categories were combined in meaningful and valid ways. In order to determine if the contingency tables have been collapsed, you sometimes must compare the degrees of freedom used with the chi square analysis as reported at the bottom of the table (or in the text) and the degrees of freedom you compute based on the printed contingency table.

Chi square analyses are not done with fewer than 20 subjects, primarily because of the old expected values requirement. A good rule of thumb in planning a chi square analysis is to have five to 10 possible subjects for every cell of the table. When fewer than 20 subjects are included and $df = 1$, Fisher's exact test (see Chapter 19) is more appropriate.

Finally, a fundamental assumption of the chi square test of independence is that all observations are independent. Thus, pre- and posttest scores on a group of subjects or observations that are matched cannot be analyzed using the chi square test of independence. It would produce an inflated test statistic by doubling n and could easily lead to a type I error. In these situations, the chi square goodness of fit test may be appropriate. It is discussed later in this chapter.

Correction for Continuity

When a chi square analysis has $df = 1$ and between 20 and 40 subjects or any expected values less than 10, the correction for continuity (also called the Yates correction) must be used. This merely subtracts .5 from the difference between the observed and expected frequencies in *each* of the cells. Without the correction, the resulting χ^2 statistic might be too high and you would make a type I error.

The 2 × 2 Table

A special version of the chi square formula is used with a 2 × 2 contingency table, if n is less than 40 or any expected frequency is less than 10. It is easier to use than the regular procedure because only one division is necessary and fewer decimals are involved. It also includes the correction for continuity. (The formula without the correction is presented as formula 18.9 later in the chapter. It can be used with $n > 40$.) The formula is as follows:

$$\chi^2 = \frac{\left(n\,|AD - BC| - \dfrac{n}{2}\right)^2}{(A + B)(C + D)(A + C)(B + D)} \qquad (18.4)$$

where A, B, C, and D are the observed frequencies in the cells of the following contingency table:

A	B
C	D

and $df = 1$

Note that the absolute value (which ignores plus or minus signs) of $AD - BC$ is used. The denominator is simply the product of the row and column totals.

Suppose we want to be able to say, specifically, that the two experimental groups were significantly different from the control group. For the sake of illustration, assume we do not care about a difference between the two experimental groups. We therefore decide to do a 2 × 2 analysis between groups 1 and 3. Our 2 × 2 table is given in Exhibit 18.8. To compute the χ^2 statistic, we use formula 18.4 because the expected frequency in one of the cells is less than 10:

$$\chi^2 = \frac{43\,(|(10)(2) - (13)(18)| - {}^{43}\!/\!_2)^2}{(10 + 13)\,(18 + 2)\,(10 + 18)\,(13 + 2)} = \frac{43\,(|20 - 234| - {}^{43}\!/\!_2)^2}{(23)(20)(28)(15)}$$

$$= \frac{43\,(214 - 21.5)^2}{193{,}200} = \frac{43\,(192.5)^2}{193{,}200} = \frac{43\,(37{,}056.25)}{193{,}200} = \frac{1{,}593{,}418.7}{193{,}200} = 8.24$$

Using the χ^2 table, the critical value for $df = 1$, $\alpha = .05$, is 3.8. At $\alpha = .01$, the critical value for $df = 1$ is 6.6. Therefore, groups 1 and 3 are significantly different at $p < .01$.

When using a 2 × 2 table, if n is between 20 and 40, the chi square test may be used if *all* expected frequencies are 5 or more. If the smallest expected frequency is less than 5, Fisher's exact test should be used. When n is less than 20, Fisher's exact test must also be used; it is described in Chapter 19.

Exhibit 18-8. 2 × 2 table for experimental condition and stabilization.

		Stabilization	
		No	Yes
Experimental Condition	Group 1	10	13
	Group 3	18	2

The chi square test is usually two-tailed; however, when $df = 1$, a one-tailed test is possible. In that case, the critical value is obtained from the chi square table by *doubling* the alpha level. In our example, we expected fewer controls to stabilize; thus, we might have used a one-tailed test. In the table in Exhibit 18.6, then, we would have found the critical value at $\alpha = .05$, by using $\chi^2_{.90}$. This value is 2.7 as compared to 3.8 for a two-tailed test.

Chi Square Goodness of Fit, or One-Sample Test

Occasionally, chi square is used with just one variable. Suppose it has been established that 65 percent of hypertensive patients stabilize within 6 months. We would then compare these figures with the observed frequencies to see if a clinic population varied from the general population. For this we would use the chi square **goodness of fit** test. Instead of computing expected frequencies for each cell we would use the values found in the population.

Suppose 36 patients came to the clinic on March 3 and 25 had not stabilized. To test whether the clinic population was typical of the general population, we would use the population values. The expected frequency for the stabilization cell would be 65 percent of 36 or 23.4, and the expected frequency for the no stabilization cell would be 35 percent of 36 or 12.6. We would use the correction for continuity, which subtracts .5 from the difference between observed and expected frequencies for each cell, because the n is less than 40 and $df = 1$. The calculations are shown below:

$$\chi^2 = \Sigma \frac{(O - E - .5)^2}{E} = \frac{(25 - 12.6 - .5)^2}{12.6} + \frac{(11 - 23.4 - .5)^2}{23.4}$$

$$= \frac{(11.9)^2}{12.6} + \frac{(-12.9)^2}{23.4} = \frac{141.61}{12.6} + \frac{166.41}{23.4} = 11.23 + 7.11 = 18.34$$

The chi square statistic, using the correction for continuity, would be 18.34 at $df = 1$. This is significant at $p < .01$.

The goodness-of-fit test cannot be used when n is less than 20. When n is between 20 and 40, the correction for continuity must be used. Expected values for $1 \times k$ tables can be as low as 1. Sometimes the degrees of freedom are reduced if in order to get population values, means and standard deviations must be computed. In this case, the degrees of freedom would equal the number of cells minus 3.

Post Hoc Tests for Contingency Tables*

As stated in the discussion of $k \times m$ contingency tables, significant differences between more than two categories of a variable require additional post hoc

---

*Just as χ^2 can be partitioned, separate χ^2 analyses can be combined in which the test statistic and df are the sum of the values for each contingency table being added. Discussion of the procedures for doing this may be found in McNemar [3].

tests. Three methods are presented here. The first partitions χ^2 into a number of independent (i.e., orthogonal) 2×2 tables equal to the number of degrees of freedom and can be used for $k \times m$ tables. The values of each 2×2 table sum to the overall value of χ^2, and thus there is no need to adjust the alpha level. The second method, designed for $2 \times k$ tables, partitions into nonindependent 2×2 tables, and thus the α level must be adjusted before determining the statistical significance of the χ^2 test statistic. It is especially useful when comparing several experimental groups with a control group. The last method presents a simple way to determine the contribution of each cell to the overall χ^2 statistic.

Partitioning k × m *Tables into Independent 2 × 2 Tables*

The first method for partitioning χ^2 allows as many smaller 2×2 tables as there are degrees of freedom; moreover, the χ^2 values calculated for each table sum to the overall χ^2 value. Therefore, there are rules on how the 2×2 tables are formulated. These rules are beyond the scope of this book except to say that the first 2×2 can involve whichever four cells you wish as long as two values of each variable are included. The next 2×2 table, however, must then include the first values, compressed over one variable (and therefore comprising two cells) and only two new cells. This continues until all possible tables are developed. Those wishing further detail may consult Kimball [2].

Exhibit 18-9. Partitioning χ^2 into independent 2×2 tables.

Given: A 2×3 contingency table where the cells are labeled U, V, W, X, Y, and Z; row totals are labeled R_1, R_2, and R_3; column totals are labeled C_1 and C_2; and $N = $ total number of subjects.

Experimental Condition	Stabilization		Row
	No	Yes	
Group 1	Cell $U = 10$	Cell $V = 13$	$R_1 = 23$
Group 2	Cell $W = 03$	Cell $X = 15$	$R_2 = 18$
Group 3	Cell $Y = 18$	Cell $Z = 02$	$R_3 = 20$
	$C_1 = 31$	$C_2 = 30$	$N = 61$

(1) To compare groups 1 and 2:

$$\chi^2_1 = \frac{N^2[UX - WV]^2}{C_1C_2R_1R_2(R_1 + R_2)} \quad \text{and} \quad df = 1 \tag{18.5}$$

(2) To compare group 3 with groups 1 and 2 combined:

$$\chi^2_2 = \frac{N^2[Y(V + X) - Z(U + W)]^2}{C_1C_2R_3(R_1 + R_2)(R_1 + R_2 + R_3)} \quad \text{and} \quad df = 1 \tag{18.6}$$

Exhibit 18.9 presents formulas for partitioning a 2×3 table. It can be used as a pattern for developing 2×2 comparisons. Formula 18.5 compares groups 1 and 2, or cells $U, V, W,$ and X. Formula 18.6 then compares group 3 with groups 1 and 2 combined, or cells $U + W, V + X, Y$ and Z. If a fourth group (and thus a fourth row) were included, the next comparison would be group 4 (with cells A and B) with groups 1, 2, and 3 combined (cells $U + W + Y, V + X + Z, A$ and B) and the formula would be as follows:

$$\chi^2_3 = \frac{N^2 \left[A \left(V + X + Z \right) - B \left(U + W + Y \right) \right]^2}{C_1 C_2 R_4 \left(R_1 + R_2 + R_3 \right) \left(R_1 + R_2 + R_3 + R_4 \right)} \tag{18.7}$$

where $A =$ no stabilization cell for group 4
       $B =$ stabilization cell for group 4
       $R_4 =$ row total for group 4

This same partitioning would apply if there were three categories of stabilization. The decision when to compare these levels would of course depend on your research hypothesis. The formula for partitioning χ^2 when both variables have more than two categories is somewhat cumbersome. For those wishing it, refer to Kimball [2].

Using the data displayed in Exhibit 18.9 (which is the data used at the beginning of the chapter to illustrate $k \times m \ \chi^2$ analysis), we can compare groups 1 and 2 with formula 18.15:

$$\chi^2_1 = \frac{(61)^2 [150 - 39]^2}{(31)(30)(23)(18)(41)} = \frac{(3,721)(12,321)}{15,785,820} = 2.9$$

The critical value of χ^2 for $df = 1$ at $\alpha = .05$ is 3.8 for a two-tailed test and 2.7 for a one-tailed test. Thus, the two experimental conditions are significantly different only if a directional hypothesis is tested. To test the difference between groups 1 and 2 combined and group 3, the control group, the second formula, 18.6, is used:

$$\chi^2_2 = \frac{(61)^2 [504 - 26]^2}{(31)(30)(20)(41)(61)} = \frac{(3,721)(228,484)}{46,518,600} = 18.276$$

The value of χ^2 indicates that the experimental and control conditions are clearly different. Also note that $18.276 + 2.9 = 21.176$, which equals the overall χ^2 value of 21.172 reported in Exhibit 18.7, given rounding error for that computation.

The formulas presented in Exhibit 18.9 do not include the correction for continuity. If it is needed, it can be applied in the usual way by subtracting $(n \div 2)$ from the numerator difference (in brackets) before it is squared. When the correction is used, the $2 \times 2 \ \chi^2$ values do not exactly sum to the overall χ^2 value, although the discrepancy is negligible.

This second method for partitioning χ^2 is appropriate when one of several groups is a control group against which *each* of the experimental groups are compared. Because the 2 × 2 tables are no longer independent (i.e., orthogonal), the α level must be adjusted downward, depending on the number of comparisons, $k - 1$, made. To determine the alpha level for obtaining the critical value of χ^2, the following formula is used:

$$\hat{\alpha} = \frac{\alpha}{2(k - 1)}$$

where $\hat{\alpha}$ = adjusted alpha
α = alpha for the overall test
k = number of categories for the second variable

Thus, if an α of .05 were used for the overall test and there were three categories (as in our example) of k, the adjusted α would be:

$$\hat{\alpha} = \frac{.05}{2(3 - 1)} = \frac{.05}{4} = .0125$$

Entering Table F, Appendix III, we find that the critical value of χ^2 at $df = 1$ and $\alpha = .01$ is 6.6 for a two-tailed test and 5.0 for a one-tailed test. It is against this value that our test statistic must be compared if we are to maintain the .05 level of significance. In this case a .01 critical value is used for an α level of .05.

The formula for computing each 2 × 2 χ^2 is that presented as formula 18.4 for the 2 × 2 table. Formula 18.4 includes the correction for continuity. The formula without the correction for continuity is as follows:

$$\chi^2 = \frac{n(|AD - BC|)^2}{(A + B)(C + D)(A + C)(B + D)} \tag{18.9}$$

where A, B, C, and D are the observed frequencies in the cells of the following contingency table:

A	B
C	D

and $df = 1$

Because, in our example, the correction for continuity is needed, we must use formula 18.4 instead of formula 18.9. To compare each of the two experimental conditions with those in the control group (Group 3), the following calculations are involved:

(1) For Group 1 versus Group 3:

$$\chi^2 = \frac{61 \, (|20 - 234| - 6\frac{1}{2})^2}{(23)(20)(28)(15)} = \frac{61 \, (33{,}672.25)}{193{,}200} = 10.63$$

(2) For Group 2 vs. Group 3:

$$\chi^2 = \frac{61 \, (|6 - 270| - 6\frac{1}{2})^2}{(18)(20)(21)(17)} = \frac{61 \, (54{,}522.25)}{128{,}520} = 25.878$$

Comparing these test statistics with the critical values, we find that they are significant at $p < .05$. In fact, if an alpha of .01 had been used, the adjusted alpha would have been:

$$\hat{\alpha} = \frac{.01}{2 \, (3 - 1)} = \frac{.01}{4} = .0025$$

The critical values for χ^2 when $df = 1$ and $\alpha = .001$ is 10.8 two-tailed and somewhat smaller, one-tailed. (Most tables do not present this value.) Clearly, these post hoc tests are significant at $p < .01$.

Partitioning According to Cell Contributions to χ^2

The last method is the most simple. It does not provide an inferential test *per se,* however. For each cell, the $(O - E)^2/E$ is divided by the value of χ^2. This yields the percent contribution of that cell to χ^2. Exhibit 18.10 presents the contributions of the cells from our example. It is clear from Exhibit 18.10 that groups 2 and 3 contributed most to χ^2. This corroborates our earlier analysis. In this example, partitioning according to cell contribution does not really yield any information of interest. However, in nonexperimental designs, this approach may provide more useful information, such as sex differences under varying conditions, when there is a theoretical basis for partitioning the sample itself.

Exhibit 18-10. Percentage contributions of cells to χ^2.

Group	Cell	$\dfrac{(O - E)^2}{E}$	Percentage of χ^2
1	U	0.243	1.0
	V	0.252	1.0
2	W	4.130	19.5
	X	4.269	20.0
3	Y	6.036	28.5
	Z	6.242	29.0

Note: Percentages may not sum to 100 due to rounding error.

Nominal Measures of Relationship

The chi square test of independence, if significant, declares that two variables are related or correlated. However, the chi square statistic does not describe the extent or *amount* of the relationship. If you wish to describe the correlation between two nominal level variables or calculate a magnitude estimate for χ^2, a simple additional calculation is necessary. This value, can then be placed at the bottom of the table along with the χ^2 value, *df*, and the probability level when you are reporting results.

The Contingency Coefficient (C)

The most widely used measure of association between two nominal level variables is Pearson's coefficient of contingency, better known as the **contingency coefficient.** It is calculated by the following formula:

$$C = \sqrt{\frac{\chi^2}{\chi^2 + N}} \tag{18.10}$$

If you wanted to describe the relationship between experimental condition and stabilization in the 2 × 3 contingency table from Exhibit 18.7, you would use this formula. The calculations would be:

$$C = \sqrt{\frac{21.172}{21.172 + 61}} = \sqrt{\frac{21.172}{82.172}} = \sqrt{.2576} = .5075 = .51$$

Although the contingency coefficient is widely used, it cannot be interpreted as indicating the same degree of relationship as an ordinary coefficient like the Pearson *r*. It does not take into account the number of cells in the table. Therefore, its upper limit varies. The upper limit for a 2 × 2 table is $\sqrt{½}$ or .71; for a 3 × 3 table is $\sqrt{⅔}$ or .82; and for a 4 × 4 is $\sqrt{¾}$ or .87. For a *k* × *k* table, the upper limit is $\sqrt{(k - 1)/k}$. The exact upper limits for rectangular tables, such as 2 × 3, are unknown. Also, *C* can never be negative. Two contingency coefficients are never comparable unless they result from tables of the same size. Because *C* is widely used, it is wise to include it along with one of the two following measures of association which are better.

The Phi Coefficient (φ)

The **phi coefficient** (ϕ), also known as the **fourfold point correlation coefficient,** is used for 2 × 2 tables only. It can vary between zero and one, and its calculation is also simple:

$$\phi = \sqrt{\frac{\chi^2}{N}} \tag{18.11}$$

The phi coefficient is like a Pearson *r* between two dichotomous variables. Therefore, it can be interpreted similarly. It ranges from zero to one but is never negative.

If we wanted to describe the relationship between experimental condition and stabilization for data in Exhibit 18.8, we would calculate a phi as follows:

$$\phi = \sqrt{\frac{\chi^2}{N}} = \sqrt{\frac{8.24}{43}} = \sqrt{.1916} = .4377 = .44$$

Phi is .44 out of a possible range of 0 to 1. A contingency coefficient for this same table would have been .40, out of a range of 0 to .71. The phi is decidedly easier to interpret.

Cramer's Phi (φ')

Cramer's phi, also known as Cramer's *V*, is used with $k \times m$ tables. It ranges from zero to one just as does the phi for 2×2 tables. The formula is as follows:

$$\phi' = \sqrt{\frac{\chi^2}{N(L-1)}}$$

where L = the smaller of the number of rows or number of columns

To compute a ϕ' for the 2×3 table in Exhibit 18.7, the procedure is as follows:

$$\phi' = \sqrt{\frac{21.172}{61(2-1)}} - \sqrt{\frac{21.172}{61}} - \sqrt{.347} = .58$$

Recall, the *C* for this table was .51 with an unknown upper limit.

The interpretation of ϕ' is unclear. It cannot be used to discuss shared variances because the variables are not interval level or dichotomous. It is used simply as a descriptor, as is *C*, and because its upper limit is 1, it is far superior to *C*. When the difference between observed and expected frequencies is held constant over increasing numbers of cells, ϕ' decreases. This is not true of *C*. For example, a 2×3 table might have a *C* of .30 and a ϕ' of .32 for a given value of a chi square statistic. If a 3×3 table had the same *chi* square value, the *C* would remain at .30 but the ϕ' would drop from .32 to .22. This is because, as stated previously, *C* does not take into account the number of cells. It is therefore important to be suspicious of studies using larger tables that report values only for C. Not only may the upper limit be unknown, but they may be misleading in terms of suggesting a greater relationship than really exists.

Power Analysis for Chi Square

Many times researchers do not find significance and therefore discontinue their research. Other times, researchers or readers of research reports mistakenly conclude that there is no difference or relationship when the null hypothesis is accepted. Therefore, it is useful to know the probability of a type II error, the failure to reject your null hypothesis when you should have.

Table D, Appendix IV, enables you to estimate the probability of having made a type II error when the value of χ^2 did not reach statistical significance. It assumes an *a priori* α level of .05. To enter the table you use sample size (n), degrees of freedom (df), and effect size (ES). The ES is simply your chi square test statistic divided by your sample size:

$$ES = \frac{\chi^2}{N} \tag{18.13}$$

For example, if you have 30 subjects, one df, and a nonsignificant chi square statistic of 2.1, the ES equals 2.1 ÷ 30 or .07. Using the table you find that the probability of type II error is 69 percent. This is very high. Therefore, you decide to repeat your study using a larger sample. In no event do you conclude that there is *no relationship* or no difference between your two variables.

Suppose you have a chi square statistic of 2.68 for $n = 33$ with $df = 2$. Your ES = 2.68 ÷ 33 or .0812. In order to use the table you must find the probability levels for ES = .08, $df = 2$, $n = 30$ and ES = .08, $df = 2$, $n = 35$. They are 73 percent and 69 percent. Because $n = 33$ is about halfway between 30 and 35, you find the probability level halfway betwen 69 percent and 73 percent. It is 71 percent.

What constitutes a high probability of type II error? Certainly any probability over 50 percent is suspect. As stated in the preceding chapters, researchers generally agree that a 20 percent probability of type II error is acceptable. Therefore, when your probabilities are higher, you should be suspicious of your results. If your probability level is excessive, it should be reported along with your results and the suggestion that the research be repeated using a larger sample and some of the other techniques associated with accepting a null hypothesis (see Chapter 15).

Multivariate Chi Square Analysis

Often researchers will have more than two nominal level variables of interest. For instance, suppose that in our example we were also interested in whether the sex of the subject related to stabilization. In this case, all women would have been randomly assigned *equally* to one of the three groups, and then men would have also been equally assigned to each group. Separate contingency tables for each sex would then have been subjected to χ^2 analysis. If one was significant and the other was not, we would find that the experimental variable was differentially effective according to sex. It would be more effective for men if that χ^2 was significant and the χ^2 for women was not. Even if both were significant, partitioning of χ^2 might result in group 1's being more effective for women and group 2's being more effective for men. The possibilities are endless.

Adding additional variables to χ^2 analysis often provides more useful information. This procedure of using three or more variables is known as **analysis of crossbreaks.** As variables are added, however, the number of subjects required is also increased. Interpretation of results may also become difficult as with contingency tables with more than five categories. When planning contingency tables *before* you gather data, consider all possible outcomes. How will you interpret or explain each?

Vocabulary

Analysis of crossbreaks	Goodness of fit
Cell	Observed frequency
Collapsing cells	One-sample χ^2
Contingency coefficient (C)	Partitioning χ^2
Contingency table	Phi (ϕ) coefficient
Correction for continuity	Row total
Cramer's phi (ϕ')	Test of independence
Expected frequency	Upper limits

References

1. Everitt, B. S. *The Analysis of Contingency Tables.* New York: Wiley, 1977.
2. Kimball, A. W. Short-cut formula for the exact partition of χ^2 in contingency tables. *Biometrics* 10:452, 1954.
3. McNemar, Q. *Psychological Statistics* (4th ed.). New York: Wiley, 1969.

An entire chapter was devoted to chi square analysis because it is by far the most frequently used nonparametric statistical test. It is not only the most versatile of the nonparametric tests, it is also involved in other tests, some of which are included in this chapter. Chi square analysis is a very helpful and useful technique to include in your repertoire. So, too, are the nonparametric tests presented in this chapter. However, it is not necessary to remember all the details of each as long as you remember where to find them when you need them. These tests are relatively simple to compute, as is chi square, given sufficient directions. For these reasons, the computational procedures for each are presented as Exhibits, while the textual material in this chapter discusses them in terms of their use and interpretation.

Nonparametric procedures, recall, are not as powerful as parametric procedures. That is, under the same conditions you would be more likely to make a type II error with a nonparametric test than you would with a parametric test. However, it is possible that, if one of the assumptions for a parametric test (e.g., equivariance or normality) is *seriously* violated, the corresponding nonparametric test could be just as powerful. For some of the nonparametric tests **power efficiency** percentages have been developed. For example, for the Wilcoxon Matched-Pairs Signed-Ranks test, power efficiency is 95 percent of that of the t test for dependent groups. This means that to have the same power (hence type II error rate) as t, the Wilcoxon test would have to use 100 subjects for every 95 (or 20 for every 19) used with the t test. Thus, to avoid having to meet some of the assumptions of parametric tests without increasing the probability of type II error, you could simply use a nonparametric test and increase your n by using the power efficiency percentage if it is available. Furthermore, to determine the probability of type II error after accepting the null hypothesis of a nonparametric test, you can use the type II error probability table for the corresponding parametric test by entering it at the value of n that corresponds to the power efficiency percentage for the test you are using. If you accepted a null hypothesis as a result of the Wilcoxon test using an n of 40, you would use the type II error probability table for t as if you had an n of 38. Whenever the power efficiency percentages of the tests in this chapter are known, they are included. If you decide to use one of the procedures for which a power efficiency percentage is not given, consult the professional journals that publish the results of research in mathematical statistics. A value may have been derived since preparation of this chapter.

Another point requires exploration. We have just finished stating that *increasing n* can make nonparametric procedures as powerful as parametric procedures. How is this equated with the fact that nonparametric are often more appropriate than parametric procedures with very *small* sample sizes? It does seem contradictory. Parametric procedures often have higher minimum sample size requirements than their corresponding nonparametric procedures. Thus,

Exhibit 19-1. Nonparametric tests for small sample sizes.

Test	Level of Measurement	Minimum N	Special Conditions
Two Independent Groups			
Fisher's Exact Probability Test	Nominal	6	2 × 2 table
Mann-Whitney U Test	Ordinal	6*	No group < 2
Median Test	Ordinal	6	2 × 2 table
Two Dependent (or Related) Groups			
Binomial Test	Nominal	5 pairs*	Considers change regardless of direction
McNemar Test for the Significance of Changes	Nominal	5 pairs*	2 × 2 table
Wilcoxon Matched-Pairs Signed-Ranks Test	Ordinal	6 pairs	Pairs with no differences dropped from analysis; Underlying continuous distribution; Need capacity to compute magnitude of difference between pairs
Sign Test	Ordinal	5 pairs*	Underlying continuous distribution; Pairs with no change are dropped from the analysis
Three or More Independent Groups			
Kruskal-Wallis One-way Analysis of Variance by Ranks	Ordinal	6*	Always two-tailed; If $k > 3$, must be five cases in each k group
Extension of the Median Test	Ordinal	20	Underlying continuous distribution; This test is essentially a χ^2 test and requires that the assumptions of χ^2 be met
Three or More Dependent Groups			
Cochran Q Test (for Nominal Data)	Nominal	~ 10 pairs	Always two-tailed
Friedman Two-way Analysis of Variance by Ranks	Ordinal	3 pairs*	Always two-tailed

*Tables yield probabilities (rather than critical values) for small sample sizes.

when a sample size is especially small, say 6 or 7, the nonparametric tests are the *only* ones available. Exhibit 19.1 lists the tests described in this chapter that can be used for very small samples. For example, the t test requires a minimum of 10, while the nonparametric tests corresponding to it, the median test and Mann-Whitney U test, allow an n of 6. Neither is very powerful with such small n. However, at least there is a test that can be used when n is between 6 and 10 and from which you can infer differences if the observed differences are sufficiently large. With small samples such as 6, moreover, the level of significance is usually increased to at least .10 in order to increase power. In addition, the exact probability level that was observed is reported, if at all possible, in order to give the reader more detail for use in evaluating the results.

One assumption, an **underlying continuous distribution,** is made for some of the nonparametric tests for ordinal level data. This assumption results in greater power for the test. The requirement is that there be a continuum underlying the observed scores, although the actual scores may fall into categories. Pass-fall categories have an underlying continuum. Education categories of grade school, high school, and college graduates have an underlying continuum, although the categories themselves may not include equal amounts of education. Young adult, middle age, and old age is another example. Prognosis and severity of disease have underlying continua, but disease diagnosis, even if rank-ordered according to severity by experts, does not. Whenever this assumption is made by a test in this chapter, an alternate, generally less powerful test is included for use when your data do not meet this assumption.

The tests in this chapter, all comparative, are grouped first according to the four types of independent variables they may be using:

Tests for two independent groups
Tests for two dependent or related groups
Tests for three or more (k) independent groups
Tests for three or more (k) dependent groups

Within each of the categories, the tests are grouped according to the level of measurement for the dependent variable—**nominal** or **ordinal.** If two tests are suggested for the *same* level of measurement and type of comparison, the preferred or more powerful test is introduced first. Note that for many of the tests H_0 is rejected when the test statistic is equal to or *less* than the critical value. This is different from most parametric tests.

Tests for Two Independent Groups

The tests in this group correspond to the parametric t test for independent groups (or one-way ANOVA with two groups). Independent groups result when subjects are randomly assigned to either an experimental or a control group. They also result when two categories of a variable are compared, such as men and women or children and adults. The three procedures presented in this section test whether two independent groups differ in location or central tendency. On the other hand, chi square, when more than two levels of the dependent variable are considered, tests for *all* differences including location, dispersion, and skewness. If dispersion is of interest with ordinal data, another test not included in this book, the two-tailed Kolmogarov-Smirnov test [2], might be more appropriate. Procedures that test for *all* differences combine them in such a way that you cannot tell the effects of any single factor. If H$_0$ is rejected, you can conclude that the two groups differ, but you cannot say in which specific ways they differ. Of the two procedures presented for ordinal data, the Mann-Whitney *U* test is more powerful than the Median test and should be used whenever possible. All procedures presented in this section can be **one-** or **two-tailed,** because only two groups are being compared, and they can be used with unequal group sizes.

Nominal Data

Chi Square Test of Independence

This test was described in detail as the $k \times m$ test in Chapter 18. It gets its name from the null hypothesis (H$_0$), which states that the two variables represented by k and m are independent, not related. Under H$_0$, group membership, which is the first or k variable, is not related to the second or m variable. Hence, the two groups do not differ with respect to the second variable. If the H$_0$ is rejected, then you conclude that either the two groups are significantly different or the two variables are related. The title of this statistical test is confusing to many because of the inclusion of the word *independence*. Perhaps that is why most researchers rarely use it in reports of research, preferring the more simple label of *chi square test* or *chi square analysis*.

Fisher's Exact Probability Test

Fisher's exact test, as it is commonly called, is useful when the expected frequency assumptions of χ^2 cannot be met and is appropriate for sample sizes as small as 6. It is used with nominal data that are summarized into a 2×2 table for two independent groups. The test determines if either two groups differ significantly in location (central tendency) on the other variable or two dichotomous variables are related. The procedure presented in this text is for samples ranging in size from 6 to 30. If it is necessary to use Fisher's exact test rather than χ^2 with larger samples, consult Siegel [2] for the procedure. Using Exhibit 19.2, let us compute p for the following 2×2 table:

2	7
3	2

First, $A + B = 2 + 7 = 9$ and $C + D = 3 + 2 = 5$ are computed. Next, we consult Table G in Appendix III. We locate our values in the table including a 7

Exhibit 19-2. Fisher's exact probability test.

---

1. Organize data into a 2 × 2 table where the cells are labeled as follows:

A	B
C	D

2. Determine the values of $A + B$ and $C + D$. (*Note:* To use the method in this book, neither $A + B$ nor $C + D$ can be greater than 15. If they exceed 15, invert the table so that $B + D$ becomes $A + B$ and $A + C$ becomes $C + D$. If either still exceeds 15, refer to Siegel [2] for an alternate computational procedure.)
3. Turn to Table G in Appendix III. Find the value of $A + B$ under the heading "Totals in the right margin." Locate the value of $C + D$ under the same heading. For the value of $C + D$, locate the value of B in the second column. (If the value of B is not included, use the value of A.)
4. Compare your value of D (use C if you used A in step 3) with the critical value listed under your level of significance. If D is *equal to or less than* the critical value, the H_0 is rejected.
5. If you have accepted H_0 by a very narrow margin, consult Siegel [2] for an alternate procedure. Significance levels in Table G are approximate and tend to be conservative.

---

for value B. The critical value shown for D is zero. Because our $D = 2$, it is *greater than* the critical value, and therefore, H_0 is accepted.

Ordinal Data

Mann-Whitney *U* Test

The Mann-Whitney U, one of the most powerful nonparametric tests, tests a hypothesis that the medians of two groups are significantly different. It is sometimes better than the t test when parametric assumptions are violated. It is useful with sample sizes as small as 6 when there are at least two in the smaller group. It has a power efficiency of about 95 percent as compared with t for moderate and larger-sized samples. Ties in ranks have only a slight effect. Research has shown that even when over 90 percent of the observations involved ties, the effect was negligible. However, when many of the ties involve four or more observations, it is wise to apply a correction factor (described by Siegel [2]), which will tend to increase the Z statistic, making it significant at a lower probability of type I error. Exhibit 19.3 presents the computational procedures for this test. Using the computational procedure with the data presented in Exhibit 19.4, we calculate:

$$R_1 = 12 + 9.5 + 9.5 + 7 + 6 = 44$$

$$\hat{U} = n_1 n_2 + \frac{n_1(n_1 + 1)}{2} - R_1 = (5)(7) + \frac{(5)(6)}{2} - 47.5 = 35 + 15 - 47.5 = 2.5$$

$$U' = n_1 n_2 - \hat{U} = (5)(7) - 6 = 35 - 6 = 29$$

Exhibit 19-3. Mann-Whitney U test.

1. Let n_1 = number of observations in the smaller group and n_2 = number of observations in the larger group.
2. Combine scores of both groups, and rank in order of magnitude (the lowest algebraic score assigned a rank of 1). Label from which group each rank comes.
3. Compute R_1, which is the sum of ranks assigned to group n_1.
4. Calculate

$$\hat{U} = n_1 n_2 + \frac{n_1(n_1 + 1)}{2} - R_1$$

5. Calculate

$$U' = n_1 n_2 - \hat{U}$$

6. Select the smaller value of $\hat{U}$ or U' as U.
7. For $n_2 \leq 8$, use Table H in Appendix III for the one-tailed probability. If a two-tailed test is desired, double the probability in the table.
8. When n_2 is between 9 and 20, use Table I in Appendix III for the critical value at your level of significance. If U *equals or is less than* the critical value, H_0 is rejected.
9. If $n_2 > 20$, the sampling distribution approaches normal, and the Z statistic should be calculated:

$$Z = \frac{U - n_1 n_2 / 2}{\dfrac{\sqrt{(n_1 n_2)(n_1 + n_2 + 1)}}{12}}$$

10. The sign of Z depends on whether U' or $\hat{U}$ was used. Therefore, use the absolute value. If Z *equals or is greater than* 1.96 (two-tailed) or 1.643 (one-tailed), H_0 is rejected at $p < .05$. If Z *equals or is greater than* 2.58 (two-tailed) or 2.33 (one-tailed), H_0 is rejected at $p < .01$.

Using Table H, Appendix IV, for $n_2 = 7$, $n_1 = 5$, and $U = 6.0$, we find a probability of 0.037 one-tailed and p $< .074$ for a two-tailed test. H_0 is rejected only if a directional hypothesis was used.

The Median Test

The Median test also tests for differences in central tendency but is less powerful with small and moderately sized samples than the Mann-Whitney U because it uses less information. It notes only whether scores are above or below the median, while the U statistic also considers the distance in number of ranks. For very small samples, say 6, it is preferable to the Mann-Whitney U because its power efficiency is about 95 percent of t. The power efficiency of the Median test decreases to about 63 percent as sample size increases. Exhibit 19.5 presents

Exhibit 19-4. Fictitious data for examples.

Group 1	Group 2	Rank-Ordered Scores	Rank	Group
14	13	14	12	1
13	13	13	9.5	2
13	10	13	9.5	2
12	10	13	9.5	1
11	10	13	9.5	1
	10	12	7	1
$n = 5$	9	11	6	1
		10	3.5	2
	$n = 7$	10	3.5	2
		10	3.5	2
		10	3.5	2
		9	1	2

Exhibit 19-5. Median test (for ordinal data).

1. Combine scores for both groups, and determine the median of all scores.
2. Develop a 2 × 2 table for scores above and below the median and for groups 1 and 2:

	Group 1	Group 2
Scores above median	A	B
Scores below median	C	D

3. When several scores fall at the median, they can be dichotomized by considering only those which *exceed* the median as above the median.
4. Compute chi square or Fisher's exact probability test.

the computational procedures for this test. Using the data from Exhibit 19.4, the median for all scores is 11.5. By considering the lowest ranking six scores as below the median and the highest six as above, we develop the following 2 × 2 table:

	Group 1	Group 2
Scores Above $\bar{X}$	4	2
Scores Below $\bar{X}$	2	4

To compute Fisher's exact test for this data, we first refer to Exhibit 19.2 and compute the following:

(1) $A + B = 4 + 2 = 6$

(2) $C + D = 1 + 4 = 5$

Next, we turn to Table G, Appendix III. Entering the table for $A + B = 6, C + D = 5, A = 4$ (the value of $B = 2$ is not in the table), we extract a critical value of 0; C must be equal to or less than this value in order for us to declare statistical significance. Because $C = 2$, H_0 is accepted. According to the Median test, the two medians are not significantly different. Thus, the Mann-Whitney Test is clearly more powerful than the Median test, which uses much less information (i.e., the sum of actual ranks is ignored and only a frequency count is used.)

Tests for Two Dependent or Related Groups

The tests in this group correspond to the parametric t test for correlated or dependent measures. Perhaps the most obvious example of related groups (or measures) is the single group pretest-posttest design. Related groups could include comparison of parent and child pairs or patients who have been rank ordered according to cognitive ability (or capacity for self-care) and are then paired according to the two highest ranks, the next two highest ranks, the next two highest ranks, and so on before random assignment of one member of each pair to the experimental group and the other to the control group. Analysis of the *same* patient's assessment of the quality of care in two different clinical settings is yet another application of these tests.

Of the three procedures presented in this section, only the McNemar test for the Significance of Changes does not assume an underlying continuous distribution. It is useful when this assumption cannot be met and when data on both the pretest and posttest can be dichotomized, such as Nurse A or Nurse B, aspirin or Tylenol, lobster or steak, halter monitor or sphygmomanometer and stethoscope, and so forth. On the other hand, if scores within each pair can be ranked such that one score in the pair is *less than* the other score in the pair (e.g., pass-fail, satisfied-unsatisfied, older-younger, compliant-noncompliant, painful-painless, radical or simple mastectomy), the Sign test is appropriate. Unfortunately ties within pairs must be dropped from Sign test analysis, thereby reducing sample size. Finally, if scores from the entire sample can be rank ordered, the Wilcoxon Matched-Pairs Signed-Ranks test should be used. When parametric assumptions are met, the Sign test has a power efficiency of about 95 percent for samples as small as 6 and it declines to about 63 percent as sample size increases. The Wilcoxon, on the other hand, maintains a power efficiency of about 95 percent for all sample sizes.

As with all analyses involving only two groups of data, tests can be either one-tailed or two-tailed. Because groups are related, groups, of course, have equal n. All tests in this section are concerned with differences in the *direction* or **magnitude of change.** None concerns whether change actually occurred because all pairs for which no change or difference is observed are dropped from the analysis. If $N < 25$ pairs and you wish to ascertain whether a significant change occurred, regardless of direction, use the **binomial test,** which assumes that the probability of P (change) + probability of Q (no change) = 50 percent. Enter Table J, Appendix III, with x = the smaller of the number of changes or no-changes, to extract the one-tailed probability that this proportion (x/N) would occur by chance alone. If a two-tailed probability is desired, double the tabled value. If $N > 25$, see Siegel [2] for the binomial test.

Nominal Data

The McNemar Test for the Significance of Changes

The McNemar Test involves developing a 2 × 2 table in which the two cells representing change on a dichotomous variable, such as a choice between Hospital A and Hospital B, are of interest. Thus the H_0 is that the probability of Change A (from selecting Hospital A to selecting Hospital B) is the same as Change B (from Hospital B to Hospital A). Those who do not change their selection are not considered in this analysis. The power efficiency of the McNemar Test is about 95 percent of t when $N = 6$ and decreases to about 63 percent as N increases. Exhibit 19.6 presents the computational procedures for this test. Using the data presented in Exhibit 19.7, let us compute this test. Suppose these data represented stress levels, and values of 8 and above were considered at risk. The following 2 × 2 table can then be developed according to the directions in Exhibit 19.6:

		Posttest	
		Below 8 ($-$)	8 and Above ($+$)
Pretest	$\geq 8\,(+)$	3	2
	$< 8\,(-)$	3	2

E is calculated as follows:

$$E = \tfrac{1}{2}(A + D) = \tfrac{1}{2}(3 + 2) = 2.5$$

Since E is less than 5, the binomial test is appropriate. Recall that we wish to determine if a significant change has occurred. Using Table J, Appendix III, with $N = A + D = 5$ and $x = 2$, we find the probability is 0.50, one-tailed, and 1.00, two-tailed. Clearly, according to the McNemar test, a significant change has not occurred.

Exhibit 19-6. McNemar test for significance of changes (for nominal data).

1. Set up a 2 × 2 table to represent two categories of before and after measures, where cells $A + D$ represent change:

		After −	After +
Before	+	*A*	*B*
	−	*C*	*D*

2. Determine the expected frequency of cells $A + D$:

$$E = \tfrac{1}{2}(A + D)$$

3. If $E < 5$, the binomial test is appropriate. Use Table J, Appendix III, with $N = A + D$ and $x =$ the smaller of the observed frequencies of either *A* or *D*. The one-tailed probability is given in Table J. For the two-tailed case, double the probability given in the table.
4. If $E \geq 5$, compute χ^2, using the following formula:

$$\chi^2 = \frac{(|A - D| - 1)^2}{A + D} \quad \text{with } df = 1$$

where $|A - D| =$ the absolute value of the difference between *A* and *D*.
5. Compare χ^2 with the critical value given in Table F, Appendix III. If it is *equal to or greater than* the critical value, H_0 is rejected.

Exhibit 19-7. Fictitious data for test of change.

Ss	Pretest	Postest	*d*	*d* Rank-Ordered
1	10	9	1	(+) 2.5
2	10	10	0	—
3	8	6	2	(+) 5.5
4	7	6	1	(+) 2.5
5	5	2	3	(+) 8.0
6	4	1	3	(+) 8.0
7	7	8	−1	(−) 2.5
8	7	8	−1	(−) 2.5
9	8	6	2	(+) 5.5
10	8	5	3	(+) 8.0

Ordinal Data

The Wilcoxon Matched-Pairs Signed-Ranks Test

The Wilcoxon test, as stated previously, assumes an underlying continuous distribution. It is more powerful than the Sign test because it uses the magnitude of change as well as the direction. There is one drawback, however: the nature of this test involves assessing the magnitude of a change in rank between pre- and post-measures. When no change occurs, the pair is dropped from the analysis thereby decreasing sample size. Tied scores when the total sample of observations are rank-ordered are retained, however, and given the average of the tied ranks. It is only when no change between pairs is observed that the two observations are dropped. The power efficiency of the Wilcoxon test is about 95 percent of t for all sample sizes. Exhibit 19.8 presents the computational procedures for this test. Using the data given in Exhibit 19.7 for which d has been computed and rank ordered, the sum of pluses and minuses is computed:

$$+ s = 2.5 + 5.5 + 2.5 + 8 + 8 + 5.5 + 8 = 40$$

$$- s = 2.5 + 2.5 = 5$$

T, the smaller of the sums, is 5, and N is 9, the number of pairs. One pair (subject 2) is dropped from the analysis because no change occurred. Since T is less than 25, Table K, Appendix III, is entered to retrieve the critical value for T, which is 6 (two-tailed). Because our T of 5 is less than the critical value, H_0 is rejected. A significant change has occurred (toward less anxiety).

Exhibit 19-8. Wilcoxon matched-pairs signed-ranks test (for ordinal data).

---

1. Compute d for the difference between X_1 and X_2 for each pair of scores, taking care to assign a plus or minus sign to each d. If $d = 0$, the pair is dropped from the analysis and N is reduced.
2. Ignoring signs (but not separating them from their d's), rank the d values in order of magnitude, with the lowest algebraic score assigned a rank of 1. If some d's are tied, assign the average of the ranks [e.g., $(2 + 3 + 4)/3 = 3$] to each d.
3. Sum the d's for all the pluses and all the minuses. Let $T =$ the smaller sum and $N =$ the number of pairs.
4. If $T \leq 25$, enter Table K, Appendix III, for the critical value of T. If T *equals or is less than* the critical value, H_0 is rejected.
5. If $T > 25$, the sampling distribution approaches normal, and a Z test is:

$$Z = \frac{T - \dfrac{N(N + 1)}{4}}{\sqrt{\dfrac{N(N + 1)(2N + 1)}{24}}}$$

6. If $Z \geq 1.96$ (two-tailed) or 1.643 (one-tailed), H_0 is rejected at $p < .05$. If $Z \geq 2.58$ (two-tailed) or 2.33 (one-tailed), H_0 is rejected at $p < .01$.

Exhibit 19-9. Sign test (for ordinal data).

---

1. Each matched pair is observed for a plus ($+$) or minus ($-$) change in direction. (If a pair has no change, it is dropped from the analysis.)
2. Count the number of pluses and minuses.
3. For $N \leq 25$, let N = number of pairs and X = the number of *fewer* signs (smaller of either the sum of pluses or the sum of minuses). Enter Table J, Appendix III, based on the binomial expansion, for the one-tailed probability. If a two-tailed test is desired, double the probability given in Table J.
4. If $N > 25$, the sampling distribution approaches normal; therefore, the Z statistic is appropriate. Again, let N = the number of pairs and X = the smaller of either the sum of pluses or the sum of minuses.

$$Z = \frac{(X + 0.5) - \frac{1}{2}N}{\frac{1}{2}\sqrt{N}}$$

where $X + 0.5$ is used when $X < \frac{1}{2}N$ and $X - 0.5$ is used when $X > \frac{1}{2}N$.
5. If the value of Z *equals or is greater than* 1.96 (two-tailed) or 1.643 (one-tailed), H_0 is rejected at $p < .05$. If Z *equals or is greater than* 2.58 (two-tailed) or 2.33 (one-tailed), H_0 is rejected at $p < .01$.

The Sign Test

The Sign test, like the Wilcoxon, also assumes an underlying continuous distribution and is especially good for small sample sizes. In this analysis, also, a pair is dropped from the analysis if no change or difference occurs. Thus, H_0 states that, of those pairs where change occurred, changes in the one direction were equal to changes in the other direction. The Sign test requires ranking only within pairs and is useful when responses can be considered rank data (e.g., yes, uncertain, or no) but not scores. However, it is less powerful than the Wilcoxon. The power efficiency of the Sign test is 95 percent of t for $N = 6$, and it declines to 63 percent as N increases. Exhibit 19.9 presents the computational procedures for the Sign test. Still using the data from Exhibit 19.7, let us compute the Sign test. In this test, we count only the numbers of pluses and minuses. There are 7 pluses and 2 minuses. One pair is dropped because no change occurred. Because $N = 9$, Table J, Appendix III, is used. For $X = 2$, the number of fewer signs, the probability is .02 (one-tailed) and .04 (two-tailed). The H_0 is therefore rejected (at $\alpha = .05$).

Tests for Three or More Independent Groups

The procedures presented here correspond to the F ratio in one-way analysis of variance (ANOVA). Three or more groups are often compared, such as AD, Diploma, and Baccalaureate nurses. Somtimes a second control group is used to receive the added time and attention of the experimental group without actually being exposed to the independent variable. Of the two tests appropriate for ordinal data, the Kruskal-Wallis one-way analysis of variance by ranks is the most efficient, because it converts scores to ranks making use of the magnitude of the scores, while the Extension of the Median test converts them only to pluses or minuses. The Kruskal-Wallis test has a power efficiency of about 95 percent of F and assumes an underlying continuous distribution. The Extension of the Median test requires *only* ordinal data and has power efficiency equal to chi square. It is, essentially, a χ^2 test and therefore requires that the χ^2 expected frequencies assumptions be met. Both tests use tied ranks, the Kruskal-Wallis having a correction for them. As with the F ratio and χ^2, both allow unequal group sizes.

All tests are two-tailed because more than two groups are involved. In addition, because three or more groups are involved, if H_0 is rejected you can conclude only that the groups differ. To specify which group differs from the other(s), additional post hoc tests must be performed in such a way as not to increase the probability of type I error.

Nominal Data

Chi Square Test of Independence

This is the same test mentioned in the comparison of two independent samples and is described in detail in Chapter 18. If more then two categories of the dependent (or criterion) variable are used, chi square tests differences in dispersion together with differences in central tendency or location.

Ordinal Data

The Kruskal-Wallis One-Way Analysis of Variance (ANOVA) by Ranks

If the assumption of an underlying continuous distribution can be met, the Kruskal-Wallis is the most powerful of the tests in this category. Its power efficiency equals 95 percent of F. Exhibit 19.10 presents computational procedures. The H_0 states that there is no difference among groups in central tendency. Using the data presented in Exhibit 19.11, we compute a Kruskal-Wallis test. The scores have already been rank-ordered (across groups) and ranks assigned to scores in each group. We then sum the ranks and record n for each group:

Group 1: $\quad R_1 = 1 + 2 + 10 + 6 = 19; n_1 = 4$

Group 2: $\quad R_2 = 3 + 4.5 + 11 + 8 = 26.5; n_2 = 4$

Group 3: $\quad R_3 = 4.5 + 7 + 12 + 9 = 32.5; n_3 = 4$

Next, we compute E, which is the sum of each R squared divided by its n:

$$E = \frac{(19)^2}{4} + \frac{(26.5)^2}{4} + \frac{(32.5)^2}{4} = \frac{361}{4} + \frac{702.25}{4} + \frac{1056.25}{4}$$

$$= 90.25 + 175.56 + 264.06 = 529.87$$

H is then computed:

$$H = \frac{12}{12\,(12 + 1)}\,(529.87) - 3\,(12 + 1) = \frac{12}{156}\,(529.87) - 39$$

$$= .0769\,(529.87) - 39 = 40.75 - 39 = 1.75$$

Exhibit 19-10. Kruskal-Wallis one-way
analysis of variance by ranks (for ordinal data).

---

1. Let N = the number of observations in the *total* sample of k independent groups.
2. Combine scores from all groups, and rank in order of magnitude (with lowest algebraic score assigned a rank of 1).
3. List the rank of each score in columns designated for each of the k groups.
4. Let n_1 = number of observations in group 1, n_2 = number of observations in group 2, n_3 = number of observations in group 3, and so on.
5. Sum the ranks in each column. Let R_1 = sum of group 1, R_2 = sum of group 2, R_3 = sum of group 3, and so on.
6. Compute E:

$$E = \Sigma \frac{R^2}{n}$$

   where $\dfrac{R^2}{n}$ = squared sum of ranks divided by n observations in each group

   $\Sigma \dfrac{R^2}{n}$ = sum of R^2/n for each group

7. Compute H:

$$H = \frac{12}{N(N + 1)}(E) - 3(N + 1)$$

8. If more than 25 percent of the observations involved ties, correct H by dividing it by

$$1 - \frac{\Sigma T}{N^3 - N}$$

   where $T = t^3 - t$ (when t is the number of observations involved in a single given tie)
   ΣT = sum of all T values corresponding to each tie
   N = number of observations in the *total* sample of k groups

9. When there are five or more observations in *each* group, the sampling distribution for H approaches a chi-square distribution for $df = k - 1$. Therefore, use Table F, Appendix III, to extract the critical value of H. If H *equals or is greater than* the critical value, H_0 is rejected.
10. When $k = 3$ and the number of cases in each group is less than 5, use Table L, Appendix III, for the two-tailed probability associated with H.
11. If ties were less than 25 percent and H_0 was very close to being rejected, apply the correction in step 8 and enter the table again.

Exhibit 19-11. Fictitious data for computation
of the Kruskal-Wallis test (for ordinal data).

Group 1	Rank-Order of Scores	Group 2	Rank-Order of Scores	Group 3	Rank-Order of Scores
46	1	52	3	54	4.5
50	2	54	4.5	58	7
65	10	71	11	73	12
55	6	59	8	63	9
ΣR	19		26.5		32.5

Because fewer than 25 percent of the observations involved ties (only 2 out of 12 or 17 percent did), we do not need to apply the correction factor for ties. We go on to use Table L, Appendix III, to extract the probability (of type I error) for H. Entering the table for sample sizes equal to 4, 4, and 4, we see that the value of H at .10 is 4.50 and at .05 is 5.65. Clearly, our H of 1.75 is not significant.

Extension of the Median Test

The Extension of the Median test also determines if the k groups are different in central tendency. It is easier to compute than the Kruskal-Wallis test and does not require an underlying continuous distribution. However, it does require that the assumptions of χ^2 be met. Suppose a nurse researcher wanted to study the differences among three groups of mothers, grouped according to their terminal level of education (i.e., grade school, high school, college), in the number of visits to a well-baby clinic. Because one cannot make a half or a quarter visit to the clinic, visits are discrete rather than continuous measures. The Extension of the Median test is therefore appropriate. The power of this test corresponds to that of chi square. Exhibit 19.12 describes its computation. Because the Median test extension is essentially a χ^2 test, its computation will not be illustrated here. Refer to Chapter 18.

Tests for Three or More Related Samples

The two tests presented in this section correspond to the F ratio in the parametric Repeated Measures ANOVA test. They are, of course, two-tailed. The most obvious research example would involve a group of patients being measured at three or more intervals over time. Others include patient assessment of a k series of nurse actions or patient responses at three or more consecutive visits. Siegel suggests, further, that k items on a test of knowledge might be analyzed for difficulty by using data consisting of pass-fail information on each of the k items for N individuals. The k items or groups would be considered matched because the same individual answered all items. On the

---

Exhibit 19-12. Extension of the Median test.

---

1. Combine scores for all groups, and determine the median of all scores.
2. Label scores in each group by assigning a plus sign to scores that exceed the median and a minus sign to scores that fall at or below the median.
3. Develop a $k \times 2$ table, where the numbers in the table represent the frequencies of pluses and minuses in each of the k groups:

	Group A	Group B	Group C
Pluses			
Minuses			

4. Compute chi square for the contingency table at $df = k - 1$. (When data do not meet the expected-frequency assumptions of χ^2, combine cells or use another test.) Use Table F, Appendix III, to get the two-tailed critical value. If χ^2 *equals or is greater than* the critical value, H_0 is rejected.

---

other hand, one item might be analyzed comparing responses of N subjects under different k conditions. Here the matching would be achieved by having the same Ss in each k condition. The H_0 would be that the responses to the conditions were equal. Another example of matching might be three matched sets of patients (on some relevant variable like diagnosis) who are interviewed under three different conditions (e.g., at home before surgery, during hospitalization, and at home after surgery), members of each set having been randomly assigned to a condition. The type of response as well as sample size would determine whether the Cochran Q test or Friedman Two-way ANOVA test is appropriate.

The Cochran test uses only dichotomous responses (e.g., satisfied-unsatisfied, compliant-noncompliant, pass-fail, physician-nurse) and requires only nominal level data. The Friedman test makes use of scores, although an assumption of an underlying continuous distribution is not specified. Scores for *each set* of matched pairs or repeated measures are rank ordered. The Friedman test appears to be more powerful. It can also be used with few matched samples ($n = 3$). The Cochran test, on the other hand, is not suitable when the number of matched groups or samples is small, although Cochran does not define "small." It seems reasonable to assume, however, because this test uses the χ^2 distribution, that the number of pairs should be at least 10.

Nominal Data

The Cochran Q Test

The Cochran test uses dichotomous responses that do not even need to be ordinal or continuous in nature. H_0 states that the k related groups will be equal in their plus or minus responses. Its power efficiency is not known. Exhibit 19.13 describes computation of the Cochran Q test, and Exhibit 19.14 presents

Exhibit 19-13. Cochran Q test (for nominal data).

1. All observations are dichotomized as pluses or minuses.
2. Develop a two-way table ($k \times N$) consisting of N rows (one row for each subject or matched observation) and k columns (one column for each measurement condition) in which each dichotomous response is recorded.
3. Add the number of pluses in each column, and let them each be G_1, G_2, G_3, and so on to G_k.
4. Add the sum of pluses in each column to compute ΣG.
5. Square the sum of pluses in each column, and let them each be $G_1{}^2, G_2{}^2, G_3{}^2$, and so on to $G_k{}^2$.
6. Add the squared sums of column pluses (e.g., $G_1{}^2 + G_2{}^2 + G_3{}^2 + \cdots + G_k{}^2$) to compute ΣG^2.
7. Add the number of pluses in each row, and let each be L_1, L_2, L_3, and so on to L_n.
8. Add the sum of pluses in each row to compute ΣL.
9. Square the sum of pluses in each row, and let each be $L_1{}^2, L_2{}^2, L_3{}^2$, and so on to $L_n{}^2$.
10. Add the squared sums of row pluses (e.g., $L_1{}^2 + L_2{}^2 + L_3{}^2 + \cdots + L_k{}^2$) to compute ΣL^2.
11. Compute Q:

$$Q = \frac{(k-1)[k(\Sigma G^2) - (\Sigma G)^2]}{k\,\Sigma L - \Sigma L^2}$$

12. Enter Table F, Appendix III, based on the χ^2 distribution, for the critical value at $df = k - 1$.

Exhibit 19-14. Satisfaction data for three patient visits.

Ss	Visit 1	+/−	Visit 2	+/−	Visit 3	+/−	ΣL	ΣL^2
01	6	+	8	+	10	+	3	9
02	8	+	9	+	4	−	2	4
03	4	−	5	+	4	−	1	1
04	3	−	8	+	9	+	2	4
05	7	+	10	+	9	+	3	9
06	9	+	7	+	5	+	3	9
07	8	+	8	+	8	+	3	9
08	7	+	8	+	7	+	3	9
09	5	+	3	−	4	−	1	1
10	2	−	3	−	3	−	0	0
ΣG		7		8		6		
ΣG^2		49		64		36		

Note: Patient is considered satisfied if ratings are 5 or above.

data to illustrate its computation. The sum of pluses has already been computed and squared for columns and rows in Exhibit 19.14. Therefore, we are ready to compute the sums for the rows and columns:

(1) $\Sigma G^2 = 49 + 64 + 36 = 149$

(2) $\Sigma L^2 = 9 + 4 + 1 + 4 + 9 + 9 + 9 + 9 + 1 = 55$

(3) $\Sigma G = 7 + 8 + 6 = 21$

(4) $\Sigma L = 3 + 2 + 1 + 2 + 3 + 3 + 3 + 3 + 1 = 21$

We are now ready to compute Q:

$$Q = \frac{(3 - 1)[3(149) - (21)(21)]}{(3)(21) - 55} = \frac{2(447 - 441)}{63 - 55} = \frac{12}{8} = 1.5$$

Entering the chi square distribution table, Table F in Appendix III, for $df = k - 1 = 2$, we find a critical value of 5.99 at $\alpha = .05$. These repeated measures of patient satisfaction show no change over successive patient visits.

Ordinal Data

The Friedman Two-Way Analysis of Variance (ANOVA) by Ranks

The Friedman test makes use of the magnitude (from 1 to k) of responses in each matched set of observations. Therefore, it is more likely to reject H_0 than

---

Exhibit 19-15. Friedman two-way analysis of variance by ranks (for ordinal data).

1. Develop a two-way table ($k \times n$) for n rows and k columns with scores for each subject or matched group (n) entered under each condition.
2. Separately rank-order the scores in each *row*. Let the lowest algebraic score be assigned a rank of 1. Give equal scores the average of the tied ranks [e.g., $(2 + 3 + 4)/3 = 3$].
3. Develop a second two-way table ($k \times n$), entering the rank order of scores in each row.
4. Add the ranks in each *column*, and square this sum to get ΣR^2 for each column.
5. Add the squared sum of ranks in each column to compute $\Sigma\Sigma R^2$.
6. Compute

$$\chi_r^2 = \frac{12}{nk(k + 1)}(\Sigma\Sigma R^2) - 3n(k - 1)$$

where n = number of rows and k = number of columns.

7. If $k = 3$ and $n = 3$ to 9, or $k = 4$ and $n = 2$ to 4, use Table M, Appendix III, for the probability.
8. If k and n are larger, use Table F, Appendix III, based on the chi-square distribution, for critical values of χ_r^2 with $df = k - 1$. If χ_r^2 *equals or is greater than* the critical value, H_0 is rejected.

Exhibit 19-16. Data organization for the Friedman two-way ANOVA by ranks.

Ss	Visit 1	Visit 2	Visit 3	
01	1	2	3	
02	2	3	1	
03	1.5	3	1.5	
04	1	2	3	
05	1	3	2	
06	3	2	1	
07	2	2	2	
08	1.5	3	1.5	
09	3	1	2	
10	1	2.5	2.5	
ΣR	17	23.5	19.5	
$(\Sigma R)^2$	289	552.25	380.25	$\Sigma\Sigma R^2 = 1221.5$

the Cochran test, given the same set of responses. The Friedman test is approximately equal in power efficiency to the F test when $\alpha = .05$ and slightly less (85 percent) when $\alpha = .01$. The computational procedure for the Friedman test is presented in Exhibit 19.15. Using data presented in Exhibit 19.14, Exhibit 19.16 shows the data organization for the Friedman test. Scores have been rank-ordered within each row and the column ranks summed and squared. These have then been added to yield $\Sigma\Sigma R^2$. We can now compute the test statistic:

$$\chi_r^2 = \frac{12}{(10)(3)(3 + 1)} (1221.5) - (3)(10)(3 + 1)$$

$$= \frac{12}{120} (1221.5) - 120 = 122.15 - 120 = 2.15$$

Since $n = 10$, we can use Table F, Appendix III, to retrieve the critical value at $df = k - 1 = 2$. It is 5.99 at $\alpha = .05$ and therefore H_0 is accepted.

This concludes our discussion of other nonparametric tests. If you wish to pursue this further, refer to Siegel [2]. For yet another approach to non-parametric procedures that is gaining in popularity, refer to Mosteller and Tukey [1] and Tukey [3].

Vocabulary

Binominal test

Chi square test of independence

Cochran Q test

Extension of the Median test

Fisher's exact probability test

Friedman two-way ANOVA by ranks

H_0 (null hypothesis)

Independent groups

Kruskall-Wallis one-way ANOVA by ranks

McNemar test for the significance of
changes
Magnitude of change
Mann-Whitney U test
Matched groups
Median test
Nominal level data
Nonparametric test
One-tailed

Ordinal level data
Power efficiency
Related groups
Sign test
Two-tailed
Underlying continuous distribution
Wilcoxon matched-pairs signed-ranks
test

References

1. Mosteller, F., and Tukey, J. W. *Data Analysis and Regression: A Second Course in Statistics.* Reading, Mass.: Addison-Wesley, 1977.
2. Siegel, S. *Nonparametric Statistics for the Behavioral Sciences.* New York: McGraw-Hill, 1956.
3. Tukey, J. W. *Exploratory Data Analysis.* Reading, Mass.: Addison-Wesley, 1977.

Multivariate analysis or statistics has a sophisticated ring to it—even an ominous one. Actually, most multivariate procedures are just alternate versions of procedures you already know, much as one-way analysis of variance (ANOVA [in Chap. 17]) involves computing three versions of a variance that was a basic procedure (from Chap. 6) that you already knew.

Human beings, if viewed holistically, are complex indeed. Many variables must be considered at the same time. Multivariate analysis enables this. There are two definitions of multivariate statistics. In this book it means that three or more variables are used together in the data analysis. These can be two independent variables (e.g., an intervention and patient diagnosis) and one dependent variable or one independent variable and two dependent variables. The second definition, which is used less often, limits multivariate statistics to research designs in which two or more *dependent* variables are involved. This chapter presents a limited discussion of some computational procedures for four kinds of multivariate analyses and then conceptually presents some of the more advanced procedures.

Partial Correlation

Partial correlation provides a single measure of correlation between two variables while at the same time adjusting for their correlations to one or more additional variables. For example, in a study of the relationship between presurgical anxiety and recovery rate, you may wish to control the effects due to age or other variables like prior surgeries or general physical condition. Some of this, of course, is done via a **sampling protocol** in which only patients meeting certain criteria, like no prior surgeries, are admitted to the study. Other variables remain, however, if sample size is to be adequate. Thus, partial correlation can be a very useful tool.

The procedure when only one variable is being **partialed out** is fairly simple. First, three simple or **one-way Pearson *r* correlations** are computed between each pair of variables. All the assumptions of a Pearson *r* correlation must be met, of course. Then, these three correlations are used in the following formula, which yields the partial correlation coefficient.

$$r_{ab.c} = \frac{r_{ab} - r_{ac}r_{bc}}{\sqrt{1 - r_{ac}^2}\sqrt{1 - r_{bc}^2}}$$

(20.1)

where $r_{ab.c}$ = the partial correlation coefficient

c = the variable being partialed out

r_{ab}, r_{bc}, r_{ac} = the one-way Pearson *r* correlations between all pairs

Interpretation is similar to that of a one-way correlation (between only two variables), except that the partial correlation reflects the relationship between the two variables *after* all the overlap or factors *each* have in common with the third variable have been removed from the analysis. The correct interpretation of a partial *r* is "with the effects due to variable *c held constant*, a relationship between variable *a* and variable *b* was found." This is a good way to control a confounding variable that cannot be controlled by your research design or sampling procedure.

Partial correlation can also be used to uncover **spurious** (i.e., inflated) **relationships.** For example, suppose a high correlation is found between mothers and daughters in compliance for well-baby checkups. You could erroneously conclude that this runs in families. However, if the variance due to educational level is partialed out, it is possible that the original *r* would be reduced. This would mean that the original *r* was misleading or spurious. Instead, the more significant variable related to compliance is educational level.

It is possible to partial out more than one variable. The analysis then becomes more complex, and therefore a computer should be used. Partial correlation can also be done with ordinal level data. Kendall's tau is perhaps the best known procedure, although there are procedures for some of the other ordinal level correlations, such as Somers' D. At the nominal level, separate contingency tables are developed for each level of the third variable that is to be partialed out. Chi square values or the measures of association for each table can then be compared to determine differences attributable to the third variable. This is known as **analysis of crossbreaks.** Power analysis for partial correlation follows the same procedures as those used with multiple regression. Refer to the power analysis section in the discussion of multiple regression.

Multiple Regression

Much correlational research involves prediction. For example, large sums of money have been spent trying to predict reenlistment in military service according to the personal characteristics of new recruits. In this way maximum training efforts can be directed toward those who remain in service; the money spent in training therefore reaches a higher level of "payoff." Similarly, some research has been directed at predicting job performance or job satisfaction from the characteristics of job applicants.

Suppose we wanted to predict job performance of baccalaureate nursing graduates, using grade point average, faculty assessment of each graduate's clinical performance, the subject's attitude toward nursing as a profession, the subject's attitude toward the effects on children of working mothers, and the subject's degree of willingness to work evening and weekend shifts. **Multiple regression** would be an appropriate statistical analysis procedure if the **criterion variable,** job performance, was measured at the interval level. Generally, the **predictor variables** (i.e., all the other variables) are also interval level measures, although dichotomous "dummy" variables (e.g., gender) can also be used. Another assumption of multiple regression is that the predictors are not correlated with each other, although this assumption is often violated.*

In our example of predicting the job performance of nurses, assume that all the predictor measures were recorded during the last semester of school. Three years later questionnaires were mailed to a random sample of graduates. Follow-up letters yielded a 95 percent return rate, with only three persons no longer working as nurses. The questionnaire included an interval level measure of job performance completed by supervisors as well as other information such as salary, marital status, and so forth.

For purposes of our prediction problem, only the original variables measured during the last semester of school are considered possible predictors. The criterion variable is the job performance scale completed by supervisors 3 years later. Now, how do we find out what the predictors are? That is easy. We use principles from simple correlation and partial correlation. First, a simple correlation (which meets the assumptions for a Pearson r) is computed between the criterion and *each* of the predictors. Whichever one is largest is the first predictor. Next, this r is squared and subtracted from 1 in order to find out how much variance is left unexplained by the first predictor $(1 - R^2)$. Each of the leftover predictors is then correlated with the criterion. These correlations, called **part correlations,** are similar to partial correlations in that the effects (or variance) due to the first predictor, in this case faculty assessment of clinical performance, are removed from the other predictors. The predictor with the highest correlation to the criterion is chosen, and it becomes the second predictor. In our example, the second predictor is attitude toward the effects on children of working mothers. The procedure continues, each time removing (via a part correlation) the effects or variance due to all the predictors that have already been established or *entered*.

A capital R, instead of a small r, is used in multiple regression. Usually, about three to five predictors (or about half of those you start with) are the most efficient in accounting for most of the predicted variance. Additional predictors ordinarily account for very little additional variance (i.e., often no statistically significant additions) and are therefore not used unless, as in rare occasions, theory requires it or the data are pilot test variables that require further study.

The final "product" in the multiple regression procedure is a formula, often called a **prediction equation,** which allows you to predict a person's score on the criterion measure if you know his or her scores on the predictors. The method for determining this formula when only one predictor is used was explained in Chapter 7. When more predictors are used, it is wise to use one of the computer programs available for this purpose.

Many researchers stop at this point. However, an additional step called **cross-**

---

*When some or all predictors are highly intercorrelated, the situation is called *multicollinearity*. It is not good. It results in a large *shrinkage of R*. See the discussion in the following pages.

validation is necessary. The prediction equation should be tested using another sample. Because the R you get when you develop the equation is based on the best possible fit for the sample you are using, most of the time the R yielded when you test the equation on another sample is lower. This is known as **shrinkage of R** and is the reason why cross-validation is an essential step in multiple regression. Further, error resulting in even more shrinkage of R is present to the extent that predictor variables were correlated with each other. **Multicollinearity** is said to exist when predictors are highly correlated. It is not good, although, as stated previously, some intercorrelation among predictors is almost always present in behavioral research.

Cross-validation simply involves computing a correlation between **observed scores** and **predicted scores** (using the equation) in a new sample and comparing it to the original R. When you have only one sample, it is best to divide it in half and use half for developing the equation and half for testing the equation. Sometimes, this requires reducing the number of predictors, because a good rule of thumb in determining sample size for a regression design is never to use fewer than 10 or 15 subjects for each variable in the study, although 30 subjects per variable is more defensible. Moreover, no fewer than 100 subjects should ever be used, even if the number of predictors is few. Violation of these rules results in a larger shrinkage of R.

Five to nine predictors are usually adequate to start with, and those you select should be the best ones reported in the literature you review or the theory that guides your research. Just as with r, interpretation of R is based on R^2, the amount of variance in the criterion that is explained by all the predictors in the final prediction equation.

When your criterion is at the nominal level of measurement (e.g., group membership), another procedure, *discriminant analysis*, is used. Its outcome is the prediction of group membership. This procedure is more complicated mathematically and is also best accomplished by using a computer. It also yields a formula that should be tested on another sample to give its ratio of "hits and misses." It does not yield an R as such.

Kinds of Regression Procedures

There are several methods that can be used to select predictors for a regression analysis. The one you select depends on the purpose of your research.

1. Forward stepwise. The forward stepwise procedure was the procedure used in the example of predicting job performance of nursing graduates. The first predictor is selected on the basis of its correlation to the criterion, the second is selected on the basis of its correlation to the residual, and so forth. When predictors fail to add a statistically significant amount (via an ANOVA F ratio) to the regression, the analysis is generally considered completed. A possible weakness in this approach is that when predictors are correlated, variables entered at a later stage may weaken the usefulness of variables entered earlier. This situation can be assessed at each step via most computer printouts, however, and appropriate steps can be taken, such as deleting the variable that is most difficult to measure.

2. Backward elimination. The backward stepwise procedure enters all predictors and then deletes variables one at a time, each time assessing whether the loss to R is statistically significant.

3. General solution. The general solution involves entering predictors in a predesignated order according to theory or some special research situation. (Groups of variables can also be entered at the same time, in a specified order.) An example might involve a research setting in which predictor variables are measured over a period of time. Predictors might therefore be entered in the order they are measured to determine when additional information or measures are no longer necessary. This method is used in cross-lag panel designs (see Chap. 5) in order to first control for (i.e., partial out) specified variables.

Regression with Two Predictors   It is possible to compute an R by hand when there are two predictors entered simultaneously. This procedure is called **multiple correlation** rather than multiple regression if prediction is not involved and the purpose is simply to correlate two variables with a third variable. Just as with partial correlation, one-way Pearson r correlations are first computed between each of the variables. Then, the following formula is used:

$$R_{c.ab} = \sqrt{\frac{r_{ca}^2 + r_{cb}^2 - 2\,r_{ca}r_{cb}r_{ab}}{1 - r_{ab}^2}}$$

(20.2)

where $R_{c.ab}$ = the multiple R for predicting c from a and B
r_{ca}, r_{cb}, r_{ab} = one-way correlations between each pair of the three variables

If more than the value of R is desired, that is, if a prediction equation is desired, a computer program is best used.

The Prediction Equation   Recall that in Chapter 7, a prediction equation was given as

$$\hat{Y} = a + bX$$

where $\hat{Y}$ = predicted value of Y
$\quad X$ = a person's score on X
$\quad a$ = a constant
$\quad b$ = a weight for score X

If only two variables are involved, a constant and a weight for the predictor score are all that are needed to predict $\hat{Y}$. Chapter 7 presented the method for determining the constant and weight for the bivariate situation. When more than two predictor variables are involved, this calculation becomes considerably more complex, and therefore a computer is used for the computations. When two predictors are used to predict Y, the equation is as follows:

$$\hat{Y} = a + b_1X_1 + b_2X_2$$

It simply adds a second predictor, X_2, and its weight, b_2. When three variables are used, the equation adds a third variable and its weight:

$$\hat{Y} = a + b_1X_1 + b_2X_2 + b_3X_3$$

As more predictors are added to the equation, they are simply added to the string. Finally, when the number of predictors is uncertain, it is signified by using a k (or similar letter) as follows:

$$\hat{Y} = a + b_1X_1 + b_2X_2 + \cdots + b_kX_k$$

Computerized Multiple Regression

Exhibit 20.1 presents typical data output from a forward stepwise multiple regression analysis run on a computer. It uses data from a hypothetical research study in which prediction of assertiveness was tested using the personality variables of complacency, rigidity, and dependence. Each step is separated from the others. Moreover, within each step output is usually divided into three parts. The first deals with the value of R at that step and the ANOVA table that tests the significance of R. (The mean square values are not included in Exhibit 20.1 because of space limitations.) The standard error of estimate (SEe) is also presented. Recall from Chapter 7 that the SEe allows you to place confidence intervals around the value of $\hat{Y}$, your predicted value of Y. In step 1 of Exhibit 20.1, the SEe is 13.8. Therefore, you can be about 68 percent certain that Y, the real Y score, will fall within the range from ($\hat{Y} - 13.8$) to ($\hat{Y} + 13.8$). If you wish to know the confidence interval for 95 percent, 1.96 standard errors above and below $\hat{Y}$ must be used. You can be 95 percent certain Y will fall within the range from ($\hat{Y} - 27$) to ($\hat{Y} + 27$). In this example prediction of assertiveness from dependence is not very certain, even though the correlation between the two variables, $-.427$, is better than many correlations found in behavioral research. The confidence intervals become much better (i.e., smaller) as more predictors are added in steps 2 and 3.

The second part of the computer output for *each* of the steps is called *variables in the equation*. It gives information needed for the prediction equation. From Exhibit 20.1, the value of the constant in step 1 is 46.168 and the weight for dependence, X_1, is $-.185$. The negative sign for the weight signifies a negative relationship between the two variables. On most computer printouts two values for a variable's weights are given. The **B weight** is for use with raw scores and the **beta weight*** is used when raw scores have been converted to z scores. They are equally valid in the prediction equation. The **standard error of B,** SE_B, is also given. This allows you to place confidence intervals around the B, *not beta*, weights themselves. Obviously, the larger SE_B, the less certain you can be about your prediction and the fact that a weight of like value would emerge if you replicated your regression study with a different sample. Finally the second part of step 1 presents the statistical significance of the predictor's contribution via an ANOVA F ratio at 1 and 212 degrees of freedom, *df*. On the first step this is the same as the F in the ANOVA table to test the significance of R, which was given in the first part of the output. However, in subsequent steps, each F pertains only to a single predictor, thereby allowing determination of whether or not the variables contribute significantly to the prediction equation. In forward stepwise regression, when predictors fail to make statistically significant contributions, recall, the analysis is usually stopped.

The third part of the computer output for each of the steps is called *variables not in equation*. These are listed with their correlations to the residual. When only one predictor is partialed out, these correlations are called **first order partials;** when two are partialed out, they are called **second order partials;** and so forth. Note that the numerator *df* for the F ratio increase by one and the denominator *df* decrease by one for every additional predictor that is partialed out. The F ratio in this section tests the statistical significance of the part correlations. The highest is selected for inclusion as the next predictor at the next step.

Step 2 in Exhibit 20.1 increases R to .63 and decreases SEe slightly. The SE_B of the weights remains good. When the SE_B of the weights approaches one-third to one-half the value of the B weight itself, there are problems with the analysis. The prediction equation will probably not be replicated. The negative value of the weights indicates a negative correlation between the predictors and criterion, and to accommodate these the constant is correspondingly increased.

Step 3 yields a dramatically lowered SEe and ever increasing R^2. Because no other predictors are available, the analysis is finished. At this point some researchers attempt to decide which is the "best predictor" in the prediction equation. There is no foolproof way to do this. Some compare the *beta* weights at the last step. This, of course, does not consider the various standard errors of the weights. There are special formulae for making these comparisons, but each also has drawbacks. In Exhibit 20.1, it appears just by inspection that dependence is the "best" predictor because (1) it has a larger *beta* weight and (2) its SE_B is smaller for the raw scores, which, in this example, are all on the same scale. If they were not, the various SE_B would not be comparable.

Power Analysis for Multiple Regression

Power analysis for partial correlation and multiple regression involves two steps before the table (Table E, Appendix IV) can be entered. The first step involves

---

*The *beta* weight is often used, instead of R, in reporting the results of cross-lag panel designs as described in Chapter 5.

Exhibit 20-1. Computer output for a forward stepwise regression analysis.

Dependent (criterion) variable: Assertiveness

Step 1

Variable entered: Dependence

	Source	df	SS	F
Multiple *R*: .427	Regression	1	8,980.5	47.37
R^2: .182	Residual	212	40,189.8	
SEe: 13.788				

Variables in the equation:

Variable	*B*	Beta	SE_B	$F (df = 1;212)$
Dependence	−.185	−.427	.026	47.372
Constant	46.168			

Variables not in equation:

Variable	First-Order Partial	$F (df = 2;211)$
Rigidity	−.514	75.91
Complacence	−.487	65.60

Step 2

Variable entered: Rigidity

	Source	df	SS	F
Multiple *R*: .631	Regression	2	19,614.00	70.01
R^2: .398	Residual	211	29,556.33	
SEe: 11.835				

Variables in the equation:

Variable	*B*	Beta	SE_B	$F (df = 2;211)$
Dependence	−.296	−.68	.026	125.62
Rigidity	−.465	−.53	.053	75.91
Constant	77.249			

Variables not in equation:

Variable	Second-Order Partial	$F (df = 3;210)$
Complacence	−.784	336.93

Step 3

Variable entered: Complacence

	Source	df	SS	F
Multiple R: .877	Regression	3	37,821.92	233.29
R^2: .769	Residual	210	11,348.42	
SEe: 7.351				

Variables in the equation:

Variable	B	Beta	SE_B	$F(df = 3;210)$
Dependence	−0.677	−1.560	.026	654.80
Rigidity	−0.657	−0.749	.034	357.31
Complacence	−0.644	−1.002	.035	336.93
Constant	142.050			

Variables not in the equation:

Variable	Third-Order Partial	F
None		

computing effect size (ES):

$$ES - \frac{R^2}{1 - R^2} \tag{20.3}$$

Because the power tables yield values for ANOVA F ratios testing the proportion of variance in Y accounted for by g predictor variables comprising R^2, H is computed in order to enter the power table:

$$H = ES(N - g - 1)$$

where $(N - g - 1) = df$ for error (or denominator df for the F ratio)
g = number of predictor variables (or numerator df)

When Table E in Appendix IV is used to determine sample size, for a power of .20 and designated ES, you retrieve H but not N. To change H to a value for N, first divide H by the ES and then add $(g + 1)$ to this value.

Factorial ANOVA

One-way ANOVA, which was presented in Chapter 17, is limited to looking at the effects of only one independent variable at a time. Often, we have information on other independent variables, like sex or diagnosis. If we use one-way ANOVA, we must look at each separately, and this can then present problems in terms of **family type I Error** (see Chap. 17) as well as power to achieve statistical significance. For each separate one-way ANOVA, the other independent variables, part of the error sum of squares, could actually act as confounding variables that contribute to accepting the null hypothesis. Therefore, groups of procedures exist, the family name of which is **factorial ANOVA,** whereby different kinds of independent variables are considered simultaneously in various kinds of combinations—each with a different name and slightly different sums of squares and *df* to compute. In a few of the more complex designs, moreover, the denominator of the *F* ratio is not the error mean square. This chapter will illustrate one of the more simple factorial designs in which manipulated and blocking independent variables are used. This type of design has already been described conceptually in Chapter 4.

Suppose we were investigating the effects of a newly developed patient education program on recovery of surgical patients. Our review of literature, moreover, indicates that patient coping strategy may be a factor that influences the success or failure of many patient education programs. Therefore, in addition to the experimental variable of education that we can manipulate, we add another independent variable, coping strategy, which is broken down into information seekers and information avoiders. There will be experimental and control groups within which, by random assignment, half of the Ss are avoiders and half are seekers, as determined by a structured interview prior to inception of the study (in which patients are asked about their illness, surgery, the postoperative course, and whether or not they sought information from others). Recovery, on the other hand, is assessed by a composite score of indicators in which a higher score means *better* recovery. Therefore, the layout for this design investigating the effects of two independent variables, each with two categories, is called a 2 × 2 ANOVA. The 2s stand for the number of categories or levels in each variable. If, say, a third variable with four categories were also included, the design would be called 4 × 2 × 2 ANOVA.

Assume that we carried out the experiment investigating the effects of coping strategy and patient education on recovery. Applying factorial ANOVA would enable us to find (1) whether there was a significant difference between the recovery of the subjects who were information seekers and those who were information avoiders, (2) whether there was a significant difference in recovery of the subjects given the patient education program and those who were not, and (3) whether or not the two variables, coping strategy and patient education, had a combined effect on recovery. The effects investigated by the first and second analysis are called **main effects.** They are, essentially, two experiments combined into one. The third analysis is referred to as the **interaction** effect. This is the bonus you get by combining the two experiments rather than doing them separately as two one-way ANOVAs. An interaction might tell you, for example, that only with information seekers is there a significant difference between the education program group and the control group; or it might tell

Exhibit 20-2. Fictitious recovery data for two categories of personality under two conditions of patient education.

	Coping Strategy		
	Information Seekers	Information Avoiders	Total
Patient education	*Group 1:*	*Group 2:*	
	10	7	
	9	6	$\Sigma X_E = 71$
	9	5	
	8	5	$\bar{X}_E = 7.1$
	8	4	
	$\Sigma X_{ES} = 44$	$\Sigma X_{EA} = 27$	$SD_E = 2.02$
	$\bar{X}_{ES} = 8.8$	$\bar{X}_{EA} = 5.4$	
	$SD_{ES} = .84$	$SD_{EA} = 1.14$	
No patient education	*Group 1:*	*Group 2:*	
	8	6	
	7	6	$\Sigma X_C = 59$
	7	5	
	6	5	$\bar{X}_C = 5.9$
	5	4	
	$\Sigma X_{CS} = 33$	$\Sigma X_{CA} = 26$	$SD_C = 1.20$
	$\bar{X}_{CS} = 6.6$	$\bar{X}_{CA} = 5.2$	
	$SD_{CS} = 1.14$	$SD_{CA} = .84$	
Total			
	$\Sigma X_S = 77$	$\Sigma X_A = 53$	
	$\bar{X}_S = 7.7$	$\bar{X}_A = 5.3$	
	$SD_S = 1.49$	$SD_A = 0.95$	

you that only with patient education is there a significant difference in recovery between avoiders and seekers.

The end product of these analyses would be three *F* ratios, two of which indicate the significance of the two main effects and one that indicates the significance of the interaction effect. For your inspection, the raw data and summary statistics are presented in Exhibit 20.2.

The 2 × 2 ANOVA Table
Exhibit 20.3 presents the 2 × 2 ANOVA table for our 2 × 2 design. It also presents one-way ANOVA tables that would result if, instead of the factorial

Exhibit 20-3. ANOVA table for coping strategy
and patient education effects on recovery.

(a) ANOVA Table for Coping strategy and patient education effects on recovery

Source	Sum of Squares	df	Mean Square	F	p
A (Coping Strategy)	28.8	2 − 1 = 1	28.8	28.8	.000
B (Pt. Education)	7.2	2 − 1 = 1	7.2	7.2	.016
AB (Interaction)	5.0	(2 − 1)(2 − 1) = 1	5.0	5.0	.040
Error	16.0	20 − (2 × 2) = 16	1.0	—	—
Total	57.0	20 − 1 = 19			

(b) ANOVA Table for Coping Strategy on Recovery

Source	Sum of Squares	df	Mean Square	F	p
Coping	28.8	1	28.8	18.38	.0004
Error	28.2	18	1.6	—	—
Total	57.0	19			

(c) ANOVA Table for Patient Education on Recovery

Source	Sum of Squares	df	Mean Square	F	p
Education	7.2	1	7.2	2.6	.124
Error	49.8	18	2.8	—	—
Total	57.0	19			

design, two separate studies had been conducted using these same data, one using coping strategy as an independent variable and the other using patient education. In examination of the sum of squares for each of the independent variables, it is readily apparent that they are the same regardless of whether a one-way or two-way ANOVA is conducted. However, the error sum of squares changes dramatically. In the one-way ANOVAs, the sum of squares due to the second (not included) independent variable and the interaction are included in the error sum of squares. (Similarly, their *df* are part of the *df* for error.) This results in a larger mean square for error, which in turn contributes to a smaller *F* ratio. In fact, the *F* ratio for patient education in the one-way ANOVA is not statistically significant owing to the larger error term (i.e., error variance). Thus, the advantages of factorial ANOVA are apparent. Variables (and their interactions) that might have confounded one-way ANOVA analysis and lowered power or the probability of rejecting null hypotheses are controlled when they are added as additional variables in the analysis. There are, of course, special rules for making these additions, and these will be presented later in this chapter.

This discussion does not present the computational procedures involved in computing the sums of squares and *df* for the 2 × 2 design (Table A of Exhibit 20.3). They are similar to the one-way analyses except that additional computations are involved because of the additional *F* ratios. Table A, the factorial ANOVA table of Exhibit 20.3, yields three *F* ratios whose statistical significance is ascertained using the same *F* table that was used for one way ANOVA in Chapter 17 (see Table E, Appendix III). Some computer programs do not print out the significance level, although those printed for Exhibit 20.3 did so. To enter this table, use the number of *df* associated with the variable's mean square (i.e., numerator of the *F* ratio) and the number of *df* associated with the error mean square (i.e., denominator of the *F* ratio). For example, the coping *F* ratio is 28.8. Consulting the *F* table for 1 and 16 *df* and $\alpha = .05$, the critical value is 4.49. Because the test statistic is greater than the critical value, it is, obviously, statistically significant—even at $\alpha = .01$ where the critical value is 8.53. Note, also, that the *F* ratios for this 2 × 2 design are computed in the usual way by dividing the mean square for each variable by the mean square for error. Thus, the mean square for error is used as the denominator in all three *F* ratios.

Interpretation of a 2 × 2 ANOVA Table

To interpret, or find meaning, in the results of a factorial ANOVA table, you must look at the means for the various groups. Because the results for a 2 × 2 ANOVA are easiest to interpret (i.e., do not require additional *post hoc* tests like those presented in Chap. 17 for three or more means), let us consider five possible results of such an analysis. They are presented in Exhibit 20.4. Interpretation involves looking at comparing **row means** for main effects due to variable *Y* (i.e., $\bar{X}_{Y1}$ and $\bar{X}_{Y2}$), column means for main effects due to variable *X* (i.e., $\bar{X}_{X1}$ and $\bar{X}_{X2}$), and cell means for interaction effects of *X* and *Y* (i.e., $\bar{X}_{11}, \bar{X}_{12}, \bar{X}_{21},$ and $\bar{X}_{22}$).

Example A of Exhibit 20.4 clearly has no main or interaction effects, because all means are equal. Even if they varied by two or three points they would probably not be statistically significant unless the sample size was very large. Examples B and C, on the other hand, have significant main effects but no interaction effects, because the cell means differ in the same way as the row and column means. Example B has a significant main effect due to $Y (X_{Y1} = 40$ vs. $X_{Y2} = 20)$ and example C has a significant main effect due to $X(X_{x1} = 40$ versus $X_{x2} = 20)$. These are readily apparent and reasonably straightforward in interpretation. For example B, level 1 of variable *Y* is greater (or higher) than level 2. For example C, level 1 of variable *X* is greater (or higher) than level 2. If variable *X* represents coping style with category 1 being information seekers and category 2 being information avoiders, and if variable *Y* represents the experimental variable with group 1 receiving patient education and group 2 being the controls, your conclusions are also straightforward—unless you are aware of some rival hypotheses. Assuming the absence of rival hypotheses, you conclude for example B that patient education enhances recovery and that no interaction or

Exhibit 20-4. Possible 2 × 2 ANOVA results.

(a)

X

	1	2	
Y 1	$X_{11} = 30$	$X_{12} = 30$	$\overline{X}_{Y1} = 30$
2	$X_{21} = 30$	$X_{22} = 30$	$\overline{X}_{Y2} = 30$
	$X_{X1} = 30$	$X_{X2} = 30$	

Source	MS	F	p
X	.000	.000	1.00
Y	.000	.000	1.00
XY	.000	.000	1.00
Error	6.250		
Total			

(b)

X

	1	2	
Y 1	$X_{11} = 40$	$X_{12} = 40$	$\overline{X}_{Y1} = 40$
2	$X_{21} = 20$	$X_{22} = 20$	$\overline{X}_{Y2} = 20$
	$X_{X1} = 30$	$X_{X2} = 30$	

Source	MS	F	p
X	2000.000	216.216	.000
Y	0.000	0.000	1.000
XY	0.000	0.000	1.000
Error	9.250		
Total			

(c)

X

	1	2	
Y 1	$X_{11} = 40$	$X_{12} = 20$	$\overline{X}_{Y1} = 30$
2	$X_{21} = 40$	$X_{22} = 20$	$\overline{X}_{Y2} = 30$
	$X_{X1} = 40$	$X_{X2} = 20$	

Source	MS	F	p
X	2000.000	216.216	.000
Y	0.000	0.000	1.000
XY	0.000	0.000	1.000
Error	9.250		
Total			

(d)

X

	1	2	
Y 1	$X_{11} = 40$	$X_{12} = 20$	$\overline{X}_{Y1} = 30$
2	$X_{21} = 20$	$X_{22} = 40$	$\overline{X}_{Y2} = 30$
	$X_{X1} = 30$	$X_{X2} = 30$	

Source	MS	F	p
X	0.000	0.000	1.000
Y	0.000	0.000	1.000
XY	2000.000	216.216	.000
Error	9.250		
Total			

(e)

X

	1	2	
Y 1	$X_{11} = 50$	$X_{12} = 30$	$\overline{X}_{Y1} = 40$
2	$X_{21} = 10$	$X_{22} = 30$	$\overline{X}_{Y2} = 20$
	$X_{X1} = 30$	$X_{X2} = 30$	

Source	MS	F	p
X	0.000	0.000	1.000
Y	2000.000	149.533	.000
XY	2000.000	149.533	.000
Error	13.375		
Total			

main effects due to coping style were found. In example C, on the other hand, you conclude that patients whose coping styles involve seeking information recover better than those who avoid information and that no effects due to patient education or its interaction with coping style were supported. You can then discuss implications for practice and future research based on your conclusions.

Examples D and E, on the other hand, are somewhat more involved. They both have effects due to the interaction of X and Y. When a 2×2 ANOVA, or any factorial ANOVA, has a significant interaction, you must interpret it *prior to interpreting the main effects*. This is because its interpretation often renders significant main effects useless, because of its greater detail and specificity.

Example D of Exhibit 20.4 has an interaction effect but no main effects. It can be looked at two ways—from the point of view of variable X or the point of view of variable Y. With variable Y as our point of view we say that among those receiving patient education, information seekers benefit most in terms of recovery, while among those not receiving the experimental variable, the avoiders do better. Because "better" is 40 for both groups, we cannot compare them. From the point of view of variable X, we say that among information seekers patient education *causes* better recovery and among information avoiders patient education *retards* recovery. Avoiders appear to do worse than if they were left alone. Our point of view, of course, is determined by our hypothesis. Our conclusion, on the other hand, is the same regardless of point of view. We conclude that, although patient education (as defined in this research) helps seekers, it may actually harm avoiders. If no rival hypotheses are present to modify our conclusions, the implications for practice and future research are clear.

Example E of Exhibit 20.4 presents both main and interactive effects. Therefore, we look at the interactive effects first. We see that among information seekers, patient education has greater benefit while among avoiders there is neither benefit nor harm derived from this particular patient education program. We conclude that patient education is helpful for information seekers and suggest that, in clinical practice, first coping style be assessed and then, to save costs, patient education in the form that was tested in this research be given only to information seekers. Or, a well advertised program might attract information seekers while allowing avoiders to pass. When you communicate these findings, you would, of course, compare them to similar research studies and speculate on why your results conflict with others, if they do. This would then lead logically to suggestions for further research.

Returning to example E of Exhibit 20.4, there is also a highly significant main effect due to patient education. Would you also interpret this (i.e., patient education enhances recovery) and draw corresponding conclusions? No. The effects due to Y are included with more precision in your interpretation of the interaction. Not only would conclusions based on this be repetitive, they would conflict with the finding of no effects among avoiders.

Now that the basic elements of interpreting a 2 × 2 ANOVA table are clear, return to Exhibit 20.2 and use it to interpret the results of Table A in Exhibit 20.3. Do you conclude that patient education should be given to everyone regardless of coping style because of the significant *F* ratio of 7.2? Why or why not? For more practice in interpreting factorial design results, return to Exhibit 20.4. Define variables *X* and *Y* and their levels differently. Then, interpret results, draw conclusions, and suggest implications for practice and future research. You might draw from topics in which you are familiar with the literature so that you can consider rival hypotheses and the results of similar research as you draw conclusions and suggest implications for practice.

Using Factorial ANOVA

The use of factorial ANOVA is of great value in the study of questions that are inherently complex in nature. These techniques enable us to analyze the combined effects of two or more independent variables in relation to a dependent variable. With the widespread use of computers, any number of independent variables may now be incorporated into factorial designs, although interpretation of complex interactions is often impossible.

An additional point should be considered in regard to factorial ANOVA: cell sizes should be about equal or proportional. In fact, cell sizes must be equal or proportional in order to follow the usual computational routines. When cell sizes differ, more complex procedures may still allow you to do the analysis. However, it is much easier to make cell sizes equal. *Plan ahead* the number of subjects to be randomly assigned to each cell. Even so, mortality may reduce some cell sizes, thereby making them unequal. In this case, if you started with a fairly large sample size, you could follow the usual computational procedures after randomly selecting for removal from each cell enough subjects to again make cells equal or proportional.

Beginning researchers often discover factorial ANOVA midway during their first research project. That is, they learn that it is not as complicated as they had thought it was, and that, in addition, it tends to reduce error variance and provide an opportunity to examine interactions. Therefore, they decide to use it. Suppose in the patient education one-way ANOVA example of Exhibit 20.3, which used two levels of education as an independent variable, researchers had decided to investigate the main and interactive effects of coping style on the dependent variable *after* the subjects were assigned to experimental and control groups. The chances are that there would be uneven numbers of seekers and avoiders in each of the groups. This would produce uneven cell sizes. Because the number of seekers and avoiders was not determined ahead of time and half of each randomly assigned as experimental or control, cell size is unequal. This in turn can require more complicated analysis, which is sometimes difficult to interpret, especially in terms of the interaction.

Perhaps, after you gather data, you decide to control for the confounding effects of age. In order to keep cell sizes nearly equal, you divide the sample into older and younger using the age mean or median of your sample as a cutting point. You have just caused another problem! Age has now become a *random effects variable* because the cutting point between older and younger was decided on the basis of your sample characteristics rather than in advance. Again, the computation of your F ratio becomes more difficult, because you often cannot use the error mean square as the denominator. Unequal cell sizes and random effect variables are becoming less of a problem as more people have access to high-speed computers for the more complex analyses they require. Nevertheless, careful planning and blocking ahead (on variables like coping style) result in stronger studies whose results can be more easily interpreted.

One more word must be said about interactions. Because of the smaller n in the cells involved in the interaction analysis, many statisticians including Cohen [1] believe larger α levels, such as .10 rather than .05, should be used to test the F ratios of interactions. The increase in power, they believe, offsets the price paid in credibility when an interaction H_0 is rejected at .10 rather than .05.

Other Factorial ANOVA Designs

We have barely scratched the surface of the variety of factorial designs available. Additional independent variables can be added, of course, although the interactions that result from more than three independent variables, especially if each has more than three levels or categories, are almost impossible to interpret. In fact, some computer routines allow you to ignore interactions of more than three variables. Consider a three-variable (or three-factor) ANOVA. It would result in three main effects and four interactions (e.g., AB, AC, BC, ABC) or 7 F ratios. By adding just one more variable, you have 4 main effects and 11 interactions (e.g., AB, AC, AD, BC, BD, CD, ABC, BCD, ACD, ABD, ABCD) or 15 F ratios. Although these complex designs have great appeal in describing complex human behavior, they also require more subjects, just as do additional cells in chi square analysis. The exact number, of course, can be calculated using power analysis (see Table C, Appendix IV).

In addition to adding independent variables, like coping style, on which you are able to block ahead, other factors can be repeated measures, as described in Chapter 17, in which subjects are measured more than once. This certainly helps to reduce error variance in designs that allow repeated testing. There are also special designs, called nested, that compare to sampling units and their elements as described in Chapter 10. This removes from error variance any effects due to subjects coming from the same hospital, say, when patients from several hospitals are sampled. Only one other ANOVA procedure will be presented in this chapter—analysis of covariance (ANCOVA). For the other more complex factorial designs, you may wish to take a more advanced statistical course. Whole semester courses, called something like design of experiments, are offered, which do nothing but study the various ANOVA designs. Others, of course, study nothing but multiple regression, and still others study other multivariate procedures. In using any of these, the procedure is only as good as the data—which emphasizes again the need for excellence in operationally defining variables.

As usual, an ES must be computed in order to perform power analysis for factorial ANOVA. It is the same as that for one-way ANOVA.

$$ES = \sqrt{\frac{SS_{between}}{SS_{error}}} \tag{20.5}$$

However, since the SS error includes error due to all factors and interactions, it is necessary to adjust the n for entering Table C, Appendix IV, as follows:

$$\hat{n} = \frac{df \text{ for } MS_{error}}{(df \text{ for } E) + 1} + 1 \tag{20.6}$$

where E = the effect or interaction being interpreted

When using Table C, Appendix IV, to determine sample size prior to implementing a research design for a power of .20, α = .05, and designated ES, you retrieve $\hat{n}$ instead of n. To change $\hat{n}$ to a value for n, in a two-factor case, use the following formula for a main effect:

$$n = \hat{n}(p - 1) + pq \tag{20.7}$$

where p = number of categories in the main effect of interest
q = number of categories in the other main effect

In a two-factor design when you want to determine n for the interaction, the following formula can be used after $\hat{n}$ is retrieved from the table:

$$n = \hat{n}(p - 1)(q - 1) + pq \tag{20.8}$$

where p and q = number of categories in each of the two factors

Similarly, in a three-factor design, n can be calculated for main effects by the following formula:

$$n = \hat{n}(p - 1) + pqk \tag{20.9}$$

where p = number of categories in the main effect of interest
q and k = number of categories in the other two factors

The formula for retrieving n from $\hat{n}$ for the interaction of the three factors is as follows:

$$n = \hat{n}(p - 1)(q - 1)(k - 1) + pqk \tag{20.10}$$

where p, q, and k = number of categories of the three factors

For the more complex ANOVA designs or other values of α, refer to Cohen [1].

Analysis of Covariance (ANCOVA)

When we began the discussion of simple one-way ANOVA in Chapter 17, we stated that the object was to get a large between groups (i.e., the experimental variable) mean square as compared to the error mean square. This would then yield a larger F ratio. We have also said that you can get a larger F ratio if you *reduce* error variance (i.e., the error mean square) by removing from it the effects of confounding variables. In using factorial ANOVA, the effects due to the second independent variable are removed from error mean square and used as a separate variable. Thus, you reduce the MS error, which is the denominator of the F ratio, and increase your chances for reaching statistical significance.

There is yet another way of reducing error variance. This is by using analysis of covariance, ANCOVA, which is another version of ANOVA. Suppose you were investigating the effects of three kinds of contraceptives on urinary tract infection (UTI) (as defined by number of days in a year with symptoms, corroborated by positive cultures of more than 100,000 colonies) among sexually active women ages 18 to 30. A one-way ANOVA yielded no significant effects. A colleague then suggested that frequency of intercourse may be a confounding variable. Therefore, you decide to remove from the analysis the effects due to frequency of sexual intercourse. Your reason for not considering it as a second independent variable is that even if it were significant or an interaction were found, a successful intervention to change the frequency would be unlikely, if not ethically indefensible. Besides, the focus of the research is the efficacy of various contraception methods in regard to prevention of UTI. Therefore, in order to remove the effects of intercourse frequency, you use ANCOVA. In this case, you would be using each subject's frequency of activity in the *same way you would use a pretest*. The basic ANOVA still tests the differences among the three groups on UTI, but this time with the variance due to frequency of intercourse removed. While the effects due to frequency of intercourse had been randomly distributed to all contraceptive groups and included in error, now these are singled out as a **covariate.** This results, among other things, in reducing error variance. It has the same effect as partialing out variables has in multiple regression when you correlate new predictors with the residual.

In addition to all the ANOVA assumptions discussed when one-way ANOVA was presented in Chapter 17, ANCOVA has three others. A basic assumption of classical ANCOVA, of course, is that the covariate is measured at the interval level of measurement. When it is not, factorial ANOVA is used. Another assumption of this procedure is that frequency of intercourse, the covariate, and UTI, the dependent variable, are correlated. There must be a *linear* correlation, usually around .60 but never below .30, between the covariate and the dependent variable. If not, use factorial ANOVA because ANCOVA will do little to reduce error. A third assumption of covariance is that of **homogeneity of regression**. This means that the linear regression lines between the covariate and dependent variable for *each* of the groups (i.e., cells) must be parallel if they are all placed on the same graph. When homogeneity of regression is not present, another procedure can be used. Violation of the homogeneity of regression assumption increases the chance of a type I error.

ANCOVA can never be used to make intact groups equal. Quite often less knowledgeable researchers try to do this. A basic assumption in using ANCOVA is that the effects due to the covariate have fallen randomly to all groups. (Thus, random assignment to groups is advisable.) You will find in the journal literature occasional cases where ANCOVA has been used in an attempt to equalize intact groups. For example, perhaps two pediatric wards are compared to determine the relative effectiveness of two methods designed to reduce patient anxiety before surgery. The mean age of one ward is 9.2 and the mean age of the other ward is 4.5. Clearly, they are very different in age, and because age could affect anxiety, the researchers decide to equalize the groups with ANCOVA by removing the effects due to age. This cannot be done. These two intact groups are simply not equal or even nearly equal. This research cannot be done using this design and these subjects. In order to be a covariate, age must be distributed about equally in both groups.

Often, researchers cannot decide if it is better to use factorial ANOVA or ANCOVA. The first consideration hinges on whether the potential covariate and the dependent variable show significant departures from linear relations. If they do, then factorial ANOVA must be used. Then, there should be an opportunity to block ahead of time if you are going to use factorial ANOVA. Otherwise, cell sizes will be unequal. Third, if you are interested in interactions, or a main effect due to a potential covariate, only factorial ANOVA will give you this. Therefore, if the two variables are linearly related and you are not interested in main effects or interactions due to the potential covariate, the extent to which they are correlated might make your decision. If the relationship between the dependent variable and potential covariate is .60 or more, a good rule of thumb is to use ANCOVA. If the relationship is less than .30, you will have more power by using factorial ANOVA.

The two advantages of ANCOVA are that the *df* for error are not reduced as much as they are when you use factorial ANOVA. This means that a *slightly* smaller *F* is required to reach statistical significance. Second, in covariance you are using more information—individual scores versus, for example, high, medium, and low categories for the same scores. Whenever you use more precise measures, you are likely to reduce error variance more.

ANCOVA must be used with care in a research design. Just as with partial correlation, it is possible to *remove* statistical significance from an *F* ratio when a covariate is used. Thus, the theoretical or conceptual basis for using a covariate should be clear before it is employed. Know the literature in your topic area thoroughly. The reason for suspecting a variable as a confounder and therefore using it as a covariate should make sense logically.

Another area of concern is that scores on the covariate are not influenced by the dependent or experimental variables. For this reason, it is generally advisable to measure the covariate at the onset of the research. If frequency of sexual intercourse as a covariate were measured after an education program in which frequency of intercourse and kind of contraceptive used were presented as related to UTI, you would hardly expect "clean," uncontaminated data for the covariate.

Interpreting ANCOVA

Essentially, ANCOVA asks, "Do the groups differ after the effects of the covariate are removed?" In computational terms, the first step in ANCOVA is like the first step in multiple regression, where the variability in the dependent measure that is shared by the covariate is removed. Then, ANOVA is performed on the residual scores of the dependent variable to see if group differences are present. Therefore, when a significant ANCOVA *F* ratio is interpreted, raw score group means must be adjusted to allow for the variance due to the covariate that has been partialed out.

Exhibit 20.5 presents a series of three ANOVA tables based on the same data. The fictitious example in Exhibit 20.5 was deliberately contrived so that a nonsignificant *F* ratio resulted from the one-way ANOVA (Table A) and a significant one resulted from the ANCOVA (Tables B and C). However, there is no reason why similar results cannot be obtained from a *well-conceptualized* ANCOVA design based on real data. Table B represents typical output from a computer run. As is apparent, there is a considerable amount of redundancy although there would be less if several independent variables and several covariates had been used, because the sources labeled *covariates* and *main effects* would be the sum of all the covariates and independent variables, respectively. The source labeled *explained*, moreover, is the sum of the covariate and main effect, and what remains, in this case misleadingly labeled *residual*, is error (or within). Table C in Exhibit 20.5 represents what you would actually present in a research report if space limitations allowed inclusion of the table. Some authors might even omit the sum of squares for the covariate and the *p*-value column because a reader could easily compute it given the other information.

Elsewhere on the computer printout is printed the correlation between the covariate and dependent variable, the grand mean, constants to be added or subtracted from the grand mean to yield adjusted group means, and miscellaneous nonessential information. In our example, the grand mean is 17.30, and the constant for group 1 (the pill) is $+5$, group 2 (condom, foam, or both) is -5, and group 3 (IUDs or diaphragms) is $+4$. Thus, the adjusted means are 22.3 for group 1, 12.3 for group 2, and 21.3 for group 3. To be perfectly safe, one can perform one of the post hoc group tests presented in Chapter 17 to establish a significant difference between adjusted means. Such tests would reveal that groups 1 and 2 as well as groups 2 and 3 are different. Interpretation of results is then undertaken.

Recall that results are interpreted with the caveat that "when effects due to the covariate are removed, . . ." Therefore, for our fictitious example, when the effects due to the frequency of sexual intercourse are removed, there exists a

Exhibit 20-5. Comparison of ANOVA and ANCOVA results.

(*a*)

Source	SS	df	MS	F	p
Between (Contraceptives)	550	2	275	.70	.8429
Error	22,300	57	391.22		
Total	22,850	59			

(*b*)

Source	SS	df	MS	F	p
Covariate	10,753	1	10,753	61.445*	.0001
Frequency	10,753	1	10,753	61.445*	.0001
Main effects	2,265	2	1,132.5	6.471	.0186
Contraceptives	2,265	2	1,132.5	6.471	.0186
Explained	13,018	3	4,439.34	25.376	
Residual (Error)	9,832	56	175		
Total	22,850	59			

(*c*)

Source	SS	df	MS	F	p
Covariate	10,753	1	—		—
Contraceptive	2,265	2	1,132.5	6.47	.0186
Error	9,832	56	175		
Total	22,850	59			

*While a significant F ratio for the covariate means it did indeed remove a significant amount of variance, it is ignored in a discussion of the research.

difference in the days per year with diagnosed UTI among users of different contraceptives. Those using either the pill, an IUD, or a diaphragm were infected more often than those using foam, condoms, or a combination of these. At this point you discuss design flaws and rival hypotheses, if any, and then draw conclusions. You might conclude that foam, condoms, or a combination of these *prevent* UTI. You can relate your findings to existing literature, if appropriate, and point out implications for practice and future research.

Power Analysis for ANCOVA

Power analysis for ANCOVA is conducted the same way as that for factorial ANOVA. Please consult that section of the factorial ANOVA discussion.

Other Multivariate Procedures

This book, of course, cannot possibly introduce all the various statistical procedures available to you. It can only whet your appetite and, most importantly, provide you with the basic concepts (e.g., mean, sums of squares, variance, linear correlation and regression, standard error, power) on which the more advanced and complex measures are based. As presented in the discussion of factorial ANOVA, whole courses are devoted to each of these procedures. Whole books are also. Therefore little can be done in this chapter except to name some of the other procedures and describe them so briefly that they may be done a disservice.

Before doing so, I wish to emphasize (1) the importance of your personally becoming acquainted with as many of these procedures as possible rather than relying on a statistician consultant for this and (2) that all statistical techniques be used only to support research in which their use is conceptually based in theory or empirical evidence. It is not uncommon for a researcher to fall in love with multiple regression or another procedure and then force-fit all her research into multiple regression designs, totally ignoring the theoretical underpinnings of the research topic that may call for, say, factorial ANCOVA designs. Let your research topic guide selection of your research designs. On the other hand, some leaders in the health professions believe that health researchers need only know their subject matter—which *does not* include a knowledge of statistical procedures at all. They argue that statistician consultants can be hired at the appropriate times to help in the design and analysis. The author believes this is rather short-sighted. No statistician can know your specialty area as well as you do. This consultant must be guided by what *you* impart about your research purpose, theoretical basis, and hypotheses, and therefore he or she can only suggest methods based on what you present. This may be acceptable in some cases, particularly if the topic area is well developed. However, research in health behavior is in its infancy. Theory is not highly developed and creativity is needed in developing designs to address emerging issues and questions. Therefore, only a researcher knowledgeable in both the statistical options available (although perhaps not all the fine points required for execution) and the literature related to a health specialty area will be in a position to develop creative, rather than mundane, designs that address the more complex (and interesting) questions arising from a more consumer and self-care oriented approach to health care delivery.

Finally, some statistical procedures are sophisticated indeed. And, if you enter data, a computer will grind through the numbers and give you output. However, your output is going to be only as good as the numbers or data you enter. If you have failed to meet assumptions or, more probably, the numbers you present are loaded with measurement error, the output you receive will be meaningless or, even worse, misleading or wrong. Pay special attention to the quality of your measures and demand excellence in instrument credentials. The operational definition of behavioral variables in health care is not nearly as well developed or sophisticated as the statistical design procedures that use these measures. Look at your raw data. Do they make sense? What is the observed range of scores and how are they distributed?

Factor Analysis

Factor analysis was first introduced in Chapter 13, in describing an approach to testing the construct validity of an instrument. It is a most useful procedure in measurement. It is also appropriate in some research settings. Briefly, factor analysis clusters a larger set of measures or items into a much smaller number of "factors," thereby reducing the number of variables being considered by combining those in the original set. About 25 subjects are required for each variable or item in the larger initial set, although as few as 15 have been used for pilot work. Whole courses and books are devoted to this topic, which relies heavily on correlation principles. There are spin-off procedures based on the same principles as factor analysis (e.g., principle components analysis), on which whole books and courses are also based.

Discriminant Analysis

Discriminant analysis was first mentioned in the discussion of multiple regression earlier in this chapter as an alternative to multiple regression when the criterion variable was at the nominal rather than the interval level of measurement. Essentially, it is used to predict (from a set of predictor variables) group membership, or to which category of a dependent variable an individual belongs. It could be very useful in health research where prediction of categoric, or even ordinal, outcomes is of interest.

Canonical Correlation

Have you ever wondered if there was a way to have more than one criterion variable in multiple regression? CANON, a shortened name for canonical correlation, allows just that. Essentially it correlates one set of variables with another set. Interpreting results in terms of the individual variables involved can be difficult, so learn more about this procedure before you base a design on it.

Multivariate Analysis of Variance (MANOVA)

What CANON does for multiple regression, MANOVA does for ANOVA. That is, in ANOVA or ANCOVA there is only one dependent variable. In MANOVA or MANCOVA, there are two or more dependent variables. If these multiple dependent variables can be defensible as a single composite score, more power is gained than when each dependent variable is subjected to a separate analysis. Multimodal compliance measures lend themselves to MANOVA when sample size is large enough.

Meta-analysis

Because large bodies of literature, particularly conflicting or ambiguous literature, develop around topical areas like patient education, weight control, patient compliance, and psychotherapy, an approach to integrating and making sense out of it has emerged. This is called meta-analysis. Briefly, the results presented in several hundred journal articles are systematically combined statistically to make a state-of-the-art statement about knowledge in the field. Some researchers initially view this as an easier approach than gathering their own data, because they are using data reported in journal articles. In the end most find that it is more work and effort. Therefore, let your research purpose be your guide. If you really wish to integrate a body of knowledge, meta-analysis is a handy tool. Do not confuse meta-analysis with *secondary analysis*, which involves subjecting someone else's quantitative data to additional statistical analysis in order to test new hypotheses.

O*ther Advanced Procedures*

These last two research procedures are really not multivariate or entirely quantitative. They are presented because they represent still other approaches to generating new knowledge about which you should be aware. Whole courses and books are devoted to each of the topics, also.

Ethnographic Methods

This broad group includes historical and anthropologic research that is non-quantitative in the sense that quantitative methods were presented in this book. It is sometimes called qualitative research. First described in Chapter 11, in the discussion of observational techniques, the ethnographic approach appears subjective rather than objective. This leads some to conclude erroneously that it is softer, easier, and less valuable than quantitative methods. This, of course, is far from the truth. Good ethnographic research requires the same rigor and objectivity found in quantitative research. To achieve it, even greater effort is required than with quantitative, because there is greater opportunity to become subjective and biased, thereby introducing error. For this reason, ethnographic researchers must have thorough training in the *easier* quantitative methods before attempting the qualitative.

Cluster Analysis

Cluster analysis groups subjects according to their profile of scores on a number of variables. (Of course, variables could be grouped also, but this is done less often.) To group subjects, you must consider whether your major interest is (1) the shape of the profile (e.g., body measurement proportions for wrist, bust, waist, hip, and ankle regardless of their absolute values) or (2) similarities in absolute values of scores, even if some are greater and others lesser than another subject in the cluster. In the first case, *correlational* clustering algorithms are used and in the second case *distance* clustering techniques are appropriate.

Many kinds of cluster analysis (e.g., hierarchical, iterative) are available. Because there are no inferential statistics or p values used, there are also no rigid rules. You could even have more variables than subjects. Because of the many approaches, some of which are questionable, and the absence of inferential rules, results of cluster analysis must always be cross-validated or replicated using different kinds of cluster analysis on the same data before they can be published. It is one of the most subjective of procedures, because you must decide via inspection of the computer printout how many clusters to use. There are as yet no significant tests to aid you. Nevertheless, this approach has wide applicability to health research and is among the least mathematically complex of the multivariate procedures.

Vocabulary

Analysis of crossbreaks	Main effects
ANCOVA	MANOVA
B weight	Meta-analysis
Backward elimination regression	Multicollinearity
Beta weight	Multiple correlation
Cannonical correlation	Multiple regression
Cell	Multivariate statistics
Cluster analysis	Observed scores
Covariate	One-way Pearson r
Criterion variable	Part correlation
Cross-validation	Partial correlation
Discriminant analysis	Partialed out
Effect size	Predicted scores
Ethnographic methods	Prediction equation
Factor analysis	Predictor variables
Factorial ANOVA	Residual
Family type I error	Sampling protocol
First order partial	Second order partial
Forward stepwise regression	Shrinkage of R
General solution regression	Spurious relationship
Homogeneity of regression	Standard error of B
Interaction effects	

Reference

1. Cohen, J. *Statistical Power Analysis for the Behavioral Sciences* (rev. ed.). New York: Academic, 1977.

VII: *Interpreting Results and Communicating Findings*

Chapters 21 and 22 help pull together all we have discussed so far. They do not have vocabulary words per se because they use those that have already been presented. Chapter 21 presents a series of research studies, which must be interpreted. You can try your hand at these and then look up the answers at the end of the chapter. Perhaps you can bring another study like those in this chapter to class.

Chapter 22 should be read in its entirety, because points made earlier in the chapter are not repeated, although they may equally apply to, say, theses as well as journal articles. Think about how you will communicate the results of the research you have undertaken. In addition, how might articles from a recent journal be converted into a poster?

21: *Interpreting Results*

Mary L. Wolfe

An instructor taught two sections of an undergraduate course in nursing research. One section met on Monday afternoons from 1 PM to 4 PM; the other section met on Friday mornings from 9 AM to noon. Friday's class met in a spacious, well-ventilated room, while Monday's class was crammed into quarters designed for a much smaller group. Analysis of data from the midterm examination scores of the two classes revealed that the Monday section's scores were, on the average, significantly lower than those of the Friday section. Monday's students did, in fact, complain that they felt that they were "packed in like sardines" and were sure they did not perform nearly as well as they were capable of doing. The instructor made a mental note to reserve a larger classroom for the final examination for the Monday section.

Clearly, the instructor based her decision on what she perceived to be a causal relationship between the crowded condition and subsequent discomfort of the Monday class and their relatively poor performance on the midterm examination. Although it is possible, indeed, that such a cause and effect relationship existed, there are several *plausible rival hypotheses,* or competing explanations, for the observed difference between the performances of the two classes. To begin with, all sections of the research course were given a common examination. Although instructors are generally quite careful to avoid any security leaks (and although students are generally conscientious about not transmitting information about examination questions to students in other sections) some leakage may be inevitable and probably quite unintentional. Students relaxing over a cola after a difficult examination are likely to blurt out remarks like, "I didn't think the last five questions were fair at all!" and then, with a little prompting, provide just enough cues to enable their peers who have yet to take the test to focus their studying more sharply, thus improving their chances for a better grade.

Cook and Campbell [1] would probably identify this phenomenon as a threat to internal validity known as *history*. The observed effect (the superior performance of Friday's class) may have been due to an event (the communication of information about some of the examination questions, followed by specific preparation by Friday's students for those questions) that is not related to the independent variable (classroom size). In laboratory research this threat is controlled by insulating respondents from outside influences; unfortunately, field researchers (which is what many of us are much of the time) do not have this luxury.

There is another rival hypothesis: students are likely to be much more alert in the morning than they are in the afternoon. It is possible that the Monday section had already taken one examination, or had spent the morning in a clinic, or had engaged in some other equally tiring activity. If, following the morning's activity, the students had eaten lunch, they probably felt more like taking a nap than an examination. *Maturation* (a threat to internal validity when an observed effect might be due to the respondents' growing older, wiser, or just more tired) is clearly a rival hypothesis in this instance.

Last but not least, this particular instructor had adopted a policy of giving students the option of taking the midterm and final examinations either with the section to which they were officially assigned or with the other section she taught. Thus, a Friday student might choose to take the examination with Monday's class, or vice versa. So, even though students were originally randomly assigned to sections in approximately equal numbers, at examination time there could have been a substantial influx of Monday's students into the Friday class. These students may have been more conscientious than usual and may have used the extra few days of studying time to carry out a really thorough review of the course material, thereby giving them an advantage over their classmates who took the examination at the regularly scheduled time. *Selection* is a threat to internal validity when an effect (better examination performance) may be due to the difference between the kinds of people in one group as opposed to another. The group taking the examination on Friday may have been better motivated, on the average, than the Monday group; and this difference was very likely reflected in better performance on the examination.

As professionals in the health care field, you will often read reports of research studies; in many of these studies, the researchers will attempt to demonstrate that a causal relationship exists between two or more variables. Sometimes these causal inferences are justified; however, more often than not, conclusions are drawn on the basis of studies that were improperly designed or data that have been inappropriately analyzed. If such is the case, there will be rival hypotheses, or competing explanations, for the observed effect, and one's confidence in the purported causal relationship among the relevant variables is diminished.

Research results (statistical tests, tables, graphs, and so on) must be *interpreted* in terms of the research design, the measures used to gather data, confounding variables, sampling, and generalization from the sample to the accessible population and from the accessible population to the target population. These results then yield *findings*—that is, modified results—from which conclusions can be drawn and implications made for practice and future research. This chapter focuses on interpreting research results to yield the actual findings of the researcher.

This chapter has been written for nursing students and practitioners who want to improve their ability to identify plausible rival hypotheses in research studies they read. It contains a series of exercises, each consisting of two parts. The first part is a summary of a research study and the conclusions drawn from it. Although the studies themselves are fictitious, they were each suggested by research actually carried out in real-life settings. In each case, there is at least one plausible rival hypothesis that may account for the effect observed by the researcher. Your assignment is to identify these errors in interpreting results.

The second part of each exercise consists of the solution. The solutions are placed at the end of the chapter in order to minimize the temptation to look at the answer before you have had a chance to figure it out on your own. Those of you who are interested in trying your hand at some more examples may want to read Huck and Sandler [2].

Research Examples

Problem 1: Math Anxiety

Facility in mathematics and statistics is assuming increasing importance in the health sciences, including nursing—an area traditionally regarded as "feminine." Quantitative competence, in fact, has been referred to as the "critical filter" that may determine the occupational mobility of workers in a number of fields. Although fear and dislike of mathematics and statistics are fairly prevalent among students of both sexes, studies show that women are more likely to be affected than men by these negative attitudes.

A study was conducted a few years ago involving 25 female nursing students enrolled in a beginning graduate course in descriptive and inferential statistics. A 20-item inventory was constructed to measure "statistics anxiety." The inventory consisted of the phrase "Whenever I think about studying statistics, I feel   ." followed by a series of adjectives, such as *tense, secure, nervous, comfortable,* and so on. Next to each adjective were five blank spaces in which students were asked to indicate, on a scale from 1 to 5, the extent to which each adjective described their feelings about statistics. The inventory was given to the students on the first day of class (the pretest) and again on the last day of class (the posttest) right after the final examination. A total statistics anxiety score was computed for each student on each testing occasion. Because of the small sample size, simple descriptive statistics (mean and standard deviation) were used to examine pretest-to-posttest changes in measured anxiety. Four students dropped the course before the end of the semester; thus, posttest anxiety was measured for only 21 students.

The researcher found a substantial decrease—nearly 10 scale points—in the mean anxiety score from the beginning to the end of the semester, and concluded that this effect was due to a sort of "desensitization" that had occurred during the semester. That is, having met the beast (statistics) and wrestled with it, more or less successfully, students no longer feared it quite as much.

The author's interpretation of her findings may well be correct. There is no doubt that repeated, gradual exposure to an aversive stimulus under supportive conditions often results in a reduction of its aversiveness. However, there may be an alternative explanation for the decrease in statistics anxiety from the beginning to the end of the semester. What is the most plausible rival hypothesis in this study?

Problem 2: A Little Intervention Goes a Long Way—or Does It?

Colleges and universities have been paying more attention recently to the necessity and importance of providing remediation in the basic skills—reading, writing, and computation. Many otherwise capable students fail to achieve a satisfactory level of performance in college courses because of deficiencies in those essential "tool" subjects. In fields such as nursing, in which critical shortages still exist, it is in the public interest for professional schools to make sure that students with the potential for productive careers are not lost because of correctable gaps in their linguistic or arithmetic competence.

A pilot study of the effectiveness of remedial mathematics workshops for senior nursing students was conducted a few years ago at a large eastern university. All sections of the nursing research course (an introduction to research design and statistics) were given a 25-item pretest of basic arithmetic and mathematics skills on the first day of class. Students who appeared to need remediation were identified and invited to attend a series of six math workshops covering such topics as the basic operations (addition, subtraction, multiplication, and division); fractions; negative numbers; decimals; exponents; and roots. Following the workshops, a posttest (an alternative form of the pretest) was given to all students in the nursing research course. Scores for those 20 students who attended the workshops showed a significant pretest-to-posttest gain; moreover, the mean gain scores for this group were significantly higher than the mean gain scores for the students who did not attend the workshops. The investigator concluded that the math workshops had a beneficial effect on students' basic computational skills and should be continued.

It is possible that the extra attention and effort expended on the small group of students needing remedial work did, indeed, pay off in terms of improved performance. However, there are at least three competing explanations for the results observed by the investigator. Can you identify them?

Problem 3: Out With the Old, In With the New

Ever since interest in adult education was aroused over half a century ago, much attention has been given to the differences between it and the education of the young. Various approaches to adult education have been used; the most common one makes a distinction between the characteristics of young and mature students. A common assumption is that the adult learner is self-directed, with a reservoir of experience that becomes a rich resource for learning.

Registered nurse (RN) students—students with a nursing diploma who are returning to school for a baccalaureate degree—are increasingly found in university-affiliated schools of nursing. These students generally fit the model of the adult learner. They vary widely in age and professional experience and usually have very different goals and needs than the young students fresh out of high school or junior college. These mature students, it is believed, should be encouraged to identify their own learning objectives, select appropriate educational experiences, and evaluate the outcomes of their own learning. The role of the faculty member is to serve as mentor or guide.

Some educators have been experimenting in the education of RN students using adult learning principles. At the school of nursing at a large midwestern university, a study was undertaken to see whether RN students could achieve nursing course clinical objectives in their own work setting without the presence of a clinical instructor. This approach was designated as the flexible clinical scheduling (FCS) approach. Sixty registered nurses participated in the study. They were taught by a total of six instructors in small groups ranging in size from ten to twelve. Within each group, approximately half the students elected to participate in the FCS program; the remaining students were enrolled in the traditional curriculum. All 60 students participated in large group sessions, clinical conferences, and individual instructor–student conferences. Each student spent 15 hours a week in a clinical setting providing nursing care to selected clients. At the end of each week, each student submitted nursing process records for each patient to the instructor responsible for his or her evaluation. These records served as the basis for the students' final achievement scores in the course. The critical feature distinguishing students in the FCS program from those in the traditional clinical curriculum was the absence of the instructor in the clinical setting.

At the end of the term, final achievement scores for the FCS and traditional groups were compared. The former was found to be significantly higher, on the average, than the latter. The researchers concluded that the FCS approach resulted in enhanced learning for RN students and recommended that it be implemented as a permanent feature of the curriculum. Can you think of at least one competing explanation for the apparent superiority of the experimental FCS approach?

Problem 4: Lullaby and Goodnight

The goal of the nurse responsible for giving care to the hospitalized aged should be to restore functional capacity to the point at which the elderly person can live in his environment with a minimum of dependency. An understanding of the aging central nervous system is essential, particularly when it comes to the administration of sleep medication. Many authorities feel that sleep medication for the aged should be given relatively early in the evening in order to give it time to act. Because the gastrointestinal absorption process in older people is slower, sleep medication takes effect more slowly than in a young person, and its effects may carry over into the morning. As a result, the elderly person's social behavior and functioning may be adversely affected.

An investigation of the effect of shifting the administration of sleep medication to an earlier time was conducted with 30 hospitalized patients between the ages of 65 and 90. A staff nurse who worked on the day shift rated the social behavior of each patient on a 10-point scale while the patient was getting sleep medication at the traditional time (between 9:30 PM and 10 PM). The patients were then given sleep medication at 8 PM for four consecutive evenings. The same nurse then repeated the social behavior assessment, using the same 10-point scale, on the morning following the fourth early administration of sleep medication. A correlated *t* test performed on the two sets of ratings showed a significant increase in social behavior scores following the shift to early administration of sleep medication. The researchers concluded that the shift was beneficial and recommended that early administration of sleep medication be implemented on a regular basis. Can you think of a rival hypothesis that could explain the observed improvement in social behavior?

Problem 5: Insulin Therapy and Wound Healing

Because of the increasing number of hospitalized elderly patients, most of whom have multiple health problems, decubitus ulcers—their prevention and treatment—are a major concern in nursing. Studies have shown that the topical application of insulin is of value in the healing of wounds, probably by facilitating the formation of collagen.

A pilot study was conducted to determine whether topical insulin therapy would facilitate the healing of decubitus ulcers. The subjects were residents of a nursing home who had a variety of medical problems and who had developed one or more decubiti within 2 weeks of participation in the study. Twenty subjects ranging in age from 40 to 95 were randomly assigned to experimental and control groups. The mean age for experimental subjects was 60.0; for control subjects, 85.2.

A pretest-posttest control group design was used. All subjects in both groups received routine supportive nursing care from the staff; in addition, subjects in the experimental group received insulin therapy twice daily for two weeks right after the morning and evening meals. Healing rate was operationally defined as the amount of decrease in the area of the ulcer per day. Statistical analysis showed that the healing rate for patients in the experimental group was significantly higher than that for the control group, and the researchers concluded that topical application of insulin was effective. Do you agree, or do you think there is another explanation for the observed effect?

Problem 6: Sex and the Mentally Handicapped

The fears surrounding marriage and procreation in mentally retarded persons have created uncertainty among professionals as to the advisability of providing any form of sex education to them. However, physical sexual development occurs in the majority of the mentally handicapped, and they need to learn how to handle heterosexual relationships. Indeed, the retarded need more help than do normal individuals in understanding themselves and their bodies.

Nurses and other health professionals may be called upon to provide counseling in all areas of sexual behavior. Attitudes toward sexuality may be of particular importance in assessing the readiness of the nurse to take an active role in providing the guidance the retarded need to make informed decisions regarding marriage, contraception, and parenthood.

In a study involving 100 respondents randomly selected from the population of all senior nursing students at a large eastern university, attitudes toward various aspects of sexuality in the mentally retarded were examined. A 26-item Likert scale assessing attitudes toward dating, sexual education, contraception, marriage, reproduction, and voluntary sterilization was administered to the sample. Analysis of the data revealed that the respondents agreed that the mentally retarded should date, be provided with sex education, and be permitted to marry. However, contraception and sterilization—even voluntary sterilization—were looked on with disfavor. The researchers concluded that the nursing students are likely to be negatively biased toward such issues as contraception and sterilization in the retarded and thus may not provide the impartial guidance that these handicapped clients need. Do you agree with this conclusion?

Problem 7: This Hurts Me More Than It Hurts You

Patients' emotional reactions to certain procedures in health care processes compose a major area of concern for practicing nurses and nurse researchers. A number of studies have suggested that nursing interventions aimed at meeting patients' emotional needs reduce patient anxiety. Some of these studies have investigated the relationships between cognitive processes and anxiety, with results indicating that emotional responses can in fact be altered by cognitive restructuring. These studies have led to the hypothesis that a lack of congruence between expected and experienced sensations during a threatening event lead to increased stress and anxiety in the patient. If this is the case, then nursing intervention aimed at reducing that lack of congruence should result in greater psychological and physical comfort for the patient.

In a study involving adolescent females, researchers hypothesized that discrepancies between expected and experienced physical sensations during a pelvic examination would result in distress. Fifteen patients between the ages of 12 and 17, none of whom had previously undergone a pelvic examination, were randomly assigned in equal numbers to three groups: a control group that was given no information about the procedure; a group that was given factual information about the procedure (that is, the various steps were described), and a group that was given information about the physical sensations that could be expected during the procedure. Patients were observed by the researcher for behavioral signs of distress during the pelvic examination and were rated on a three-point scale, with 1 indicating no signs of distress, 2 indicating minor distress, and 3 indicating major distress. One-way analysis of variance (ANOVA) showed no significant differences among the three groups, and the researchers concluded that providing information about the procedures or sensations involved in a pelvic examination did not alter the patients' experience of distress. Do you agree?

Problem 8: Problem 7 Revisited

The researchers who conducted the study described in Problem 7 were a conscientious group and took the criticisms outlined in the solution to Problem 7 to heart. They obtained a modest grant, which enabled them to develop a reliable and valid 50-item measure of patient distress and to replicate their study with a convenience sample of 600 Hispanic adolescent female patients. Once again, patients were randomly assigned to the treatment conditions outlined in Problem 7, and measures of distress were obtained on each patient. ANOVA, followed by appropriate post hoc tests, showed that there were significant differences among the groups. The "sensory information" group had the lowest distress score, with a mean of 20.3, while the control group had the highest distress score, with a mean of 22.3. The researchers recommended that health care practitioners responsible for giving first-time pelvic examinations to adolescent girls routinely provide detailed information about the physical sensations to be expected, thereby alleviating the distress that accompanies such examinations. Do you agree?

Solutions

Solution to Problem 1: Math Anxiety

The most plausible rival hypothesis associated with this study is *mortality*. This term does not mean the literal death of any of the students participating in the research. Rather, it refers to the fact that subject dropout between the pretest and posttest may make it appear that the independent variable (exposure to a semester of statistics) was effective in reducing anxiety, when it really was not. The four students who dropped the course did so because they were having unusual difficulty with it. Had they struck it out until the bitter end, their responses might have substantially altered the pretest-to-posttest change pattern. A somewhat stronger research design would have resulted if the investigator had also given the anxiety inventory to a comparison group—perhaps one similar to her own class in size and relevant demographic characteristics but taking a course in a subject less threatening than statistics.

Solution to Problem 2: A Little Intervention Goes a Long Way—or Does It?

The most obvious rival hypothesis in this study is *regression*. Remember, regression is a purely statistical effect whereby a group selected on the basis of extremely low or high scores on some measure will tend to have less extreme scores when tested again on the same measure or one related to it. The 20 students who attended the math workshops had, on the average, much lower scores on the basic math skills pretest than did those who did not attend. Even if they had not attended any of the workshops (or if the workshops had been ineffective) their scores on the posttest would, on the average, have shown some improvement.

Another possible explanation for the apparent effectiveness of the math workshops is the phenomenon known as *testing* (that is, the effect of taking a pretest on posttest scores). There is usually a gain of a few points when the same test, or an alternate form of it, is taken on a second testing occasion. The students who did poorly on the pretest may have been so concerned about their performance that they did some brushing up on their own before the posttest, which could have accounted for their improved performance.

A third possible explanation for the observed result is *selection*: the bias in the method for obtaining comparison groups. Students were *invited,* not required, to attend the math workshops; it is possible that the 20 students who did attend were especially highly motivated to improve their computational skills.

The fact that the average pretest-to-posttest gain scores for this group of students were significantly higher than those for students who did not attend the workshops could simply have been because of the fact that the former group tried a lot harder than the latter.

The study could have been improved somewhat by using a pretest-posttest control group design. Those students in need of remediation would be randomly assigned to experimental (workshop) and control (no workshop) groups. If the workshops proved to be effective, the control group could have been given the opportunity to participate later on during the semester.

Even with this design, the possible reactivity of the pretest remains a problem. However, because the pretest is necessary in order to identify those students who need the treatment, we will simply have to learn to live with it. In the real world, it is rarely possible to resolve all of our research design dilemmas at once!

Solution to Problem 3: Out With the Old, In With the New

The most obvious competing explanation for the superior performance of students in the FCS program is *selection*. Recall, students *chose* this curriculum; chances are that these RNs were, to begin with, better motivated, more self-directed, and more venturesome than those choosing the more conventional curriculum. That being the case, their nursing process records were probably more detailed, more perceptive, and generally better written, resulting in higher final achievement scores.

Another possible explanation for the observed difference is *history*. Extraneous events occurring during the course of the semester might have contributed to the apparent enhanced learning of students in the FCS program. Bear in mind that these students were fulfilling their clinical course requirements in their own work settings without the presence of a clinical instructor. The researcher could not have exerted any sort of control over the environment of these students, or over their activities, in these settings. It is possible that the FCS students' milieu may have been richer in learning experiences than that to which the students in the traditional curriculum were exposed.

The study would have been somewhat improved by randomly assigning students to the flexible and traditional curricula; this approach would have controlled for selection bias. History, unfortunately, would remain an uncontrolled threat to internal validity, because the essential feature of the experiment—the absence of the clinical instructor in the work setting for the FCS students— would make it impossible to rule out those extraneous influences that would be likely to affect learning during the course of the semester.

Solution to Problem 4: Lullaby and Goodnight

Although the one-group pretest-posttest design used in this study is usually chock-full of threats to internal validity, the most obvious threat is undoubtedly instrumentation; that is, changes in the measuring device during its use, resulting in different scores for equivalent characteristics. The measuring device may be a paper and pencil tool or a human observer (in this case, the staff nurse who rated the elderly patients' social behavior before and after the treatment). In the latter case, the observer may improve with practice, with the result that subsequent observations are actually made with a different "instrument," so to speak. A check on intrarater reliability should help to reduce the likelihood of this threat to internal validity.

Another possible explanation for the observed improvement in social behavior is experimenter bias. Despite the best of intentions, most of us who do research in health care have a strong desire to demonstrate that a particular intervention *actually works*! This strong desire may result in an often unconscious bias in our observations. Experimenter bias can be minimized by training others to act as observers and data collectors and by keeping them in the dark about the expected outcome of the research.

Solution to Problem 5: Insulin Therapy and Wound Healing

The flaw in this study is not due to faulty design as such; rather, it demonstrates quite dramatically that random assignment to comparison groups does not *guarantee* that those groups will be equivalent on all relevant variables prior to treatment. The two groups differed significantly in age, a variable known to be related to the rate of wound healing. The experimental group, with a mean age of 60.0, would be likely to have a faster rate of healing than the control group, with a mean age of 85.2, even in the absence of treatment. Analysis of covariance (ANCOVA), a statistical procedure that provides some measure of control for pretreatment differences, would have strengthened this study. Age would, of course, be the covariate of choice.

Solution to Problem 6: Sex and the Mentally Handicapped

It is possible that nursing students in general, by virtue of their special training, have a particular reverence for human life—even potential human life—and thus may be more likely to regard contraception and sterilization as unwarranted interference in the sexual lives of the mentally retarded. In this particular study, examination of the demographic data revealed that 40 percent of the students in the sample were members of the Roman Catholic church. Given that church's traditional opposition to any artificial form of birth control, it is not surprising that contraception and sterilization were looked on with disfavor.

The researchers, in interpreting the results of their study, have made the rather common error of generalizing from the *study population* (all senior nursing students at a particular school) to the *target population* (nursing students in general). It is possible that entirely different results would be obtained with samples of students drawn from institutions located in the midwest, the far west, or the deep south. The study should, in fact, be replicated with samples of students from a variety of geographic regions before any conclusions can be drawn about nursing students' biases about contraception and sterilization in the mentally retarded.

Solution to Problem 7: This Hurts Me More Than It Hurts You

One major problem with this study has to do with the issue of statistical conclusion validity: Is the procedure used to test the hypothesis sensitive enough, or powerful enough, to detect relationships among the variables of interest? The power of an inferential procedure is the likelihood of detecting an effect, or relationship, that is "really there" in the population from which the samples were drawn. Power is influenced by several factors, such as the actual magnitude of the effect, the significance level chosen by the researcher, and the sample size. It is the last of these factors that should cause concern in this study. Other things being equal, the larger the samples, the more powerful the test. For example, if providing information about the physical sensations to be expected during a pelvic examination really does reduce the distress experienced by the patient undergoing the examination, the researcher has a better chance of detecting this effect with larger comparison groups. Had the researchers in this study determined the power of their statistical procedures, they would have found that the probability of committing a type II error (that is, of retaining a false null hypothesis) was relatively large owing to the small samples involved in their study. A power analysis to determine the sample size required for detecting an effect of a given magnitude would enable the researchers to redesign their study in the hope that it would result in a more powerful test of the research hypothesis.

Another threat to statistical conclusion validity is posed by the dependent measure—the three-point scale used to assess patient distress. Measures with low reliability cannot be counted on to indicate true differences, and a single measure with only three scale points is almost guaranteed to have low reliability. The researchers could improve the reliability of their distress index by developing a scale with a number of items, rather than just a single item, and constructing each item so that it involves a five- or seven-point rather than a three-point scale.

Finally, the researchers provide us with no information about the validity of their distress measure—that is, how certain can you be that behavioral observations of apparent distress actually measure distress? Multiple measures of distress—behavioral, physiological, and psychological—should be used and tested to see whether they intercorrelate to an acceptable degree.

Solution to Problem 8: Problem 7 Revisited

In the solution to Problem 7, it was pointed out that very small sample sizes may result in failing to reject a null hypothesis when it should have been rejected. The other side of the coin, so to speak, is the fact that very small effects will be statistically significant, given large enough samples. The researchers, in replicating their study, are to be commended for their diligence in refining their measure of distress and replicating their study with a large sample. However, from a purely practical point of view, one must question whether a decrease of 2.0 scale points on a 50-point distress scale, although statistically significant, is really large enough to warrant the increased cost in terms of staff time and effort that would result if the recommended treatment were implemented. The authors should reexamine their independent variable and determine whether there were problems with its operational definition or its implementation that could have resulted in such small differences in distress scores.

An additional problem lies in the fact that the sample of 600 Hispanic adolescent females was quite clearly a convenience sample, and as such, hardly representative of adolescent females in general. The research design, although internally valid, lacked *external validity:* any cause and effect relationship inferred from the significant differences between the groups' distress scores could not be generalized beyond the particular sample in which it was observed.

The authors would be well advised to identify a study population that is as representative as possible of the target population of, say, adolescents in the United States. Stratified random sampling, followed by random assignment to treatment groups, would permit them to generalize the results they observed beyond the sample itself and would justify their recommendations that treatment, if found effective, should be implemented routinely.

References

1. Cook, T. D., and Campbell, D. T. *Quasi-Experimentation: Design and Analysis Issues for Field Settings.* Chicago: Rand McNally, 1979.
2. Huck, S. W., and Sandler, H. M. *Rival Hypotheses: Alternative Interpretations of Data Based Conclusions.* New York: Harper & Row, 1979.

Communicating the findings of research to others is a vital link in the research process. If communication is missing, there really is little reason to have done the research. This becomes apparent each time you search the literature to gain greater insights into your research topic. If others had not communicated their findings, you would have no literature to review. Basically, communication to other researchers and experts in your topic area takes the form of journal articles and oral or visual presentations at professional meetings. For students, it might also involve a written thesis. These are the four kinds of communications that are discussed in this chapter.

There are two other kinds of communication, however, which should not be overlooked. One is a final or technical report to a funding agency. This tends to resemble a thesis more than a journal article because of its length and the detail that is included. Its nature and format usually are determined by the funding agent, who spells out exactly what must be included. The other kind of communication involves speeches and articles in popular journals or magazines for lay audiences who are also interested in research findings. There is more variety than similarity in this category, so it is difficult to make generalizations regarding its composition and format. This category is often overlooked by researchers who do not consider it scholarly or a candidate for inclusion in their vitae or resumes. This is unfortunate, because it may be the most effective means of achieving implementation of research findings in the clinical or practice setting.

If you have never communicated the findings of research and are seeking an easy recipe for doing so, you will be disappointed. Success in this area is partly art, and it depends on your skills not only as a researcher, but also as a writer and a storyteller. As with most things, it takes practice. The first thing to do is to find examples of successful communications and study them, carefully considering the content, format, and style. For example, as you search the literature, identify journals publishing articles in your content area. Study the various articles and read the manuscript requirements for each journal. These requirements are usually printed near the inside of either the front or back cover. Decide for which journal you will write your article. Then, study several issues of the journal more closely. What percentage of space, on the average, is devoted to a literature review or to the discussion of results? In what style are references presented (e.g., American Psychological Association [1]; Turabian [8]; University of Chicago [9])? Look very closely at figures and tables. Begin by constructing similar figures and tables for your article. Then develop an outline of the major sections of your article, based on the kinds of subtopics generally found in the articles you are studying and modify it to fit your topic. Under each section jot down the main points and relevant information you wish to include. You are now ready to write. Begin writing to get your ideas on paper quickly. Do not worry about spelling or punctuation or choosing just the right word. This comes later when you edit and polish your copy. Once a rough draft is written, your hardest work is over. It is much easier to edit and modify than it is to generate new material. After you have polished your product, give it for critiquing to someone else, preferably someone who has already published and definitely someone who will not fear giving you negative feedback. With this information, rewrite. You can then either have someone else critique it or submit it to the journal. You must be the judge—again.

Journal Articles

Journal articles are generally divided into four major parts: introduction, method, results, and discussion. Most also have an abstract, which precedes the actual article. Some nursing journals add a fifth part, a review of literature (or theoretical framework), which comes after the introduction and before the method. This, presumably, is because of the current emphasis on theory development in nursing and the perceived need of some reviewers for detailed linkage of your research to that preceding it, thereby building a nomological network as a percursor to full-blown theory. The practice of including extensive literature reviews is becoming less prevalent, however, as research becomes more sophisticated and printing costs mount. In other journals, readers are presumed to know the literature and the network of interrelationships among variables, so that only a brief overview of the literature (i.e., involving citations of three to eight of the most relevant studies) is included in the introduction. There are still other journals, particularly in medicine, that have little or no literature review in the introduction and, instead, introduce other research as part of the discussion when it relates to a result of the study being reported. Thus, it is important to study articles in the journal to which you will submit your manuscript to determine the appropriate format.

Unlike a thesis, a journal article must be as brief as possible while still providing enough information for readers to replicate the research if desired. Printing costs are astronomic and unnecessary words and tables are unaffordable. A very helpful guide to concise writing is *Why Not Say It Clearly* by L. King [6]. To keep length down while still providing sufficient detail, researchers who are using new instruments often either use a footnote to indicate that copies of a measure are available from the author or incorporate the items into a table presenting results (e.g., item means and standard deviations, item means for each of two or more subgroups). Sometimes additional tables are made available from the author.*

Introduction

The introduction to an article states the problem area and presents evidence that your research met the so-what test. It tells how your research contributes to a

---

*There are journals that expect an author to pay for the printing of tables. This should be indicated in the journal's manuscript requirements.

solution of the problem and presents the logic or theory that led to your hypotheses or research questions. This logic or theory usually, but not always, includes references to other research. As indicated in Chapter 1, it might be based on clinical practice.

Once the rationale for and purpose of your question(s) have been provided, research literature is presented that has already shed some light on your questions. Do not cite all studies you have reviewed. Only those with direct bearing on your research questions are appropriate. Each study is critiqued in such a manner as to demonstrate the strengths you have replicated and the weaknesses you have not. You may need to justify replicating weaknesses or failing to replicate strengths found in these studies. Finally, any important assumptions on which your research was based should be presented.

Some journal editors like to have the introduction end with statements of the hypotheses or research questions that guided the research. It should be readily apparent to the reader at this point why these particular questions were researched and in what way their answers will contribute to new knowledge and the problem area being studied. Their appearance here should be the logical outcome of the introductory material.

Method

This section is considerably easier to write than the introduction or discussion. For anyone experiencing writer's block, this may be the place to begin writing. Once a flow of words has begun, the section can easily be completed and the writer can return to the introduction.

The method section should be as brief as possible while still allowing sufficient detail for replication. It generally includes at least three subsections: sample, instrumentation, and procedures. It begins with two or three sentences presenting an overview of the design (e.g., experimental, correlational), kind of subjects (e.g., nursing students, children hospitalized for tonsillectomies), and measures of research variables. The ordering of the three subheadings is sometimes changed to describe the research better (e.g., complex experimental designs may require presentation of the procedures section first).

Sample

The sample section describes the number of subjects and how they were solicited, the sampling method used, and the study population. Methods for obtaining informed consent can be presented here or in the procedures section, depending on whether or not consent was given prior to or at the time the research design was executed. Selected demographic characteristics of subjects are presented. The number refusing to participate and their reasons, if available, should also be given. For example, if seven of ten institutions approached refused your research, it should be reported here. Are the three who cooperated different from the other seven? Sometimes comparison of response rates with known standards are made, particularly if large deviations from norms occurred in the study.

Instrumentation

This section describes how all research variables were operationally defined and, in some cases, your reasons for doing so. It also presents the credentials of each instrument, including reliability and validity data based on this research sample. Depending on the journal, some researchers may present correlations between measures here, particularly if multimodal measurement was used.

Instruments should be discussed in some detail. The number and nature of items on a scale or categories of an observation code would be presented. Sample items or categories of unfamiliar instruments might be included if the entire measure cannot be parsimoniously worked into a table. The time it took subjects to complete scales and the manner in which they responded (e.g., one-to-one, take-home) might be included.

Procedures

This section describes the research design in "living color." If the design is complex, a figure might be included as a graphic presentation on which to base the textual discussion. All events to which subjects were exposed must be presented, including those that were unanticipated. Possible rival hypotheses that actually occurred should be reported. A timetable of events might be appropriate for more complex designs.

Researchers often forget a very important part of the procedures section or describe it inadequately. This is the operational definition of the independent or experimental variable. Remember, enough detail must be provided so that replication is possible. If it is not, the reader may well wonder if the independent variable remained the same for all subjects. Evidence of its reliability, if appropriate, may also be presented in this section.

And, the time and setting in which the research occurred may be described. The location, environmental factors, and even travel distances for subjects might be reported, if appropriate.

Results

Before beginning to write the results section, the researcher is well advised to develop in tabular form the results to be included. Not all results will be presented, of course. Now that computers are available, researchers often run additional analyses besides those called for by the hypotheses. If they are earth-shattering, they may become the core of a separate article. If not, they are rarely included in an article testing other hypotheses unless they also relate to the purpose in some very relevant way. It is in this section that beginning researchers make their worst mistake—including too many data.

The results section usually begins with a description of how the data were analyzed statistically. The results of these analyses are then presented, including means and standard deviations of each measure. This section can be very short when only one research question or hypothesis is addressed. Then again, with surveys or designs yielding large amounts of nominal level data, the results can encompass many tables. When you have voluminous data to present, it is appropriate to consult other articles in the journal to observe how many tables are generally included and the methods for handling large amounts of data that were used by other authors in the journal.

Typically (but not always), this section presents results without comment. Interpretation is reserved for the discussion section.

Discussion

The discussion section pulls it all together. It is the final act and, as such, should relate back to the introductory material to confirm or disaffirm it. The two must flow together. Basically, the results are explored in terms of the limitations of the study and the presence of any rival hypotheses. Given these, the hypotheses or research questions are then addressed. Finally, these findings are amplified by comparison with the research presented in the introduction and implications for practice (or theory) and further research are presented. In essence, you describe how this study has advanced knowledge and speculate about where to go from there.

This section is the most difficult to write, because it allows interpretation and speculation by the author. Having adhered to facts and nothing but the facts for the rest of the article, you may find it difficult to let loose and speculate, especially because peer readers will not hesitate to disagree.

In conclusion, the entire article centers around the purpose or hypotheses of the study. Any material that does not relate to the purpose weakens the article. It is not uncommon for first drafts of an article to proceed without much problem through about one-third of the discussion, at which point only tangentially related material is launched with vigor and explored to the end of the article. The reader is then left with a vague feeling that a major point was never made.

Abstract

The abstract actually precedes your article, but it is best written last. There are usually word limitations placed on the abstract. As concisely as possible, state the purpose of the study, hypotheses or research questions tested, method used, results, and conclusions.

Theses

Almost everything presented in the previous section applies to theses, with the exception of brevity. The classical thesis, which is what is described here, is very repetitious and inclusive of a fair amount of tangential material. This is apparent when one observes how easily a 100-page thesis can be converted to a 10-page or shorter journal article. That is, however, the way things are, and there is a reason for this. It centers around the fact that the thesis is the scholarly treatise a student presents as evidence of obtained knowledge and expertise. It is the final product of course work and, if accepted, facilitates earning of an academic degree. Therefore, evidence of expertise in related areas is presented along with the crucial material relating directly to the purpose.

Like journal articles, theses come with a variety of subtle (and sometimes not so subtle) differences. With articles, the format depends largely on the journal policy and somewhat on the preferences of the editor. With theses, the format depends largely upon your thesis chairperson and somewhat on the rest of the committee. If you have chosen your committee intelligently (i.e., by selecting a chairperson who is known to be helpful and effective and then allowing the chairperson to strongly influence committee membership), the format for your thesis should not be difficult to determine. Committee members usually defer to the chairperson's wishes. A good approach is to ask your committee for copies of theses that are worthy of emulation.

This discussion, like that for journal articles, does not pretend to present the components of a thesis as carved in stone. They can easily vary according to the topic of your research as well as your committee's wishes. To begin with, theses usually (but not always) have five chapters as well as an abstract:

Chapter 1: Introduction
Chapter 2: Review of related literature
Chapter 3: Methodology
Chapter 4: Results
Chapter 5: Discussion, conclusions, and interpretation of results

In the classical thesis, each chapter begins with an introductory paragraph describing the purpose of the study in one or two sentences and what will be presented in that chapter. Each chapter ends, moreover, with a full summary of what was presented in the chapter, a brief review of what was presented in previous chapters, and a brief overview of what will be presented in the following chapters. Perhaps this practice evolved in order to help absent-minded professors. At any rate, when the reader finishes the thesis, there is little doubt that the purpose and major components will be forgotten.

Most colleges and universities publish a thesis style manual, which describes how references and footnotes are written, the inclusion and ordering of the preface, author's vita, table of contents, appendices, width of margins, the appropriate kind of paper, and so forth. Follow this exactly. Do not let a comma or column be out of place. Part of writing a thesis involves, apparently, self-discipline and following directions. Be creative in your thinking and the design of your research. It is unwise to be creative with footnote style or column width. A successful scholar knows when to conform.

Chapter 1: Introduction

The introduction begins with an introductory paragraph like that of an article. It goes on to include many of the following subheadings in varying order depending on the nature of the research: (1) statement of the problem area, (2) purpose of the study, (3) theoretical background and/or rationale (or theoretical considerations), (4) significance of the study, (5) hypotheses or research questions, (6) definition of terms, (7) assumptions of the study, and, of course, (7) summary.

Statement of the Problem Area

This section presents the problem area in a social context. It demonstrates that there indeed is a need for your research. For example, if you are studying patient compliance among diabetics, you would discuss the extent of noncompliance in the population and its ramifications in terms of the nation's health and the health care system. Economic costs as well as human costs might be cited. The unique aspects of noncompliance among diabetics would also be presented.

Purpose of the Study

This section tells just what you investigated. It is, essentially, your hypotheses or research questions presented in a different form. It should be clear, at this point, how your purpose relates to the larger problem area. In other words, you are describing the piece of the problem area you took for further study.

Theoretical Background and Rationale

This section describes the logic, evidence, and theory that led you to hypothesize relationships as you have. In essence, you observed an important problem area, studied theory that purports to explain the phenomenon under scrutiny, and, based on this theory, generated research hypotheses. Sometimes rival theories exist. In this case, your purpose may be to find out which one can be supported by your research. In other cases, there may be no theory at all—only a series of research findings, beliefs of experts, and your educated guesses based on your own clinical experience as a professional. In this event, this section may be labeled *Theoretical Considerations*. It would present the various pieces of evidence or speculation as well as the logical links among them that led to your hypothesis. You would be creating your own nomological network.

Significance of the Study

How your study will enhance practice is the primary focus of this section. It also shows how this research contributes to the problem area presented earlier in the chapter. If your research is more basic, the benefits to future research may be cited. This section lays the groundwork for the implications for practice section in Chapter 5 of the thesis.

Hypotheses or Research Questions

This section formally presents the research hypotheses or questions that guide the research.

Definition of Terms

Any terms used in the hypotheses that may have more than a single definition should be included here to avoid any misunderstandings. Although I do not advocate it, some committees like not only to have almost every variable defined, regardless of need, but also the operational definition of each variable presented in a sentence or two. It is wise to discuss with your committee which definitions are needed and whether or not operational definitions should also be mentioned.

Assumptions of the Study

Some committees like to include obvious assumptions, such as that the subjects answer truthfully and the sample is repesentative of the study and target populations. Others handle them under limitations or ignore them. Most reserve this section for more unique assumptions; for instance, if patient compliance is being studied, assumptions might be (1) compliance to the therapeutic regimen results in improved health or (2) the disease is in a stable state so that the appearance of noncompliance is not the result of disease instability. It is sometimes prudent to gather data or evidence from which to infer that your assumptions are based in fact. When doing so, you usually present the evidence along with the assumption. Furthermore, because assumptions often undergird theory, or vice versa, a clear presentation of the theory can provide evidence for the assumptions.

Chapter 2: Review of Related Literature

Unlike journal articles, a thesis has a review of literature that includes tangentially related areas. Therefore, the chapter is divided according to various content subtopics of your problem area. For example, in a study relating adolescent attitudes and knowledge about contraception with contraceptive practice, Ashton [2] divided her review of literature into research related to (1) adolescent cognitive development, (2) sexual development and sexuality, (3) sexual knowledge and sexuality, and (4) contraceptive practice. In a different study, which focused on the patient-provider relationship as it correlated with patient compliance, Davis [3] divided her review of the compliance research literature according to (1) the relationship between patient and provider, (2) provider style as nonauthoritarian or authoritarian, (3) the matching of patient and provider style preferences, and (4) current research emphasis. In still another study, Walleck [10], when investigating the effects of purposeful touch on intracranial pressure, reviewed (1) touch, (2) studies on the meaning of touch, and (3) touching behaviors and intracranial pressure.

As a rule, this chapter includes research literature rather than essays by experts. If some of these essays must be included, they should be kept to a minimum unless the nature of your thesis is different from the usual research study in which hypotheses are tested. In one such unusual thesis, Stephens [7] tested the reliability and some aspects of the validity of a newly developed multidimensional scale to assess biopsychosocial system functioning as described by a specific theory of human development. The entire review of literature, therefore, centered around presentation of the theory, which is complex and not particularly well known. The subsections of Chapter 2 were (1) historical development of the theory, (2) characteristics of the systems, (3) transitions from one system to another, (4) open, closed, and arrested system functioning, (5) applications and tests of the theory, (6) comparison to other theories, (7) state of the art in assessing biopsychosocial systems, and (8) summary.

It is especially important, early in the production of a thesis, to meet with your committee to decide the nature of Chapter 2. It is particularly important for everyone to set and agree on limits about how much literature will be reviewed, because it could be virtually endless. For example, if your topical area is stress, you might limit your review of research to human subjects, thereby ignoring animal research. Moreover, except for very famous or classic studies, most reviews are limited in the number of years back the coverage extends. Generally it is between 3 and 10 years—usually 5. Your search of the literature usually involves several computerized information retrieval systems for published research and other indices designed to reference work in progress (see Appendix II). If you and your committee can agree on which ones you will use (and others you will not be expected to use), and if the number of years backward is determined, the end is in sight.

When there is an extensive body of literature in an area, it is sometimes helpful to make charts or tables to summarize all work and then present in the text only the more relevant studies. If your committee agrees and you are interested in this approach, you may wish to observe how this was accomplished in the Haynes, Taylor, and Sackett [4] book on patient compliance and in the Haynes and Wilson [5] book on behavioral assessment. If these seem complex, remember that anything can be handled if approached systematically. Exhibit 22.1 presents one version of a standardized form that might be completed as each relevant study is reviewed. After your review is completed, these sheets can be sorted according to whatever subcategories you are using and ordered even further, say, according to when they will be presented.

The literature review should have a point of view. There is nothing worse than a lengthy narrative that simply describes the findings, sample, and sometimes design of a series of studies without one interpretative or reflective remark from the author. The thesis review of literature demonstrates what a magnificent scholar you are. A thoughtful and thorough review in which strengths and weaknesses of previous work are *diplomatically* presented is impressive. Moreover, you should use the strengths and weaknesses of other research when you design yours. That is, as you review studies with obvious weaknesses, point out how you overcame them in your research. As you present strengths, point out how you emulated them. In addition, do not forget to present a good rationale for not emulating strengths or improving on weakness in the research you reviewed.

It is, of course, very important to acknowledge the contributions of others to your topic area. Therefore, you should show the logical continuity of content (findings) between previous work and yours. A point of view might be that the series of studies complement each other with respect to covering design flaws but are limited to a specific target population. You are focusing on a different

---

Exhibit 22-1. Review form for research articles.

Bibliographic Citation:

Purpose or Hypotheses: (Underline measured variables)

Design and Procedure: (Define independent variable, if any)

Sample: n = _____ Sampling Method: _____
   Characteristics:

Instrumentation: (Measures and their credentials)

Statistical Procedures:

Findings: (Include ES or values of test statistics, *df,* and correlations)

Unique Aspects:

Strengths:

Weaknesses:

Conclusions: (You can live with)

---

target population. Another point of view may be weakness in measures or conflicting results. Perhaps the conflicting results can be accounted for by something that your research considers.

Another point of view might be that correlations between the variables being studied have been weak in previous research studies. These studies, however, did not control certain confounding variables you believe were present. Present your evidence for this as you review the studies. Note how none considered this and say you are going to do just that. To find your point of view, reflect on all the studies you have reviewed. What can you conclude from them? Perhaps they simply point out the need for your research. Why and in what way?

In conclusion, it should be obvious from the preceding discussion that your review of literature must be completed before your research is implemented. Not only does it save you work at a time when you are busy with data analysis, it prevents errors in your design that can be avoided when you have read certain articles earlier. Literature published after your research begins, on the other hand, must also be included. However, it is obvious your design could not have benefited from it. These studies, if any, are therefore usually introduced in the discussion in Chapter 5 as, "In an interesting study published after this research began, so-and-so (198*X*) found . . ." These new findings can then be incorporated into the discussion that leads to the conclusion and implications for practice and future research.

Chapter 3: Methodology

Except for the minor additions like the introductory paragraph and summary, this chapter includes the same material presented as the method section of a journal article. Sometimes a subsection on setting is separated out from the procedures section. Moreover, copies of all instruments are provided as an appendix, which is cited in the instrumentation section. In addition, another section, limitations of the study, is added when appropriate. Although some committees prefer that the limitations be presented in Chapter 1, it seems more logical to present them after the methodology has been discussed, because the limitations generally deal with design or sampling (i.e., construct validity) problems.

The first three chapters usually constitute the research proposal that is prepared and approved by your committee prior to actual implementation of the research. The major difference between the proposal and thesis is usually in verb tense. The future tense is used in some parts of your proposal and the past tense is used in the thesis.

Chapter 4: Results

Like the methodology chapter, the results chapter presents the same material included as the results section of a journal article but does not have the same constraints regarding figures and tables. When you begin writing this chapter, it is especially important to begin by developing tables to summarize most of your results. These should be as concise as possible. For more information on how to develop these, you may wish to consult the *Publication Manual* of the American Psychological Association [1] or the University of Chicago's *A Manual of Style* [9]. Once you have your tables, arrange them in order of their presentation. As you organize for writing, you may find that some of your tables are better placed in an appendix because they are not directly related to your hypotheses.

Chapter 4 almost always has subheadings, just as do the other chapters. As in Chapter 2 these subheadings depend on the nature of the material to be presented. Demographic data are usually presented first. When several hypotheses or questions are involved, each is often given a separate section and the chapter is divided accordingly. Additional findings are presented as a separate section at the end of the chapter.

Chapter 5: Discussion, Conclusions, and Interpretation of Results

This chapter has five sections: summary, discussion, conclusions, implications for practice, and recommendations for further research. When a reader has time to read only one chapter, this is the chapter that is read. Therefore it must, so to speak, stand by itself. In this chapter you can be more creative and speculative as you interpret the results according to your perceptions and judgment and anticipate the impact of the findings for nursing and future research. As long as the ideas are logical and based on the facts (i.e., results) as you perceive them, you are free to do your own thing.

Summary

Instead of the usual introductory paragraph, this chapter begins with a summary of the first four chapters. It can be two or three typed (double-spaced) pages long. This is easy to write if you have adequately summarized each of the chapters. Borrow heavily from each of those summaries and end with the results.

Discussion

The discussion centers around why you got your results and how they relate to the existing body of knowledge. Were there problems in distribution of scores? Were there rival hypotheses that were not expected? Did an assumption turn out to be false? Are there additional limitations? Are there design flaws that make cause and effect conclusions unjustifiable? Are correlations misleading because of the distribution of scores? When a null hypothesis is accepted, does power analysis to determine the probability of type II error support a null conclusion? Were the research variables ambiguously defined operationally? Are the statistical results practically significant? All factors that might affect how the statistical results are viewed and interpreted should be considered. Do not overdo the negative aspects, however. No research is perfect. There is still knowledge to be gained and implications for practice and future research to be inferred. Point out the strengths of the research also. From the bare-bones *results* interpreted against these strengths and weaknesses emerge the *findings*.*

Next, given the preceding discussion, the findings are discussed in terms of the related research literature. Do they support or flow from the work of others or are there contradictions? Include any relevant studies published after your research was implemented. Just what is the state of the art in this topic area *now*? How did your work contribute to this body of knowledge?

Conclusions

This section is usually brief. It states, simply, the conclusions you can draw (new knowledge) from your research, given the material presented in the discussion section. It should flow naturally from that section. Usually (but not always) your conclusions are presented without your reasons or rationale for them. However, if your reasoning is not readily apparent as a result of a well-written discussion section, you may wish to add a sentence or two stating your rationale. This section should relate back to the theoretical background section of Chapter 1. Have you supported the theory on which the research was based?

Implications for Practice

What implications do your conclusions have for practice? This section should relate to the significance of the study section of Chapter 1.

---

*Many researchers do not distinguish between *results* and *findings*. The distinction is used here as an aid to the thinking process. The distinction is not, however, inviolate.

Recommendations for Further Research

Where should work in your topic area go from here? Generate ideas for future research that will continue and expand upon your research in order to enlarge the body of knowledge and address any gaps or inconsistencies that were presented in the discussion section of this chapter.

Abstract

After the thesis is complete you are ready to write a 500-word or so (the limit varies with institutions) abstract of your research. The summary and conclusions sections of Chapter 5 can act as the material from which you extract the "pearls" that in turn become your abstract. It does not generally include reference to your literature review.

Presentations at Professional Meetings

Presentations at professional meetings can be in two forms. The traditional methods involve presenting your research orally, called a *paper,* or visually, called a *poster*. The emphasis of both is on your method and results. Little, if any, literature is reviewed when the focus is reporting your research findings; time constraints do not allow it, and the assumed expertise of the audience makes it unnecessary. If these presentations had to be described in a few words, they would have to be known as "here is what we are doing" presentations. They usually precede publication of the research in journals and are given different titles so that the authors are given additional publications and presentations credit by their institutions and in their vitae or resumes. Often they are progress reports rather than final reports. Sometimes only preliminary data analysis is reported. More is promised and delivered at the next meeting.

Published work, when presented at conventions, is usually presented with quite a different point of view than the straightforward reporting of research. It might be (1) presentation of a model (or your methodology) to be used for a specific type of research or (2) presentation of the credentials of a new instrument (part of which came from your research project). Once in a while, as in journal articles, it might involve generation of research needs and ideas as a result of a thoughtful state-of-the-art literature review. These types of presentations are infrequently presented by students and beginning researchers.

The privilege of presenting at a professional meeting is usually granted by a program committee that reviews abstracts of presentations submitted by potential presenters. A carefully developed abstract, therefore, is the first step toward presenting at a meeting. This abstract is written before the actual paper. These abstracts vary considerably. It is important to follow directions for the submission carefully and, if possible, secure the assistance of a successful applicant in reviewing your abstract. Papers and posters at professional meetings help you to become known. They also help you get to know researchers working in your area and provide an excellent opportunity to have your work critiqued prior to journal submission. Strengths and weaknesses that you might have missed can be incorporated into your articles as a result.

The Paper

Oral presentations are referred to as *papers*. That is because they are usually written out and read to the audience by the author or a designate. They generally include some kind of visual presentation like slides or handouts. This is often the first version of what eventually becomes a journal article. Questions and comments from the audience help clarify points and are often incorporated into the paper. Sometimes various versions (with different titles) are presented at a number of professional meetings, each with different audiences who have interest in the research. This is an excellent way to meet people and establish cooperative relationships with other professionals working in your area.

The conference committee usually establishes time limits and groups presenters according to similarity of topics. Sometimes it requests minor changes in your approach or format (e.g., change of a paper to part of a seminar or a panel discussion presentation). The committee also designates a session chairperson, who introduces speakers and keeps time. When you have used your allotted time, you will be interrupted and asked to stop. Therefore, if you want a lengthy question-and-answer period after your presentation, make your remarks short enough. The reverse is also true!

Traditionally, papers have been written. This allows their presentation by others when the author, for instance, cannot afford travel expenses or is otherwise occupied. It also allows publication in the proceedings* of a conference, so that those unable to attend can learn the latest developments and news. It also helps when you are nervous. Nevertheless, some particularly gifted or relaxed speakers prefer to speak extemporaneously, using only an outline on note cards to guide them. Even better, some speakers use a series of slides or transparencies as guides. These presentations are usually more fun to attend, and, if an actual paper does not have to be provided for proceedings, it may be your preferred method of presentation.

Posters

Poster sessions are becoming more popular. They allow many researchers to present their work in a relatively short period of time. The poster itself varies in size, depending on program committee negotiations with the hotel or building staff in which the meetings are held. At large meetings, a portable bulletin board is provided. However, it is usually safer to have assembled your display on a large poster board prior to the session. Sometimes, however, this must be transported in parts if large distances are to be traveled to get to the meeting.

Typically, the poster session lasts 1 hour and is held in a large ballroom that has been filled with rows of bulletin boards. The researcher stands in front of the poster informally and talks about the research with viewers who walk by.

---

*Most conference proceedings do not copyright the papers themselves and therefore researchers are free to publish the same material as journal articles. However, it is always best to check this first.

Sometimes a handout with an abstract or tables is distributed by the researcher. Posters may be presented as a shortened version of a paper; however, rather than consisting of just typed pages, the presentation is enhanced by the use of color in graphs, tables, charts, and pictures. The material needs to be readable from a distance of several feet. Viewers have usually been given a list of the poster titles and authors, each of which is numbered in some systematic way. This is an excellent, nonthreatening way to share your results and meet other people interested in your topic area.

Begin by attending poster sessions at meetings where you intend to present. Study the poster presentations that seem most successful, even taking notes, and emulate them.

References

1. American Psychological Association. *Publication Manual* (3rd ed.). Washington: American Psychological Association, 1983.
2. Ashton, R. S. Teenage girls' knowledge and attitudes of reproduction, sexual activity, and the utilization of contraception. University of Maryland at Baltimore Master's Thesis, 1981.
3. Davis, P. D. Patient-provider interaction and compliance among diabetic patients. University of Maryland at Baltimore Master's Thesis, 1979.
4. Haynes, R. B., Taylor, D. W., and Sackett, D. L., (eds.). *Compliance in Health Care*. Baltimore: Johns Hopkins Press, 1979.
5. Haynes, S. N., and Wilson, C. C. *Behavioral Assessment*. San Francisco: Jossey Bass, 1979.
6. King, L. S. *Why Not Say It Clearly: A Guide to Scientific Writing*. Boston: Little, Brown, 1978.
7. Stephens, N. E. Reliability and validity testing of a multidimensional instrument to assess biopsychosocial systems according to Clare W. Graves' theory. University of Maryland at Baltimore Master's Thesis, 1981.
8. Turabian, K. A. *A Manual for Writers of Term Papers, Theses, and Dissertations* (4th ed.). Chicago: University of Chicago Press, 1973.
9. University of Chicago. *A Manual of Style* (13th ed.). Chicago: University of Chicago Press, 1982.
10. Walleck, C. A. The effect of purposeful touch on intracranial pressure. University of Maryland at Baltimore Master's Thesis, 1982.

Appendixes

Appendix I: *Critiquing Research Reports*

The ultimate goal of this book is to equip you to critique reports of research as well as conduct it. We hope you will have had experience conducting research as you read this book. (It seems to temper the tendency toward excessively negative critiques that is unleashed by newly found knowledge of quantitative methods.) Critiquing reports of research does not mean reviewing an author's literary style and grammar—although, of course, clarity in writing is essential for all reports. Critiquing does not mean counting the number of references and noting their age, either, or does it mean counting the number of pages. Critiquing means deciding *if* a piece of new knowledge has been generated, *why,* and *how* it fits with existing knowledge. The author of a research report, of course, is presenting a case for this. You must decide if you agree and why.

By the time you finish this text, you will know how to deal with almost any statistical outcome. For example, if you are dealing with a descriptive study, you can place confidence intervals around the mean. If a statistical test is reported as significant, you can compute a magnitude estimate to judge better the impact of the independent variable by estimating the amount of variance in the dependent variable that is accounted for by the independent variable. If no statistical significance is found, you can do power analysis to determine the type II error rate, and when it exceeds 20 percent, you expect the research to be continued with more effort devoted to isolating confounding variables and reducing measurement error.

Moreover, when differences or correlations are reported, you will look at the actual data, via reported means, standard deviations, and other summary statistics, to see if the interpretation of results is valid. For example, if a researcher reports a correlation between sexual liberalism–conservatism and comfort in conducting a sexual interview with myocardial infarction patients and then concludes that therefore conservative health care providers are uncomfortable conducting the interview, is it really true? If the group mean for sexual liberalism–conservatism is reported as 72 with a standard deviation of 4.5 on a scale with a possible range from 16 to 96, obviously high scorers will be liberal. However, low scores in the group will be moderate, not conservative. A conclusion involving conservative health care providers would be inappropriate, because the sample did not include conservative providers—only moderate ones! Moreover, suppose comfort was measured on a five-point self-report scale on which 1 was "extremely uncomfortable," 3 was "somewhat comfortable and somewhat uncomfortable," and 5 was "extremely comfortable." If the researcher reports a mean of 4.1 for comfort and a standard deviation of .34, there are few, if any, providers in the sample who are uncomfortable with conducting a sexual interview. Instead, the range is from somewhat comfortable/uncomfortable to extremely comfortable. Thus the conclusion that conservative providers are uncomfortable is doubly wrong, because the sample included no conservative or uncomfortable providers. A correct conclusion would address liberal providers as comfortable and moderate providers as somewhat comfortable/

uncomfortable; or you might conclude that among health care providers there is a relationship between increased liberalism and increased comfort. Thus, besides considering all rival hypotheses and threats to validity, we must always take a good look at the data themselves. The use of fancy statistical procedures and computers must never obscure the real meaning of our data.

Finally, having completed the foregoing quantitative analysis of the *researcher's* quantitative analysis, you will have derived findings and conclusions of *your own* about the research. These (plus the researcher's suggestions) will then lead you to the most important questions about the research:

1. What piece of new knowledge, if any, has been generated here?
2. How does it relate to existing theory and knowledge?
3. What are the implications for practice? (In some cases there is none.)
4. And, how might this research be extended or improved? (Don't forget replications.) What related questions need answers?

The research outline presented on the following pages of this appendix is meant to help you make an analysis of research you review. It is meant as a guide, not as a standard against which all reports must be measured in every detail. Some parts of the outline may not apply to a report you are reviewing, and there may be some other aspects of a report that are not covered by the outline.

A good written critique of research is short (two or three pages at most) and does not discuss, point by point, each applicable part of the research outline—although this might well have been part of the process of preparing to write a critique. Instead, in a sentence or two the research is summarized. Then, the major strengths are discussed and followed by a discussion of major weaknesses. In this discussion, your knowledge of quantitative methods should be apparent. The research outline is intended to help you write this discussion in a knowledgeable and professional way. Your discussion presents your "evidence," on which are based your conclusions about the research. Finally, you conclude your critique by focusing on the preceding four questions. Namely, just what piece of new knowledge, if any, was generated, and where do we go from here?

Research Outline

I. Research questions
   A. What is the researcher trying to find out?
   B. Are relationships being examined? What kind (causal or correlational)?
   C. Are there any hypotheses being tested? Do they evolve naturally from the literature review and theoretical framework, if any?

II. Rationale and significance of the study
   A. What is the purpose of the study?
   B. Why is the researcher considering this research question?
   C. Will the answer meet the so-what test?
   D. Have similar studies been conducted? Does the researcher appear to have a good command of related literature?
III. Methodology
   A. How is the researcher answering the research question (or gathering evidence to prove or disprove a hypothesis)? Consider the following:
      1. Variables
         a. Just what are the characteristics, traits, elements, actions, responses, and so forth that are being studied?
         b. What are their constitutive definitions (i.e., definitions using words)?
         c. What are the independent and dependent variables? Predictor/criterion variables?
         d. Can any variables be modified or manipulated by the researcher?
      2. Operational definitions of variables
         a. How is a measure, value, or category level given to each of the research variables described in 1 above? Is mulitmodal measurement used?
         b. What are the reliability and validity of this number? What additional instrument credentialing is needed?
         c. What kind of number is it (e.g., frequency count for each category, rank, or score)?
         d. If this is a new measure, was it adequately pretested?
         e. How was the instrument developed and with what target population? Are accuracy and precision concerns?
      3. Sampling
         a. Who are the subjects and how were they selected (i.e., random, stratified random, convenience sampling)?
         b. From what study population does this sample come? Were they prelisted?
         c. How many subjects were solicited? How many actually participated? Is the sample size adequate? Did anyone refuse to participate?
         d. How were the rights of human subjects protected? What constituted informed consent?
      4. Research design
         a. Is this study longitudinal, cross-sectional, or retrospective?
         b. What type of study is this (e.g., comparative, correlational, experimental, or a combination of these)?
         c. Are subjects randomly assigned to groups? If not, how are they

assigned? Is there a control group? Are intact groups used? Is there a comparison group? How is equivalency of groups argued?

   d. Are subjects measured more than once? How many variables per subject are measured?

   e. What relationships between variables, if any, are being examined?

   f. What threats to internal, construct, and external validity are inherent in the design? Which ones are controlled?

   g. Are blind, double-blind, or placebo techniques used?

5. Procedure

   a. How is the research design implemented? What methods are used to gather data? Where? When?

   b. Who is gathering the data and what are the subjects told?

6. Data analysis

   a. How is the accuracy of the data verified? Is the scoring scheme, if any, apparent?

   b. How are missing data handled?

   c. How are cutting points established? Do they seem reasonable?

   d. What summary statistics are given (i.e., frequencies, measures of central tendency and dispersion)?

   e. What is the level of significance (*alpha*)?

   f. What statistical tests are computed? Are they appropriate to the research design and type of operational definitions?

   g. Are there threats to statistical conclusion validity?

   h. Was power analysis performed for null findings?

7. Rival hypotheses

   a. What confounding or intervening variables were present?

   b. Did the researcher control for them? How?

   c. Were any not controlled?

IV. Results (findings)

  A. What are the "facts and figures" as a result of this study?

  B. Do tables and graphs adequately summarize the results?

V. Interpretation of results and conclusions

  A. Are the results of statistical tests interpreted correctly?

  B. How does the researcher explain the results of this study?

  C. Are there any implied or stated basic assumptions that might affect the results and conclusions?

  D. What are the limitations of the study?

  E. Are there any confounding variables present that affect interpretation of results and conclusions?

  F. What conclusions are drawn? Are they justified?

  G. To what target population are results generalized? Is this appropriate?

  H. Are suggestions made for further research, including replication?

  I. What suggestions are made for implementation of the results?

VI. Critique

    A. What do you think of this study?

    B. What are its strengths and weaknesses? (Consider sections I through V above.)

    C. How could this study be improved? What changes could be made in design or operationalization of replications in order to enhance construct validity?

    D. Where do we go from here?

Appendix II: *The Literature Search*

Research, development of *new* knowledge, depends to a large extent on what knowledge already exists. This is just plain common sense. Therefore, as we said in Chapter 1, when we have a research idea one of the first things we do is *search the literature* to find out what is known about our topic. A good literature search tells us the state of the art, or what is known and what needs to be learned, in our topic area. When we know this, we are ready to begin pushing forward the frontier of knowledge by filling gaps and otherwise generating new information. This is not the only role the literature search plays in research, however. From reports of related research, we get ideas for research designs, ways of measuring our variables, selecting study populations, data anaysis, ways to develop tables and figures to display our results, and clues about possible pitfalls we can then try to avoid. We also learn what magnitude of differences or relationships we can expect (i.e., effect size) and this helps us determine the size of our sample and the need for additional independent variables. From theory or research results, moreover, we often can derive more specificity for our hypothesis, such as which group will do better than others. As we proceed with the research process, therefore, we continue to search the literature. Not only do we keep current on the very latest developments in our field but we also get ideas for better ways to execute each step of the research process. To repeat, the literature search is continuing. It is not just a step we can complete and consider finished.

Kinds of Information

In Chapter 1, the information we encounter as a result of the literature search was grouped into three categories—theory, results of research, and clinical experience. These are usually the most relevant to research. However, you will encounter much published material that does not fit any of these categories precisely. Therefore, it may be helpful to expand the kinds of information available as follows:

1. Textbooks, encyclopedias, and reviews of literature present an overview of existing knowledge. They may be objective reports or they may be quite biased if the author has an axe to grind. As a rule, publications in this category are objective, very general summaries of a topic. They lack the detail required by researchers. However, they are a good place to start learning about a topic.

2. Think pieces are articles that present an author's beliefs about a topic. Because of this, they are sometimes called *this-I-believe* essays. This category of information includes a wide range of material that must be sifted through and evaluated for accuracy and objectivity. It can range from value-laden, subjective, even hysterical writing to excellent presentations of theories and conceptual frameworks reflecting the very best of scholarship. To determine the usefulness of think pieces, first investigate the author. What is the author's reputation as an expert and scholar in this area? On what basis does the author claim expertise in the topic? Is it years of research and experience or is it a quick review/interview typical of many journalists? Second, consider the fit between a think piece and your overview of the topic. Is is a logical outcome or just someone's opinion? Never assume all published material is true or good just because it is published. Except for theoretical formulations or syntheses of existing knowledge presented by scholars, your literature review will include few articles from this category.

3. Research reports describe the results of investigations to generate new knowledge. Your literature review is focused on this type of information. Here, too, you must judge the *quality* of the research and the researcher's credentials as you determine the usefulness or even accuracy of the new knowledge that is reported. Appendix I presents guidelines for critiquing research reports.

4. Statistical data include census bureau reports and other data. Even this category of information can have errors, so you must still evaluate its accuracy and usefulness.

5. Clinical case studies are detailed descriptions by experts of single cases and fall somewhere between think pieces and research reports. They must also be evaluated and not just accepted as truth because they are published.

These five kinds of information are not mutually exclusive, nor is this framework the only way information can be viewed. However, it does provide one way of categorizing and then evaluating information you encounter as you review the literature.

Primary and Secondary Sources

Another consideration when searching the literature is whether or not an article is a primary or secondary source. A primary source is the original article. Research reports are primary sources for the research being reported. Secondary sources are descriptions or summaries of articles rather than the original article itself. Because secondary sources can possibly introduce bias from the author of the secondary source, it is best to read the original.

Bibliographic Indices

Early in our schooling we all learned to use the card catalog and *Readers Guide to Periodicals* in the library. We also used many of the reference books, such as the major encyclopedias, in the reference room. These are still sources for locating literature appropriate to a topic. However, they rarely include or cite primary-source research reports and clinical case studies, which are very important for the research literature search. There are a number of indices, abstracting services, and other retrieval mechanisms available for locating this kind of information, which is usually found in scholarly journals (as opposed to magazines) like *Nursing Research,* the *New England Journal of Medicine, Research in Nursing and Health,* the *Journal of Behavioral Medicine,* and many, many others. Below is a list of indices that are especially useful for retrieving citations of health-related research. They are all computerized and available at most university libraries. In libraries without the computer service, printed volumes corresponding to most of the computerized indices are available. These are included below in the descriptions of the indices. Fees for the computerized search vary, with off-line, nonprime time being less costly.

1. Medline (also called Medlars) is produced by the United States National Library of Medicine and is one of the major sources for citations in the biomedical literature. It includes three printed indices: *Index Medicus, Index to Dental Literature,* and *International Nursing Index.* Additional citations are also included on the topics of communication disorders and population/reproductive biology. Abstracts taken directly from published articles are available (for a fee) for about 40 percent of the citations since 1975. Medline indexes articles from 3,200 journals published in over 70 countries. Citations to chapters or articles from selected monographs are included from May 1976 through 1981.

2. A comprehensive **Dissertation Index** gives subject, title, and author citations for 99 percent of American dissertations accepted at accredited institutions since 1861, when academic doctoral degrees were first granted in the United States. Selected Master's theses have been indexed since 1962. Many Canadian and other foreign dissertations are also increasingly indexed. Citations are also included in University Microfilms International printed publications: *Dissertation Abstracts International, American Doctoral Dissertations, Comprehensive Dissertation Index,* and *Masters Abstracts.* Abstracts of the citations are available. This is an especially good source for related citations because most dissertations include comprehensive reviews of related literature.

3. Excerpta Medica indexes literature on human medicine and related disciplines dating from June 1974. Abstracts are available for about 60 percent of the citations. Each citation is classified and indexed by medical research specialists who assign terms and codes. An outstanding feature of this index is its coverage of drugs. It indexes more than 3,500 journals from 110 countries.

4. Health Planning and Administration, also produced by the United States National Library of Medicine, contains citations since 1975 of the nonclinical aspects of health care delivery. It corresponds to the printed *Hospital Literature Index* and includes additional citations from Medline and the American Hospital Association. Selected entries from monographs are also included. In the future, technical reports will be added by the National Health Planning Information Center of the Health Resources Administration. About 20 percent of the citations include author abstracts.

5. ERIC, produced by the National Institute of Education, collects and indexes many document types, such as research reports, evaluation studies, curriculum guides, lesson plans, bibliographies, course descriptions, theses, journal articles, and pamphlets. All noncopyrighted items can be purchased from the ERIC Document Reproduction Service. Approximately 650 locations have collections of ERIC microfiche. It includes two subfiles: *Resources in Education* and *Current Index to Journals in Education,* an index of more than 700 periodicals. It dates back to 1966.

6. IRL Life Sciences Collection, produced by Information Retrieval Ltd., corresponds to a printed series of 15 IRL abstracting journals. It contains abstracts and citations from over 5,000 worldwide journals in major areas of biology, medicine, biochemistry, ecology, and microbiology, and in some aspects of agriculture and veterinary science. It also contains selective data on books, conference reports, patents, and statistical publications. It dates from January 1978.

7. PSYC INFO, produced by the American Psychological Association, covers the world's literature in psychology and related behavioral and social sciences such as psychiatry, sociology, anthropology, education, and pharmacology. Over 950 periodicals, technical reports, and monographs are scanned every year. It includes citations since 1967 from the printed *Psychological Abstracts* as well as selected citations from *Dissertation Abstracts* and others.

8. Sociological Abstracts, which corresponds to the printed index of the same name, dates from 1963 and covers the world's literature in sociology and related disciplines, including women's studies. Each year the staff of Sociological Abstracts, Inc. scans 1,200 journals. Before 1973, some monographs were included.

9. SSIE (Smithsonian Social Science Information Exchange) used to be the major source for *ongoing research* citations. However, it was not updated in 1982 and 1983 because of funding cuts. All federally funded research was included, as well as some other research. Abstracts, names of principal investigators, and funding levels were usually available. Ask about whether or not this valuable (albeit expensive) resource has been reactivated when you visit your librarian.

10. Cancerlit (formerly called Cancerline), sponsored by the International Cancer Research Data Bank Program of the National Cancer Institute, covers citations since 1963 from *Carcinogenesis Abstracts* and *Cancer Therapy Abstracts* and since 1977 from all other cancer-related articles, proceedings from meetings, government reports, and so forth. Author abstracts are available. Although most articles are medical or physiological, some behavioral articles are also included.

11. SSCI, which corresponds to the printed *Social Science Citation Index,* is a multidisciplinary index of significant items since 1972 from the 1,000 most important social science journals throughout the world and social science articles selected from 2,200 additional journals in the natural, physical, and biomedical sciences. Important monographs are included as well. SSCI is a unique information retrieval technique because, in addition to the usual methods, you can search by way of an author's cited references. That is, if you have an older article that directly relates to your topic, you can secure citations for all the more recent articles that have cited it in their references or bibliographies. It is an excellent way to trace classic (or just old) references when there seems to be a paucity of literature in your area.

12. Scisearch, which corresponds to the printed *Science Citation Index,* is a multidisciplinary index like *Social Science Citation Index,* which, instead of focusing on social science, focuses on the literature of science and technology since 1974. It has the same unique retrieval capacity as SSCI.

13. NTIS is produced by the National Technical Information Service of the United States Department of Commerce, which is the central source for sale and dissemination of government-sponsored research. The data base includes government-sponsored research, development, and engineering reports as well as other reports prepared by government agencies, their contractors, and grantees since 1964. It corresponds to several printed publications, like *Government Reports Announcements and Index,* and 26 abstract newsletters. It represents reports from the Departments of Energy and Defense, NASA, and others. It is likely to include material in the behavioral sciences that may not be available elsewhere.

14. SDILINE is another unique source. It is a monthly current awareness service from the National Library of Medicine's computer data bases of Medline, Cancerlit, and Toxline. It covers over 3,000 English and foreign biomedical journals and selected monographs. Articles in SDILINE are available one month before publication of the printed *Index Medicus.* Each month subscribers are mailed a computer-generated bibliography on their topics as a means of helping them to keep abreast of current developments in their fields. Printouts can be tailored to your specifications to include author, title, source, abstract, reprint source, or language.

In addition to using appropriate indices from the above list, consult your librarian to make sure you have exhausted all possible avenues for a complete bibliography. Some indices may be printed but not computerized (e.g., *Cumulative Index to Nursing Literature*). Librarians are usually aware of not only their own services but also services available elsewhere, particularly those of the Health Sciences Library Network in the United States. They will also know of special topic books that describe how to conduct a comprehensive literature search for a given topic, like Winifred Sewell's *Guide to Drug Information* published by Drug Intelligence Publications, Inc. of Hamilton, Illinois in 1976. Finally, if there are scholarly journals that seem to specialize in your topic area, skim them to see if additional articles are available that were missed by the indexing services. (If certain key words are not selected for an article, it will not appear on bibliographic searches using those key words.) Many journals, such as the *Journal of Sex Research,* periodically publish indexes for articles in their journals as well.

Scope of the Search

Generally, a literature search includes citations for the previous 5 years plus any classics in the field. In areas such as stress, for which citations could number in the thousands, the search is further limited to such things as only English language, human subjects, specific target populations like cancer patients, and so forth. This is usually done before your computerized search through the indices in order to save both money and the time it would take for you to read all the useless citations. It is best to begin narrowly and then widen the search as needed. Your librarian will help you with this.

Organize for Survival

Many of us look up the relevant titles on our printout of citations and xerox them. Before we know it we are up to our ears in piles of journal articles—all our own. If we manage to read them all, we soon feel overwhelmed and disorganized, even if we underscore major passages. What we need is organization.

One of the many ways to organize is by subtopics and use of article summary sheets. Chapter 22 discusses various methods for organizing (and writing) a literature review and also presents an article summary sheet (see Exhibit 22.1), which can be used to note major aspects of each article. Summary sheets can then be sorted into subtopic piles according to how you have decided to present your review. The sooner you can decide on your organization and how you will implement it (e.g., summary sheets), the smoother and easier will be your literature review.

Appendix III: *Statistical Tables*

Table A. Random five-digit numbers

12367	23891	31506	90721	18710	89140	58595	99425	22840	08267
38890	30239	34237	22578	74420	22734	26930	40604	10782	80128
80788	55410	39770	93317	18270	21141	52085	78093	85638	81140
02395	77585	08854	23562	33544	45796	10976	44721	24781	09690
73720	70184	69112	71887	80140	72876	38984	23409	63957	44751
61383	17222	55234	18963	39006	93504	18273	49815	52802	69675
39161	44282	14975	97498	25973	33605	60141	30030	77677	49294
80907	74484	39884	19885	37311	04209	49675	39596	01052	43999
09052	65670	63660	34035	06578	87837	28125	48883	50482	55735
33425	24226	32043	60082	20418	85047	53570	32554	64099	52326
72651	69474	73648	71530	55454	19576	15552	20577	12124	50038
04142	32092	83586	61825	35482	32736	63403	91499	37196	02762
85226	14193	52213	60746	24414	57858	31884	51266	82293	73553
54888	03579	91674	59502	08619	33790	29011	85193	62262	28684
33258	51516	82032	45233	39351	33229	59464	65545	76809	16982
75973	15957	32405	82081	02214	57143	33526	47194	94526	73253
90638	75314	35381	34451	49246	11465	25102	71489	89883	99708
65061	15498	93348	33566	19427	66826	03044	97361	08159	47485
64420	07427	82233	97812	39572	07766	65844	29980	15533	90114
27175	17389	76963	75117	45580	99904	47160	55364	25666	25405
32215	30094	87276	56896	15625	32594	80663	08082	19422	80717
54209	58043	72350	89828	02706	16815	89985	37380	44032	59366
59286	66964	84843	71549	67553	33867	83011	66213	69372	23903
83872	58167	01221	95558	22196	65905	38785	01355	47489	28170
83310	57080	03366	80017	39601	40698	56434	64055	02495	50880
64545	29500	13351	78647	92628	19354	60479	57338	52133	07114
39269	00076	55489	01524	76568	22571	20328	84623	30188	43904
29763	05675	28193	65514	11954	78599	63902	21346	19219	90286
06310	02998	01463	27738	90288	17697	64511	39552	34694	03211
97541	47607	57655	59102	21851	44446	07976	54295	84671	78755
82968	85717	11619	97721	53513	53781	98941	38401	70939	11319
76878	34727	12524	90642	16921	13669	17420	84483	68309	85241
87394	78884	87237	92086	95633	66841	22906	64989	86952	54700
74040	12731	59616	33697	12592	44891	67982	72972	89795	10587
47896	41413	66431	70046	50793	45920	96564	67958	56369	44725
87778	71697	64148	54363	92114	34037	59061	62051	62049	33526
96977	63143	72219	80040	11990	47698	95621	72990	29047	85893
43820	13285	77811	81697	29937	70750	02029	32377	00556	86687
57203	83960	40096	39234	65953	59911	91411	55573	88427	45573
49065	72171	80939	06017	90323	63687	07932	99587	49014	26452
94250	84270	95798	13477	80139	26335	55169	73417	40766	45170
68148	81382	82383	18674	40453	92828	30042	37412	43423	45138
12208	97809	33619	28868	41646	16734	88860	32636	41985	84615
88317	89705	26119	12416	19438	65665	60989	59766	11418	18250
56728	80359	29613	63052	15251	44684	64681	42354	51029	77680
07138	12320	01073	19304	87042	58920	28454	81069	93978	66659
21188	64554	55618	36088	24331	84390	16022	12200	77559	75661
02154	12250	88738	43917	03655	21099	60805	63246	26842	35816
90953	85238	32771	07305	36181	47420	19681	33184	41386	03249
80103	91308	12858	41293	00325	15013	19579	91132	12720	92603

Table B. Standardized normal distribution

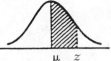

z	.00	.01	.02	.03	.04	.05	.06	.07	.08	.09
.0	.0000	.0040	.0080	.0120	.0160	.0199	.0239	.0279	.0319	.0359
.1	.0398	.0438	.0478	.0517	.0557	.0596	.0636	.0675	.0714	.0753
.2	.0793	.0832	.0871	.0910	.0948	.0987	.1026	.1064	.1103	.1141
.3	.1179	.1217	.1255	.1293	.1331	.1368	.1406	.1443	.1480	.1517
.4	.1554	.1591	.1628	.1664	.1700	.1736	.1772	.1808	.1844	.1879
.5	.1915	.1950	.1985	.2019	.2054	.2088	.2123	.2157	.2190	.2224
.6	.2257	.2291	.2324	.2357	.2389	.2422	.2454	.2486	.2517	.2549
.7	.2580	.2611	.2642	.2673	.2704	.2734	.2764	.2794	.2823	.2852
.8	.2881	.2910	.2939	.2967	.2995	.3023	.3051	.3078	.3106	.3133
.9	.3159	.3186	.3212	.3238	.3264	.3289	.3315	.3340	.3365	.3389
1.0	.3413	.3438	.3461	.3485	.3508	.3531	.3554	.3577	.3599	.3621
1.1	.3643	.3665	.3686	.3708	.3729	.3749	.3770	.3790	.3810	.3830
1.2	.3849	.3869	.3888	.3907	.3925	.3944	.3962	.3980	.3997	.4015
1.3	.4032	.4049	.4066	.4082	.4099	.4115	.4131	.4147	.4162	.4177
1.4	.4192	.4207	.4222	.4236	.4251	.4265	.4279	.4292	.4306	.4319
1.5	.4332	.4345	.4357	.4370	.4382	.4394	.4406	.4418	.4429	.4441
1.6	.4452	.4463	.4474	.4484	.4495	.4505	.4515	.4525	.4535	.4545
1.7	.4554	.4564	.4573	.4582	.4591	.4599	.4608	.4616	.4625	.4633
1.8	.4641	.4649	.4656	.4664	.4671	.4678	.4686	.4693	.4699	.4706
1.9	.4713	.4719	.4726	.4732	.4738	.4744	.4750	.4756	.4761	.4667
2.0	.4772	.4778	.4783	.4788	.4793	.4798	.4803	.4808	.4812	.4817
2.1	.4821	.4826	.4830	.4834	.4838	.4842	.4846	.4850	.4854	.4857
2.2	.4861	.4864	.4868	.4871	.4875	.4878	.4881	.4884	.4887	.4890
2.3	.4893	.4986	.4898	.4901	.4904	.4906	.4909	.4911	.4913	.4916
2.4	.4918	.4920	.4922	.4925	.4927	.4929	.4931	.4932	.4934	.4936
2.5	.4938	.4940	.4941	.4943	.4945	.4946	.4948	.4949	.4951	.4952
2.6	.4953	.4955	.4956	.4957	.4959	.4960	.4961	.4962	.4963	.4964
2.7	.4965	.4966	.4967	.4968	.4969	.4970	.4971	.4972	.4973	.4974
2.8	.4974	.4975	.4976	.4977	.4977	.4978	.4979	.4979	.4980	.4981
2.9	.4981	.4982	.4982	.4983	.4984	.4984	.4985	.4985	.4986	.4986
3.0	.4987	.4987	.4987	.4988	.4988	.4989	.4989	.4989	.4990	.4990

Table C. Critical values of Pearson's *r* for five significance levels

$n - 2$	.10	.05	.02	.01	.001
1	.98769	.99692	.999507	.999877	.9999988
2	.90000	.95000	.98000	.990000	.99900
3	.8054	.8783	.93433	.95873	.99116
4	.7293	.8114	.8822	.91720	.97406
5	.6694	.7545	.8329	.8745	.95074
6	.6215	.7067	.7887	.8343	.92493
7	.5822	.6664	.7498	.7977	.8982
8	.5494	.6319	.7155	.7646	.8721
9	.5214	.6021	.6851	.7348	.8471
10	.4973	.5760	.6581	.7079	.8233
11	.4762	.5529	.6339	.6835	.8010
12	.4575	.5324	.6120	.6614	.7800
13	.4409	.5139	.5923	.6411	.7603
14	.4259	.4973	.5742	.6226	.7420
15	.4124	.4821	.5577	.6055	.7246
16	.4000	.4683	.5425	.5897	.7084
17	.3887	.4555	.5285	.5751	.6932
18	.3783	.4438	.5155	.5614	.6787
19	.3687	.4329	.5034	.5487	.6652
20	.3598	.4227	.4921	.5368	.6524
25	.3233	.3809	.4451	.4869	.5974
30	.2960	.3494	.4093	.4487	.5541
35	.2746	.3246	.3810	.4182	.5189
40	.2573	.3044	.3578	.3932	.4896
45	.2428	.2875	.3384	.3721	.4648
50	.2306	.2732	.3218	.3541	.4433
60	.2108	.2500	.2948	.3248	.4078
70	.1954	.2319	.2737	.3017	.3799
80	.1829	.2172	.2565	.2830	.3568
90	.1726	.2050	.2422	.2673	.3375
100	.1638	.1946	.2301	.2540	.3211

Source: From Fisher and Yates, *Statistical Tables for Biological, Agricultural and Medical Research.* Published by Longman Group Ltd., London (previously published by Oliver & Boyd Ltd., Edinburgh) and by permission of the authors and publishers.

Table D. The t distribution

df	Alpha Level (Directional)					
	.10	.05	.025	.01	.005	.0005
	Alpha Level (Nondirectional)					
	.20	.10	.05	.02	.01	.001
1	3.078	6.314	12.706	31.821	63.657	636.619
2	1.886	2.920	4.303	6.965	9.925	31.598
3	1.638	2.353	3.182	4.541	5.841	12.924
4	1.533	2.132	2.776	3.747	4.604	8.610
5	1.476	2.015	2.571	3.365	4.032	6.869
6	1.440	1.943	2.447	3.143	3.707	5.959
7	1.415	1.895	2.365	2.998	3.499	5.408
8	1.397	1.860	2.306	2.896	3.355	5.041
9	1.383	1.833	2.262	2.821	3.250	4.781
10	1.372	1.812	2.228	2.764	3.169	4.587
11	1.363	1.796	2.201	2.718	3.106	4.437
12	1.356	1.782	2.179	2.681	3.055	4.318
13	1.350	1.771	2.160	2.650	3.012	4.221
14	1.345	1.761	2.145	2.624	2.977	4.140
15	1.341	1.753	2.131	2.602	2.947	4.073
16	1.337	1.746	2.120	2.583	2.921	4.015
17	1.333	1.740	2.110	2.567	2.898	3.965
18	1.330	1.734	2.101	2.552	2.878	3.922
19	1.328	1.729	2.093	2.539	2.861	3.883
20	1.325	1.725	2.086	2.528	2.845	3.850
21	1.323	1.721	2.080	2.518	2.831	3.819
22	1.321	1.717	2.074	2.508	2.819	3.792
23	1.319	1.714	2.069	2.500	2.807	3.767
24	1.318	1.711	2.064	2.492	2.797	3.745
25	1.316	1.708	2.060	2.485	2.787	3.725
26	1.315	1.706	2.056	2.479	2.779	3.707
27	1.314	1.703	2.052	2.473	2.771	3.690
28	1.313	1.701	2.048	2.467	2.763	3.674
29	1.311	1.699	2.045	2.462	2.756	3.659
30	1.310	1.697	2.042	2.457	2.750	3.646
40	1.303	1.684	2.021	2.423	2.704	3.551
60	1.296	1.671	2.000	2.390	2.660	3.460
120	1.289	1.658	1.980	2.358	2.617	3.373
∞	1.282	1.645	1.960	2.326	2.576	3.291

Source: From Fisher and Yates, *Statistical Tables for Biological, Agricultural and Medical Research*. Published by Longman Group Ltd., London (previously published by Oliver & Boyd Ltd., Edinburgh) and by permission of the authors and publishers.

Table E. The *F* distribution

df_2	α	1	2	3	4	5	6	8	12	24	∞
1	.001	405284	500000	540379	562500	576405	585937	598144	610667	623497	636619
	.01	4052	4999	5403	5625	5764	5859	5981	6106	6234	6366
	.05	161.45	199.50	215.71	224.58	230.16	233.99	238.88	243.91	249.05	254.32
	.10	39.86	49.50	53.59	55.83	57.24	58.20	59.44	60.70	62.00	63.33
	.20	9.47	12.00	13.00	13.73	14.01	14.26	14.59	14.90	15.24	15.58
2	.001	998.5	999.0	999.2	999.2	999.3	999.3	999.4	999.4	999.5	999.5
	.01	98.49	99.00	99.17	99.25	99.30	99.33	99.36	99.42	99.46	99.50
	.05	18.51	19.00	19.16	19.25	19.30	19.33	19.37	19.41	19.45	19.50
	.10	8.53	9.00	9.16	9.24	9.29	9.33	9.37	9.41	9.45	9.49
	.20	3.56	4.00	4.16	4.24	4.28	4.32	4.36	4.40	4.44	4.48
3	.001	167.5	148.5	141.1	137.1	134.6	132.8	130.6	128.3	125.9	123.5
	.01	34.12	30.81	29.46	28.71	28.24	27.91	27.49	27.05	26.60	26.12
	.05	10.13	9.55	9.28	9.12	9.01	8.94	8.84	8.74	8.64	8.53
	.10	5.54	5.46	5.39	5.34	5.31	5.28	5.25	5.22	5.18	5.13
	.20	2.68	2.89	2.94	2.96	2.97	2.97	2.98	2.98	2.98	2.98
4	.001	74.14	61.25	56.18	53.44	51.71	50.53	49.00	47.41	45.77	44.05
	.01	21.20	18.00	16.69	15.98	15.52	15.21	14.80	14.37	13.93	13.46
	.05	7.71	6.94	6.59	6.39	6.26	6.16	6.04	5.91	5.77	5.63
	.10	4.54	4.32	4.19	4.11	4.05	4.01	3.95	3.90	3.83	3.76
	.20	2.35	2.47	2.48	2.48	2.48	2.47	2.47	2.46	2.44	2.43
5	.001	47.04	36.61	33.20	31.09	29.75	28.84	27.64	26.42	25.14	23.78
	.01	16.26	13.27	12.06	11.39	10.97	10.67	10.29	9.89	9.47	9.02
	.05	6.61	5.79	5.41	5.19	5.05	4.95	4.82	4.68	4.53	4.36
	.10	4.06	3.78	3.62	3.52	3.45	3.40	3.34	3.27	3.19	3.10
	.20	2.18	2.26	2.25	2.24	2.23	2.22	2.20	2.18	2.16	2.13
6	.001	35.51	27.00	23.70	21.90	20.81	20.03	19.03	17.99	16.89	15.75
	.01	13.74	10.92	9.78	9.15	8.75	8.47	8.10	7.72	7.31	6.88
	.05	5.99	5.14	4.76	4.53	4.39	4.28	4.15	4.00	3.84	3.67
	.10	3.78	3.46	3.29	3.18	3.11	3.05	2.98	2.90	2.82	2.72
	.20	2.07	2.13	2.11	2.09	2.08	2.06	2.04	2.02	1.99	1.95
7	.001	29.22	21.69	18.77	17.19	16.21	15.52	14.63	13.71	12.73	11.69
	.01	12.25	9.55	8.45	7.85	7.46	7.19	6.84	6.47	6.07	5.65
	.05	5.59	4.74	4.35	4.12	3.97	3.87	3.73	3.57	3.41	3.23
	.10	3.59	3.26	3.07	2.96	2.88	2.83	2.75	2.67	2.58	2.47
	.20	2.00	2.04	2.02	1.99	1.97	1.96	1.93	1.91	1.87	1.83
8	.001	25.42	18.49	15.83	14.39	13.49	12.86	12.04	11.19	10.30	9.34
	.01	11.26	8.65	7.59	7.01	6.63	6.37	6.03	5.67	5.28	4.86
	.05	5.32	4.46	4.07	3.84	3.69	3.58	3.44	3.28	3.12	2.93
	.10	3.46	3.11	2.92	2.81	2.73	2.67	2.59	2.50	2.40	2.29
	.20	1.95	1.98	1.95	1.92	1.90	1.88	1.84	1.83	1.79	1.74
9	.001	22.86	16.39	13.90	12.56	11.71	11.13	10.37	9.57	8.72	7.81
	.01	10.56	8.02	6.99	6.42	6.06	5.80	5.47	5.11	4.73	4.31
	.05	5.12	4.26	3.86	3.63	3.48	3.37	3.23	3.07	2.90	2.71
	.10	3.36	3.01	2.81	2.69	2.61	2.55	2.47	2.38	2.28	2.16
	.20	1.91	1.94	1.90	1.87	1.85	1.83	1.80	1.76	1.72	1.67

Table E (continued)

df_2 \ df_1	α	1	2	3	4	5	6	8	12	24	∞
10	.001	21.04	14.91	12.55	11.28	10.48	9.92	9.20	8.45	7.64	6.76
	.01	10.04	7.56	6.55	5.99	5.64	5.39	5.04	4.71	4.33	3.91
	.05	4.96	4.10	3.71	3.48	3.33	3.22	3.07	2.91	2.74	2.54
	.10	3.28	2.92	2.73	2.61	2.52	2.46	2.35	2.28	2.18	2.06
	.20	1.88	1.90	1.86	1.83	1.80	1.78	1.75	1.72	1.67	1.62
11	.001	19.69	13.81	11.56	10.35	9.58	9.05	8.35	7.63	6.85	6.00
	.01	9.65	7.20	6.22	5.67	5.32	5.07	4.74	4.40	4.02	3.60
	.05	4.84	3.98	3.59	3.36	3.20	3.09	2.95	2.79	2.61	2.40
	.10	3.23	2.86	2.66	2.54	2.45	2.39	2.30	2.21	2.10	1.97
	.20	1.86	1.87	1.83	1.80	1.77	1.75	1.72	1.68	1.63	1.57
12	.001	18.64	12.97	10.80	9.63	8.89	8.38	7.71	7.00	6.25	5.42
	.01	9.33	6.93	5.95	5.41	5.06	4.82	4.59	4.16	3.78	3.36
	.05	4.75	3.88	3.49	3.26	3.11	3.00	2.85	2.69	2.50	2.30
	.10	3.18	2.81	2.61	2.48	2.39	2.33	2.24	2.15	2.04	1.90
	.20	1.84	1.85	1.80	1.77	1.74	1.72	1.69	1.65	1.60	1.54
13	.001	17.81	12.31	10.21	9.07	8.35	7.86	7.21	6.52	5.78	4.97
	.01	9.07	6.70	5.74	5.20	4.86	4.62	4.30	3.96	3.59	3.16
	.05	4.67	3.80	3.41	3.18	3.02	2.92	2.77	2.60	2.42	2.21
	.10	3.14	2.76	2.56	2.43	2.35	2.28	2.20	2.10	1.98	1.85
	.20	1.82	1.83	1.78	1.75	1.72	1.69	1.66	1.62	1.57	1.51
14	.001	17.14	11.78	9.73	8.62	7.92	7.43	6.80	6.13	5.41	4.60
	.01	8.86	6.51	5.56	5.03	4.69	4.46	4.14	3.80	3.43	3.00
	.05	4.60	3.74	3.34	3.11	2.96	2.85	2.70	2.53	2.35	2.13
	.10	3.10	2.73	2.52	2.39	2.31	2.24	2.15	2.05	1.94	1.80
	.20	1.81	1.81	1.76	1.73	1.70	1.67	1.64	1.60	1.55	1.48
15	.001	16.59	11.34	9.34	8.25	7.57	7.09	6.47	5.81	5.10	4.31
	.01	8.68	6.36	5.42	4.89	4.56	4.32	4.00	3.67	3.29	2.87
	.05	4.54	3.68	3.29	3.06	2.90	2.79	2.64	2.48	2.29	2.07
	.10	3.07	2.70	2.49	2.36	2.27	2.21	2.12	2.02	1.90	1.76
	.20	1.80	1.79	1.75	1.71	1.68	1.66	1.62	1.58	1.53	1.46
16	.001	16.12	10.97	9.00	7.94	7.27	6.81	6.19	5.55	4.85	4.06
	.01	8.53	6.23	5.29	4.77	4.44	4.20	3.89	3.55	3.18	2.75
	.05	4.49	3.63	3.24	3.01	2.85	2.74	2.59	2.42	2.24	2.01
	.10	3.05	2.67	2.46	2.33	2.24	2.18	2.09	1.99	1.87	1.72
	.20	1.79	1.78	1.74	1.70	1.67	1.64	1.61	1.56	1.51	1.43
17	.001	15.72	10.66	8.73	7.68	7.02	6.56	5.95	5.32	4.63	3.85
	.01	8.40	6.11	5.18	4.67	4.34	4.10	3.79	3.45	3.08	2.65
	.05	4.45	3.59	3.20	2.96	2.81	2.70	2.55	2.38	2.19	1.96
	.10	3.03	2.64	2.44	2.31	2.22	2.15	2.06	1.96	1.84	1.69
	.20	1.78	1.77	1.72	1.68	1.65	1.63	1.59	1.55	1.49	1.42
18	.001	15.38	10.39	8.49	7.46	6.81	6.35	5.76	5.13	4.45	3.67
	.01	8.28	6.01	5.09	4.58	4.25	4.01	3.71	3.37	3.00	2.57
	.05	4.41	3.55	3.19	3.93	2.77	2.66	2.51	2.34	2.15	1.92
	.10	3.01	2.62	2.42	2.29	2.20	2.13	2.64	1.93	1.81	1.66
	.20	1.77	1.76	1.71	1.67	1.64	1.62	1.58	1.53	1.48	1.40
19	.001	15.08	10.16	8.28	7.26	6.61	6.18	5.59	4.97	4.29	3.52
	.01	8.18	5.93	5.01	4.50	4.17	3.94	3.63	3.30	2.92	2.49
	.05	4.38	3.52	3.13	2.90	2.74	2.63	2.48	2.31	2.11	1.88
	.10	2.99	2.61	2.40	2.27	2.18	2.11	2.02	1.91	1.79	1.63
	.20	1.76	1.75	1.70	1.66	1.63	1.61	1.57	1.52	1.46	1.39

Table E (continued)

df_2	α	1	2	3	4	5	6	8	12	24	∞
20	.001	14.82	9.95	8.10	7.10	6.46	6.02	5.44	4.82	4.15	3.38
	.01	8.10	5.85	4.94	4.43	4.10	3.87	3.56	3.23	2.86	2.42
	.05	4.35	3.49	3.10	2.87	2.71	2.60	2.45	2.28	2.08	1.84
	.10	2.97	2.59	2.38	2.25	2.16	2.09	2.00	1.89	1.77	1.61
	.20	1.76	1.75	1.70	1.65	1.62	1.60	1.56	1.51	1.45	1.37
21	.001	14.59	9.77	7.94	6.95	6.32	5.88	5.31	4.70	4.03	3.26
	.01	8.02	5.78	4.87	4.37	4.04	3.81	3.51	3.17	2.80	2.36
	.05	4.32	3.47	3.07	2.84	2.68	2.57	2.42	2.25	2.05	1.81
	.10	2.96	2.57	2.36	2.23	2.14	2.08	1.95	1.88	1.75	1.59
	.20	1.75	1.74	1.69	1.65	1.61	1.59	1.55	1.50	1.44	1.36
22	.001	14.38	9.61	7.80	6.81	6.19	5.76	5.19	4.58	3.92	3.15
	.01	7.94	5.72	4.52	4.31	3.99	3.76	3.45	3.12	2.75	2.31
	.05	4.30	3.44	3.05	2.82	2.66	2.55	2.41	2.23	2.03	1.78
	.10	2.95	2.56	2.35	2.22	2.13	2.06	1.97	1.86	1.73	1.57
	.20	1.75	1.73	1.68	1.64	1.61	1.58	1.54	1.49	1.43	1.35
23	.001	14.19	9.47	7.67	6.69	6.08	5.65	5.09	4.48	3.82	3.05
	.01	7.88	5.66	4.76	4.26	3.94	3.71	3.41	3.07	2.70	2.26
	.05	4.28	3.42	3.03	2.80	2.64	2.53	2.38	2.20	2.00	1.76
	.10	2.94	2.55	2.34	2.21	2.11	2.05	1.95	1.84	1.72	1.55
	.20	1.74	1.73	1.68	1.63	1.60	1.57	1.54	1.49	1.42	1.34
24	.001	14.03	9.34	7.55	6.59	5.98	5.55	4.99	4.39	3.74	2.97
	.01	7.82	5.61	4.72	4.22	3.99	3.67	3.39	3.03	2.66	2.21
	.05	4.26	3.40	3.01	2.78	2.62	2.51	2.31	2.18	1.98	1.73
	.10	2.93	2.54	2.33	2.19	2.10	2.04	1.94	1.53	1.70	1.53
	.20	1.74	1.72	1.67	1.63	1.59	1.57	1.53	1.48	1.42	1.33
25	.001	13.88	9.22	7.45	6.49	5.88	5.46	4.91	4.31	3.66	2.89
	.01	7.77	5.57	4.65	4.18	3.89	3.63	3.32	2.99	2.62	2.17
	.05	4.24	3.38	2.99	2.76	2.60	2.49	2.34	2.16	1.96	1.71
	.10	2.92	2.53	2.32	2.18	2.09	2.02	1.93	1.82	1.69	1.52
	.20	1.73	1.72	1.66	1.62	1.59	1.56	1.52	1.47	1.41	1.32
26	.001	13.74	9.12	7.36	6.41	5.80	5.38	4.83	4.24	3.59	2.82
	.01	7.72	5.53	4.64	4.14	3.82	3.59	3.29	2.96	2.58	2.13
	.05	4.22	3.37	2.98	2.74	2.59	2.47	2.32	2.15	1.95	1.69
	.10	2.91	2.52	2.31	2.17	2.08	2.01	1.92	1.81	1.68	1.50
	.20	1.73	1.71	1.66	1.62	1.58	1.56	1.52	1.47	1.40	1.31
27	.001	13.61	9.02	7.27	6.33	5.73	5.31	4.76	4.17	3.52	2.75
	.01	7.68	5.49	4.60	4.11	3.78	3.56	3.26	2.93	2.55	2.10
	.05	4.21	3.35	2.96	2.73	2.57	2.46	2.30	2.13	1.93	1.67
	.10	2.90	2.51	2.30	2.17	2.07	2.00	1.91	1.80	1.67	1.49
	.20	1.73	1.71	1.66	1.61	1.58	1.55	1.51	1.46	1.40	1.30
28	.001	13.50	8.93	7.19	6.25	5.66	5.24	4.69	4.11	3.46	2.70
	.01	7.64	5.45	4.57	4.07	3.75	3.53	3.23	2.90	2.52	2.06
	.05	4.20	3.34	2.95	2.71	2.56	2.44	2.29	2.12	1.91	1.65
	.10	2.89	2.50	2.29	2.16	2.06	2.00	1.90	1.79	1.66	1.48
	.20	1.72	1.71	1.65	1.61	1.57	1.55	1.51	1.46	1.39	1.30
29	.001	13.39	8.85	7.12	6.19	5.59	5.18	4.64	4.05	3.41	2.64
	.01	7.60	5.42	4.54	4.04	3.73	3.50	3.20	2.87	2.49	2.03
	.05	4.18	3.33	2.93	2.70	2.54	2.43	2.28	2.10	1.90	1.64
	.10	2.89	2.50	2.28	2.15	2.06	1.99	1.89	1.78	1.65	1.47
	.20	1.72	1.70	1.65	1.60	1.57	1.54	1.50	1.45	1.39	1.29

Table E (continued)

df_2	α	1	2	3	4	5	6	8	12	24	∞
30	.001	13.29	8.77	7.05	6.12	5.53	5.12	4.58	4.00	3.36	2.59
	.01	7.56	5.39	4.51	4.02	3.70	3.47	3.17	2.84	2.47	2.01
	.05	4.17	3.32	2.92	2.69	2.53	2.42	2.27	2.09	1.89	1.62
	.10	2.88	2.49	2.28	2.14	2.05	1.98	1.88	1.77	1.64	1.46
	.20	1.72	1.70	1.64	1.60	1.57	1.54	1.50	1.45	1.38	1.28
40	.001	12.61	8.25	6.60	5.70	5.13	4.73	4.21	3.64	3.01	2.23
	.01	7.31	5.18	4.31	3.83	3.51	3.29	2.99	2.66	2.29	1.80
	.05	4.08	3.23	2.84	2.61	2.45	2.34	2.18	2.00	1.79	1.51
	.10	2.84	2.44	2.23	2.09	2.00	1.93	1.83	1.71	1.57	1.38
	.20	1.70	1.68	1.62	1.57	1.54	1.51	1.47	1.41	1.34	1.24
60	.001	11.97	7.76	6.17	5.31	4.76	4.37	3.87	3.31	2.69	1.90
	.01	7.08	4.98	4.13	3.65	3.34	3.12	2.82	2.50	2.12	1.60
	.05	4.00	3.15	2.76	2.52	2.37	2.25	2.10	1.92	1.70	1.39
	.10	2.79	2.39	2.18	2.04	1.95	1.87	1.77	1.66	1.51	1.29
	.20	1.68	1.65	1.59	1.55	1.51	1.48	1.44	1.38	1.31	1.18
120	.001	11.38	7.31	5.79	4.95	4.42	4.04	3.55	3.02	2.40	1.56
	.01	6.85	4.79	3.95	3.48	3.17	2.96	2.66	2.34	1.95	1.38
	.05	3.92	3.07	2.68	2.45	2.29	2.17	2.02	1.83	1.61	1.25
	.10	2.75	2.35	2.13	1.99	1.90	1.82	1.72	1.60	1.45	1.19
	.20	1.66	1.63	1.57	1.52	1.48	1.45	1.41	1.35	1.27	1.12
∞	.001	10.83	6.91	5.42	4.62	4.10	3.74	3.27	2.74	2.13	1.00
	.01	6.64	4.60	3.78	3.32	3.02	2.80	2.51	2.18	1.79	1.00
	.05	3.84	2.99	2.60	2.37	2.21	2.09	1.94	1.75	1.52	1.00
	.10	2.71	2.30	2.08	1.91	1.85	1.77	1.67	1.55	1.38	1.00
	.20	1.64	1.61	1.55	1.50	1.46	1.43	1.35	1.32	1.23	1.00

Source: From Fisher and Yates, *Statistical Tables for Biological, Agricultural and Medical Research*. Published by Longman Group Ltd., London (previously published by Oliver & Boyd Ltd., Edinburgh) and by permission of the authors and publishers.

Table F. The chi square distribution

	Alpha Level					
df	.20	.10	.05	.02	.01	.001
1	1.642	2.706	3.841	5.412	6.635	10.827
2	3.219	4.605	5.991	7.824	9.210	13.815
3	4.642	6.251	7.815	9.837	11.345	16.266
4	5.989	7.779	9.488	11.668	13.277	18.467
5	7.289	9.236	11.070	13.388	15.086	20.515
6	8.558	10.645	12.592	15.033	16.812	22.457
7	9.803	12.017	14.067	16.622	18.475	24.322
8	11.030	13.362	15.507	18.168	20.090	26.125
9	12.242	14.684	16.919	19.679	21.666	27.877
10	13.442	15.987	18.307	21.161	23.209	29.588
11	14.631	17.275	19.675	22.618	24.725	31.264
12	15.812	18.549	21.026	24.054	26.217	32.909
13	16.985	19.812	22.362	25.472	27.688	34.528
14	18.151	21.064	23.685	26.873	29.141	36.123
15	19.311	22.307	24.996	28.259	30.578	37.697
16	20.465	23.542	26.296	29.633	32.000	39.252
17	21.615	24.769	27.587	30.995	33.409	40.790
18	22.760	25.989	28.869	32.346	34.805	42.312
19	23.900	27.204	30.144	33.687	36.191	43.820
20	25.038	28.412	31.410	35.020	37.566	45.315
21	26.171	29.615	32.671	36.343	38.932	46.797
22	27.301	30.813	33.924	37.659	40.289	48.268
23	28.429	32.007	35.172	38.968	41.638	49.728
24	29.553	33.196	36.415	40.270	42.980	51.179
25	30.675	34.362	37.652	41.566	44.314	52.620
26	31.795	35.563	38.885	42.856	45.642	54.052
27	32.912	36.741	40.113	44.140	46.963	55.476
28	34.027	37.916	41.337	45.419	48.278	56.893
29	35.139	39.087	42.557	46.693	49.588	58.302
30	36.250	40.256	43.773	47.962	50.892	59.703

Source: From Fisher and Yates, *Statistical Tables for Biological, Agricultural and Medical Research*. Published by Longman Group Ltd., London (previously published by Oliver & Boyd Ltd., Edinburgh) and by permission of the authors and publishers.

Table G. Critical values of D (or C)* in the Fisher exact probability test

Totals in right margin		B (or A)	Level of significance			
			.05	.025	.01	.005
$A + B = 3$	$C + D = 3$	3	0	—	—	—
$A + B = 4$	$C + D = 4$	4	0	0	—	—
	$C + D = 3$	4	0	—	—	—
$A + B = 5$	$C + D = 5$	5	1	1	0	0
		4	0	0	—	—
	$C + D = 4$	5	1	0	0	—
		4	0	—	—	—
	$C + D = 3$	5	0	0	—	—
	$C + D = 2$	5	0	—	—	—
$A + B = 6$	$C + D = 6$	6	2	1	1	0
		5	1	0	0	—
		4	0	—	—	—
	$C + D = 5$	6	1	0	0	0
		5	0	0	—	—
		4	0	—	—	—
	$C + D = 4$	6	1	0	0	0
		5	0	0	—	—
	$C + D = 3$	6	0	0	—	—
		5	0	—	—	—
	$C + D = 2$	6	0	—	—	—
$A + B = 7$	$C + D = 7$	7	3	2	1	1
		6	1	1	0	0
		5	0	0	—	—
		4	0	—	—	—
	$C + D = 6$	7	2	2	1	1
		6	1	0	0	0
		5	0	0	—	—
		4	0	—	—	—
	$C + D = 5$	7	2	1	0	0
		6	1	0	0	—
		5	0	—	—	—
	$C + D = 4$	7	1	1	0	0
		6	0	0	—	—
		5	0	—	—	—
	$C + D = 3$	7	0	0	0	—
		6	0	—	—	—
	$C - D = 2$	7	0	—	—	—

Table G (continued)

Totals in right margin		B (or A)	Level of significance			
			.05	.025	.01	.005
A + B = 8	C + D = 8	8	4	3	2	2
		7	2	2	1	0
		6	1	1	0	0
		5	0	0	—	—
		4	0	—	—	—
	C + D = 7	8	3	2	2	1
		7	2	1	1	0
		6	1	0	0	—
		5	0	0	—	—
	C + D = 6	8	2	2	1	1
		7	1	1	0	0
		6	0	0	0	—
		5	0	—	—	—
	C + D = 5	8	2	1	1	0
		7	1	0	0	0
		6	0	0	—	—
		5	0	—	—	—
	C + D = 4	8	1	1	0	0
		7	0	0	—	—
		6	0	—	—	—
	C + D = 3	8	0	0	0	—
		7	0	0	—	—
	C + D = 2	8	0	0	—	—
A + B = 9	C + D = 9	9	5	4	3	3
		8	3	3	2	1
		7	2	1	1	0
		6	1	1	0	0
		5	0	0	—	—
		4	0	—	—	—
	C + D = 8	9	4	3	3	2
		8	3	2	1	1
		7	2	1	0	0
		6	1	0	0	—
		5	0	0	—	—
	C + D = 7	9	3	3	2	2
		8	2	2	1	0
		7	1	1	0	0
		6	0	0	—	—
		5	0	—	—	—

Table G (continued)

Totals in right margin		B (or A)	Level of significance			
			.05	.025	.01	.005
$A + B = 9$	$C + D = 6$	9	3	2	1	1
		8	2	1	0	0
		7	1	0	0	—
		6	0	0	—	—
		5	0	—	—	—
	$C + D = 5$	9	2	1	1	1
		8	1	1	0	0
		7	0	0	—	—
		6	0	—	—	—
	$C + D = 4$	9	1	1	0	0
		8	0	0	0	—
		7	0	0	—	—
		6	0	—	—	—
	$C + D = 3$	9	1	0	0	0
		8	0	0	—	—
		7	0	—	—	—
	$C + D = 2$	9	0	0	—	—
$A + B = 10$	$C + D = 10$	10	6	5	4	3
		9	4	3	3	2
		8	3	2	1	1
		7	2	1	1	0
		6	1	0	0	—
		5	0	0	—	—
		4	0	—	—	—
	$C + D = 9$	10	5	4	3	3
		9	4	3	2	2
		8	2	2	1	1
		7	1	1	0	0
		6	1	0	0	—
		5	0	0	—	—
	$C + D = 8$	10	4	4	3	2
		9	3	2	2	1
		8	2	1	1	0
		7	1	1	0	0
		6	0	0	—	—
		5	0	—	—	—
	$C + D = 7$	10	3	3	2	2
		9	2	2	1	1
		8	1	1	0	0
		7	1	0	0	—
		6	0	0	—	—
		5	0	—	—	—

Table G (continued)

Totals in right margin		B (or A)	Level of significance			
			.05	.025	.01	.005
$A + B = 10$	$C + D = 6$	10	3	2	2	1
		9	2	1	1	0
		8	1	1	0	0
		7	0	0	—	—
		6	0	—	—	—
	$C + D = 5$	10	2	2	1	1
		9	1	1	0	0
		8	1	0	0	—
		7	0	0	—	—
		6	0	—	—	—
	$C + D = 4$	10	1	1	0	0
		9	1	0	0	0
		8	0	0	—	—
		7	0	—	—	—
	$C + D = 3$	10	1	0	0	0
		9	0	0	—	—
		8	0	—	—	—
	$C + D = 2$	10	0	0	—	—
		9	0	—	—	—
$A + B = 11$	$C + D = 11$	11	7	6	5	4
		10	5	4	3	3
		9	4	3	2	2
		8	3	2	1	1
		7	2	1	0	0
		6	1	0	0	—
		5	0	0	—	—
		4	0	—	—	—
	$C + D = 10$	11	6	5	4	4
		10	4	4	3	2
		9	3	3	2	1
		8	2	2	1	0
		7	1	1	0	0
		6	1	0	0	—
		5	0	—	—	—
	$C + D = 9$	11	5	4	4	3
		10	4	3	2	2
		9	3	2	1	1
		8	2	1	1	0
		7	1	1	0	0
		6	0	0	—	—
		5	0	—	—	—

Table G (continued)

Totals in right margin		*B* (or *A*)	Level of significance			
			.05	.025	.01	.005
A + *B* = 11	*C* + *D* = 8	11	4	4	3	3
		10	3	3	2	1
		9	2	2	1	1
		8	1	1	0	0
		7	1	0	0	—
		6	0	0	—	—
		5	0	—	—	—
	C + *D* = 7	11	4	3	2	2
		10	3	2	1	1
		9	2	1	1	0
		8	1	1	0	0
		7	0	0	—	—
		6	0	0	—	—
	C + *D* = 6	11	3	2	2	1
		10	2	1	1	0
		9	1	1	0	0
		8	1	0	0	—
		7	0	0	—	—
		6	0	—	—	—
	C + *D* = 5	11	2	2	1	1
		10	1	1	0	0
		9	1	0	0	0
		8	0	0	—	—
		7	0	—	—	—
	C + *D* = 4	11	1	1	1	0
		10	1	0	0	0
		9	0	0	—	—
		8	0	—	—	—
	C + *D* = 3	11	1	0	0	0
		10	0	0	—	—
		9	0	—	—	—
	C + *D* = 2	11	0	0	—	—
		10	0	—	—	—
A + *B* = 12	*C* + *D* = 12	12	8	7	6	5
		11	6	5	4	4
		10	5	4	3	2
		9	4	3	2	1
		8	3	2	1	1
		7	2	1	0	0
		6	1	0	0	—
		5	0	0	—	—
		4	0	—	—	—

Table G (continued)

Totals in right margin		B (or A)	Level of significance			
			.05	.025	.01	.005
A + B = 12	C + D = 11	12	7	6	5	5
		11	5	5	4	3
		10	4	3	2	2
		9	3	2	2	1
		8	2	1	1	0
		7	1	1	0	0
		6	1	0	0	—
		5	0	0	—	—
	C + D = 10	12	6	5	5	4
		11	5	4	3	3
		10	4	3	2	2
		9	3	2	1	1
		8	2	1	0	0
		7	1	0	0	0
		6	0	0	—	—
		5	0	—	—	—
	C + D = 9	12	5	5	4	3
		11	4	3	3	2
		10	3	2	2	1
		9	2	2	1	0
		8	1	1	0	0
		7	1	0	0	—
		6	0	0	—	—
		5	0	—	—	—
	C + D = 8	12	5	4	3	3
		11	3	3	2	2
		10	2	2	1	1
		9	2	1	1	0
		8	1	1	0	0
		7	0	0	—	—
		6	0	0	—	—
	C + D = 7	12	4	3	3	2
		11	3	2	2	1
		10	2	1	1	0
		9	1	1	0	0
		8	1	0	0	—
		7	0	0	—	—
		6	0	—	—	—

Table G (continued)

Totals in right margin		B (or A)	Level of significance			
			.05	.025	.01	.005
A + B = 12	C + D = 6	12	3	3	2	2
		11	2	2	1	1
		10	1	1	0	0
		9	1	0	0	0
		8	0	0	—	—
		7	0	0	—	—
		6	0	—	—	—
	C + D = 5	12	2	2	1	1
		11	1	1	1	0
		10	1	0	0	0
		9	0	0	0	—
		8	0	0	—	—
		7	0	—	—	—
	C + D = 4	12	2	1	1	0
		11	1	0	0	0
		10	0	0	0	—
		9	0	0	—	—
		8	0	—	—	—
	C + D = 3	12	1	0	0	0
		11	0	0	0	—
		10	0	0	—	—
		9	0	—	—	—
	C + D = 2	12	0	0	—	—
		11	0	—	—	—
A + B = 13	C + D = 13	13	9	8	7	6
		12	7	6	5	4
		11	6	5	4	3
		10	4	4	3	2
		9	3	3	2	1
		8	2	2	1	0
		7	2	1	0	0
		6	1	0	0	—
		5	0	0	—	—
		4	0	—	—	—
	C + D = 12	13	8	7	6	5
		12	6	5	5	4
		11	5	4	3	3
		10	4	3	2	2
		9	3	2	1	1
		8	2	1	1	0
		7	1	1	0	0
		6	1	0	0	—
		5	0	0	—	—

Table G (continued)

Totals in right margin		B (or A)	Level of significance			
			.05	.025	.01	.005
A + B = 13	C + D = 11	13	7	6	5	5
		12	6	5	4	3
		11	4	4	·3	2
		10	3	3	2	1
		9	3	2	1	1
		8	2	1	0	0
		7	1	0	0	0
		6	0	0	—	—
		5	0	—	—	—
	C + D = 10	13	6	6	5	4
		12	5	4	3	3
		11	4	3	2	2
		10	3	2	1	1
		9	2	1	1	0
		8	1	1	0	0
		7	1	0	0	—
		6	0	0	—	—
		5	0	—	—	—
	C + D = 9	13	5	5	4	4
		12	4	4	3	2
		11	3	3	2	1
		10	2	2	1	1
		9	2	1	0	0
		8	1	1	0	0
		7	0	0	—	—
		6	0	0	—	—
		5	0	—	—	—
	C + D = 8	13	5	4	3	3
		12	4	3	2	2
		11	3	2	1	1
		10	2	1	1	0
		9	1	1	0	0
		8	1	0	0	—
		7	0	0	—	—
		6	0	—	—	—
	C + D = 7	13	4	3	3	2
		12	3	2	2	1
		11	2	2	1	1
		10	1	1	0	0
		9	1	0	0	0
		8	0	0	—	—
		7	0	0	—	—
		6	0	—	—	—

Table G (continued)

Totals in right margin		B (or A)	Level of significance			
			.05	.025	.01	.005
$A + B = 13$	$C + D = 6$	13	3	3	2	2
		12	2	2	1	1
		11	2	1	1	0
		10	1	1	0	0
		9	1	0	0	—
		8	0	0	—	—
		7	0	—	—	—
	$C + D = 5$	13	2	2	1	1
		12	2	1	1	0
		11	1	1	0	0
		10	1	0	0	—
		9	0	0	—	—
		8	0	—	—	—
	$C + D = 4$	13	2	1	1	0
		12	1	1	0	0
		11	0	0	0	—
		10	0	0	—	—
		9	0	—	—	—
	$C + D = 3$	13	1	1	0	0
		12	0	0	0	—
		11	0	0	—	—
		10	0			
	$C + D = 2$	13	0	0	0	—
		12	0	—	—	—
$A + B = 14$	$C + D = 14$	14	10	9	8	7
		13	8	7	6	5
		12	6	6	5	4
		11	5	4	3	3
		10	4	3	2	2
		9	3	2	2	1
		8	2	2	1	0
		7	1	1	0	0
		6	1	0	0	—
		5	0	0	—	—
		4	0	—	—	—

Table G (continued)

Totals in right margin		B (or A)	Level of significance			
			.05	.025	.01	.005
$A + B = 14$	$C + D = 13$	14	9	8	7	6
		13	7	6	5	5
		12	6	5	4	3
		11	5	4	3	2
		10	4	3	2	2
		9	3	2	1	1
		8	2	1	1	0
		7	1	1	0	0
		6	1	0	—	—
		5	0	0	—	—
	$C + D = 12$	14	8	7	6	6
		13	6	6	5	4
		12	5	4	4	3
		11	4	3	3	2
		10	3	3	2	1
		9	2	2	1	1
		8	2	1	0	0
		7	1	0	0	—
		6	0	0	—	—
		5	0	—	—	—
	$C + D = 11$	14	7	6	6	5
		13	6	5	4	4
		12	5	4	3	3
		11	4	3	2	2
		10	3	2	1	1
		9	2	1	1	0
		8	1	1	0	0
		7	1	0	0	—
		6	0	0	—	—
		5	0	—	—	—
	$C + D = 10$	14	6	6	5	4
		13	5	4	4	3
		12	4	3	3	2
		11	3	3	2	1
		10	2	2	1	1
		9	2	1	0	0
		8	1	1	0	0
		7	0	0	0	—
		6	0	0	—	—
		5	0	—	—	—

Table G (continued)

Totals in right margin		B (or A)	Level of significance			
			.05	.025	.01	.005
$A + B = 14$	$C + D = 9$	14	6	5	4	4
		13	4	4	3	3
		12	3	3	2	2
		11	3	2	1	1
		10	2	1	1	0
		9	1	1	0	0
		8	1	0	0	—
		7	0	0	—	—
		6	0	—	—	—
	$C + D = 8$	14	5	4	4	3
		13	4	3	2	2
		12	3	2	2	1
		11	2	2	1	1
		10	2	1	0	0
		9	1	0	0	0
		8	0	0	0	—
		7	0	0	—	—
		6	0	—	—	—
	$C + D = 7$	14	4	3	3	2
		13	3	2	2	1
		12	2	2	1	1
		11	2	1	1	0
		10	1	1	0	0
		9	1	0	0	—
		8	0	0	—	—
		7	0	—	—	—
	$C + D = 6$	14	3	3	2	2
		13	2	2	1	1
		12	2	1	1	0
		11	1	1	0	0
		10	1	0	0	—
		9	0	0	—	—
		8	0	0	—	—
		7	0	—	—	—
	$C + D = 5$	14	2	2	1	1
		13	2	1	1	0
		12	1	1	0	0
		11	1	0	0	0
		10	0	0	—	—
		9	0	0	—	—
		8	0	—	—	—

Table G (continued)

Totals in right margin		B (or A)	Level of significance			
			.05	.025	.01	.005
A + B = 14	C + D = 4	14	2	1	1	1
		13	1	1	0	0
		12	1	0	0	0
		11	0	0	—	—
		10	0	0	—	—
		9	0	—	—	—
	C + D = 3	14	1	1	0	0
		13	0	0	0	—
		12	0	0	—	—
		11	0	—	—	—
	C + D = 2	14	0	0	0	—
		13	0	0	—	—
		12	0	—	—	—
A + B = 15	C + D = 15	15	11	10	9	8
		14	9	8	7	6
		13	7	6	5	5
		12	6	5	4	4
		11	5	4	3	3
		10	4	3	2	2
		9	3	2	1	1
		8	2	1	1	0
		7	1	1	0	0
		6	1	0	0	—
		5	0	0	—	—
		4	0	—	—	—
	C + D = 14	15	10	9	8	7
		14	8	7	6	6
		13	7	6	5	4
		12	6	5	4	3
		11	5	4	3	2
		10	4	3	2	1
		9	3	2	1	1
		8	2	1	1	0
		7	1	1	0	0
		6	1	0	—	—
		5	0	—	—	—

Table G (continued)

Totals in right margin		B (or A)	Level of significance			
			.05	.025	.01	.005
A + B = 15	C + D = 13	15	9	8	7	7
		14	7	7	6	5
		13	6	5	4	4
		12	5	4	3	3
		11	4	3	2	2
		10	3	2	2	1
		9	2	2	1	0
		8	2	1	0	0
		7	1	0	0	—
		6	0	0	—	—
		5	0	—	—	—
	C + D = 12	15	8	7	7	6
		14	7	6	5	4
		13	6	5	4	3
		12	5	4	3	2
		11	4	3	2	2
		10	3	2	1	1
		9	2	1	1	0
		8	1	1	0	0
		7	1	0	0	—
		6	0	0	—	—
		5	0	—	—	—
	C + D = 11	15	7	7	6	5
		14	6	5	4	4
		13	5	4	3	3
		12	4	3	2	2
		11	3	2	2	1
		10	2	2	1	1
		9	2	1	0	0
		8	1	1	0	0
		7	1	0	0	—
		6	0	0	—	—
		5	0	—	—	—
	C + D = 10	15	6	6	5	5
		14	5	5	4	3
		13	4	4	3	2
		12	3	3	2	2
		11	3	2	1	1
		10	2	1	1	0
		9	1	1	0	0
		8	1	0	0	—
		7	0	0	—	—
		6	0	—	—	—

Table G (continued)

Totals in right margin		B (or A)	Level of significance			
			.05	.025	.01	.005
A + B = 15	C + D = 9	15	6	5	4	4
		14	5	4	3	3
		13	4	3	2	2
		12	3	2	2	1
		11	2	2	1	1
		10	2	1	0	0
		9	1	1	0	0
		8	1	0	0	—
		7	0	0	—	—
		6	0	—	—	—
	C + D = 8	15	5	4	4	3
		14	4	3	3	2
		13	3	2	2	1
		12	2	2	1	1
		11	2	1	1	0
		10	1	1	0	0
		9	1	0	0	—
		8	0	0	—	—
		7	0	—	—	—
		6	0	—	—	—
	C + D = 7	15	4	4	3	3
		14	3	3	2	2
		13	2	2	1	1
		12	2	1	1	0
		11	1	1	0	0
		10	1	0	0	0
		9	0	0	—	—
		8	0	0	—	—
		7	0	—	—	—
	C + D = 6	15	3	3	2	2
		14	2	2	1	1
		13	2	1	1	0
		12	1	1	0	0
		11	1	0	0	0
		10	0	0	0	—
		9	0	0	—	—
		8	0	—	—	—
	C + D = 5	15	2	2	2	1
		14	2	1	1	1
		13	1	1	0	0
		12	1	0	0	0
		11	0	0	0	—
		10	0	0	—	—
		9	0	—	—	—

Table G (continued)

Totals in right margin		B (or A)	Level of significance			
			.05	.025	.01	.005
$A + B = 15$	$C + D = 4$	15	2	1	1	1
		14	1	1	0	0
		13	1	0	0	0
		12	0	0	0	—
		11	0	0	—	—
		10	0	—	—	—
	$C + D = 3$	15	1	1	0	0
		14	0	0	0	0
		13	0	0	—	—
		12	0	0	—	—
		11	0	—	—	—
	$C + D = 2$	15	0	0	0	—
		14	0	0	—	—
		13	0	—	—	—

*When B is entered in the middle column, the significance levels are for D. When A is used in place of B, the significance levels are for C.

Source: Adapted from Finney, The Fisher-Yates test of significance in 2 × 2 contingency tables. *Biometrika* 35:149, 1948. This abridgement is reproduced from Table I in Siegel, *Nonparametric Statistics for the Behavioral Sciences.* New York: McGraw-Hill, 1956.

Table H. Probabilities associated with values as small as observed values of U in the Mann-Whitney test*

$n_2 = 3$

U \ n_1	1	2	3
0	.250	.100	.050
1	.500	.200	.100
2	.750	.400	.200
3		.600	.350
4			.500
5			.650

$n_2 = 4$

U \ n_1	1	2	3	4
0	.200	.067	.028	.014
1	.400	.133	.057	.029
2	.600	.267	.114	.057
3		.400	.200	.100
4		.600	.314	.171
5			.429	.243
6			.571	.343
7				.443
8				.557

$n_2 = 5$

U \ n_1	1	2	3	4	5
0	.167	.047	.018	.008	.004
1	.333	.095	.036	.016	.008
2	.500	.190	.071	.032	.016
3	.667	.286	.125	.056	.028
4		.429	.196	.095	.048
5		.571	.286	.143	.075
6			.393	.206	.111
7			.500	.278	.155
8			.607	.365	.210
9				.452	.274
10				.548	.345
11					.421
12					.500
13					.579

Table H (continued)

$n_2 = 6$

U \ n_1	1	2	3	4	5	6
0	.143	.036	.012	.005	.002	.001
1	.286	.071	.024	.010	.004	.002
2	.428	.143	.048	.019	.009	.004
3	.571	.214	.083	.033	.015	.008
4		.321	.131	.057	.026	.013
5		.429	.190	.086	.041	.021
6		.571	.274	.129	.063	.032
7			.357	.176	.089	.047
8			.452	.238	.123	.066
9			.548	.305	.165	.090
10				.381	.214	.120
11				.457	.268	.155
12				.545	.331	.197
13					.396	.242
14					.465	.294
15					.535	.350
16						.409
17						.469
18						.531

$n_2 = 7$

U \ n_1	1	2	3	4	5	6	7
0	.125	.028	.008	.003	.001	.001	.000
1	.250	.056	.017	.006	.003	.001	.001
2	.375	.111	.033	.012	.005	.002	.001
3	.500	.167	.058	.021	.009	.004	.002
4	.625	.250	.092	.036	.015	.007	.003
5		.333	.133	.055	.024	.011	.006
6		.444	.192	.082	.037	.017	.009
7		.556	.258	.115	.053	.026	.013
8			.333	.158	.074	.037	.019
9			.417	.206	.101	.051	.027
10			.500	.264	.134	.069	.036
11			.583	.324	.172	.090	.049
12				.394	.216	.117	.064
13				.464	.265	.147	.082
14				.538	.319	.183	.104
15					.378	.223	.130

Table H (continued)

$n_2 = 7$

U \ n_1	1	2	3	4	5	6	7
16					.438	.267	.159
17					.500	.314	.191
18					.562	.365	.228
19						.418	.267
20						.473	.310
21						.527	.355
22							.402
23							.451
24							.500
25							.549

$n_2 = 8$

U \ n_1	1	2	3	4	5	6	7	8	t	Normal
0	.111	.022	.006	.002	.001	.000	.000	.000	3.308	.001
1	.222	.044	.012	.004	.002	.001	.000	.000	3.203	.001
2	.333	.089	.024	.008	.003	.001	.001	.000	3.098	.001
3	.444	.133	.042	.014	.005	.002	.001	.001	2.993	.001
4	.556	.200	.067	.024	.009	.004	.002	.001	2.888	.002
5		.267	.097	.036	.015	.006	.003	.001	2.783	.003
6		.356	.139	.055	.023	.010	.005	.002	2.678	.004
7		.444	.188	.077	.033	.015	.007	.003	2.573	.005
8		.556	.248	.107	.047	.021	.010	.005	2.468	.007
9			.315	.141	.064	.030	.014	.007	2.363	.009
10			.387	.184	.085	.041	.020	.010	2.258	.012
11			.461	.230	.111	.054	.027	.014	2.153	.016
12			.539	.285	.142	.071	.036	.019	2.048	.020
13				.341	.177	.091	.047	.025	1.943	.026
14				.404	.217	.114	.060	.032	1.838	.033
15				.467	.262	.141	.076	.041	1.733	.041
16				.533	.311	.172	.095	.052	1.628	.052
17					.362	.207	.116	.065	1.523	.064
18					.416	.245	.140	.080	1.418	.078
19					.472	.286	.168	.097	1.313	.094
20					.528	.331	.198	.117	1.208	.113

Table H (continued)

$n_2 = 8$

U	1	2	3	4	5	6	7	8	t	Normal
21						.377	.232	.139	1.102	.135
22						.426	.268	.164	.998	.159
23						.475	.306	.191	.893	.185
24						.525	.347	.221	.788	.215
25							.389	.253	.683	.247
26							.433	.287	.578	.282
27							.478	.323	.473	.318
28							.522	.360	.368	.356
29								.399	.263	.396
30								.439	.158	.437
31								.480	.052	.481
32								.520		

*Tables probabilities are one-tailed. For two-tailed probabilities, double the value in the table.
Source: From Mann and Whitney, On a test of whether one of two random variables is stochastically larger than the other. *Ann. Math. Statistics* 18:52, 1947. This is reproduced from Table J in Siegel, *Nonparametric Statistics for the Behavioral Sciences.* New York: McGraw-Hill, 1956.

Table I. Critical values of the U statistic of the Mann-Whitney test

$\alpha = .002$ (two-tailed) and $.001$ (one-tailed)

n_1 \ n_2	9	10	11	12	13	14	15	16	17	18	19	20
1												
2												
3										0	0	0	0
4		0	0	0	1	1	1	2	2	3	3	3
5	1	1	2	2	3	3	4	5	5	6	7	7
6	2	3	4	4	5	6	7	8	9	10	11	12
7	3	5	6	7	8	9	10	11	13	14	15	16
8	5	6	8	9	11	12	14	15	17	18	20	21
9	7	8	10	12	14	15	17	19	21	23	25	26
10	8	10	12	14	17	19	21	23	25	27	29	32
11	10	12	15	17	20	22	24	27	29	32	34	37
12	12	14	17	20	23	25	28	31	34	37	40	42
13	14	17	20	23	26	29	32	35	38	42	45	48
14	15	19	22	25	29	32	36	39	43	46	50	54
15	17	21	24	28	32	36	40	43	47	51	55	59
16	19	23	27	31	35	39	43	48	52	56	60	65
17	21	25	29	34	38	43	47	52	57	61	66	70
18	23	27	32	37	42	46	51	56	61	66	71	76
19	25	29	34	40	45	50	55	60	66	71	77	82
20	26	32	37	42	48	54	59	65	70	76	82	88

$\alpha = .02$ (two-tailed) and $.01$ (one-tailed)

n_1 \ n_2	9	10	11	12	13	14	15	16	17	18	19	20
1												
2					0	0	0	0	0	0	1	1
3	1	1	1	2	2	2	3	3	4	4	4	5
4	3	3	4	5	5	6	7	7	8	9	9	10
5	5	6	7	8	9	10	11	12	13	14	15	16
6	7	8	9	11	12	13	15	16	18	19	20	22
7	9	11	12	14	16	17	19	21	23	24	26	28
8	11	13	15	17	20	22	24	26	28	30	32	34
9	14	16	18	21	23	26	28	31	33	36	38	40
10	16	19	22	24	27	30	33	36	38	41	44	47
11	18	22	25	28	31	34	37	41	44	47	50	53
12	21	24	28	31	35	38	42	46	49	53	56	60

Table I (continued)

$\alpha = .02$ (two-tailed) and .01 (one-tailed)

n_1 \ n_2	9	10	11	12	13	14	15	16	17	18	19	20
13	23	27	31	35	39	43	47	51	55	59	63	67
14	26	30	34	38	43	47	51	56	60	65	69	73
15	28	33	37	42	47	51	56	61	66	70	75	80
16	31	36	41	46	51	56	61	66	71	76	82	87
17	33	38	44	49	55	60	66	71	77	82	88	93
18	36	41	47	53	59	65	70	76	82	88	94	100
19	38	44	50	56	63	69	75	82	88	94	101	107
20	40	47	53	60	67	73	80	87	93	100	107	114

$\alpha = .05$ (two-tailed) and .025 (one-tailed)

n_1 \ n_2	9	10	11	12	13	14	15	16	17	18	19	20
1												
2	0	0	0	1	1	1	1	1	2	2	2	2
3	2	3	3	4	4	5	5	6	6	7	7	8
4	4	5	6	7	8	9	10	11	11	12	13	13
5	7	8	9	11	12	13	14	15	17	18	19	20
6	10	11	13	14	16	17	19	21	22	24	25	27
7	12	14	16	18	20	22	24	26	28	30	32	34
8	15	17	19	22	24	26	29	31	34	36	38	41
9	17	20	23	26	28	31	34	37	39	42	45	48
10	20	23	26	29	33	36	39	42	45	48	52	55
11	23	26	30	33	37	40	44	47	51	55	58	62
12	26	29	33	37	41	45	49	53	57	61	65	69
13	28	33	37	41	45	50	54	59	63	67	72	76
14	31	36	40	45	50	55	59	64	67	74	78	83
15	34	39	44	49	54	59	64	70	75	80	85	90
16	37	42	47	53	59	64	70	75	81	86	92	98
17	39	45	51	57	63	67	75	81	87	93	99	105
18	42	48	55	61	67	74	80	86	93	99	106	112
19	45	52	58	65	72	78	85	92	99	106	113	119
20	48	55	62	69	76	83	90	98	105	112	119	127

Table I (continued)

$\alpha = .10$ (two-tailed) and $.05$ (one-tailed)

n_2\\n_1	9	10	11	12	13	14	15	16	17	18	19	20
1											0	0
2	1	1	1	2	2	2	3	3	3	4	4	4
3	3	4	5	5	6	7	7	8	9	9	10	11
4	6	7	8	9	10	11	12	14	15	16	17	18
5	9	11	12	13	15	16	18	19	20	22	23	25
6	12	14	16	17	19	21	23	25	26	28	30	32
7	15	17	19	21	24	26	28	30	33	35	37	39
8	18	20	23	26	28	31	33	36	39	41	44	47
9	21	24	27	30	33	36	39	42	45	48	51	54
10	24	27	31	34	37	41	44	48	51	55	58	62
11	27	31	34	38	42	46	50	54	57	61	65	69
12	30	34	38	42	47	51	55	60	64	68	72	77
13	33	37	42	47	51	56	61	65	70	75	80	84
14	36	41	46	51	56	61	66	71	77	82	87	92
15	39	44	50	55	61	66	72	77	83	88	94	100
16	42	48	54	60	65	71	77	83	89	95	101	107
17	45	51	57	64	70	77	83	89	96	102	109	115
18	48	55	61	68	75	82	88	95	102	109	116	123
19	51	58	65	72	80	87	94	101	109	116	123	130
20	54	62	69	77	84	92	100	107	115	123	130	138

Source: From Auble, Extended tables for the Mann-Whitney statistic. *Bull. Inst. Educ. Res. Indiana Univ.* 1, No. 2; 1953. This abridgement is reproduced from Table K in Siegel, *Nonparametric Statistics for the Behavioral Sciences.* New York: McGraw-Hill, 1956.

Table J. Probabilities associated with values as small as observed values of x in the binomial test*

N \ x	0	1	2	3	4	5	6	7	8	9	10	11	12	13	14	15
5	031	188	500	812	969	†										
6	016	109	344	656	891	984	†									
7	008	062	227	500	773	938	992	†								
8	004	035	145	363	637	855	965	996	†							
9	002	020	090	254	500	746	910	980	998	†						
10	001	011	055	172	377	623	828	945	989	999	†					
11		006	033	113	274	500	726	887	967	994	†	†				
12		003	019	073	194	387	613	806	927	981	997	†	†			
13		002	011	046	133	291	500	709	867	954	989	998	†	†		
14		001	006	029	090	212	395	605	788	910	971	994	999	†	†	
15			004	018	059	151	304	500	696	849	941	982	996	†	†	†
16			002	011	038	105	227	402	598	773	895	962	989	998	†	†
17			001	006	025	072	166	315	500	685	834	928	975	994	999	†
18			001	004	015	048	119	240	407	593	760	881	952	985	996	999
19				002	010	032	084	180	324	500	676	820	916	968	990	998
20				001	006	021	058	132	252	412	588	748	868	942	979	994
21				001	004	013	039	095	192	332	500	668	808	905	961	987
22					002	008	026	067	143	262	416	584	738	857	933	974
23					001	005	017	047	105	202	339	500	661	798	895	953
24					001	003	011	032	076	154	271	419	581	729	846	924
25						002	007	022	054	115	212	345	500	655	788	885

*To save space, decimal points are omitted in the ps of the table; p values given are one-tailed. For two-tailed tests, double the tabled value.
†1.0 or approximately 1.0.
Source: From Walker and Lev, *Statistical Inference*. New York: Holt, Rinehart & Winston, 1953. This adaptation is reproduced from Table D in Siegel, *Nonparametric Statistics for the Behavioral Sciences*. New York: McGraw-Hill, 1956.

Table K. Critical values of T in the Wilcoxon matched-pairs signed-ranks test

	Level of significance for one-tailed test		
	.025	.01	.005
	Level of significance for two-tailed test		
N	.05	.02	.01
6	0	—	—
7	2	0	—
8	4	2	0
9	6	3	2
10	8	5	3
11	11	7	5
12	14	10	7
13	17	13	10
14	21	16	13
15	25	20	16
16	30	24	20
17	35	28	23
18	40	33	28
19	46	38	32
20	52	43	38
21	59	49	43
22	66	56	49
23	73	62	55
24	81	69	61
25	89	77	68

Source: From Wilcoxon, *Some Rapid Approximate Statistical Procedures.* New York: American Cyanamid Co, 1949. This adaptation is reproduced from Table G in Siegel, *Nonparametric Statistics for the Behavioral Sciences.* New York: McGraw-Hill, 1956.

Table L. Probabilities associated with values as large as observed values of H in the Kruskal-Wallis one-way analysis of variance by ranks test

Sample sizes					Sample sizes				
n_1	n_2	n_3	H	p	n_1	n_2	n_3	H	p
2	1	1	2.7000	.500	4	3	2	6.4444	.008
2	2	1	3.6000	.200				6.3000	.011
2	2	2	4.5714	.067				5.4444	.046
			3.7143	.200				5.4000	.051
3	1	1	3.2000	.300				4.5111	.098
3	2	1	4.2857	.100				4.4444	.102
			3.8571	.133	4	3	3	6.7455	.010
3	2	2	5.3572	.029				6.7091	.013
			4.7143	.048				5.7909	.046
			4.5000	.067				5.7273	.050
			4.4643	.105				4.7091	.092
3	3	1	5.1429	.043				4.7000	.101
			4.5714	.100	4	4	1	6.6667	.010
			4.0000	.129				6.1667	.022
3	3	2	6.2500	.011				4.9667	.048
			5.3611	.032				4.8667	.054
			5.1389	.061				4.1667	.082
			4.5556	.100				4.0667	.102
			4.2500	.121	4	4	2	7.0364	.006
3	3	3	7.2000	.004				6.8727	.011
			6.4889	.011				5.4545	.046
			5.6889	.029				5.2364	.052
			5.6000	.050				4.5545	.098
			5.0667	.086				4.4455	.103
			4.6222	.100	4	4	3	7.1439	.010
4	1	1	3.5714	.200				7.1364	.011
4	2	1	4.8214	.057				5.5985	.049
			4.5000	.076				5.5758	.051
			4.0179	.114				4.5455	.099
4	2	2	6.0000	.014				4.4773	.102
			5.3333	.033	4	4	4	7.6538	.008
			5.1250	.052				7.5385	.011
			4.4583	.100				5.6923	.049
			4.1667	.105				5.6538	.054
4	3	1	5.8333	.021				4.6539	.097
			5.2083	.050				4.5001	.104
			5.0000	.057	5	1	1	3.8571	.143
			4.0556	.093	5	2	1	5.2500	.036
			3.8889	.129				5.0000	.048
								4.4500	.071
								4.2000	.095
								4.0500	.119

Table L (continued)

Sample sizes					Sample sizes				
n_1	n_2	n_3	H	p	n_1	n_2	n_3	H	p
5	2	2	6.5333	.008				5.6308	.050
			6.1333	.013				4.5487	.099
			5.1600	.034				4.5231	.103
			5.0400	.056	5	4	4	7.7604	.009
			4.3733	.090				7.7440	.011
			4.2933	.122				5.6571	.049
5	3	1	6.4000	.012				5.6176	.050
			4.9600	.048				4.6187	.100
			4.8711	.052				4.5527	.102
			4.0178	.095	5	5	1	7.3091	.009
			3.8400	.123				6.8364	.011
5	3	2	6.9091	.009				5.1273	.046
			6.8218	.010				4.9091	.053
			5.2509	.049				4.1091	.086
			5.1055	.052				4.0364	.105
			4.6509	.091	5	5	2	7.3385	.010
			4.4945	.101				7.2692	.010
5	3	3	7.0788	.009				5.3385	.047
			6.9818	.011				5.2462	.051
			5.6485	.049				4.6231	.097
			5.5152	.051				4.5077	.100
			4.5333	.097	5	5	3	7.5780	.010
			4.4121	.109				7.5429	.010
5	4	1	6.9545	.008				5.7055	.046
			6.8400	.011				5.6264	.051
			4.9855	.044				4.5451	.100
			4.8600	.056				4.5363	.102
			3.9873	.098	5	5	4	7.8229	.010
			3.9600	.102				7.7914	.010
5	4	2	7.2045	.009				5.6657	.049
			7.1182	.010				5.6429	.050
			5.2727	.049				4.5229	.099
			5.2682	.050				4.5200	.101
			4.5409	.098	5	5	5	8.0000	.009
			4.5182	.101				7.9800	.010
5	4	3	7.4449	.010				5.7800	.049
			7.3949	.011				5.6600	.051
			5.6564	.049				4.5600	.100
								4.5000	.102

Source: From Kruskal and Wallis, Use of ranks in one-criterion variance analysis. *J. Am. Statist. Assoc.* 47:614 and 48:910, 1952. This abridgement is reproduced from Table O in Siegel, *Nonparametric Statistics for the Behavioral Sciences.* New York: McGraw-Hill, 1956.

Table M. Probabilities associated with values as large as observed values of χ_r^2 in the Friedman two-way analysis of variance by ranks test

$k = 3$

$N = 2$		$N = 3$		$N = 4$		$N = 5$	
χ_r^2	p	χ_r^2	p	χ_r^2	p	χ_r^2	p
0	1.000	.000	1.000	.0	1.000	.0	1.000
1	.833	.667	.944	.5	.931	.4	.954
3	.500	2.000	.528	1.5	.653	1.2	.691
4	.167	2.667	.361	2.0	.431	1.6	.522
		4.667	.194	3.5	.273	2.8	.367
		6.000	.028	4.5	.125	3.6	.182
				6.0	.069	4.8	.124
				6.5	.042	5.2	.093
				8.0	.0046	6.4	.039
						7.6	.024
						8.4	.0085
						10.0	.00077

$N = 6$		$N = 7$		$N = 8$		$N = 9$	
χ_r^2	p	χ_r^2	p	χ_r^2	p	χ_r^2	p
.00	1.000	.000	1.000	.00	1.000	.000	1.000
.33	.956	.286	.964	.25	.967	.222	.971
1.00	.740	.857	.768	.75	.794	.667	.814
1.33	.570	1.143	.620	1.00	.654	.889	.865
2.33	.430	2.000	.486	1.75	.531	1.556	.569
3.00	.252	2.571	.305	2.25	.355	2.000	.398
4.00	.184	3.429	.237	3.00	.285	2.667	.328
4.33	.142	3.714	.192	3.25	.236	2.889	.278
5.33	.072	4.571	.112	4.00	.149	3.556	.187
6.33	.052	5.429	.085	4.75	.120	4.222	.154
7.00	.029	6.000	.052	5.25	.079	4.667	.107
8.33	.012	7.143	.027	6.25	.047	5.556	.069
9.00	.0081	7.714	.021	6.75	.038	6.000	.057
9.33	.0055	8.000	.016	7.00	.030	6.222	.018
10.33	.0017	8.857	.0084	7.75	.018	6.889	.031
12.00	.00013	10.286	.0036	9.00	.0099	8.000	.019
		10.571	.0027	9.25	.0080	8.222	.016
		11.143	.0012	9.75	.0048	8.667	.010
		12.286	.00032	10.75	.0024	9.556	.0060
		14.000	.000021	12.00	.0011	10.667	.0035

Table M (continued)

N = 6		N = 7		N = 8		N = 9	
χ_r^2	p	χ_r^2	p	χ_r^2	p	χ_r^2	p
				12.25	.00086	10.889	.0029
				13.00	.00026	11.556	.0013
				14.25	.000061	12.667	.00066
				16.00	.0000036	13.556	.00035
						14.000	.00020
						14.222	.000097
						14.889	.000054
						16.222	.000011
						18.000	.0000006

k = 4

N = 2		N = 3		N = 4			
χ_r^2	p	χ_r^2	p	χ_r^2	p	χ_r^2	p
.0	1.000	.2	1.000	.0	1.000	5.7	.141
.6	.958	.6	.958	.3	.992	6.0	.105
1.2	.834	1.0	.910	.6	.928	6.3	.094
1.8	.792	1.8	.727	.9	.900	6.6	.077
2.4	.625	2.2	.608	1.2	.800	6.9	.068
3.0	.542	2.6	.524	1.5	.754	7.2	.054
3.6	.458	3.4	.446	1.8	.677	7.5	.052
4.2	.375	3.8	.342	2.1	.649	7.8	.036
4.8	.208	4.2	.300	2.4	.524	8.1	.033
5.4	.167	5.0	.207	2.7	.508	8.4	.019
6.0	.042	5.4	.175	3.0	.432	8.7	.014
		5.8	.148	3.3	.389	9.3	.012
		6.6	.075	3.6	.355	9.6	.0069
		7.0	.054	3.9	.324	9.9	.0062
		7.4	.033	4.5	.242	10.2	.0027
		8.2	.017	4.8	.200	10.8	.0016
		9.0	.0017	5.1	.190	11.1	.00094
				5.4	.158	12.0	.000072

Source: From Friedman, The use of ranks to avoid the assumption of normality implicit in the analysis of variance. *J. Am. Statist. Assoc.* 32:688, 1937. This adaptation is reproduced from Table N in Siegel, *Nonparametric Statistics for the Behavioral Sciences.* New York: McGraw-Hill, 1956.

Table N. Fisher's *Z* transformation function for Pearson's coefficient

r	Z	r	Z	r	Z	r	Z	r	Z
.000	.000	.200	.203	.400	.424	.600	.693	.800	1.099
.005	.005	.205	.208	.405	.430	.605	.701	.805	1.113
.010	.010	.210	.213	.410	.436	.610	.709	.810	1.127
.015	.015	.215	.218	.415	.442	.615	.717	.815	1.142
.020	.020	.220	.224	.420	.448	.620	.725	.820	1.157
.025	.025	.225	.229	.425	.454	.625	.733	.825	1.172
.030	.030	.230	.234	.430	.460	.630	.741	.830	1.188
.035	.035	.235	.239	.435	.466	.635	.750	.835	1.204
.040	.040	.240	.245	.440	.472	.640	.758	.840	1.221
.045	.045	.245	.250	.445	.478	.645	.767	.845	1.238
.050	.050	.250	.255	.450	.485	.650	.775	.850	1.256
.055	.055	.255	.261	.455	.491	.655	.784	.855	1.274
.060	.060	.260	.266	.460	.497	.660	.793	.860	1.293
.065	.065	.265	.271	.465	.504	.665	.802	.865	1.313
.070	.070	.270	.277	.470	.510	.670	.811	.870	1.333
.075	.075	.275	.282	.475	.517	.675	.820	.875	1.354
.080	.080	.280	.288	.480	.523	.680	.829	.880	1.376
.085	.085	.285	.293	.485	.530	.685	.838	.885	1.398
.090	.090	.290	.299	.490	.536	.690	.848	.890	1.422
.095	.095	.295	.304	.495	.543	.695	.858	.895	1.447
.100	.100	.300	.310	.500	.549	.700	.867	.900	1.472
.105	.105	.305	.315	.505	.556	.705	.877	.905	1.499
.110	.110	.310	.321	.510	.563	.710	.887	.910	1.528
.115	.116	.315	.326	.515	.570	.715	.897	.915	1.557
.120	.121	.320	.332	.520	.576	.720	.908	.920	1.589
.125	.126	.325	.337	.525	.583	.725	.918	.925	1.623
.130	.131	.330	.343	.530	.590	.730	.929	.930	1.658
.135	.136	.335	.348	.535	.597	.735	.940	.935	1.697
.140	.141	.340	.354	.540	.604	.740	.950	.940	1.738
.145	.146	.345	.360	.545	.611	.745	.962	.945	1.783
.150	.151	.350	.365	.550	.618	.750	.973	.950	1.832
.155	.156	.355	.371	.555	.626	.755	.984	.955	1.886
.160	.161	.360	.377	.560	.633	.760	.996	.960	1.946
.165	.167	.365	.383	.565	.640	.765	1.008	.965	2.014
.170	.172	.370	.388	.570	.648	.770	1.020	.970	2.092
.175	.177	.375	.394	.575	.655	.775	1.033	.975	2.185
.180	.182	.380	.400	.580	.662	.780	1.045	.980	2.298
.185	.187	.385	.406	.585	.670	.785	1.058	.985	2.443
.190	.192	.390	.412	.590	.678	.790	1.071	.990	2.647
.195	.198	.395	.418	.595	.685	.795	1.085	.995	2.994

Source: From Edwards, *Statistical Methods*. New York: Holt, Rinehart & Winston, 1967. This adaptation is reproduced from Appendix F in Bruning and Kintz, *Computational Handbook of Statistics,* (2nd ed.). Glenview, Ill.: Scott, Foresman Co., 1977.

Table O. Significant studentized ranges for Newman-Keul's and Tukey multiple comparison tests

Error df	α	Number of means or number of steps between ordered means									
		2	3	4	5	6	7	8	9	10	11
5	.05	3.64	4.60	5.22	5.67	6.03	6.33	6.58	6.80	6.99	7.17
	.01	5.70	6.98	7.80	8.42	8.91	9.32	9.67	9.97	10.24	10.48
6	.05	3.46	4.34	4.90	5.30	5.63	5.90	6.12	6.32	6.49	6.65
	.01	5.24	6.33	7.03	7.56	7.97	8.32	8.61	8.87	9.10	9.30
7	.05	3.34	4.16	4.68	5.06	5.36	5.61	5.82	6.00	6.16	6.30
	.01	4.95	5.92	6.54	7.01	7.37	7.68	7.94	8.17	8.37	8.55
8	.05	3.26	4.04	4.53	4.89	5.17	5.40	5.60	5.77	5.92	6.05
	.01	4.75	5.64	6.20	6.62	6.96	7.24	7.47	7.68	7.86	8.03
9	.05	3.20	3.95	4.41	4.76	5.02	5.24	5.43	5.59	5.74	5.87
	.01	4.60	5.43	5.96	6.35	6.66	6.91	7.13	7.33	7.49	7.65
10	.05	3.15	3.88	4.33	4.65	4.91	5.12	5.30	5.46	5.60	5.72
	.01	4.48	5.27	5.77	6.14	6.43	6.67	6.87	7.05	7.21	7.36
11	.05	3.11	3.82	4.26	4.57	4.82	5.03	5.20	5.35	5.49	5.61
	.01	4.39	5.15	5.62	5.97	6.25	6.48	6.67	6.84	6.99	7.13
12	.05	3.08	3.77	4.20	4.51	4.75	4.95	5.12	5.27	5.39	5.51
	.01	4.32	5.05	5.50	5.84	6.10	6.32	6.51	6.67	6.81	6.94
13	.05	3.06	3.73	4.15	4.45	4.69	4.88	5.05	5.19	5.32	5.43
	.01	4.26	4.96	5.40	5.73	5.98	6.19	6.37	6.53	6.67	6.79
14	.05	3.03	3.70	4.11	4.41	4.64	4.83	4.99	5.13	5.25	5.36
	.01	4.21	4.89	5.32	5.63	5.88	6.08	6.26	6.41	6.54	6.66
15	.05	3.01	3.67	4.08	4.37	4.59	4.78	4.94	5.08	5.20	5.31
	.01	4.17	4.84	5.25	5.56	5.80	5.99	6.16	6.31	6.44	6.55
16	.05	3.00	3.65	4.05	4.33	4.56	4.74	4.90	5.03	5.15	5.26
	.01	4.13	4.79	5.19	5.49	5.72	5.92	6.08	6.22	6.35	6.46
17	.05	2.98	3.63	4.02	4.30	4.52	4.70	4.86	4.99	5.11	5.21
	.01	4.10	4.74	5.14	5.43	5.66	5.85	6.01	6.15	6.27	6.38
18	.05	2.97	3.61	4.00	4.28	4.49	4.67	4.82	4.96	5.07	5.17
	.01	4.07	4.70	5.09	5.38	5.60	5.79	5.94	6.08	6.20	6.31
19	.05	2.96	3.59	3.98	4.25	4.47	4.65	4.79	4.92	5.04	5.14
	.01	4.05	4.67	5.05	5.33	5.55	5.73	5.89	6.02	6.14	6.25
20	.05	2.95	3.58	3.96	4.23	4.45	4.62	4.77	4.90	5.01	5.11
	.01	4.02	4.64	5.02	5.29	5.51	5.69	5.84	5.97	6.09	6.19
24	.05	2.92	3.53	3.90	4.17	4.37	4.54	4.68	4.81	4.92	5.01
	.01	3.96	4.55	4.91	5.17	5.37	5.54	5.69	5.81	5.92	6.02
30	.05	2.89	3.49	3.85	4.10	4.30	4.46	4.60	4.72	4.82	4.92
	.01	3.89	4.45	4.80	5.05	5.24	5.40	5.54	5.65	5.76	5.85
40	.05	2.86	3.44	3.79	4.04	4.23	4.39	4.52	4.63	4.73	4.82
	.01	3.82	4.37	4.70	4.93	5.11	5.26	5.39	5.50	5.60	5.69
60	.05	2.83	3.40	3.74	3.98	4.16	4.31	4.44	4.55	4.65	4.73
	.01	3.76	4.28	4.59	4.82	4.99	5.13	5.25	5.36	5.45	5.53
120	.05	2.80	3.36	3.68	3.92	4.10	4.24	4.36	4.47	4.56	4.64
	.01	3.70	4.20	4.50	4.71	4.87	5.01	5.12	5.21	5.30	5.37
∞	.05	2.77	3.31	3.63	3.86	4.03	4.17	4.29	4.39	4.47	4.55
	.01	3.64	4.12	4.40	4.60	4.76	4.88	4.99	5.08	5.16	5.23

Source: From Table 29 of Pearson and Hartley, *Biometrika Tables for Statisticians.* (3rd ed.). Cambridge: Cambridge University Press, 1966. Vol. 1.

Table O (continued)

number of means or number of steps between ordered means

12	13	14	15	16	17	18	19	20	α	Error df
7.32	7.47	7.60	7.72	7.83	7.93	8.03	8.12	8.21	.05	5
10.70	10.89	11.08	11.24	11.40	11.55	11.68	11.81	11.93	.01	
6.79	6.92	7.03	7.14	7.24	7.34	7.43	7.51	7.59	.05	6
9.48	9.65	9.81	9.95	10.08	10.21	10.32	10.43	10.54	.01	
6.43	6.55	6.66	6.76	6.85	6.94	7.02	7.10	7.17	.05	7
8.71	8.86	9.00	9.12	9.24	9.35	9.46	9.55	9.65	.01	
6.18	6.29	6.39	6.48	6.57	6.65	6.73	6.80	6.87	.05	8
8.18	8.31	8.44	8.55	8.66	8.76	8.85	8.94	9.03	.01	
5.98	6.09	6.19	6.28	6.36	6.44	6.51	6.58	6.64	.05	9
7.78	7.91	8.03	8.13	8.23	8.33	8.41	8.49	8.57	.01	
5.83	5.93	6.03	6.11	6.19	6.27	6.34	6.40	6.47	.05	10
7.49	7.60	7.71	7.81	7.91	7.99	8.08	8.15	8.23	.01	
5.71	5.81	5.90	5.98	6.06	6.13	6.20	6.27	6.33	.05	11
7.25	7.36	7.46	7.56	7.65	7.73	7.81	7.88	7.95	.01	
5.61	5.71	5.80	5.88	5.95	6.02	6.09	6.15	6.21	.05	12
7.06	7.17	7.26	7.36	7.44	7.52	7.59	7.66	7.73	.01	
5.53	5.63	5.71	5.79	5.86	5.93	5.99	6.05	6.11	.05	13
6.90	7.01	7.10	7.19	7.27	7.35	7.42	7.48	7.55	.01	
5.46	5.55	5.64	5.71	5.79	5.85	5.91	5.97	6.03	.05	14
6.77	6.87	6.96	7.05	7.13	7.20	7.27	7.33	7.39	.01	
5.40	5.49	5.57	5.65	5.72	5.78	5.85	5.90	5.96	.05	15
6.66	6.76	6.84	6.93	7.00	7.07	7.14	7.20	7.26	.01	
5.35	5.44	5.52	5.59	5.66	5.73	5.79	5.84	5.90	.05	16
6.56	6.66	6.74	6.82	6.90	6.97	7.03	7.09	7.15	.01	
5.31	5.39	5.47	5.54	5.61	5.67	5.73	5.79	5.84	.05	17
6.48	6.57	6.66	6.73	6.81	6.87	6.94	7.00	7.05	.01	
5.27	5.35	5.43	5.50	5.57	5.63	5.69	5.74	5.79	.05	18
6.41	6.50	6.58	6.65	6.73	6.79	6.85	6.91	6.97	.01	
5.23	5.31	5.39	5.46	5.53	5.59	5.65	5.70	5.75	.05	19
6.34	6.43	6.51	6.58	6.65	6.72	6.78	6.84	6.89	.01	
5.20	5.28	5.36	5.43	5.49	5.55	5.61	5.66	5.71	.05	20
6.28	6.32	6.45	6.52	6.59	6.65	6.71	6.77	6.82	.01	
5.10	5.18	5.25	5.32	5.38	5.44	5.49	5.55	5.59	.05	24
6.11	6.19	6.26	6.33	6.39	6.45	6.51	6.56	6.61	.01	
5.00	5.08	5.15	5.21	5.27	5.33	5.38	5.43	5.47	.05	30
5.93	6.01	6.06	6.14	6.20	6.26	6.31	6.36	6.41	.01	
4.90	4.98	5.04	5.11	5.16	5.22	5.27	5.31	5.36	.05	40
5.76	5.83	5.90	5.96	6.02	6.07	6.12	6.16	6.21	.01	
4.81	4.88	4.94	5.00	5.06	5.11	5.15	5.20	5.24	.05	60
5.60	5.67	5.73	5.78	5.84	5.89	5.93	5.97	6.01	.01	
4.71	4.78	4.84	4.90	4.95	5.00	5.04	5.09	5.13	.05	120
5.44	5.50	5.56	5.61	5.66	5.71	5.75	5.79	5.83	.01	
4.62	4.68	4.74	4.80	4.85	4.89	4.93	4.97	5.01	.05	∞
5.29	5.35	5.40	5.45	5.49	5.54	5.57	5.61	5.65	.01	

Table P. Dunnett's test: comparison of treatment means with a control

Error df	α	\multicolumn{9}{c}{r = number of treatment means, including control}
		2	3	4	5	6	7	8	9	10
5	.05	2.57	3.03	3.29	3.48	3.62	3.73	3.82	3.90	3.97
	.01	4.03	4.63	4.98	5.22	5.41	5.56	5.69	5.80	5.89
6	.05	2.45	2.86	3.10	3.26	3.39	3.49	3.57	3.64	3.71
	.01	3.71	4.21	4.51	4.71	4.87	5.00	5.10	5.20	5.28
7	.05	2.36	2.75	2.97	3.12	3.24	3.33	3.41	3.47	3.53
	.01	3.50	3.95	4.21	4.39	4.53	4.64	4.74	4.82	4.89
8	.05	2.31	2.67	2.88	3.02	3.13	3.22	3.29	3.35	3.41
	.01	3.36	3.77	4.00	4.17	4.29	4.40	4.48	4.56	4.62
9	.05	2.26	2.61	2.81	2.95	3.05	3.14	3.20	3.26	3.32
	.01	3.25	3.63	3.85	4.01	4.12	4.22	4.30	4.37	4.43
10	.05	2.23	2.57	2.76	2.89	2.99	3.07	3.14	3.19	3.24
	.01	3.17	3.53	3.74	3.88	3.99	4.08	4.16	4.22	4.28
11	.05	2.20	2.53	2.72	2.84	2.94	3.02	3.08	3.14	3.19
	.01	3.11	3.45	3.65	3.79	3.89	3.98	4.05	4.11	4.16
12	.05	2.18	2.50	2.68	2.81	2.90	2.98	3.04	3.09	3.14
	.01	3.05	3.39	3.58	3.71	3.81	3.89	3.96	4.02	4.07
13	.05	2.16	2.48	2.65	2.78	2.87	2.94	3.00	3.06	3.10
	.01	3.01	3.33	3.52	3.65	3.74	3.82	3.89	3.94	3.99
14	.05	2.14	2.46	2.63	2.75	2.84	2.91	2.97	3.02	3.07
	.01	2.98	3.29	3.47	3.59	3.69	3.76	3.83	3.88	3.93
15	.05	2.13	2.44	2.61	2.73	2.82	2.89	2.95	3.00	3.04
	.01	2.95	3.25	3.43	3.55	3.64	3.71	3.78	3.83	3.88
16	.05	2.12	2.42	2.59	2.71	2.80	2.87	2.92	2.97	3.02
	.01	2.92	3.22	3.39	3.51	3.60	3.67	3.73	3.78	3.83
17	.05	2.11	2.41	2.58	2.69	2.78	2.85	2.90	2.95	3.00
	.01	2.90	3.19	3.36	3.47	3.56	3.63	3.69	3.74	3.79
18	.05	2.10	2.40	2.56	2.68	2.76	2.83	2.89	2.94	2.98
	.01	2.88	3.17	3.33	3.44	3.53	3.60	3.66	3.71	3.75
19	.05	2.09	2.39	2.55	2.66	2.75	2.81	2.87	2.92	2.96
	.01	2.86	3.15	3.31	3.42	3.50	3.57	3.63	3.68	3.72
20	.05	2.09	2.38	2.54	2.65	2.73	2.80	2.86	2.90	2.95
	.01	2.85	3.13	3.29	3.40	3.48	3.55	3.60	3.65	3.69
24	.05	2.06	2.35	2.51	2.61	2.70	2.76	2.81	2.86	2.90
	.01	2.80	3.07	3.22	3.32	3.40	3.47	3.52	3.57	3.61
30	.05	2.04	2.32	2.47	2.58	2.66	2.72	2.77	2.82	2.86
	.01	2.75	3.01	3.15	3.25	3.33	3.39	3.44	3.49	3.52
40	.05	2.02	2.29	2.44	2.54	2.62	2.68	2.73	2.77	2.81
	.01	2.70	2.95	3.09	3.19	3.26	3.32	3.37	3.41	3.44
60	.05	2.00	2.27	2.41	2.51	2.58	2.64	2.69	2.73	2.77
	.01	2.66	2.90	3.03	3.12	3.19	3.25	3.29	3.33	3.37
120	.05	1.98	2.24	2.38	2.47	2.55	2.60	2.65	2.69	2.73
	.01	2.62	2.85	2.97	3.06	3.12	3.18	3.22	3.26	3.29
∞	.05	1.96	2.21	2.35	2.44	2.51	2.57	2.61	2.65	2.69
	.01	2.58	2.79	2.92	3.00	3.06	3.11	3.15	3.19	3.22

Source: From Dunnett, New tables for multiple comparisons with a control. *Biometrics* 20:482, 1964. This version is reproduced from Appendix L in Bruning and Kintz, *Computational Handbook of Statistics*, (2nd ed.). Glenview, Ill.: Scott, Foresman & Co, 1977.

Table Q. Critical values for Hartley's maximum F ratio significance test for homogeneity of variance

Alpha = .05 and *.01* (in italics)

df \ k	2	3	4	5	6	7	8	9	10	11	12
2	39.0	87.5	142.	202.	266.	333.	403.	475.	550.	626.	704.
	199.	*448.*	*729.*	*1036.*	*1362.*	*1705.*	*2063.*	*2432.*	*2813.*	*3204.*	*3605.*
3	15.4	27.8	39.2	50.7	62.0	72.9	83.5	93.9	104.	114.	124.
	47.5	*85.*	*120.*	*151.*	*184.*	*216.**	*249.**	*281.**	*310.**	*337.**	*361.**
4	9.60	15.5	20.6	25.2	29.5	33.6	37.5	41.1	44.6	48.0	51.4
	23.2	*37.*	*49.*	*59.*	*69.*	*79.*	*89.*	*97.*	*106.*	*113.*	*120.*
5	7.15	10.8	13.7	16.3	18.7	20.8	22.9	24.7	26.5	28.2	29.9
	14.9	*22.*	*28.*	*33.*	*38.*	*42.*	*46.*	*50.*	*54.*	*57.*	*60.*
6	5.82	8.38	10.4	12.1	13.7	15.0	16.3	17.5	18.6	19.7	20.7
	11.1	*15.5*	*19.1*	*22.*	*25.*	*27.*	*30.*	*32.*	*34.*	*36.*	*37.*
7	4.99	6.94	8.44	9.70	10.8	11.8	12.7	13.5	14.3	15.1	15.8
	8.89	*12.1*	*14.5*	*16.5*	*18.4*	*20.*	*22.*	*23.*	*24.*	*26.*	*27.*
8	4.43	6.00	7.18	8.12	9.03	9.78	10.5	11.1	11.7	12.2	12.7
	7.50	*9.9*	*11.7*	*13.2*	*14.5*	*15.8*	*16.9*	*17.9*	*18.9*	*19.8*	*21.*
9	4.03	5.34	6.31	7.11	7.80	8.41	8.95	9.45	9.91	10.3	10.7
	6.54	*8.5*	*9.9*	*11.1*	*12.1*	*13.1*	*13.9*	*14.7*	*15.3*	*16.0*	*16.6*
10	3.72	4.85	5.67	6.34	6.92	7.42	7.87	8.28	8.66	9.01	9.34
	5.85	*7.4*	*8.6*	*9.6*	*10.4*	*11.1*	*11.8*	*12.4*	*12.9*	*13.4*	*13.9*
12	3.28	4.16	4.79	5.30	5.72	6.09	6.42	6.72	7.00	7.25	7.48
	4.91	*6.1*	*6.9*	*7.6*	*8.2*	*8.7*	*9.1*	*9.5*	*9.9*	*10.2*	*10.6*
15	2.86	3.54	4.01	4.37	4.68	4.95	5.19	5.40	5.59	5.77	5.93
	4.07	*4.9*	*5.5*	*6.0*	*6.4*	*6.7*	*7.1*	*7.3*	*7.5*	*7.8*	*8.0*
20	2.46	2.95	3.29	3.54	3.76	3.94	4.10	4.24	4.37	4.49	4.59
	3.32	*3.8*	*4.3*	*4.6*	*4.9*	*5.1*	*5.3*	*5.5*	*5.6*	*5.8*	*5.9*
30	2.07	2.40	2.61	2.78	2.91	3.02	3.12	3.21	3.29	3.36	3.39
	2.63	*3.0*	*3.3*	*3.4*	*3.6*	*3.7*	*3.8*	*3.9*	*4.0*	*4.1*	*4.2*
60	1.67	1.85	1.96	2.04	2.11	2.17	2.22	2.26	2.30	2.33	2.36
	1.96	*2.2*	*2.3*	*2.4*	*2.4*	*2.5*	*2.5*	*2.6*	*2.6*	*2.7*	*2.7*
∞	1.00	1.00	1.00	1.00	1.00	1.00	1.00	1.00	1.00	1.00	1.00
	1.00	*1.00*	*1.00*	*1.00*	*1.00*	*1.00*	*1.00*	*1.00*	*1.00*	*1.00*	*1.00*

*Values in the column $k = 2$ and in the rows $df = 2$ and ∞ are exact. Elsewhere the third digit may be in error by a few units for $F_{.95}$ and several units for $F_{.99}$. The third-digit figures of values marked by an asterisk are the most uncertain.

Source: Table Q is taken from Table 31 of Pearson and Hartley, *Biometrika Tables for Statisticians* (3rd ed.). Cambridge: Cambridge University Press, 1966. Vol. 1. This adaptation is reproduced from Bruning and Kintz, *Computational Handbook of Statistics,* (2nd ed.). Glenview, Ill.: Scott, Foresman & Co., 1977.

Appendix IV: *Power Tables**

A. Estimated Percent Probability of Type II Error for *t* When $\alpha = .05$.
B. Estimated Percent Probability of Type II Error for Differences Between Correlation Coefficients at $\alpha = .05$.
C. Estimated Percent Probability of Type II Error for *F* When $\alpha = .05$
D. Estimated Percent Probability of Type II Error for χ^2 When $\alpha = .05$
E. Estimated Percent Probability of Type II Error for *R* When $\alpha = .05$

*The power table for *r* is presented in Chapter 15 as Exhibit 15.2. Accuracy of the tables is within 5 percent owing to rounding error. For more detailed treatment, such as *alpha* levels other than .05, please refer to Cohen, *Statistical Power Analysis for the Behavioral Sciences* (rev. ed.). New York: Academic, 1977.

Table A. Estimated percent probability of type II error for t when $\alpha = .05$

$$ES = \frac{|\,\overline{X}_1 - \overline{X}_2\,|}{SD}$$

n	tails	.10	.20	.30	.40	.45	.50	.55	.60	.65	.70	.75	.80	.85	.90	.95	1.00	1.10	1.20	1.40
8	2	95	93	91	89	87	85	83	80	77	75	73	69	66	62	58	54	47	40	27
	1	93	90	87	81	78	75	72	69	65	62	58	54	50	46	43	39	32	26	15
9	2	95	93	91	88	86	84	81	78	75	72	69	65	61	57	53	49	42	35	21
	1	93	89	85	80	77	73	70	66	62	59	55	50	46	42	38	34	28	21	*
10	2	94	93	90	87	85	82	79	76	72	69	65	61	57	53	48	44	36	29	16
	1	92	89	84	78	75	71	67	64	59	55	51	47	43	39	34	30	37	*	—
11	2	94	93	90	86	83	80	77	74	70	66	62	57	53	48	44	39	32	24	13
	1	92	88	83	77	73	69	65	61	56	52	48	43	39	35	30	*	—	—	—
12	2	94	92	89	85	82	79	76	72	67	63	59	54	49	44	40	35	28	20	*10
	1	92	88	82	75	71	67	63	59	54	49	45	40	36	32	27	*	—	—	—
13	2	94	92	89	84	81	77	73	69	64	60	55	50	45	40	36	31	24	*	—
	1	92	87	82	74	70	66	61	56	51	46	42	37	33	29	24	*	—	—	—
14	2	94	92	88	83	79	75	71	67	62	57	52	47	42	27	33	28	21	*	—
	1	92	87	81	73	69	64	59	54	48	43	39	*							
15	2	94	92	88	82	78	74	70	65	60	55	50	44	39	34	30	*	—	—	—
	1	92	87	80	72	67	62	57	52	46	41	36	*							
16	2	94	92	87	81	77	72	68	63	57	52	47	41	36	31	27	*	—	—	—
	1	91	86	79	70	65	60	55	49	43	*									
17	2	94	91	87	80	76	71	66	61	55	49	44	38	34	29	24	*	—	—	—
	1	91	86	78	69	64	58	53	47	41	*	—	—							
18	2	94	91	86	79	74	69	64	59	53	47	41	*							
	1	91	85	78	68	63	57	51	45	39	*	—	—							
19	2	94	91	85	78	73	68	62	57	51	45	39	*							
	1	91	85	77	64	59	55	49	*	—	—	—	—							
20	2	94	91	85	77	72	67	61	55	48	42	36	*							
	1	91	85	76	66	61	54	48	*	—	—	—	—							
21	2	94	90	84	76	71	65	59	53	46	40	34	*							
	1	91	84	75	64	58	52	46	*	—	—	—	—							
22	2	94	90	84	75	69	64	58	51	44	*	—	—							
	1	91	84	74	63	57	50	44	*	—	—	—	—							
23	2	94	90	83	74	68	62	56	49	42	—	—	—							
	1	90	84	74	62	56	*	—	—	—	—	—	—							
24	2	94	90	83	73	67	61	54	47	40	*	—	—							
	1	90	83	73	61	54	*	—	—	—	—	—	—							
25	2	94	89	82	72	60	53	*	—	—	—	—	—							
	1	90	83	72	65	53	*	—	—	—	—	—	—							
26	2	94	89	81	71	64	58	51	*	—	—	—	—							
	1	90	82	72	59	52	*	—	—	—	—	—	—							
27	2	94	89	81	70	63	57	50	*	—	—	—	—							
	1	90	82	71	58	51	*	—	—	—	—	—	—							

Table A (continued)

n	tails	.10	.20	.30	.40	.45	.50	.55	.60	.65	.70	.75	.80	.85	.90	.95	1.00	1.10	1.20	1.40
28	2	93	89	80	69	62	55	48	*	—	—	—	—							
	1	90	82	70	57	50	*	—	—	—	—	—	—							
29	2	93	88	80	68	61	54	47	*	—	—	—	—							
	1	90	81	70	*	—	—	—	—	—	—	—	—							
30	2	93	88	79	67	60	53	45	*	—	—	—	—							
	1	90	81	69	*	—	—	—	—	—	—	—	—							
35	2	93	87	77	62	54	*	—	—											
	1	89	79	66	*	—	—													
40	2	93	86	74	58	49	*	—	—											
	1	89	78	*	—	—	—													
50	2	92	83	68	*	—	—													
	1	88	74	*	—	—	—													
60	2	92	81	*	—	—	—													
	1	87	71	*	—	—	—													
80	2	90	76	*	—	—	—													
	1	85	*	—	—	—	—													
100	2	89	*	—	—	—	—													
	1	83	*	—	—	—	—													

*t values this large are equal to or exceed the critical value. Therefore, type II error becomes irrelevant.
Note: n values represent sample size of *one* group where groups are equal in size. When groups are unequal, enter table with harmonic mean of n in the two groups.

Table B. Estimated percent probability of type II error for the difference between correlation coefficients at $\alpha = .05$

$$ES = Zr_1 - Zr_2$$

n	tails	.10	.20	.30	.40	.45	.50	.55	.60	.65	.70	.75	.80	.85	.90	.95	1.00	1.10	1.20	1.40
8	2	95	94	92	90	89	88	86	84	82	80	74	76	73	70	63	65	59	52	40
	1	93	91	88	84	82	80	78	76	73	70	68	65	62	58	56	53	47	40	29
9	2	95	94	92	89	87	86	84	82	80	77	74	72	68	65	62	59	52	45	31
	1	93	90	87	83	81	78	76	73	70	67	64	60	57	53	50	46	40	33	22
10	2	95	93	91	88	87	85	83	80	77	74	73	68	65	61	58	54	47	39	25
	1	93	90	86	81	79	76	73	70	67	63	60	56	53	49	45	41	35	27	17
11	2	95	93	91	87	85	83	81	78	74	71	67	64	60	56	52	48	40	33	20
	1	93	89	85	80	77	74	71	67	64	60	56	52	48	44	40	36	30	23	*
12	2	94	93	90	86	84	81	78	75	71	68	64	60	52	52	48	44	36	28	16
	1	92	89	84	79	75	72	68	64	60	56	52	48	44	40	36	32	*	—	—
13	2	94	93	90	85	83	80	76	73	69	65	61	57	53	48	44	39	31	23	12
	1	92	88	84	77	73	70	66	62	58	53	49	44	40	36	32	28	*	—	—
14	2	94	92	89	84	81	78	74	71	67	62	57	53	49	44	40	35	28	20	*
	1	92	88	83	76	72	68	64	59	55	50	46	41	*	—	—	—	—	—	—
15	2	94	92	89	83	80	78	73	69	65	60	55	50	46	41	36	31	24	16	*
	1	92	88	82	75	71	66	62	57	52	47	43	38	*	—	—	—	—	—	—
16	2	94	92	88	83	79	75	71	67	62	57	52	47	43	38	33	28	26	14	*
	1	92	87	81	73	69	64	60	55	50	44	*	—	—	—	—	—	—	—	—
17	2	94	92	88	82	78	74	70	65	59	54	49	44	40	35	30	25	*	—	—
	1	92	87	80	72	68	63	57	52	47	42	*	—	—	—	—	—	—	—	—
18	2	94	91	87	81	77	72	67	62	57	52	47	41	37	32	27	22	*		
	1	91	86	80	71	66	61	56	50	*	—	—	—	—	—	—	—	—		
19	2	94	91	86	80	76	71	65	60	*	49	44	38	34	29	24	19	*		
	1	91	86	79	70	65	59	54	48	*	—	—	—	—	—	—	—	—		
20	2	94	91	84	79	75	70	64	58	53	47	41	35	31	26	22	17	*		
	1	91	86	78	68	65	57	52	46	*	—	—	—	—	—	—	—	—		
21	2	94	91	85	78	73	68	62	56	50	44	*	—	—	—	—	—	—		
	1	91	85	77	67	61	56	*	—	—	—	—	—	—	—	—	—	—		
22	2	94	91	85	77	72	67	61	54	48	42	*	—	—	—	—	—	—		
	1	91	85	76	66	60	54	*	—	—	—	—	—	—	—	—	—	—		
23	2	94	90	84	76	71	65	59	52	46	40	*	—	—	—	—	—	—		
	1	91	84	76	65	59	53	*	—	—	—	—	—	—	—	—	—	—		
24	2	94	90	84	75	70	64	58	51	*	—	—	—	—	—	—	—	—		
	1	91	84	75	64	58	51	*	—	—	—	—	—	—	—	—	—	—		
25	2	94	90	83	74	68	62	56	49	*	—	—	—	—	—	—	—	—		
	1	91	84	74	62	*	—	—	—	—	—	—	—	—	—	—	—	—		
26	2	94	90	82	73	67	61	54	47	*	—	—	—	—	—	—	—	—		
	1	90	83	73	61	*	—	—	—	—	—	—	—	—	—	—	—	—		
27	2	94	89	82	72	56	59	52	45	—	—	—	—	—	—	—	—	—		
	1	90	83	73	60	*	—	—	—	—	—	—	—	—	—	—	—	—		

Table B (continued)

n	tails	.10	.20	.30	.40	.45	.50	.55	.60	.65	.70	.75	.80	.85	.90	.95	1.00	1.10	1.20	1.40
28	2	94	89	81	71	65	58	51	44	*	—	—	—	—	—	—	—	—	—
	1	90	83	72	59	*	—	—	—	—	—	—	—	—	—	—	—	—	—
29	2	93	89	81	70	63	56	*	—	—	—	—	—	—	—	—	—	—	—
	1	90	82	71	58	*	—	—	—	—	—	—	—	—	—	—	—	—	—
30	2	93	89	80	69	62	55	*	—	—	—	—	—	—	—	—	—	—	—
	1	90	82	71	57	*	—	—	—	—	—	—	—	—	—	—	—	—	—
35	2	93	87	68	64	*													
	1	89	80	67	*	—													
40	2	93	86	75	59	*													
	1	89	78	64	*	—													
50	2	92	84	79	*	—													
	1	88	75	*	—	—													
60	2	92	81	64	*	—													
	1	87	72	*	—	—													
80	2	90	76	*	—	—													
	1	85	*	—	—	—													
100	2	89	*	—	—	—													
	1	83	*	—	—	—													

*z values this large are equal to or exceed the critical value. Therefore, Type II Error becomes irrelevant.

Note: n values represent sample size of one group when groups are equal in size. When groups are unequal, use

$$n = \frac{2(n_1 - 3)(n_2 - 3)}{n_1 + n_2 - 6} + 3$$

Table C. Estimated percent probability of type II error for F when $\alpha = .05$

$$ES = \sqrt{\frac{SS_{between}}{SS_{error}}}$$

n^*	df	.05	.10	.15	.20	.25	.30	.35	.40	.45	.50	.55	.60	.65	.70	.75	.80
2	1	95	95	94	94	93	93	92	91	91	90	89	88	87	86	85	84
	2	95	95	94	94	93	93	92	92	91	90	89	88	87	85	84	82
	3	95	95	94	94	93	93	92	91	90	89	88	87	85	83	82	80
	4	95	95	94	93	92	92	91	90	89	87	86	85	83	81	79	76
	5	95	95	94	93	92	92	91	90	89	87	85	83	81	79	77	74
	10	95	95	94	93	92	91	90	88	86	84	80	77	74	70	65	61
	15	95	95	94	93	92	90	88	86	83	80	76	72	67	61	55	49
3	1	95	95	94	93	92	91	90	88	86	84	82	80	77	74	71	68
	2	95	95	94	93	92	91	90	88	85	83	80	78	75	71	67	63
	3	95	95	94	93	92	91	89	87	85	82	79	75	71	67	62	58
	4	95	95	94	93	91	90	88	86	83	80	76	72	67	62	57	52
	5	95	94	94	93	91	89	87	85	82	78	73	69	64	58	53	47
	10	95	94	93	91	89	87	83	79	79	78	66	54	46	38	31	24
	15	95	94	92	89	85	80	72	63	52	42	32	22	15	8	5	2
4	1	95	94	94	93	91	89	87	84	80	77	74	70	65	61	56	52
	2	95	94	94	92	91	89	86	83	79	76	71	67	62	56	51	46
	3	95	94	93	92	90	88	85	82	78	73	67	62	56	50	44	38
	4	95	94	93	92	90	87	84	80	75	70	64	58	51	44	38	31
	5	95	94	93	92	89	86	83	78	73	67	60	53	46	39	32	25
	10	95	94	93	90	87	83	77	70	62	53	44	35	27	19	15	8
	15	95	94	92	89	85	80	82	63	53	42	32	22	15	8	5	2
5	1	95	94	93	92	89	87	84	80	76	71	66	61	55	50	45	39
	2	95	94	93	91	89	86	83	78	73	68	62	56	50	44	38	31
	3	95	94	93	91	88	85	81	76	70	64	57	50	43	36	30	24
	4	95	94	93	91	88	84	79	74	67	60	53	45	38	30	24	17
	5	95	94	93	90	87	83	78	71	64	56	48	39	32	24	18	12
	10	85	94	92	89	84	78	70	60	50	39	30	20	14	8	5	2
	15	95	93	91	87	81	73	62	50	38	26	18	9	6	2	—	—
6	1	95	94	93	91	88	85	80	76	71	65	58	53	47	40	35	29
	2	95	94	93	90	87	84	79	74	68	61	54	47	40	33	27	21
	3	95	94	93	90	87	82	77	71	63	56	48	40	33	25	20	14
	4	95	94	92	90	86	81	75	68	59	51	43	34	27	19	14	9
	5	95	94	92	89	85	79	73	65	55	46	37	28	21	14	10	6
	10	95	93	91	87	81	72	52	50	39	27	19	10	7	3	—	—
	15	95	93	90	85	77	66	53	39	27	15	10	4	—	—	—	—
7	1	95	94	92	90	86	82	77	72	66	59	52	45	39	32	27	21
	2	95	94	92	89	86	81	75	69	61	54	46	38	31	24	18	13
	3	95	94	92	89	85	79	73	65	56	48	39	31	24	17	13	8
	4	95	94	91	88	84	78	70	61	52	42	33	24	18	12	8	4
	5	95	93	91	88	82	76	67	58	47	37	28	19	14	8	7	2
	10	95	93	90	85	77	67	55	41	30	18	12	5	3	1	—	—
	15	94	93	89	82	72	59	44	29	19	8	5	1	—	—	—	—

Table C (continued)

n^*	df	.05	.10	.15	.20	.25	.30	.35	.40	.45	.50	.55	.60	.65	.70	.75	.80
8	1	95	94	92	89	85	80	74	68	60	53	46	38	32	25	20	15
	2	95	94	92	88	86	78	72	64	56	47	39	31	24	17	13	8
	3	95	93	91	88	83	76	69	60	51	41	32	28	18	11	8	4
	4	95	93	91	87	81	74	65	55	45	35	26	17	12	7	5	2
	5	95	93	91	86	80	72	62	51	40	29	21	13	8	4	3	1
	10	94	93	89	83	73	61	47	33	23	12	7	2	—	—	—	—
	15	94	92	88	79	67	52	35	21	11	4	—	—	—	—	—	—
9	1	95	93	91	88	83	78	71	64	56	48	40	32	26	20	16	12
	2	95	93	91	87	82	76	68	60	51	41	33	25	19	12	9	5
	3	95	93	91	86	81	73	64	54	44	34	26	18	13	7	5	2
	4	95	93	90	86	79	71	60	49	39	28	20	12	8	4	3	1
	5	95	93	90	85	77	68	57	45	34	23	16	8	5	2	—	—
	10	94	92	88	80	69	56	40	26	17	7	4	1	—	—	—	—
	15	94	92	86	76	62	45	28	15	9	2	—	—	—	—	—	—
10	1	95	93	91	87	82	75	68	60	51	43	35	27	21	15	11	7
	2	95	93	90	86	80	73	65	55	46	36	28	19	14	9	6	3
	3	95	93	90	85	79	70	60	49	39	29	21	13	9	4	3	1
	4	94	93	90	84	77	67	56	44	33	22	15	8	5	2	—	—
	5	94	93	89	83	75	64	52	39	28	17	11	5	3	1	—	—
	10	94	92	87	78	66	50	34	20	12	4	—	—	—	—	—	—
	15	94	91	85	73	57	39	22	10	6	1	—	—	—	—	—	—
15	1	94	92	88	82	74	64	53	43	33	24	18	11	8	4	3	1
	2	94	92	87	80	71	60	48	36	26	16	11	5	3	1	—	—
	3	94	92	87	79	68	55	41	29	20	10	6	2	—	—	—	—
	4	94	91	86	77	64	50	35	22	12	6	4	1	—	—	—	—
	5	94	91	85	75	61	45	30	18	11	4	—	—	—	—	—	—
	10	94	90	81	66	47	27	13	5	—	—	—	—	—	—	—	—
	15	94	89	77	58	35	16	5	1	—	—	—	—	—	—	—	—
20	1	94	91	85	77	66	54	41	30	21	12	8	4	3	1	—	—
	2	94	91	84	74	62	48	34	22	15	7	4	1	—	—	—	—
	3	94	90	83	72	57	41	27	15	9	3	—	—	—	—	—	—
	4	94	90	82	69	53	35	21	10	6	1	—	—	—	—	—	—
	5	94	89	80	66	48	30	16	7	4	1	—	—	—	—	—	—
	10	93	88	74	53	31	13	4	1	—	—	—	—	—	—	—	—
	15	93	86	69	43	19	5	1	—	—	—	—	—	—	—	—	—
25	1	94	90	82	71	58	44	31	20	13	6	4	1	—	—	—	—
	2	94	90	81	68	53	37	23	13	8	2	—	—	—	—	—	—
	3	94	89	79	65	47	30	16	7	4	1	—	—	—	—	—	—
	4	94	88	77	61	42	24	11	4	—	—	—	—	—	—	—	—
	5	93	88	76	57	37	19	8	2	—	—	—	—	—	—	—	—
	10	93	85	67	42	19	6	1	—	—	—	—	—	—	—	—	—
	15	93	83	60	30	9	2	—	—	—	—	—	—	—	—	—	—

Table C (continued)

n^*	df	.05	.10	.15	.20	.25	.30	.35	.40	.45	.50	.55	.60	.65	.70	.75	.80
30	1	94	89	79	66	51	36	23	13	8	3	—	—	—	—	—	—
	2	94	88	78	63	45	39	15	7	4	1	—	—	—	—	—	—
	3	93	87	75	58	39	21	10	4	—	—	—	—	—	—	—	—
	4	93	87	73	54	33	16	6	2	—	—	—	—	—	—	—	—
	5	93	86	71	49	27	12	4	1	—	—	—	—	—	—	—	—
	10	93	82	60	32	11	2	—	—	—	—	—	—	—	—	—	—
	15	92	79	51	20	4	—	—	—	—	—	—	—	—	—	—	—
35	1	93	88	76	61	45	29	17	8	5	1						
	2	93	87	74	57	38	21	10	4	—	—						
	3	93	86	71	52	31	15	6	2	—	—						
	4	93	85	69	46	25	10	3	1	—	—						
	5	93	84	66	42	20	7	2	—	—	—						
	10	92	79	53	24	6	1	—	—	—	—						
	15	91	75	43	13	2	—	—	—	—	—						
40	1	93	86	73	57	39	23	12	5	3	1						
	2	93	85	71	52	32	16	6	2	—	—						
	3	93	84	68	46	24	10	3	1	—	—						
	4	93	83	64	40	19	6	1	—	—	—						
	5	92	82	61	35	14	4	1	—	—	—						
	10	92	77	47	17	3	—	—	—	—	—						
	15	91	72	35	8	1	—	—	—	—	—						
50	1	93	84	68	48	29	15	6	2	—	—						
	2	92	82	64	42	21	8	2	1	—	—						
	3	92	81	60	35	15	4	1	—	—	—						
	4	92	79	56	29	10	2	—	—	—	—						
	5	92	78	52	24	7	1	—	—	—	—						
	10	91	70	35	8	1	—	—	—	—	—						
	15	90	64	23	3	—	—	—	—	—	—						
60	1	92	81	62	40	21	9	3	1	—	—						
	2	92	79	58	33	14	4	1	—	—	—						
	3	91	78	53	26	9	2	—	—	—	—						
	4	91	76	48	20	5	1	—	—	—	—						
	5	91	74	43	15	3	—	—	—	—	—						
	10	90	64	25	4	—	—	—	—	—	—						
	15	88	56	14	1	—	—	—	—	—	—						
80	1	91	76	52	28	11	3	1									
	2	91	72	44	18	5	1	—									
	3	90	71	39	14	3	—	—									
	4	90	68	34	9	1	—	—									
	5	89	65	28	6	1	—	—									
	10	87	52	12	1	—	—	—									
	15	85	41	5	—	—	—	—									

Table C (continued)

n^*	df	.05	.10	.15	.20	.25	.30	.35	.40	.45	.50	.55	.60	.65	.70	.75	.80
100	1	90	71	43	19	6	1	—									
	2	89	68	36	12	2	—	—									
	3	89	64	29	7	1	—	—									
	4	88	60	23	4	—	—	—									
	5	88	56	18	2	—	—	—									
	10	85	40	5	—	—	—	—									
	15	82	29	1	—	—	—	—									
120	1	89	66	35	12	3	—	—									
	2	88	62	27	6	1	—	—									
	3	87	57	20	3	—	—	—									
	4	87	53	15	1	—	—	—									
	5	86	48	11	1	—	—	—									
	10	82	31	2	—	—	—	—									
	15	79	19	—	—	—	—	—									
140	1	87	61	28	8	1	—	—									
	2	86	56	21	3	—	—	—									
	3	86	51	14	1	—	—	—									
	4	85	46	9	1	—	—	—									
	5	84	41	6	—	—	—	—									
	10	79	23	1	—	—	—	—									
	15	75	12	—	—	—	—	—									
160	1	86	56	23	5	1											
	2	85	51	15	2	—											
	3	84	45	9	1	—											
	4	83	39	6	—	—											
	5	82	34	3	—	—											
	10	76	16	—	—	—											
	15	71	8	—	—	—											
180	1	85	52	18	3	—											
	2	84	46	11	1	—											
	3	82	39	6	—	—											
	4	82	33	3	—	—											
	5	80	28	2	—	—											
	10	73	12	—	—	—											
	15	67	4	—	—	—											
200	1	84	48	14	2	—											
	2	82	41	8	—	—											
	3	81	34	4	—	—											
	4	80	28	2	—	—											
	5	77	23	1	—	—											
	10	70	8	—	—	—											
	15	63	3	—	—	—											

Table C (continued)

n^*	df	.05	.10	.15	.20	.25	.30	.35	.40	.45	.50	.55	.60	.65	.70	.75	.80
250	1	80	38	8	1	—											
	2	78	31	3	—	—											
	3	76	23	1	—	—											
	4	75	18	—	—	—											
	5	72	13	—	—	—											
	10	62	3	—	—	—											
	15	53	1	—	—	—											
300	1	77	30	4													
	2	75	22	1													
	3	72	16	—													
	4	71	11	—													
	5	67	7	—													
	10	54	1	—													
	15	44	—	—													
400	1	70	18	1													
	2	67	11	—													
	3	63	7	—													
	4	61	4	—													
	5	56	2	—													
	10	40	—	—													
	15	28	—	—													
500	1	64	11	—													
	2	60	5	—													
	3	55	2	—													
	4	51	1	—													
	5	46	—	—													
	10	28	—	—													
	15	17	—	—													

*For factorial ANOVA and ANCOVA, modify n by the following formula (n = number in *one* group):

$$\hat{n} = \left[\frac{df \text{ for MS error}}{(df \text{ for } H) + 1} \right] + 1$$

where H = the effect or interaction being interpreted

Table D. Estimated percent probability of type II error for χ^2, $\alpha = .05$

ES $= \chi^2/n$

N	df	.05	.06	.07	.08	.09	.10	.11	.12	.13	.14	.15	.16	.18	.20	.25	.30	.35	.40	.45
25	1	80	77	74	71	68	65	62	59	56	54	*	—	—	—	—	—	—	—	—
	2	84	81	79	77	75	73	70	68	66	63	61	59	54	50	*	—	—	—	—
	3	87	85	83	81	79	77	74	72	70	68	66	64	60	56	47	38	*	—	—
	4	88	86	84	82	80	79	77	75	73	71	69	67	63	60	51	43	35	*	—
	6	89	87	85	84	83	82	80	78	76	74	72	70	68	66	58	50	43	36	24
30	1	77	73	69	65	62	59	56	53	*	—	—	—	—	—	—	—	—	—	—
	2	82	79	76	73	70	68	65	62	59	56	53	50	46	*	—	—	—	—	—
	3	85	82	79	77	75	73	70	67	64	61	58	56	52	48	38	*	—	—	—
	4	86	84	82	80	78	76	73	70	67	65	63	61	57	53	43	34	*	—	—
	6	88	86	84	82	80	79	77	75	73	71	69	67	63	60	50	41	34	26	*
35	1	74	70	66	62	58	54	*	—	—	—	—	—	—	—	—	—	—	—	—
	2	80	76	72	69	66	63	60	57	54	51	48	42	*	—	—	—	—	—	—
	3	83	80	77	74	71	68	65	62	59	56	53	50	45	41	*	—	—	—	—
	4	85	82	79	76	74	72	69	66	63	60	57	54	50	46	36	*	—	—	—
	6	87	84	82	80	78	76	73	70	67	65	63	61	57	53	43	33	26	*	—
40	1	71	66	61	56	52	*	—	—	—	—	—	—	—	19	—	—	—	—	—
	2	77	73	69	65	61	58	55	52	49	46	*	—	—	—	—	—	—	—	—
	3	81	77	73	70	67	64	61	58	55	52	49	46	40	*	—	—	—	—	—
	4	83	80	77	74	71	68	65	62	59	56	53	50	44	40	*	—	—	—	—
	6	85	82	79	77	75	73	70	67	64	61	58	55	51	47	36	26	*	—	—
45	1	68	63	58	*	—	—	—	—	*	—	—	—	—	—	—	—	—	—	—
	2	75	70	66	62	58	54	51	48	*	—	—	—	—	—	—	—	—	—	—
	3	79	75	71	67	63	60	56	53	50	47	44	41	*	—	—	—	—	—	—
	4	81	77	73	70	67	64	61	58	55	52	49	46	40	34	*	—	—	—	—
	6	84	81	78	75	72	70	67	64	61	58	55	52	46	41	31	*	—	—	—
50	1	65	61	58	*	—	—	—	*	—	—	—	—	—	—	—	—	—	—	—
	2	73	68	63	58	54	50	46	*	—	—	—	—	—	—	—	—	—	—	—
	3	77	72	68	64	60	56	52	48	45	42	39	*	—	—	—	—	—	—	—
	4	79	75	71	67	63	60	56	52	49	46	43	40	34	*	—	—	—	—	—
	6	82	78	75	72	69	66	63	60	57	54	51	48	42	36	*	—	—	—	—
60	1	59	*	—	—	—	—	—	—	—	—	—	—	—	—	—	—	—	—	—
	2	68	62	57	52	47	*	—	—	—	—	—	—	—	—	—	—	—	—	—
	3	73	68	63	58	53	48	44	40	*	—	—	—	—	—	—	—	—	—	—
	4	76	71	66	62	58	53	49	45	41	38	35	*	—	—	—	—	—	—	—
	6	79	75	71	67	63	60	56	52	48	44	41	38	32	26	*	—	—	—	—
70	2	63	59	55	*	—	—	—	—	—	—	—	—	—	—	—	—	—	—	—
	3	68	62	56	51	46	41	*	—	—	—	—	—	—	—	—	—	—	—	—
	4	72	66	61	56	51	46	42	38	*	—	—	—	—	—	—	—	—	—	—
	6	76	71	66	61	57	53	49	45	41	37	34	31	*	—	—	—	—	—	—

Table D (continued)

N	df	.05	.06	.07	.08	.09	.10	.11	.12	.13	.14	.15	.16	.18	.20	.25	.30	.35	.40	.45
80	2	58	52	*	—	—	—	—	—	—	—	—	—	—	—	—	—	—	—	—
	3	74	66	58	50	*	—	—	—	—	—	—	—	—	—	—	—	—	—	—
	4	68	62	56	50	45	40	36	*	—	—	—	—	—	—	—	—	—	—	—
	6	73	67	62	57	52	47	43	39	35	31	28	*	—	—	—	—	—	—	—
90	2	54	48	*	—	—	—	—	—	—	—	—	—	—	—	—	—	—	—	—
	3	60	53	46	40	*	—	—	—	—	—	—	—	—	—	—	—	—	—	—
	4	64	58	52	46	40	*	—	—	—	—	—	—	—	—	—	—	—	—	—
	6	70	64	58	52	46	41	37	33	30	*	—	—	—	—	—	—	—	—	—
100	2	50	*	—	—	—	—	—	—	—										
	3	56	49	42	*	—	—	—	—	—										
	4	60	53	46	40	*	—	—	—	—										
	6	66	60	54	48	42	36	33	30	*										
120	3	36	*	—	—	—	—	—	—	—										
	4	53	46	39	*	—	—	—	—	—										
	6	60	55	50	45	40	*	—	—	—										
140	4	46	41	*	—	—	—	—	—	—										
	6	53	46	39	32	*	—	—	—	—										
160	4	40	*	—	—	—	—	—	—	—										
	6	47	40	33	*	—	—	—	—	—										
180	6	41	34	*	—	—	—	—	—	—										
200	6	36	30	*	—	—	—	—	—	—										

*χ^2 values this large are equal to or exceed the critical value. Therefore, type II error becomes irrelevant.

Table E. Estimated percent probability of type II error for R when $\alpha = .05$

$$H = \left(\frac{R^2}{1 - R^2} \right) (df_{error})$$

g^*	2	4	6	8	10	12	14	16	18	20	25	30
1	71	48	31	19	11	7	4	2	1	1	—	—
2	77	58	42	28	18	12	7	4	3	1	—	—
3	81	64	48	35	24	16	10	7	4	2	1	—
4	83	68	53	40	28	20	13	9	6	4	1	—
5	84	71	57	44	32	23	16	11	7	5	2	—
6	85	73	60	47	36	26	19	13	9	6	2	1
7	86	75	62	50	39	29	21	15	11	7	3	1
8	87	76	64	52	41	32	23	17	12	8	3	1
9	87	77	66	55	44	34	26	19	14	10	4	1
10	88	79	68	57	46	36	28	21	15	11	4	2
15	89	82	73	64	54	45	36	29	22	17	8	3
20	90	84	77	69	60	51	43	35	28	22	12	6

$^*g$ = number of predictor variables

Note: Because the tables are based on F ratios testing the proportion of variance in the dependent variable accounted for by the predictor, the ES, which is $\dfrac{R_2}{1 - R_2}$ must be multiplied by the df for error.

Index

Index